S0-EJQ-675

RICHARD J. STECKEL, M.D.

*Associate Professor of Radiological Sciences
(Diagnostic Radiology), U.C.L.A. School of Medicine,
and Director, U.C.L.A. Cancer Center, Los Angeles*

A. ROBERT KAGAN, M.D.

*Chief, Radiation Therapy Department,
Southern California Permanente Medical Group, Los Angeles,
and Associate Clinical Professor of Radiological Sciences,
(Radiation Therapy), U.C.L.A. Center for Health Sciences, Los Angeles*

DIAGNOSIS AND STAGING
OF CANCER
A Radiologic Approach

Foreword by Leo G. Rigler, M.D.

RC270
D5
1976

1976
W. B. SAUNDERS COMPANY
Philadelphia, London, Toronto

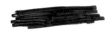

W. B. Saunders Company: West Washington Square
Philadelphia, PA   19105

1 St. Anne's Road
Eastbourne, East Sussex BN21 3UN, England

833 Oxford Street
Toronto, Ontario M8Z 5T9, Canada

Library of Congress Cataloging in Publication Data

Main entry under title:

Diagnosis and staging of cancer.

Includes bibliographical references and index.

1. Cancer—Diagnosis.   2. Diagnosis, Radioscopic.
   I. Steckel, Richard J.   II. Kagan, Arthur Robert, 1936–
   [DNLM: 1. Neoplasms—Radiography. QZ241 D536]

RC270.D5   616.9′94′0757   76–4250

ISBN 0–7216–8579–X

Diagnosis and Staging of Cancer   ISBN   0-7216-8579-X

© 1976 by the W. B. Saunders Company.   Copyright under the International Copyright
Union.   All rights reserved.   This book is protected by copyright.   No part of it may be
reproduced, stored in a retrieval system, or transmitted in any form or by any means,
electronic, mechanical, photocopying, recording or otherwise, without written permission
from the publisher.   Made in the United States of America.   Press of W. B. Saunders
Company.   Library of Congress catalog card number 76-4250.

Last digit is the print number: 9   8   7   6   5   4   3   2   1

To our wives
Julie and Jean

Contributors

HENRY M. CHERRICK, D.D.S., M.S.D.

Jaws and Alveolar Ridges
Associate Professor, School of Dentistry, University of California at Los Angeles, Los Angeles, California. Chairman, Division of Biological Dental Sciences, Center for the Health Sciences, Los Angeles, California.

J. DUNCAN CRAVEN, M.D.

Urologic Tract
Associate Professor of Radiological Sciences, School of Medicine, University of California at Los Angeles, Los Angeles, California. Chief of Diagnosis, Department of Radiological Sciences, Center for the Health Sciences, Los Angeles, California.

WYLIE J. DODDS, M.D.

Colon and Rectum
Associate Professor of Radiology and Medicine, The Medical College of Wisconsin, Milwaukee, Wisconsin. Radiologist, Milwaukee County General Hospital, Milwaukee, Wisconsin.

NEAL W. FREY, D.D.S., M.Sc.D.

Jaws and Alveolar Ridges
Associate Professor, University of Mississippi School of Dentistry, Jackson, Mississippi. Staff Member, University Hospital, University of Mississippi, Jackson, Mississippi.

GERALD W. FRIEDLAND, M.D.

Stomach; Small Bowel
Professor of Radiology, Bowman Gray School of Medicine of Wake Forest University, Winston-Salem, North Carolina. Director, Diagnostic Radiology, North Carolina Baptist Hospital Medical Center, Winston-Salem, North Carolina.

HARVEY A. GILBERT, M.D.

Female Genital Tract
Staff Radiotherapist, Southern California Permanente Medical Group, Los Angeles, California. Assistant Clinical Professor of Radiological Sciences, School of Medicine, University of California at Los Angeles, Los Angeles, California.

RICHARD H. GOLD, M.D.

Breast; Bone and Soft Tissue
Associate Professor of Radiological Sciences, School of Medicine, University of

California at Los Angeles, Los Angeles, California. Chief, Mammography Section, and Chief of Orthopedic Radiology, Center for the Health Sciences, Los Angeles, California.

HARVEY M. GOLDSTEIN, M.D.

Esophagus
Assistant Professor of Radiology, The University of Texas System Cancer Center, M.D. Anderson Hospital and Tumor Institute, Houston, Texas.

REGINALD F. GREENE, M.D.

Lung and Mediastinum
Assistant Professor of Radiology, Harvard Medical School, Boston, Massachusetts. Associate Radiologist, Massachusetts General Hospital, Boston, Massachusetts.

MICHAEL T. GYEPES, M.D.

Pediatric Neoplasms
Associate Professor of Radiological Sciences and Associate Professor of Pediatrics, School of Medicine, University of California at Los Angeles, Los Angeles, California.

A. ROBERT KAGAN, M.D.

Hodgkin's Disease; Non-Hodgkin's Lymphoma
Chief, Radiation Therapy Department, Southern California Permanente Medical Group, Los Angeles, California. Associate Clinical Professor of Radiological Sciences, Radiation Therapy, School of Medicine, University of California at Los Angeles, Los Angeles, California.

JOSEF RÖSCH, M.D.

Liver, Gallbladder, Biliary Ducts, Pancreas, and Spleen
Professor of Radiology, University of Oregon Medical School, Portland, Oregon. Director of Cardiovascular Laboratories at University of Oregon Hospitals and Clinics, Portland, Oregon.

ROBERT L. SCANLAN, M.D.

Head and Neck
Adjunct Professor of Radiological Sciences, School of Medicine, University of California at Los Angeles, Los Angeles, California.

HERVEY D. SEGALL, M.D.

Intracranial Neoplasms; Spinal Cord
Associate Professor of Radiology (Neuroradiology), University of Southern California School of Medicine, Los Angeles, California. Director of Neuroradiology, Children's Hospital of Los Angeles, and Acting Chief, Neuroradiology Section, Los Angeles County–University of Southern California Medical Center, Los Angeles, California.

LORRAINE E. SMITH, M.D.

Pediatric Neoplasms
Assistant Professor of Radiological Sciences, School of Medicine, University of California at Los Angeles, Los Angeles, California.

RICHARD J. STECKEL, M.D.

Hodgkin's Disease; Non-Hodgkin's Lymphoma
Associate Professor of Radiological Sciences (Diagnostic Radiology), School of

Medicine, University of California at Los Angeles, Los Angeles, California. Director, UCLA Cancer Center, Los Angeles, California.

STUART C. WHITE, D.D.S., Ph.D.

Jaws and Alveolar Ridges
Assistant Professor, School of Dentistry, University of California at Los Angeles, Los Angeles, California.

JAMES E. YOUKER, M.D.

Colon and Rectum
Professor and Chairman, Department of Radiology, The Medical College of Wisconsin, Milwaukee, Wisconsin.

Foreword

Despite extensive efforts to eliminate human exposure to substances that may prove to be carcinogenic, the incidence of cancer in the population is steadily increasing. The reduction or elimination of environmental factors that contribute to the causation of cancer ultimately may prove to be the best approach for controlling this group of diseases, but as long as such a large percentage of the population is or will be affected by malignant tumors, every physician will be confronted for many years to come with problems in the early diagnosis, staging, and treatment of neoplasms. The sophistication of new diagnostic and treatment methods puts an increasing burden upon the physician, but it does give him a great potential for making early diagnoses and for instituting effective therapy. Considering the nature of the disease and the history of certain types of cancer, it is not surprising that some investigators have come to believe that in treating cancer we are merely postponing the inevitable; the disease will finally overcome its host if he has not already succumbed to another disorder. Even if this *were* true, the effective prolongation of life and relief of symptoms are extraordinarily worthwhile and should be approached with as high a level of expertise as can be achieved.

The importance of diagnostic radiology in the detection of cancer in its earlier stagess, or while the neoplasm is still minimal in size, has long been recognized but is not yet universally accepted. Since a malignant tumor is microscopic in origin there is no doubt that the majority of its lifespan has already been spent by the time the lesion is sufficiently large to be detected by even the most accurate roentgenographic or other diagnostic procedure. Nevertheless, all the evidence indicates that even with such locally "advanced" lesions, if they are relatively small at the time of detection, the outlook for survival of the host with proper treatment may still be satisfactory. Unfortunately, even small, grossly evident lesions in the lungs, stomach, colon, and other organs may escape detection in a substantial percentage of cases because of inadequacies in our techniques of examination as well as in our ability to interpret the roentgen findings. The detection of a carcinoma when it is small is of such importance that it must not be left to chance, nor should detection be open to the possibilities of error that may be a consequence of inexperience or inadequate training in the interpretation of roentgenograms. A fallacy common among non-radiologists who perform and interpret their own radiographic examinations is that they can be saved from error by obtaining consultation on those cases in which they actually find an abnormality but are uncertain of its nature or significance. This is the converse of the actual situation: the diagnostic radiologist is especially trained and his experience is attuned to detect the small variations from the normal that may be in the first sign of a malignancy. Of course, the determination of the nature of a specific abnormality, once detected, may require the combined wisdom, experience, and facilities of many medical specialists.

The great value of radiographic examinations has led to their extensive use, but unfortunately has caused *abuse,* as well. Unnecessary examinations are prevalent in practice, partly because of excessive caution on the part of the physician and partly because of his ignorance of the possibilities, as well as the limitations, of a radiologic procedure. We are inclined to order radiologic examinations far too mechanically, often without proper consideration. This increases the cost to the patient, in terms of both money and radiation hazard.

Radiologic examinations encompass much more than the detection of abnormality; they may permit positive identification of the nature of a malignant process, determination of its stage or extent, and monitoring of the results of treatment. From the latter, the best course for future management can be derived. Direct roentgenographic visualization of the effects of radiation or chemotherapy upon one or more lesions may be the most important factor in effecting disease control or palliation.

With most cancers, the complexity of the disease process inevitably requires the involvement of a number of specialists. Nothing is more important than the quality of the dialogue between them. In this context the radiologist should be considered a consultant whose opinion should be sought not only in the interpretation of the roentgenographic findings after an examination but also *before* the roentgenographic study is performed in order to determine its value in a particular clinical situation and to select the proper methodology that should be used.

Newer methods of imaging, especially computer-assisted technology, may open new horizons in the diagnosis of cancer throughout the body, as has already been accomplished in the detection and identification of brain lesions. Other procedures, such as the improvement and enhancement of the roentgenographic image by television conversion and manipulation, improved methods of contrast angiography, the expansion of nuclear scanning methods, and the further development of ultrasonic echography, all give promise that the future will bring improvements in our ability to detect cancer early in its course.

The editors have assembled in this unusual book some highly authoritative and complete chapters covering most tumors by their anatomical sites. While using a unique and informative organizational approach, the material brings together the clinical, diagnostic, and staging aspects of most tumors, with particular reference to the contributions of radiology in reaching treatment decisions. The necessary correlations between various specialists are further exemplified by the organization of each chapter, which juxtaposes a brief description of the clinical problem with the potential radiologic contribution. Clearly this book brings to oncology, in all its aspects, many new ideas as well as a comprehensive view of how to achieve the best possible results from roentgenographic investigation of the cancer patient.

The great potential that the conventional diagnostic and the newer special imaging procedures have brought us may well be wasted because of small errors in technique or the improper application of available methods. The purpose of this book is to minimize the possibility of such errors of omission or commission, by bringing to the oncologist, and in fact to any physician confronted by the problems of malignancy, as much information as possible so that we may exploit our current potential for healing to the fullest. The reader of these chapters will be well rewarded.

Leo G. Rigler, M.D.

Preface and Introduction

This book is intended for the guidance of *clinicians* who treat cancer patients. It is not a radiologic text, but it may give the practicing radiologist or trainee a consultative framework for answering specific clinical questions about radiologic techniques. The emphasis is upon solving *practical clinical problems in patient diagnosis and management,* with particular attention given to the contribution of diagnostic radiology. Radionuclide scanning techniques and diagnostic ultrasound have been addressed superficially and only in the context of ways in which they might fit into the total constellation of clinical, laboratory, and pathologic findings that are considered, together with diagnostic radiologic information, in clinical decision making.

Unfortunately, there is sometimes a lack of forethought and meaningful communication between the clinician (including the radiation therapist, the medical oncologist, and the surgical oncologist) and the diagnostic radiologist, mixed occasionally with an uncritical enthusiasm for certain types of radiologic examinations. This enthusiasm may result in the repeated and inflexible use of some radiologic studies for tumor diagnosis or staging, which may waste valuable departmental resources and place unnecessary burdens upon the patient. *Cost-effectiveness* has not been addressed in this volume as such; the editors feel it is inappropriate (even if it were feasible) to assign a value to a diagnostic procedure that may affect the quality or the duration of a human life. Individual diagnostic and management decisions must be made by the patient together with his family and his "significant others," including those whom he has entrusted with his care.

The recent era of enhanced interest in cancer management (including prevention and diagnosis) has also been a time of exciting new developments in diagnostic radiology. No longer must we ask, "Do we possess an appropriate radiologic imaging study to elucidate the patient's problem?" Instead, we must be concerned with the question, "Have we controlled appropriately the choice and the sequence of radiologic studies in a given patient to maximize the clinically useful information derived from each examination?" This book addresses itself to the limitations of diagnostic radiology as well as its strengths; it is essential that the clinician perceive both the situations in which radiology will be of assistance, and those in which it has little to offer the patient. The practicing physician and the radiologist must appreciate fully the limitations in sensitivity and specificity of a diagnostic radiologic examination in the context of a given patient's problem. Patient comfort and the medical contra-indications to performing certain radiologic examinations must also be considered carefully.

Demonstrable *facts* are different from clinical judgments that ostensibly are based upon these facts. A radiologic imaging procedure may demonstrate a specific finding that is "fact," but its impact on the individual patient's care clearly depends upon a physician's judgment and the quality and relevance of the factual material that is obtained. Radiographs of poor quality, inappropriate radiographic views, inadequate correlation with other diagnostic observations, and inaccurate radiologic or clinical interpretations can all lead to faulty treatment conclusions. Consider the following examples:

1. A premenopausal patient with a history of cancer of the breast had an oöphorectomy for bilateral pulmonary nodules, which later were found to have been caused by histoplasmosis.

2. A patient with a "positive" bone scan and cancer of the prostate had a bilateral orchiectomy; the cause for the abnormal scan later was shown to be osteoarthritis.

Positive bone scans are not specific for cancer. Many benign diseases that cause a "positive" scan can be diagnosed accurately if roentgenograms are also taken of the corresponding region.

3. A 38-year-old woman with amenorrhea and galactorrhea had been followed clinically for eight years and was almost totally blind. Radiologic studies had been limited to plain skull films, which were correctly interpreted through the years as "normal." A chromophobe adenoma was found at subsequent craniotomy.

This example demonstrates the acknowledged limitations of plain skull radiographs in diagnosing small sellar tumors. The clinician should have been aware that skull films alone are an insensitive means of screening for this condition; he should have been much more aggressive diagnostically, given the persistence and worsening of the patient's clinical symptoms in the face of negative skull roentgenograms.

These brief examples illustrate treatment (or non-treatment) decisions based upon observed "facts." However, clinical judgments were made without the availability of sufficient information, essential steps in decision making were overlooked, and false conclusions were drawn from unwarranted diagnostic assumptions. Patient care decisions must never be predicated upon roentgenologic observations alone, nor on *any* isolated laboratory or physical finding.

Diagnostic radiology is capable of making important contributions at several intervention points in the clinical management of patients with cancer. (1) Radiologic studies may contribute to cancer *screening and early detection* in selected situations; (2) diagnostic radiology may be invaluable for assisting the clinician in *differential diagnosis;* (3) radiologic examinations may contribute to *staging* the extent of a known malignancy, and thereby also may assist in planning appropriate therapy and in estimating the patient's prognosis; and (4) radiologic methods are an invaluable means for *following the treated patient* in order to monitor the therapeutic response, as well as to detect tumor persistence or recurrence.

The editors have encouraged the contributing authors to address each of these four major areas of practical clinical concern. Most chapters therefore consist of a *clinical introduction* to define the problem broadly, followed by a detailed radiologic discussion addressing actual clinical problems that are encountered in the detection, differential diagnosis, staging, treatment, and post-treatment follow-up of cancer patients. Each of the contributing authors has been asked to develop a personal overview of his subject, and many legitimate areas of controversy will remain. For example, Steckel and Kagan (Chapter 1—Hodgkin's Disease) have promulgated the "classic" view in favor of obtaining an inferior venacavagram, intravenous urogram, and lymphogram in most patients with Hodgkin's disease *before exploratory laparotomy*. Although the latter view is still widely held in the United States, recent experience in Britain has suggested that these studies often may not be required.[1] Greene (Chapter 3—Lung and Mediastinum) makes the contention that most pulmonary carcinomas are centrally located, in or near the major bronchi (and hence are difficult to detect radiographically when they are small), which means that periodic chest roentgenograms for screening purposes are of limited usefulness. Rigler, on the other hand, has maintained that most pulmonary carcinomas arise peripherally but are overlooked until central (mediastinal or hilar) adenopathy, pneumonia, or atelectasis supervenes.[2] He concluded that roentgenographic screening in high-risk patients *is* worthwhile and that research (including improved radiologic imaging) should be directed toward enhancing the detection of small peripheral carcinomas.

Rösch (Chapter 9—Liver, Gallbladder, Biliary Ducts, Pancreas, and Spleen) is enthusiastic about the radiologic contribution to earlier diagnosis and improved cure rates in malignancies of the pancreas and hepatobiliary region. In surgical circles, however, consistent enthusiasm for earlier diagnosis exists only with carcinoma of the gallbladder.[3, 4] It is the editors' view that Rösch's technical and interpretative skills are matched in relatively few centers and that improved results will follow the widespread application of more exacting visceral angiographic techniques. On the other side of the spectrum, Gilbert (Chapter 12—Female Genital Tract) shows pessimism about the potential contribution of special radiologic studies such as venograms, lymphograms, or hysterosalpingograms for gynecologic malignancies; he feels these studies cannot be relied upon to reach treatment decisions for patients with gynecologic tumors. However, Gilbert's opinion is not shared by several other investigators who have taken a special interest in these radiologic studies.[5-9] Gold's viewpoint (Chapter 13—Breast) on the importance of mammography for detecting early breast carcinoma has the support of many other investigators. However, it must be emphasized that in order to achieve 90 per cent diagnostic accuracy, the radiologist doing mammography must take a special interest in each patient (including a personal examination of the patient), and he must employ exacting radiographic techniques. There must also be a continued interchange of pertinent information between the radiologist, the breast surgeon, and the pathologist. In his approach to bone tumors (Chapter 14—Bone and Soft Tissues Sarcomas), Gold correlates the appearance of bone lesions with their clinical behavior using a roentgenographic-morphologic classification. This classification differs from the traditional radiologic terminology in describing these tumors, but we feel it will provide more practical assistance to the pathologist as well as to the clinician in determining a patient's prognosis and management. In all chapters, extensive bibliographies are provided for those readers who wish to pursue certain topics, including the more controversial issues, in greater depth.

A specific illustration concerning the use of diagnostic radiology in cancer staging might serve to underline the philosophy of *interdisciplinary consultation,* which is a major premise of modern cancer diagnosis and management (a philosophy that has also prompted this book). Radiologic examinations are integral to determining the stage of many malignancies, prior to the institution of treatment. Despite acknowledged limitations, the editors have adopted the "TNM system" for cancer staging because of its practical utility and its increasingly widespread use (see accompanying table). However, the precise application of the TNM system still varies from institution to institution and (even within the same institution) from one organ to another. The TNM classification system is defined briefly as follows: T represents local tumor extent; N, regional lymph node status; and M, distant metastasis. Confusion in the use of this system still exists because some clinicians regard the TNM system solely as a means for clinical description; others use it to effect treatment decisions; and still others regard it principally as an instrument for predicting patient survival. Furthermore, in many patients (such as those with deeply situated metastatic lymph nodes from primary tumors of the breast, cervix, respiratory tract, digestive tract, colon, or prostate, with microscopic bladder wall invasion, or with splenic lymphomatous infiltration) only pathologic staging has any demonstrable validity, since clinical and roentgenographic examinations both have a wide range of error.

Proposed originally as a *clinical* staging device, the TNM system has in fact come to connote to many oncologists the employment of a much broader range of diagnostic studies beyond physical examination, including roentgenologic studies, laboratory determinations, radionuclide scanning, and (occasionally, but with increasing frequency) biopsy or surgical exploration. The editors also have favored a broader or interdisciplinary definition for TNM staging of cancer in this book. All useful diagnostic modalities, when employed judiciously *and with a potential for practical benefit to the individual patient,* are recommended to reach an accurate pretreatment assessment of the stage of the disease. Therefore, tumor staging maneuvers recommended here usually will include the use of one or more roentgenologic techniques, often with the addition of endoscopic, radionuclide, pathologic, or other contributory studies.

TNM Staging System

Tumor	
T0	No evidence of primary tumor.
TIS	Carcinoma in situ.
T1 T2 T3 T4	Progressive increase in tumor size and involvement.
TX	Tumor cannot be assessed.
Nodes	
N0	Regional lymph nodes not demonstrably abnormal.
N1 N2 N3 etc.	Increasing degrees of demonstrable abnormality of regional lymph nodes. For many primary sites the subscript "a," e.g., $N1_a$, may be used to indicate that metastasis to the node is not suspected; and the subscript "b," e.g., $N1_b$, may be used to indicate that metastasis to the node is suspected or proved.)
NX	Regional lymph nodes cannot be assessed clinically.
Metastasis	
M0	No evidence of distant metastasis.
M1 M2 M3	Ascending degrees of distant metastasis, including metastasis to distant lymph nodes.

As in the example of interdisciplinary cooperation offered by current cancer staging procedures, the repeated emphasis in this book is upon two-way communication between the diagnostic radiologist and the medical or surgical oncologist, endoscopist, radiotherapist, and pathologist. With clinical and laboratory correlation, appropriate radiologic imaging techniques may establish the correct diagnosis and tumor stage, upon which a treatment decision can then be made. In other situations, the radiologist can pinpoint a suspicious area for biopsy in the lung, bone, bronchus, mediastinum, peritoneum, retroperitoneum, liver, pleura, stomach, or colon, in order to establish the histologic diagnosis or tumor stage.

No diagnostic examination should ever be performed (or subsequently interpreted) by a radiologist in the absence of pertinent clinical information about the patient. The attitude of "let's see what the radiologist observes first without prejudicing him with our clinical findings" has absolutely no redeeming value. The diagnostic radiologist, like the radiation therapist, the medical oncologist, the surgeon, and the pathologist, is a physician first and a specialist second. He can only be expected to propose a hierarchy of *differential diagnoses* in close consultation with the patient's physician and with a full knowledge of all other pertinent physical, historic, laboratory, and pathologic findings. Like the pathologist who may be unable to interpret the significance of cytologic or histologic observations in the absence of related clinical, laboratory, and radiologic data, the radiologist is not a Delphian oracle who extracts occult meanings from stars in the heavens or from shadows on a viewbox. He is a medical consultant with a practical need for communication with the patient's physician and other consultants, to determine the need for (and the proper sequence of) individual radiologic examinations, as well as to reach a clinically useful interpretation of the results. In arriving at clinical judgments that require the use of radiologic imaging, neither the clinician nor the diagnostic radiologist is ever justified in failing to consult the other.

Finally, it should be pointed out that diagnostic radiology is undergoing rapid technical evolution at this moment. Those who surmised that the major technical advances in radiology had already been made when the fluoroscopic image amplifier was invented and the percutaneous catheter (for angiography) was adopted for clinical use had several surprises waiting for them. Computerized axial tomography ("EMI scanning") and gray-scale ultrasound techniques, virtually unknown and unappreciated as clinical imaging modalities until recently, are achieving their full stature as this book goes to press. There is little question that these and perhaps other new imaging techniques will have a revolutionary impact upon the detection, diagnosis, staging, and post-treatment follow-up of patients with cancer. In some instances the editors and contributing authors have attempted to *project* the influence of these newer technical modalities over the next several years from relatively limited data now on hand, but the situation is changing too rapidly now even for the best prognosticators. We believe that these newer imaging techniques, including "whole-body" computerized tomography, will enable the physician to visualize pathologic changes in the soft tissues and parenchymal organs that heretofore were undetectable or exceedingly difficult to demonstrate by noninvasive means. Extravagant claims that arteriography and conventional radiography are now "on their way out" are not supportable. These established radiologic methods will continue to serve essential functions in our diagnostic armamentarium and will be complementary to the newer technologies that are now on the horizon. With parallel recent technical advances in clinical endoscopy, it would seem that "in vivo" imaging is at a new crossroads and that beneficial effects upon cancer patient management will be felt strongly over the next two to three years. It is therefore incumbent upon all of us, clinical oncologists as well as diagnosticians, to remain current with the rapid advances which are taking place in imaging techniques.

RICHARD J. STECKEL, M.D.
A. ROBERT KAGAN, M.D.

References

1. A Report from the British National Lymphoma Investigation: The value of laparotomy and splenectomy in the management of early Hodgkin's disease. Clin. Radiol., 26:151–157, 1975.
2. Rigler, L. G.: Peripheral carcinoma of the lung: Incidence, possibilities for survival, methods of detection, identification. Radiologic and Other Biophysical Methods in Tumor Diagnosis. A collection of papers presented at the 18th Annual Clinical Conference on Cancer, 1973, M. D. Anderson Hosp. and Tumor Institute. Chicago, Year Book Medical Publishers Inc., 1975.
3. Solan, M. J., and Jackson, B. T.: Carcinoma of the gallbladder; a clinical appraisal and review of 57 cases. Br. J. Surg., 58:593–597, 1971.
4. Appleman, R. M., Morlock, C. G., Dahlin, D. C., et al.: Long-term survival in carcinoma of the gallbladder. Surg. Gynecol. Obstet., 117:459–464, 1963.
5. Lee, K. F., Greening, R., Kramer, S., et al.: The value of pelvic venography and lymphography in the clinical staging of carcinoma of the uterine cervix: Analysis of 105 proven cases by surgery. Am. J. Roentgenol. Radium Ther. Nucl. Med., 111:284–296, 1971.
6. Piver, M. S., Wallace, S., and Castro, J. R.: The accuracy of lymphangiography in carcinoma of the uterine cervix. Am. J. Roentgenol. Radium Ther. Nucl. Med., 111:278–283, 1971.
7. Schwartz, P. E., Kohorn, E., Knowlton, A. H., et al.: Routine use of hysterography in endometrial carcinoma and postmenopausal bleeding. Obstet. Gynecol., 45:378–384, 1975.

Contents

Chapter One

HODGKIN'S DISEASE

Richard J. Steckel, M.D., and A. Robert Kagan, M.D.

CLINICAL CONSIDERATIONS

Presenting Signs and Symptoms

The most common presentation of Hodgkin's disease is lymph node enlargement in the neck. Less common initial manifestations include severe cough or persistent "flu," nodal enlargements at sites other than the neck, an abnormal chest film on routine examination (see the section on presenting radiographic signs), severe back pain with or without long tract signs, or persistent systemic manifestations such as fever, weight loss, anemia, or pruritus. Rarely, other signs of advanced disease, such as bone pain, jaundice, or pericardial-type pain, are the first clinical symptoms.[1, 2]

Differential Diagnosis

There is no way to establish the diagnosis of Hodgkin's disease without generous tissue sampling, preferably of a palpably enlarged peripheral lymph node. When positive clinical findings are limited to intrathoracic disease, mediastinoscopy or thoracotomy may be required. Occasionally, the diagnosis is made by means of bone marrow or percutaneous liver biopsy, or by laparotomy (retroperitoneal or mesenteric lymph node biopsy, wedge liver biopsy, or splenectomy). Diagnostic difficulties may arise in distinguishing between Hodgkin's disease and other lymphomas, undifferentiated carcinomas, sarcoidosis, nonspecific or reactive inflammatory lymphadenitis, or, in the instance of unilateral mediastinal or hilar enlargement, primary tuberculous infection. Some of these differential possibilities can be eliminated by appropriate bacteriologic and serum studies, but the ultimate resolution of a differential diagnostic problem often requires the removal of one or more enlarged lymph nodes for careful histologic examination.

Therapeutic Decisions and Staging

When the diagnosis of Hodgkin's disease has been established histologically, two crucial factors affect the appropriate choice of therapy as well as the ultimate prognosis: (1) histologic subtype, and (2) stage or extent of disease.[3] The first factor will already have been elucidated through careful histologic examination of the lymph node specimen. In the Rye classification the best prognosis in all stages of disease resides with the lymphocyte-predominance subtype; the next best prognosis is for nodular sclerosis; and mixed cellularity and lymphocyte-poor subtypes signify an increasingly poorer prognosis. The second factor, that of *stage of disease,* is the one in which proper radiologic examination has much to offer

1

(see the section on radiologic considerations). The clinical stages of Hodgkin's disease are summarized in Table 1–1. Five-year survival rates, with or without active disease, usually vary inversely with the stage at initial presentation. The presence of systemic symptoms ("B" classification) also may indicate a 10 to 40 per cent diminution in the five-year survival rate for a given stage, but, in fact, the presently available statistics vary greatly in different series. This variation doubtless reflects the differences in "mix" of histologic subtypes, as well as differences in the care with which staging is carried out (in particular, the determination of the presence of infradiaphragmatic adenopathy or visceral involvement, or both). Kaplan has reported 90 per cent five-year survival rates for stages IA and IIA, 80 per cent for IB and IIB, 78 per cent for IIIA and IVA, and 47 per cent for IIIB and IVB.[4] The choice of appropriate therapy (curative radiotherapy alone; radiotherapy with chemotherapy; or chemotherapy alone) is, of course, heavily dependent upon the prompt and correct establishment of stage of disease.

Clinical Follow-up

Close clinical follow-up in treated Hodgkin's patients is critical, because of the presumed "orderly" anatomic progression of disease in many patients and the possibility of further intensive treatment, even when extension or recurrence has occurred. In addition, the physician must watch for late complications of aggressive therapy, including radiation-induced pericarditis, radiation pneumonitis, radiation enteritis, osteonecrosis, leukopenia or pancytopenia, and trans-

verse myelitis. Radiologic assistance in following the treated Hodgkin's disease patient is also of crucial importance (see later section on radiologic follow-up).

RADIOLOGIC CONSIDERATIONS

Presenting Radiographic Signs

In localized Hodgkin's disease, the most common positive radiologic finding is the presence of mediastinal or hilar adenopathy on the chest roentgenogram (Fig. 1–1).[5, 6] Usually, mediastinal adenopathy is seen in conjunction with clinically evident cervical nodes (stage II or higher), but isolated mediastinal adenopathy is not rare, particularly in young women. Initial presentation of Hodgkin's disease with parenchymal involvement of the lungs is not common, although a large proportion of patients with progressive disease develop parenchymal lung involvement at some time. In every case of untreated Hodgkin's disease presenting with lung involvement, however, mediastinal or hilar node involvement is also evident roentgenologically. Local, immediately contiguous perihilar extension of disease into the lung interstitium from involved hilar nodes (Fig. 1–2A) does not necessarily have the same grim connotation as discontinuous deposits of Hodgkin's disease in the lung parenchyma, visible as nodules or "infiltrates" on chest roentgenograms (Fig. 1–2B). This potentially important distinction has been recognized by denoting the former (*local* extension) as stage Ie or IIe, as opposed to stage IV, which is used when deposits are present in the lung fields on the chest roentgenogram.

The pulmonary manifestations of Hodgkin's disease on the chest radiograph are variable.[7, 8, 9] Ill-defined infiltrates (subsegmental, segmental, or even lobar), nodules or well-defined masses, perihilar interstitial infiltrates (see above), and even cavitating lesions have been reported, although the latter are rare.[5, 10] In addition, the differential diagnosis of pulmonary abnormalities in Hodgkin's disease can be very difficult (see below) because of the frequent concurrence of infectious complications.[11]

Other *presenting* radiologic findings in

Table 1–1 Stages of Hodgkin's Disease

Stage*	Areas Involved
I	Single site or lymphatic region
II	Two or three contiguous lymphatic regions on the same side of the diaphragm
III	Two or more noncontiguous lymphatic regions on different sides of the diaphragm
IV	Non-lymphatic (visceral, osseous, or parenchymal) involvement

*Each stage may also be classified as A or B (e.g., IA or IB): "A" indicates there are no systemic symptoms, and "B" indicates the presence of systemic symptoms.

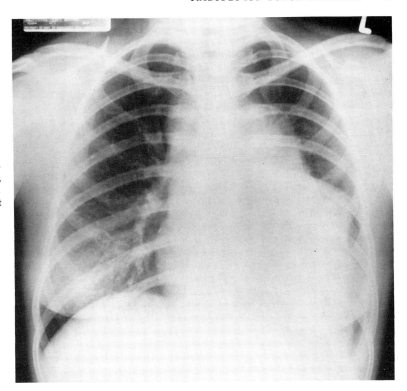

Figure 1–1 Massive mediastinal adenopathy is present, more on the left than on the right. In addition, there is a small left pleural effusion.

Hodgkin's disease include, rarely, the presence of roentgenologically visible bone lesions.[6] These are often mixed lytic lesions with sclerotic borders (Fig. 1–3); purely osteoblastic lesions are unusual. The axial skeleton is most commonly involved. It is also important to assess the bony structures on chest and abdominal roentgenograms in patients with suspected Hodgkin's disease, giving particular attention to the paraspinous soft tissues.[12] In conjunction with back pain or long tract neurologic signs, a paraspinous mass may be visible on a well-penetrated anteroposterior film after a careful search. Very rarely, hypertrophic osteoarthropathy with clubbing and periosteal elevation in the distal long bones may be seen in conjunction with intrathoracic Hodgkin's disease.[13]

Finally, certain *abdominal* plain film findings must be included in any list of presenting radiologic signs in a patient suspected to have Hodgkin's disease. These range from gross enlargement of one or both kidneys by intrarenal Hodgkin's involvement, to effacement of one or both psoas shadows, thickening of the soft tissues of the pelvic walls (denoting iliac lymph node enlargement), hepatosplenomegaly, or even a visible soft tissue mass indenting the gastric air bubble or an air-filled loop of bowel.

Radiologic *contrast studies* should also be considered for investigating puzzling abdominal symptoms or unexplained back or flank pain. Lateral displacement of the kidneys or the proximal ureters and gross periaortic lymph node enlargement on intravenous pyelography are well known. Signs of extrinsic compression of the stomach and retroperitoneal duodenum by large upper abdominal lymph nodes on the upper gastrointestinal series[14] are observed infrequently today, presumably because patients seek help at an earlier stage and the disease is diagnosed sooner. The occasional case of primary gastrointestinal Hodgkin's disease merits particular interest, however, because of its potential curability, particularly when spread to draining lymph node chains has not yet occurred or is well circumscribed. Primary Hodgkin's disease of the stomach may present as an infiltrating submucosal lesion or a submucosal mass, indistinguishable from other lymphomas or sarcomas and some inflammatory conditions, or it may be

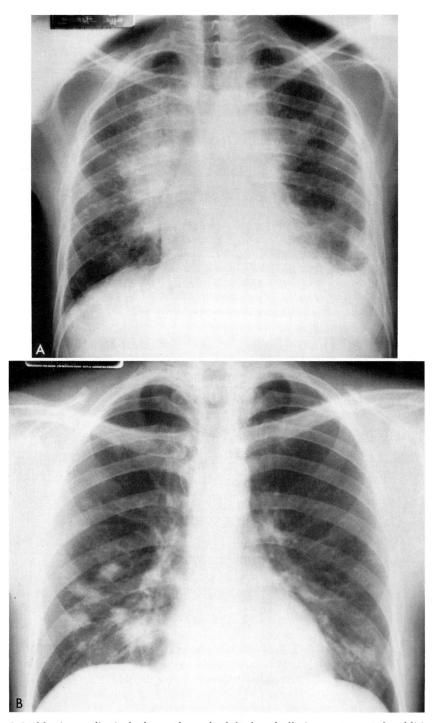

Figure 1–2   Massive mediastinal adenopathy and a left pleural effusion are present. In addition, ray-like projections of tumor extend interstitially into the adjacent portions of the lung bilaterally (*A*). *B,* In another case, irregular but discrete tumor deposits are seen near the lung bases, particularly on the right (see text).

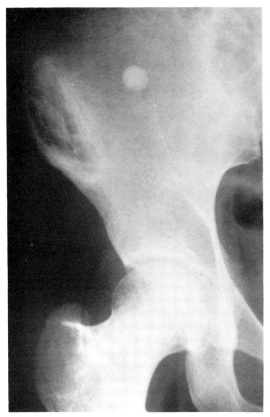

Figure 1–3 There is a "mixed" osteolytic (destructive) *and* osteoblastic (new bone-forming) lesion laterally in the right iliac bone. New bone formation has occurred at the periphery of this metastatic Hodgkin's deposit (the smooth round density overlying the midportion of the right ilium is medication in the large bowel).

an endophytic ulcerating mass mimicking primary adenocarcinoma of the stomach.[15] Hodgkin's disease in the small bowel presents like non-Hodgkin's lymphoma, with a submucosal mass or circumferential narrowing of the bowel, often involving contiguous loops in a conglomerate mass. Aneurysmal dilatation of the involved small bowel segment is probably less common than it is in lymphosarcoma. Although exceptions do occur in the lymphocyte-poor subtypes, it is helpful to conceptualize Hodgkin's disease as involving hollow viscera by way of direct extension from adjacent lymph nodes.

Differential Diagnosis

Radiologic methods are not always helpful in elucidating a *specific* diagnosis of Hodgkin's disease from a list of other differential possibilities (see earlier section on clinical considerations). Typically, Hodgkin's disease in the mediastinum involves peritracheal nodes in the anterior mediastinum and will prove to be bilateral if the contours of the mediastinum are examined carefully. Involvement of the *left* superior mediastinum is sometimes difficult for the inexperienced observer to ascertain, but effacement of the superior margin of the aortic arch or the pulmonary artery segment on the chest radiograph by enlarged left peritracheal nodes will often be visible. A *right* superior mediastinal mass usually may be easily appreciated. The interface between widened mediastinum and lungs is usually sharp and undulating or polycyclic in outline (Fig. 1–1), reflecting the nodal origin of the mediastinal enlargement. This should help to distinguish substernal thyroid masses and simple tortuosity of the great vessels from neoplastic lymph node enlargements in the superior mediastinum.

The character of *hilar* node enlargement on the chest roentgenogram can be helpful in distinguishing Hodgkin's and non-Hodgkin's lymphoma from non-neoplastic causes of hilar enlargement. First, hilar node enlargement on either side should be just as evident on the lateral film as on the posteroanterior projection. Often, superimposed pulmonary vascular structures can also be distinguished on overpenetrated posteroanterior films, and lateral films. Occasionally, hilar tomography is required to make the distinction, however. The *presence* of a clear "cleavage plane" between the inferior pole of the enlarged hilum and the adjacent border of the mediastinum, separated by normal lung tissue (Fig. 1–4), is a point in favor of the non-neoplastic origin of a hilar tumefaction (i.e., sarcoid, inflammatory nodes, and so forth). On the other hand, the presence of indistinct *outer* borders to the enlarged hilum is not particularly helpful, inasmuch as these might be seen not only with Hodgkin's disease and other lymphomas, but also in sarcoid disease with parenchymal lung involvement, bronchogenic carcinoma, and certain infectious disorders such as primary tuberculosis.

Bronchial or tracheal compression by enlarged lymph nodes is not uncommon with massive Hodgkin's involvement of the mediastinum, particularly with the nodu-

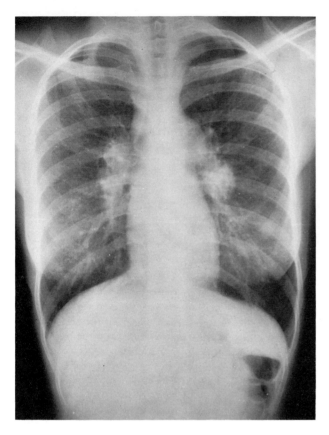

Figure 1–4 Bilateral, enlarged hilar lymph nodes are relatively well-defined and are clearly demarcated from the mediastinum (heart borders) inferiorly. This clear demarcation is suggestive of a *non*-neoplastic disorder, such as sarcoid (see text).

lar sclerosis subtype. It is extremely rare with sarcoidosis and with primary tuberculous or mycotic infection, although it may be seen in massive benign substernal goiters, large aortic aneurysms, chronic tuberculous adenitis, and, of course, bronchogenic carcinoma or mediastinal thyroid carcinoma.

Rarely, pulmonary nodules or infiltrates accompanying hilar adenopathy may be elucidated radiologically by transthoracic needle biopsy under fluoroscopic control, establishing a diagnosis of Hodgkin's disease (stage IV) without a thoracotomy. The diagnosis has also been established in three reported cases by endobronchial brush biopsy.[16]

Occasionally, other radiologic studies usually employed for *staging* Hodgkin's disease (see next section) may be helpful in the differential diagnosis as well. A fever of unknown origin, with or without back or flank pain, may be investigated by intravenous pyelography or cavography. If positive for massive para-aortic lymph node enlargement, a neoplastic disorder, often lymphomatous in type, is strongly suspected and an inflammatory origin becomes unlikely. If these studies are negative, however, no specific conclusions can (or should) be drawn. Lymphography* is even used occasionally to investigate frustrating differential diagnostic problems of this nature (i.e., persistent fever of unknown origin, with or without back pain), particularly when there is a high suspicion of Hodgkin's or non-Hodgkin's lymphoma.[17] This modality should be used with extreme reticence as a primary diagnostic test, however, because of the potentially serious complications that may be associated with lymphography in a small percentage of cases. These include oil embolism to the lungs, hypersensitivity reactions, and infectious complications. In any event, while

_____

*"Lymphogram" and "lymphangiogram" are used interchangeably throughout this book.

the presence of lymph node defects on the lymphogram may not in itself be diagnostic, the observation of gross lymph node enlargement may suggest a neoplastic problem without indicating a specific diagnosis. Furthermore, a foreign-body reaction to the injected oil in the lymph nodes might confuse subsequent histologic examination of the opacified nodes when definitive histologic examination is attempted. For these reasons, most radiologists and oncologists are reluctant to use lymphography in cases where the presence of malignancy has not already been established, except in very puzzling or difficult diagnostic situations.

Localization and Staging

Since Hodgkin's disease tends to remain confined to the lymphatic system, including the spleen, until relatively late in its course, and since localized disease is radiocurable, it is absolutely essential to establish the extent of spread as accurately as possible before proceeding with the appropriate treatment. Radiologic techniques aid in assessing localization, and therefore stage, of Hodgkin's disease in three areas: (1) the intrathoracic structures, (2) the retroperitoneal and pelvic lymph nodes, and (3) the osseous system. To a lesser extent, radiologic techniques either contribute toward or complement other means of evaluating the liver and spleen for malignant involvement (for example, scans, clinical examination, and serologic tests). Plain spine films and myelography may, in addition, be helpful in elucidating suspected extradural tumor involvement, particularly in the thoracic and lumbar areas.

CHEST

Posteroanterior and lateral chest films, with stereo or oblique views as required, confirm the relative frequency of early mediastinal or hilar lymph node involvement in Hodgkin's disease.[18, 19] Since contiguous interstitial involvement of the lung in the immediate perihilar region, together with enlarged hilar nodes (stage Ie or IIe), is thought *not* to have the same degree of ominous significance as distinct, noncontiguous nodules or infiltrates of Hodgkin's disease within the lung fields (stage

IV), careful examination of the plain chest films for local spread from enlarged hilar nodes and for separate pulmonary infiltrates or nodules is essential (Fig. 1–2,*A* and *B*). If parenchymal lung involvement is equivocal or if mediastinal or hilar lymph node enlargement cannot be established with certainty, then full chest or mediastinal tomograms (or both) should be performed.[20] A good case can be made for the performance of full chest tomograms during staging *whenever* hilar lymph node enlargement is demonstrated on plain films in Hodgkin's disease, in order to rule out parenchymal lung involvement. Since pulmonary involvement is exceedingly rare prior to treatment in the absence of visible hilar lymph node enlargement on the plain chest radiograph, it is probably not necessary to perform full chest tomograms in all cases of newly diagnosed Hodgkin's disease at the present time. Similarly, an *unequivocally negative* chest roentgenogram, in the opinion of the authors, precludes the necessity for performing "routine" mediastinal tomograms to rule out mediastinal and hilar involvement. In such cases, the added cost and effort of tomograms is rarely, if ever, rewarded.

In summary, the standard posteroanterior and lateral chest films are of critical importance in establishing the stage of newly diagnosed Hodgkin's disease, as well as in following patients with treated disease (see section on radiologic follow-up). *Routine* mediastinal or lung tomography is not indicated, in our opinion, but can be extremely helpful in diagnosing cases with equivocal findings on the plain chest projections, as well as in ruling out parenchymal lung involvement when hilar lymph node enlargement has already been demonstrated on the plain films (full chest tomograms).

ABDOMEN

The radiologic study *first* performed in establishing the presence of Hodgkin's disease involving periaortic and iliac nodes is now the bipedal lymphangiogram. Several authors have stated that, in their experience, the lymphangiogram has not changed the clincial staging in an appreciable number of cases,[21, 22] but this opinion is not borne out by the majority of investigators.[23-25] If the lymphangiogram is definitely positive in a patient with known Hodgkin's disease having unequivocally enlarged lymph nodes (Fig. 1–5A) or multiple filling defects in a typical pattern,[26] the impression of para-aortic involvement will not be altered by additional studies of the periaortic nodes, including histologic sampling. This is *not* to say that intravenous pyelography and inferior vena cavography should not be performed.[17, 27, 28] In fact, it is the authors' opinion that inferior vena cavography, with a pyelogram as part of the study, should be done in *every* case in order to investigate the possibility of renal involvement, and to investigate the high periaortic nodes above the cisterna chyli (Fig. 1–5B and C, and Fig. 1–6).[29, 30, 31] These nodes are poorly demonstrated on the average lymphangiogram, using the best of techniques. The cisterna chyli in some cases may begin as low as the third lumbar vertebra, and in these cases an inferior vena cavogram is especially important to investigate the upper para-aortic nodes. The pyelogram accompanying the cavogram may also give evidence of a horseshoe or other ectopic kidney, or an absent kidney; this may affect subsequent radiation treatment planning. Occasionally, anterior displacement of the stomach and duodenum by large upper retroperitoneal nodes may also be confirmed on an upper gastrointestinal series.

One author has recommended that a cavogram be performed as a *first* examination, and that lymphography be done only if the cavogram is negative.[32] This recommendation was based upon the observation

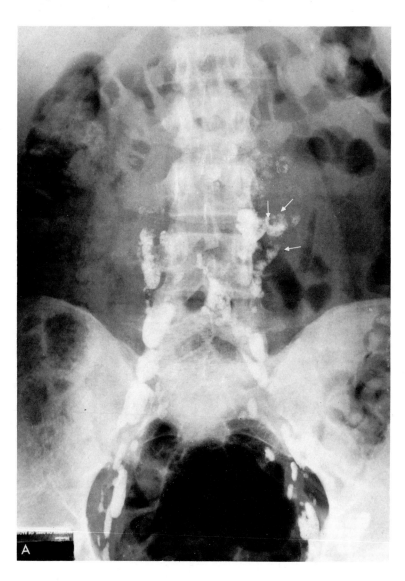

Figure 1–5 *A,* Bilateral lymphangiogram, showing partial obstruction to the para-aortic chains at the level of the third lumbar vertebra. Para-aortic lymph nodes on the patient's left side also show filling defects consistent with Hodgkin's deposits (arrows).

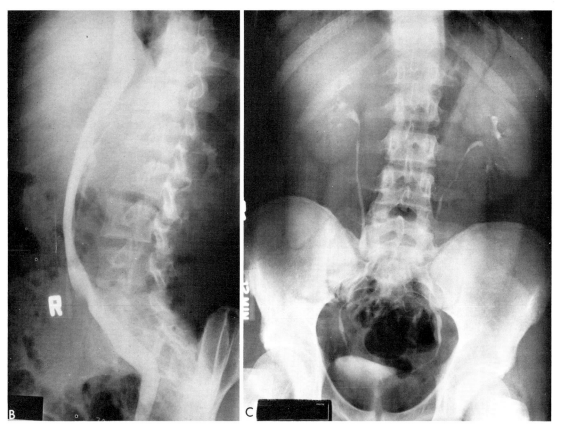

Figure 1–5 *Continued*   *B,* On the inferior vena cavogram, anterior displacement of this vessel by enlarged retroperitoneal nodes is confirmed in the same patient on an oblique view. *C,* On the intravenous pyelogram obtained following the vena cava injection, lateral displacement of both kidneys and of the proximal ureters by enlarged para-aortic nodes is demonstrated.

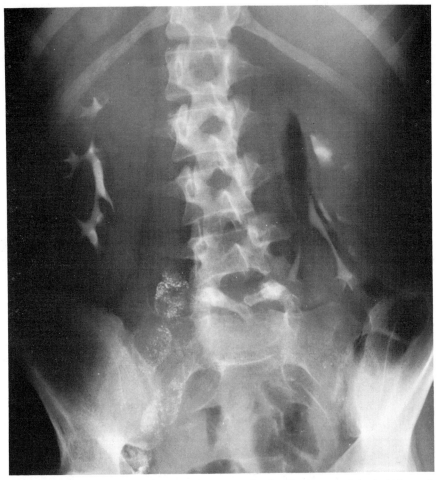

Figure 1–6 Intravenous pyelogram demonstrates generalized enlargement of both kidneys by Hodgkin's infiltrates, with stretching of the pelvocalyceal systems. Incidentally noted are enlarged lymph nodes containing Hodgkin's disease in the right iliac region, opacified from an earlier lymphangiogram.

that a *positive* cavogram is highly specific for periaortic lymph node involvement in Hodgkin's disease, and that therefore no further study is required. The same author alludes to the small potential hazard of lymphography and the possible medical and legal problems that might exist with the use of a substance not approved by the Food and Drug Administration (Ethiodol). We do not agree and feel that lymphograms should be performed in nearly every case, especially where irradiation of retroperitoneal nodes may be a potential therapeutic consideration (this dictum nevertheless would preclude the need for lymphangiography in cases with known stage IV disease at the outset). When positive, the opacification of retroperitoneal lymph nodes, in addition to giving evidence of the *presence* of Hodgkin's disease, will define the proper limits of the field for radiation therapy[17] and will also serve to opacify the nodes for continued follow-up over extended periods after initial staging and treatment. The relative contraindications to lymphography, including prior mediastinal irradiation, obstructive or restrictive lung disease, or hypersensitivity to contrast media, should of course be considered in each case.

Diagnostic laparotomy should not be necessary when *stage IV* Hodgkin's disease has already been established by clinical, laboratory, roentgenologic, or radionuclide scanning techniques. Furthermore, the present availability of laparotomy to confirm or deny the staging of diagnosed early Hodgkin's disease (stages I and II) does not alter the necessity to perform cavography and lymphography, as previously indicated. Since sampling errors are not unusual when taking specimens of retroperitoneal lymph nodes for biopsy, it is often possible for the radiologist to direct the operating surgeon to an equivocal node by prior opacification with the lymphogram. Nevertheless, it should be borne in mind that false-negative biopsy results may still occur because of sampling error, and that the presence of an unequivocally positive lymphangiogram and a "negative" retroperitoneal lymph node biopsy should not lead one to ignore the lymphogram result. Frequently, an intraoperative abdominal radiograph can assure that a "suspicious" iliac or para-aortic node *has* been biopsied.

Finally, it cannot be denied that the laparotomy may be essential, in properly selected cases, to evaluate patients for splenic and liver involvement.[33, 34] Approximately one third of cases of Hodgkin's disease classified as stage I or II before laparotomy may prove to have microscopic splenic infiltration at splenectomy, and laboratory and scan criteria are unreliable for liver involvement.[35] Unfortunately, even biopsy of the liver under visual control is subject to gross sampling error, and no ready laboratory or radiologic solution to this problem exists at the present time. Liver and spleen scanning may be of equivocal assistance;[20, 36] Hodgkin's disease within the liver is often not detectable by scan,[37] and "significant" filling defects on the liver scan may not necessarily indicate the presence of malignant involvement. Splenic enlargement observed on the lateral spleen scan has been correlated successfully with the presence of splenic involvement in Hodgkin's disease,[3] and the presence of a large focal filling defect on the spleen scan has also proved useful in several cases.[38] In addition, Castellino and associates have presented data that suggest that splenic angiography, combined with tomography in the capillary phase of the angiogram, might be useful in picking up smaller filling defects in some cases of splenic Hodgkin's disease.

Gallium-67 scanning shows promise of being a fairly sensitive, if not specific, technique for detecting Hodgkin's involvement in mediastinal and certain other lymph nodes,[39, 40] although it has limited usefulness in diagnosing abdominal or retroperitoneal disease. In addition to missing some areas of known lymph node involvement, gallium scans may often be falsely positive with inflammatory and degenerative processes. This does not preclude the use of gallium scans as a relatively sensitive means for *screening* body areas, particularly above the diaphragm, for Hodgkin's involvement during the staging procedure, as well as for detecting early recurrence or extension of disease in the post-treatment follow-up period.

BONE

Radiographic metastatic surveys of the axial skeleton should be performed in the staging of Hodgkin's disease. Even if the survey appears normal, it could serve as a useful baseline for evaluating osseous complications that might develop later. In addition, it is felt that radionuclide scanning of all the osseous structures is indicated, with additional specific roentgenologic views of equivocal or positive areas on the scan, as well as of any bones or articulations exhibiting clinical symptoms. Occasionally, tomography of an equivocally involved bone is helpful. Approximately 10 to 33 per cent of patients with Hodgkin's disease may have one or more osseous structures involved at the time of initial staging.[6, 41, 42] The most common form of roentgenologic presentation is either a lytic lesion, or, more commonly, a mixed lytic lesion with a sclerotic border (Fig. 1–3).[41, 43] The areas of most common involvement, in de-

creasing order of frequency, are the spine, ribs, sternum, and pelvis.[44, 42] Rarely, posterior mediastinal masses or metastatic para-aortic nodes may erode a vertebral body on its anterior aspect (Fig. 1–7A and B). Bone scanning, while sensitive for picking up early involvement before roentgenologic changes are evident,[45] is much less *specific* for metastatic Hodgkin's disease than roentgenologic examination.[20] Because of its high sensitivity, however, we recommend the use of total body bone scanning, a limited roentgenologic survey, and additional regional radiographic examinations (as indicated) for proper staging in all newly diagnosed cases of Hodgkin's disease. In any event, "negative" bone scans and radiographs do not obviate the necessity for performing a *marrow biopsy* as part of all staging procedures, to rule out medullary tumor infiltration.

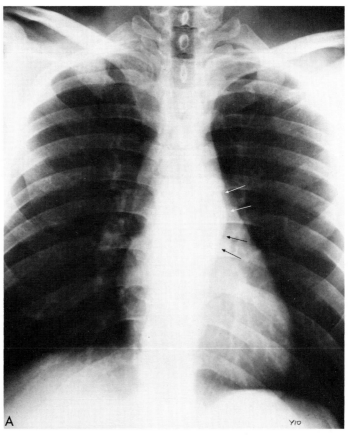

Figure 1–7   *A,* A posterior mediastinal soft tissue mass (arrows) on the patient's left is seen projecting through the upper heart shadow on this well-penetrated anteroposterior film.

OTHER RADIOLOGIC STAGING PROCEDURES

When central nervous system findings are present or suggested, a computerized axial tomographic (CAT) study or radionuclide brain scan may be indicated, possibly with additional radiologic examinations if a mass lesion is suspected. In the presence of a renal mass lesion discovered on pyelography, renal arteriography or percutaneous renal biopsy (or both) under fluoroscopic control might be used in an attempt to achieve a specific diagnosis and, it is hoped, to rule out stage IV Hodgkin's disease or another malignancy.[46, 47]

Radiologic Follow-up

The contribution of radiologic techniques to successful post-treatment follow-up of patients with Hodgkin's disease is equal in importance to its contribution in the initial staging of the disease.[48] In the absence of known disease at the termination of treatment, posteroanterior and lateral chest films and an anteroposterior abdominal film are minimal requirements for radiologic follow-up on patient return visits, preferably at quarterly intervals throughout the first two years following treatment.[49] With known or suspected persistence or recurrence of disease, more frequent and more extensive radiologic studies should be performed as indicated. It is not unusual for contrast material to remain in opacified lymph nodes, in diagnostic quantities, for periods of 9 to 24 months following lymphography. Pathologic nodes tend to retain contrast material for longer periods than normal ones. It should be noted, parenthetically, that both abnormal and normal opacified nodes tend to *decrease* slightly in size in the weeks following lymphography, and this spontaneous diminution should not be construed necessarily as reflecting patho-

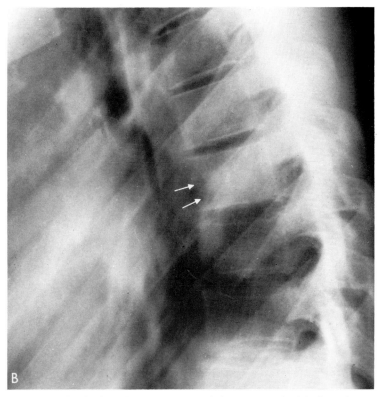

Figure 1–7 *Continued* *B,* On the lateral projection, a mid-thoracic vertebral body is shown to be eroded on its anterior aspect by the mediastinal tumor mass which was demonstrated on the anteroposterior projection (arrows).

logic involvement or a response to therapy.[50] On the other hand, seemingly minor changes in lymph node position and in the internal architecture of individual nodes may have considerable significance on follow-up (post-lymphogram) abdominal films performed after initial staging and treatment, especially when a recurrence is suspected clinically (Fig. 1–8A and B). On rare occasions, these radiographic changes may be the first and the only evidence of recurrent disease in the abdomen, or of extension of previously localized disease.

When new symptoms occur, or when findings are equivocal or "negative" on follow-up abdominal films and persistent lymph node opacification is less than optimal, a repeat lymphogram may be indicated. On most occasions, this can be performed with no greater difficulty than the original study. However, with extensive postirradiation fibrosis of the mediastinum or lung, caution must be exercised. The same indications for repeat inferior vena cavography and pyelography exist as with repeat lymphography—that is, suspected

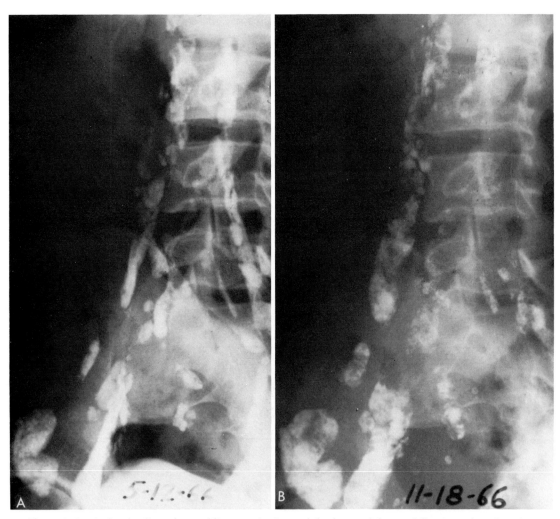

Figure 1–8 *A,* On the first of two oblique projections of the lower abdomen following a lymphangiogram, the visualized nodes are entirely normal in appearance. *B,* Six months later, without the injection of additional contrast material, residual contrast material in the nodes reveals enlargement and changes in the nodal architecture that are now consistent with involvement by Hodgkin's disease. (Courtesy of Richard Gold, M.D.)

recurrence or extension of disease beneath the diaphragm, unproved by clinical, surgical, laboratory, or plain film findings.

Gallium-67 scanning has also been advocated as a "screening procedure" in the follow-up of patients with treated Hodgkin's disease, to detect recurrence or extension of the initial lesion.[51] Although promising, the use of gallium scanning for this purpose still remains to be elucidated. Liver and spleen scanning have the same limitations as in the original staging of the disease (see above); they may be of relative assistance in directing biopsy attempts for lesions visualized as defects on the liver scan, and for suggesting the need for diagnostic splenectomy in those cases that have not been previously staged by laparotomy and that have splenic enlargement by scan.

Although routine follow-up bone scanning is not recommended at present, it should be performed when localizing symptoms are present in a given bone and should, as with initial staging, be accompanied with multiple comparison radiographs of the same symptomatic area.

Finally, routine follow-up chest radiographs are essential, as stated previously. Very careful comparison with prior films is required, as with the anteroposterior abdominal films, to detect minor changes in lymph node size in the mediastinum and in the lung hila, as well as to detect emerging lesions in the lung fields. Radiation-induced changes in the lungs, particularly in the paramediastinal and apical regions, are common. In fact, almost without exception at least minimal radiation fibrotic changes will be visible upon close inspection in the paramediastinal areas whenever adequate treatment has been given to a mantle field. When the treatment has been given through one field exclusively, as through an anterior mediastinal portal, radiation changes in the adjacent (anterior) lung may be quite marked. It is not uncommon to see acute pulmonary infiltrates on chest radiographs of the irradiated area of the lung, within approximately 8 to 12 weeks following irradiation.[52] These changes either may resolve spontaneously or may go on to produce permanent radiation fibrosis, with shrinkage and contraction of the affected lung against the mediastinum or the heart border. Interstitial fibrosis of the lungs, with contraction of the affected segments and a sharp vertical linear demarcation between the normal lung laterally and the affected lung medially, may be diagnostic of postirradiation fibrosis. In any event, the occasional problem of differentiating radiation-induced changes from recurrent tumor, drug-induced pneumonitis, or infectious complications in the lung can often be solved by careful serial comparison of chest radiographs following irradiation, and comparison in turn with the treatment portal films. *Radiation-induced fibrosis does not occur in areas of the lung that are outside the treatment portal or that have received relatively trivial doses (under 2,000 rads);* in these cases, other causes for the abnormalities in the lung fields should be sought (See also p. 67 and Fig. 3–25).

Other findings on the chest radiograph may be attributable to the treatment and not to recurrent Hodgkin's disease. Specifically, enlargement of the cardiac silhouette resulting from pericardial effusion frequently has been observed as a complication of high-dose irradiation of the mediastinum (Fig. 1–9*A* through *D*), particularly when a wide field is used or when treatment is given exclusively from an anterior portal.[52-54] An observed initial shrinkage in heart size during the course of radiation therapy might reflect poor oral intake and consequent hypovolemia. Following the initial decrease in transverse cardiac diameter, however, increasing heart size on subsequent chest radiographs, following irradiation through anterior portals, was noted in a relatively large percentage of Hodgkin's disease patients in one study.[53] It is important to recognize that a pleural effusion developing during or after treatment is rarely related to irradiation; when it does occur, pleural fluid must direct one's attention to probable Hodgkin's involvement of the pleura or the hilar-mediastinal lymph nodes.

Rarely, roentgenologic calcification of previously involved superior mediastinal and hilar nodes is seen following intensive irradiation of patients with Hodgkin's disease.[55-57] Sometimes the calcification has an "eggshell" configuration reminiscent of mediastinal lymph node involvement in silicosis. To our knowledge, roentgenologically visible lymph node calcification in the mediastinum secondary to involvement by Hodgkin's disease has never been reported in *untreated* cases.

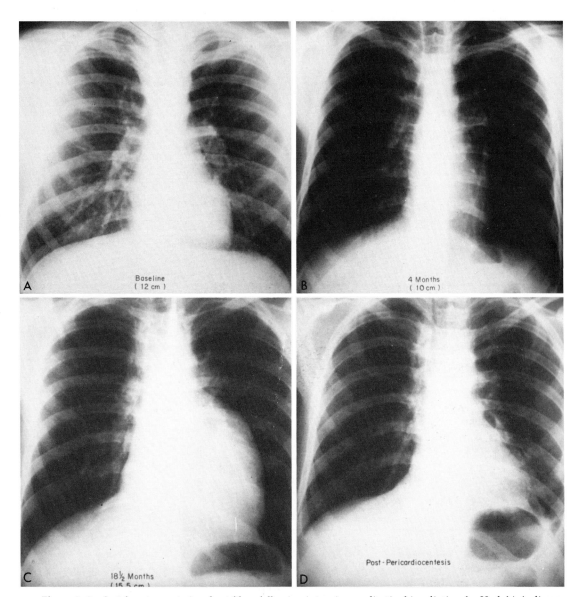

Figure 1–9 Serial posteroanterior chest films following intensive mediastinal irradiation for Hodgkin's disease. *A,* Baseline study at completion of irradiation; *B,* Four months following irradiation; *C,* Eighteen and one-half months following irradiation; *D,* Eighteen and one-half months following irradiation and also following emergency pericardiocentesis. The serial changes *(B, C)* in size of the cardiac silhouette are consistent with a developing pericardial effusion. Diagnostic and therapeutic pericardiocentesis provided symptomatic relief and failed to produce evidence of malignant cells in the effusion. Postirradiation pericarditis was diagnosed and subsequently required a pericardiectomy.

SUMMARY

Because of the apparent orderly progression of Hodgkin's disease in many patients to adjacent lymph nodes and groups of nodes, before generalization of the disease occurs, *staging* of the disease when first seen is essential to determine the appropriate treatment and the prognosis. Given the potential for sterilizing localized disease by radiotherapy and the need for tailoring radiation fields to encompass all known disease and to exclude as much normal tissue as possible, assessment of the extent or stage of the disease becomes even more crucial. Therefore, a schedule of radiologic studies to complement laboratory and clinical examinations should be planned in new cases of Hodgkin's disease. These will include, in every case, chest and abdominal radiographs, as well as a radiographic axial skeleton survey and bone scans. In most cases cavography with concomitant pyelography, lymphography, and a liver/spleen scan should also be performed. A laparotomy will then follow in appropriately selected cases. Mediastinal or full chest tomograms, or both, can be extremely helpful when the plain chest findings are equivocal, or when hilar node enlargement leads one to suspect the possibility of parenchymal lung involvement. Second only to their usefulness in staging new cases with Hodgkin's disease, radiologic techniques are also invaluable in the follow-up of previously treated cases. In particular, follow-up chest films are essential and routine plain abdominal films are equally important in the months following a lymphogram. The possible usefulness of radionuclide scanning techniques to "screen" for recurrences or extension of previously treated disease requires further exploration.

References

1. McNulty, J. G.: Diagnosis of extrahepatic jaundice in Hodgkin's disease. Br. Med. J., 4:26–27, 1971.
2. Pilcher, J., and Zubair, M.: Hodgkin's disease and pericardial effusion. Thorax, 25:631–633, 1970.
3. Smithers, D.: Hodgkin's disease: Prognosis in relation to stage and histology. Proc. R. Soc. Med., 65:61–62, 1972.
4. Kaplan, H. S.: Hodgkin's Disease. Cambridge, Harvard University Press, 1972.
5. Wolpaw, S. E., Higley, C. S., and Hauser, H.: Intrathoracic Hodgkin's Disease. Am. J. Roentgenol. Radium Ther. Nucl. Med., 52:374–387, 1944.
6. Kelly, F.: Hodgkin's disease in children. Am. Roentgenol. Radium Ther. Nucl. Med., 95: 48–51, 1965.
7. Yardumian, K., and Meyers, L.: Primary Hodgkin's disease of the lung. Arch. Intern. Med., 86: 233–244, 1950.
8. Sheinmel, A., Roswit, B., and Lawrence, L. R.: Hodgkin's disease of the lung: Roentgen appearance and therapeutic management. Radiology, 54:165–179, 1950.
9. Whitcomb, M. E., Schwarz, M. I., Keller, A. R., et al.: Hodgkin's disease of the lung. Am. Rev. Resp. Dis., 106:79–85, 1972.
10. Korbitz, B. C.: Massive cavitation of the lung in Hodgkin's disease. Chest, 58:542–545, 1970.
11. Hatfield, P. M.: Cavitating pulmonary nodules complicating Hodgkin's disease. J.A.M.A., 215:1145–1146, 1971.
12. Fayos, J. V.: Extrapulmonary intrathoracic manifestations of Hodgkin's disease. Radiol. Clin. North Am., 6:131–141, 1968.
13. Shapiro, R. F., and Zvaifler, N. J.: Concurrent intrathoracic Hodgkin's disease and hypertrophic osteoarthropathy. Chest, 63:912–916, 1973.
14. Richman, S.: Roentgen manifestations in Hodgkin's disease of retroperitoneal lymph nodes. Radiology, 50:521–524, 1948.
15. Ben-Asher, H.: The radiology corner: Hodgkin's disease of the stomach. Am. J. Gastroenterol., 56:466–471, 1971.
16. Variakojis, D., Fennessy, J. J., and Rappaport, H.: Diagnosis of Hodgkin's disease by bronchial brush biopsy. Chest, 61:326–330, 1972.
17. Viamonte, M.: Current status of lymphography. Cancer Res., 31:1731–1732, 1971.
18. Castellino, R. A., and Blank, N.: Adenopathy of the cardiophrenic angle (diaphragmatic) lymph nodes. Am. J. Roentgenol. Radium Ther. Nucl. Med., 114:509–515, 1972.
19. Fayos, J. V., and Lampe, I.: Cardiac apical mass in Hodgkin's disease. Radiology, 99:15–18, 1971.
20. Smithers, D. W.: Summary of papers delivered at the Conference on Staging in Hodgkin's Disease (Ann Arbor). Cancer Res., 31: 1869–1870, 1971.
21. Brickner, T. J., Boyer, C. W., and Perry, R. H.: Limited value of lymphangiography in Hodgkin's disease. Radiology, 90:52–56, 1968.
22. Grossman, H., Winchester, P. H., Bragg, D. G., et al.: Roentgenographic changes in childhood Hodgkin's disease. Am. J. Roentgenol. Radium Ther. Nucl. Med., 108:354–364, 1970.
23. Wiljasalo, S.: Lymphographic polymorphism in Hodgkin's disease. Correlation of lymphography to histology and duration. Acta Radiol. (Suppl.), 289:1–89, 1969.
24. Ibrahim, E., Fuller, L. M., Gamble, J. F., et al.: Stage 1 Hodgkin's disease comparison of surgical staging with incidence of new manifestations in lymphogram- and prelymphogram-studied patients. Radiology, 104:145–151, 1972.
25. Takahashi, M., and Abrams, H. L.: The accuracy of lymphangiographic diagnosis in malignant lymphoma. Radiology, 89:448–460, 1967.
26. Davidson, J. W., and Clark, E. A.: Radiographic

features of Hodgkin's disease. Lymphology, 5:95–106, 1972.

27. Viamonte, M.: Current status of lymphography. J.A.M.A., 1299–1301, 1972.

28. Sheehan, F. R., Lessmann, E. M., and Lessman, F. P.: A comparative study of intraosseous cavography and intravenous pyelography in the demonstration of retroperitoneal lymphoma. Radiology, 77:757–762, 1961.

29. Baum, S., Bron, K. M., Wexler, L., et al.: Lymphangiography, cavography, and urography. Radiology, 81:207–218, 1963.

30. Less, B. J., Nelson, J. H., and Schwarz, G.: Evaluation of lymphangiography, inferior venacavography and intravenous pyelography in the clinical staging and management of Hodgkin's disease and lymphosarcoma. N. Engl. J. Med., 271:327–337, 1964.

31. Schwarz, G., Lee, B. J., and Nelson, J. H.: Lymphography, cavography and urography in the evaluation of malignant lymphomas. Acta Radiol., 3:138–144, 1965.

32. Brower, A. C., and Seale, D. L.: A critical appraisal of radiographic studies employed in the staging of patients with Hodgkin's disease. Radiology, 110:97–101, 1974.

33. Desser, R. K., Moran, E. M., and Ultmann, J. E.: Staging of Hodgkin's disease and lymphoma diagnostic procedures including staging laparotomy and splenectomy. Med. Clin. North Amer., 57:479–498, 1973.

34. Lipton, M. J., DeNardo, G. L., Silverman, G. L., et al.: Evaluation of the liver and spleen in Hodgkin's disease: 1. The value of hepatic scintigraphy. Am. J. Med., 52:356–361, 1972.

35. Glatstein, E., Trueblood, H. W., Enright, L. P., et al.: Surgical staging of abdominal involvement in unselected patients with Hodgkin's disease. Radiology, 97:425–432, 1970.

36. Hardin, V. M., and Johnston, G. S.: Liver and spleen scintigraphy in staging Hodgkin's disease. J. Surg. Oncol., 3:109–115, 1971.

37. Milder, M. S., Larson, S. M., Bagley, C. M., et al.: Liver-spleen scan in Hodgkin's disease. Cancer, 31:826–834, 1973.

38. Castellino, R. A., Silverman, J. E., Glatstein, E., et al.: Splenic arteriography in Hodgkin's disease: A roentgenologic-pathologic study of 33 consecutive untreated patients. Am. J. Roentgenol. Radium Ther. Nucl. Med., 114:574–582, 1972.

39. Kay, D. N., and McCready, V. R.: Clinical isotope scanning using 67 Ga citrate in the management of Hodgkin's disease. Radiology, 105:740, 1972.

40. Turner, D. A., Pinsky, S. M., Gottschalk, A., et al.: The use of ^{67}Ga scanning in the staging of Hodgkin's disease. Radiology, 104:97–101, 1972.

41. Vieta, J. O., Friedell, H. L., and Craver, L. F.: A sur-vey of Hodgkin's disease and lymphosarcoma in bone. Radiology, 39:1–15, 1942.

42. Lecanet, D., Bernageau, J., Basch, A., et al.: Bone localization in Hodgkin's disease. Ann. Radiol. (Paris), 14:845–861, 1971.

43. Beachley, M. C., Lau, B. P., and King, E. R.: Bone involvement in Hodgkin's disease. Am. J. Roentgenol. Radium Ther. Nucl. Med., 114:559–563, 1972.

44. Duncan, A. W.: Calcification of the anterior longitudinal vertebral ligaments in Hodgkin's disease. Clin. Radiol., 24:394–396, 1973.

45. Harbert, J. C., and Ashburn, W. L.: Radiostrontium bone scanning in Hodgkin's disease. Cancer, 22:58–63, 1968.

46. White, A. A., and Palubinskas, A. J.: Renal Hodgkin's disease: Angiographic demonstration. Radiology, 96:551–552, 1970.

47. Williams, L. H., Anastopulos, H. P., and Presant, C. A.: Selective Renal arteriography in Hodgkin's disease of the kidney: A case report. Radiology, 93:1059–1060, 1969.

48. Castellino, R. A., Blank, N., Cassady, J. R., et al.: Roentgenologic aspects of Hodgkin's disease. II. Role of routine radiographs in detecting initial relapse. Cancer, 31:316–323, 1973.

49. Steiner, R. M., Harell, G. S., Glatstein, E., et al.: Repeat lymphangiography in Hodgkin's disease. Radiology, 97:613–618, 1970.

50. Steckel, R. J., and Camerson, T. P.: Changes in lymph node size induced by lymphangiography. Radiology, 87:753–755, 1966.

51. Henkin, R. E., Polcyn, R. E., and Quinn, J. L.: Scanning treated Hodgkin's disease with 67 Ga citrate. Radiology, 110:151–154, 1974.

52. Libshitz, H. I., Brosof, A. B., Southard, M. E., et al.: Radiographic appearance of the chest following extended field radiation therapy in Hodgkin's disease: A consideration of time-dose relationships. Cancer, 32:206–215, 1973.

53. Pierce, R. H., Hafermann, M. D., and Kagan, A. R.: Changes in the transverse cardiac diameter following mediastinal irradiation for Hodgkin's disease. Radiology, 93:619–624, 1969.

54. Kagan, A. R., Hafermann, M., Hamilton, M., et al.: Etiology, diagnosis and management of pericardial effusion after irradiation. Radiol. Clin. Biol., 41:171–182, 1972.

55. Grebbell, F. S., and Lyons, A. R.: Case report: A further case of lymph node calcification in Hodgkin's disease following radiotherapy. Br. J. Radiol., 44:720–723, 1971.

56. Whitfield, A. G. W., and Jones, E. L.: Lymph node calcification in Hodgkin's disease. Clin. Radiol., 21:259–260, 1970.

57. Wyman, S. M., and Weber, A. L.: Calcification in intrathoracic nodes in Hodgkin's disease. Radiology, 93:1021–1024, 1969.

Chapter Two

NON-HODGKIN'S LYMPHOMA

A. Robert Kagan, M.D., and Richard J. Steckel, M.D.

CLINICAL CONSIDERATIONS

Presenting Signs and Symptoms

Although other entities (particularly leukemia) are mentioned briefly, the discussion in this chapter focuses upon the diagnosis, staging, and follow-up of patients with non-Hodgkin's lymphoma. Lymphoma constitutes the sixth most common form of cancer, and the fifth most common cause of death from cancer; approximately 60 per cent of new cases of lymphoma are *non*-Hodgkin's in type.[1] The distinction between localized disease with subsequent dissemination, and multifocal or systemic neoplastic disease is less clear with non-Hodgkin's lymphoma than it is with Hodgkin's disease.[2-6] This is especially true when bone marrow, lymph nodes, and spleen appear to be involved at the outset, a condition that is unfortunately much more common in patients with non-Hodgkin's lymphoma than in those with Hodgkin's disease.[7,8] Lymphoma is somewhat different in children than in adults: unlike adults, children frequently present with involvement of mesenteric and retroperitoneal nodes, and superior vena caval syndrome with mediastinal adenopathy.[9] Approximately one third of the cases of poorly differentiated lymphocytic lymphoma in children "evolve" into leukemia.[10]

In non-Hodgkin's lymphoma, prominent respiratory symptoms caused by pulmonary infiltrations or a pleural effusion can occasionally occur without concomitant mediastinal lymphadenopathy. Ulcer-like gastrointestinal symptoms, vague but persistent abdominal distress, weight loss, malabsorption, or intermittent obstruction can result from massive mesenteric or retroperitoneal lymph node involvement, or from tumor within the gastrointestinal tract.[11] Multiple involvement at different levels of the digestive tract with viscus perforation, hemorrhage, and (rarely) complete obstruction can also occur. Other extranodal sites of clinical involvement by non-Hodgkin's lymphoma are skin, breast, and gonads (masses); nasopharynx (otitis media, discharge, stuffiness); tonsils (sore throat or neck mass); and bone (pain). Generalized hepatosplenomegaly and adenopathy associated with systemic symptoms of fever, weight loss, and anemia are poor prognostic signs.

Burkitt's lymphoma is a disease that occurs most commonly in children living in equatorial regions. It produces mandibular-maxillary (or orbital) masses, or abdominal-pelvic masses (without ascites) that involve the ovaries, kidneys, and lymph nodes.[12] Paraplegia is sometimes the initial clinical symptom.

In lymphoma other than Burkitt's, gross involvement of bone is uncommon, and spinal cord compression is rare.[13,14] The occurrence of the superior vena caval syndrome, pleural effusion, intussusception, involvement of superficial nodes, and "leukosarcoma" in the common types of non-Hodgkin's lymphoma, and their absence in Burkitt's lymphoma, are important distinguishing features. Furthermore, Burkitt's lymphoma commonly involves the ovary, but almost never affects Waldeyer's ring. In general, neoplastic involvement of most organs in non-Hodgkin's lymphoma (excluding Burkitt's) is usually more diffuse when compared to the larger localized masses in Hodgkin's disease.

Patients with acute lymphocytic leukemia, as compared to those with lymphoma, are more likely to present clinically with infection and hemorrhage (and their radiologic manifestations), but localized proliferation of leukemic cells in the bone substance and in the thorax (particularly the thymus) also may occur. Initial enlargement of the liver, spleen, and lymph nodes is a less common presentation in acute leukemia. Bone and joint pains simulating rheumatic fever occur frequently, and diffuse skeletal involvement can often be seen in acute lymphocytic leukemia in childhood (see Chapter 17). Ulcers of the gastrointestinal tract are also seen in acute leukemia, particularly monocytic leukemia. Splenomegaly is common in the acute granulocytic leukemia phase following chronic granulocytic leukemia. Destructive masses (chloromas) can also be seen in the orbit (proptosis) and sinuses; subperiosteal involvement (bone pain) and involvement of cranial nerves and spinal cord occur with leukemic extensions from the meninges within the skull and spine.[15-17] Chloromas in some bones can invade adjacent muscle; in general, they occur more often in children than in adults, however.[18]

Chronic leukemia is a disease of adults. Chronic lymphocytic leukemia may on occasion cause slow painless enlargement of superficial nodes, and moderate splenomegaly occurs early. Massive splenomegaly often occurs in granulocytic leukemia, but bone lesions occur rarely in chronic leukemia and should suggest the possibility of incipient acute leukemia. Liver enlargement occurs later in the course of chronic leukemia; marked splenomegaly, prominent clinical lymph node enlargement, anemia, thrombocytopenia, and severe lymphocytosis or myelocytosis (above 100,000 cells per cu mm) are poor prognostic signs.

Acute as well as chronic leukemia has also been described with other blood elements (megakaryocytes, erythrocytes). Splenomegaly occurs frequently in these rare types of leukemia. Myelosclerosis with myeloid metaplasia can cause striking bone changes.[19] Furthermore, this disease is associated with massive hepatosplenomegaly and can be seen as an isolated entity or in association with polycythemia vera or granulocytic leukemia.[20]

Mycosis fungoides, while primarily a skin disorder, often eventuates in systemic lymphoma or leukemia.[21] The development of lymph node enlargement connotes a poor prognosis.[22] (Multiple myeloma is discussed in Chapter 14.)

Differential Diagnosis

There are no infallible histologic criteria for distinguishing between a highly undifferentiated carcinoma and certain malignant lymphomas. Malignant histiocytic (reticulum cell sarcoma) or granulocytic or plasmocytic tumors and undifferentiated carcinomas (lung, stomach, nasopharynx) may on occasion be very difficult to distinguish histologically as well as clinically. Melanoma can metastasize to the gastrointestinal tract, brain, or lung and can also resemble a lymphocytic or pleomorphic lymphoma histologically.

The oncologist as well as the generalist must be aware that the following diseases may have clinical as well as histologic and radiologic similarities to lymphoma: (1) infectious mononucleosis and certain viral syndromes; (2) primary or miliary tuberculosis; (3) vaccination reactions; (4) reactions to Dilantin and similar drugs;[23] (5) localized benign mediastinal lymph node hyperplasia;[24-26] (6) oat cell carcinoma of the lung; and (7) thymomas and teratomas.[27]

Since the radiologist's impression of the roentgenograms may be affected by the histologic diagnosis, he too must be acutely aware that the working histologic diagnosis can sometimes be in error.[28-31] It is worth mentioning that cases of Burkitt's lymphoma were classified by Burkitt for ten years as rhabdomyosarcomas, Ewing's tumors, neuroblastomas, and other tumor types before he came to recognize this bizarre lymphoma as a separate entity.

Therapeutic Decisions and Staging

It is well to remember that non-Hodgkin's lymphoma has a greater tendency than Hodgkin's disease to disseminate early, without a predictable, orderly progression from involved lymph nodes to adjacent lymph node chains.[32] A practical clinical staging system for non-Hodgkin's lymphoma is shown in Table 2–1. (Table 2–2 contains a special system for Burkitt's lymphoma.) Each clinical stage includes "lymphatic" (nodal as well as extranodal lymphoid tissue, including Waldeyer's ring and the spleen) and "non-lymphatic" (gastrointestinal tract, lung, skin, bone, brain) sites of involvement. If lymphatic disease involves only an adjacent non-lymphatic organ in direct continuity, or if a lymphoma in a non-lymphatic organ involves a lymphatic structure in continuity, this is *not* regarded as disseminated (stage IV) disease in the staging scheme shown in Table 2–1.

The following practical clinical considerations need to be emphasized in non-Hodgkin's lymphoma, since they differ considerably from the practical considerations governing diagnosis and treatment in Hodgkin's disease:

1. Only stages I and II are truly localized (nonsystemic) disease.
2. Stage II lymphatic disease behaves more as a localized disease when the disease involvement presents *above* the level of the clavicle rather than below the clavicle.
3. Chemotherapy is less effective in non-Hodgkin's lymphoma than in Hodgkin's disease.
4. Routine exploratory laparotomy for staging is not indicated, with the data presently at hand.

In a series of cases of non-Hodgkin's lymphoma *not* staged by laparotomy, a five-year survival rate of 65 per cent can now be expected in patients with stage I disease, 35 per cent with stage II, 10 per cent with stage III, and 0 per cent with stage IV. Survival rates *may* be higher if all clinical disease is above the clavicle or if primary extranodal disease is present (skin, stomach, Waldeyer's ring), even in the presence of localized (regional) node metastases.[33] However, even when lymphoma is apparently confined to Waldeyer's ring (tonsil, pharynx, nasopharynx), occult abdominal involvement (including stomach, liver, and retroperitoneal nodes) occurs in at least two out of five patients.[34] On the other hand, nearly one out of two patients with primary gastrointestinal lymphoma will have mesenteric lymph node disease when first seen.[35] Patients with non-Hodgkin's lymphoma that involves structures on both sides of the diaphragm have a poor survival rate, even when the disease is confined to the lymph nodes.

Histopathologic findings that have a good effect on prognosis, regardless of stage, are *nodularity* and *well-differentiated lymphocytes*.[36] Paradoxically, exploratory laparotomy studies have demonstrated more intra-abdominal node involvement with nodular lymphoma than with histologically diffuse lymphoma; yet we know that patients with diffuse lymphoma have a poorer prognosis because of early massive dissemination of the disease throughout the body. The presence of systemic symptoms (fever, pruritus)

Table 2–1 Staging of Non-Hodgkin's Lymphoma

Stage	Areas Involved
I	*Single* lymphatic or non-lymphatic region
II	Multiple lymphatic or non-lymphatic regions *on one side of the diaphragm*
III	Lymphatic regions *on both sides of diaphragm**
IV	Disseminated disease; includes involvement of liver or bone marrow, or the involvement of a single extranodal lymphatic site or non-lymphatic organ, *plus* a remote lymphatic region

*Extension, in continuity, to an adjacent non-lymphatic organ is not regarded as disseminated (stage IV) disease.

Table 2–2 Staging of Burkitt's Lymphoma

Stage	Extent of Tumor
I	Single tumor mass (including tumors in facial bones)
II	Two or more separated tumor masses
III	Intrathoracic, intra-abdominal, paraspinal, or osseous tumors (excluding tumors localized to facial bones)
IV	Central nervous system involvement; may result in malignant cells in cerebrospinal fluid

has less influence on the prognosis of patients with non-Hodgkin's lymphomas than on those with Hodgkin's disease.[37]

Clinical Follow-up

Manifestations of disease recur within one year in the majority of patients with non-Hodgkin's lymphoma. Since *radiation changes* can simulate tumor, and local recurrence in the irradiated field is uncommon after 3500 to 4000 rads delivered over a period of six to eight weeks, the diagnostic radiologist must know exactly which areas have been treated, as well as the radiation dose, before he can properly interpret a follow-up chest roentgenogram.

Unlike Hodgkin's disease (except the lymphocyte-depletion type), late involvement of the gastrointestinal tract or central nervous system in non-Hodgkin's lymphoma is hematogenous and rarely constitutes local extension from retroperitoneal, mesenteric, or posterior mediastinal lymph nodes. Among drug complications, vincristine toxicity can *simulate* cranial nerve involvement by tumor, an epidural mass (peripheral neuropathy), or intestinal obstruction. It is well to remember that patients who have undergone exploratory laparotomy and splenectomy can sometimes develop intestinal obstruction from adhesions or subphrenic abscess, and thus clinical deterioration may not be caused by tumor persistence or recurrence.

Patients with pre-existing high peripheral white counts or large masses of tumor are most likely to develop uric acid nephropathy. However, renal complications that result from the deposition of uric acid crystals, particularly with vigorous antitumor therapy, can now be prevented by allopurinol. Nevertheless, xanthine stones have been reported lately, even with this drug.[38] Vomiting caused by oliguria and azotemia can be confused with that due to drug toxicity or tumor involvement of the meninges or the brain.

Any patient treated for lymphoma who has had a fever for five days should be considered a strong candidate for an occult infection. Infection is particularly probable in the patient whose white count is under 1000 per cu mm or who has been on steroids for a month or longer. Bacterial infections are common in multiple myeloma, chronic lymphocytic leukemia (hypogammaglobulinemia), and macroglobulinemia. The common viral superinfections are varicella (including zoster), vaccinia, measles, cytomegalic inclusion disease, herpes simplex, and the presumptive viral agent causing progressive leukoencephalopathy. Viral encephalitis can cause a brain mass simulating a hematopoietic neoplasm. Since viral investigations are usually not very rewarding in terms of speed or precision, any help that the radiologist can give the clinician is of potential value here.

Pseudomonas aeruginosa infection is a particular hazard in patients with ulceration of the gut, either as a primary malignant disease manifestation or as a complication of therapy. Fungal infections may occur as much as two years after diagnosis,[39] whereas they are uncommon in patients with recently diagnosed lymphoma; *Candida albicans* is the most common. *Pneumocystis carinii* is one of the few infections that occur commonly during tumor remissions. Lung infiltrates induced by methotrexate or bleomycin can be confused with pneumocystis pneumonia, bacterial pneumonia, other (nonbacterial) superinfections, or spread of tumor into the lung. A lung biopsy or bronchial aspirate may establish the diagnosis of pneumocystis, a treatable infection, but pentamidine is given on the basis of suggestive roentgenographic and clinical findings alone in some institutions.

In addition to lung infiltrates, methotrexate can induce severe bone pain with osteoporosis and fractures.[40] The roentgenographic picture can simulate scurvy. Patients with leukemia who are receiving methotrexate by intrathecal injection can develop subdural collections of cerebrospinal fluid—the so-called *double sac syndrome*. Loculation of this type prevents the medication from reaching the cerebral meninges.[41]

Finally, bleeding manifestations caused by drug-induced thrombocytopenia or liver toxicity may be confused clinically and radiologically with tumor recurrence in the post-treatment follow-up period. Soft tissue, lung, retroperitoneal, or central nervous system hematomas may simulate tumor masses, with resulting severe morbidity or a fatal outcome if blood loss is severe or a vital structure is compromised.

RADIOLOGIC CONSIDERATIONS

Presenting Radiographic Signs

The reader is referred to Chapter 1 (on Hodgkin's disease) for a basic discussion of the use of radiologic detection, diagnosis, staging, and follow-up studies in a lymphomatous disorder. Our attention in this discussion focuses upon salient differences in the indications for using radiologic techniques in non-Hodgkin's lymphoma as contrasted with Hodgkin's disease.

Involvement of the *mediastinal and hilar lymph nodes* on the chest radiograph in non-Hodgkin's lymphoma is somewhat less frequent than it is in Hodgkin's disease.[42] Nevertheless, massive lymph node enlargements in the lung hila, and occasionally in the mediastinum, are certainly not rare (Fig. 2–1A and B), and superior mediastinal compression by massive adenopathy has been reported in non-Hodgkin's lymphoma, as well as in acute childhood leukemia.[43] With the latter type of presentation, peripheral venous injection of contrast material in one or both upper extremities, with serial angiographic films to opacify the obstructed superior vena cava, may be indicated. In addition to establishing the diagnosis of caval obstruction, this study will serve as an objective baseline for subsequent tumor response to radiotherapy or chemotherapy.

In non-Hodgkin's lymphoma, metastatic deposits in the lung *parenchyma* occur more frequently and earlier than in Hodgkin's disease. These lesions may take the form of clearly circumscribed lung "masses" (Fig. 2–2), multiple "salt-and-pepper" or miliary nodules throughout the lungs, ill-defined "infiltrates," or ray-like extensions of tumor from mediastinal nodes into the perihilar lung fields (interstitial lymphangitic spread).[44]

Soft tissue films of good quality may assist in detecting or delineating *nasopharyngeal and pharyngeal masses,* and only rarely are contrast studies with barium or other agents required to add further definition to image-amplified fluoroscopy and radiography of the upper airways. On the other hand, upper gastrointestinal barium studies for the diagnosis of *stomach or small bowel involvement* are mandatory. A non-Hodgkin's lymphoma may present in the stomach as a localized mass, identical in appearance to adenocarcinoma, or it may infiltrate the stomach diffusely with massive thickening of the gastric folds (Fig. 2–3). Lymphoma in the stomach, particularly with involvement in the antral region, does not respect the pyloric barrier and often crosses the pylorus to involve the contiguous duodenal bulb. Adenocarcinoma of the stomach, on the other hand, very rarely crosses the pyloric barrier and this distinguishing sign may be very helpful in arriving at a diagnosis before operation or biopsy.

Small bowel involvement by lymphoma may cause many different patterns on barium examination. There may be localized masses involving the small bowel and causing separation of adjacent loops, often with massive ulceration of the mucosa ("aneurysmal dilatation" of the affected segment), or there may be diffuse infiltration of long segments of bowel with loss of normal markings (Fig. 2–4).[45] A "sprue-like" pattern is sometimes noted, with excess secretions in the small bowel, segmentation of the barium, and irregular dilatation and narrowing of many segments. *Colonic involvement* may also take localized or diffuse forms. A localized mass in the cecum on barium enema study may be the earliest presentation of primary extranodal lymphoma of the gastrointestinal tract.[46] Alternately, diffuse submucosal involvement of the entire colon has been reported.[47]

Plain film examination of the abdomen may be of assistance in assessing spleen, liver, and kidney size, as mentioned earlier. Diffuse tumor involvement of the *kidneys* has been reported, particularly in poorly differentiated lymphoma as well as in leukemia.[48, 49] On the other hand, hepatic or renal enlargement may occur with these diseases as a consequence of hemorrhage or nonspecific inflammation, *without* tumor involvement. Intravenous pyelography, while useful for evaluating diffuse or nodular deposits of lymphoma within the kidneys[50] and gross retroperitoneal adenopathy (Fig. 2–5A and B), is a relatively insensitive means of detecting retroperitoneal node enlargement;[51] this is not surprising in view of similar observations with Hodgkin's disease (see Chapter 1). An occasional case of unilateral renal enlargement or a lymphomatous mass lesion within the kidney may

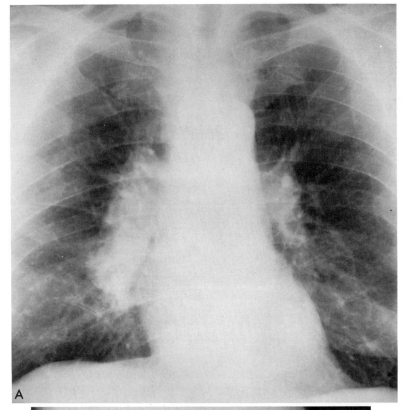

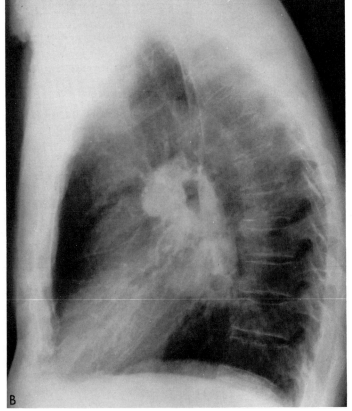

Figure 2–1   *See legend on the opposite page.*

be elucidated further by selective renal angiography, and a distinctive angiographic pattern has been reported for focal lymphomatous involvement of the kidney by several authors in anecdotal case reports.[52, 53]

As with Hodgkin's disease, the most reliable non-operative method for assessing *periaortic adenopathy* is the bipedal lymphangiogram. Depending upon the series, the lymphangiogram has been proved to be correct, by direct biopsy of lymph nodes at laparotomy, in between 92 and 98 per cent of the cases of non-Hodgkin's lymphoma examined.[42, 54] As with Hodgkin's disease also, the inferior vena cavogram may provide additional assistance in the examination of the lymph node groups at or above the celiac axis, and behind the liver.[51, 55] We recommend *both* studies in the proper staging of non-Hodgkin's lymphoma, as with Hodgkin's disease. There is nothing that distinguishes absolutely the lymphangiographic pattern of tumor involvement by non-Hodgkin's lymphoma from that of Hodgkin's disease. In general, non-Hodgkin's lymphoma may lead to diffuse involvement of all visualized nodes on the lymphangiogram, with massive enlargement and a "bubbly" pattern (Fig. 2–6A). While not seen in all cases, Hodgkin's involvement of the corresponding lymph nodes tends to cause localized filling defects in the nodes or complete replacement of a node by tumor (Fig. 2–6B).[56] Beyond these relative differences, which are of limited value in differential diagnosis, further generalizations linking histology to lymphangiographic appearance are not warranted. Benign disease including drug sensitivity, infection, and immunologic syndromes may also mimic malignant involvement of nodes in certain cases.[57, 58] Occasionally, a relative contraindication to lymphangiography (moderate pulmonary insufficiency, enormous masses extending into the middle and posterior mediastinum) or an absolute contraindication (severe pulmonary insufficiency, known sensitivity to iodinated contrast materials) may exist. In all cases, a chest film taken within two weeks of the study must be evaluated *before* undertaking a lymphangiogram, and a careful allergic history must be obtained.

Other clinical presentations in non-Hodgkin's lymphoma that may require radiologic elucidation include those involving the bones and the central nervous system. As with Hodgkin's disease, metastatic lesions in the bones from a non-Hodgkin's lymphoma are extremely uncommon in the absence of corresponding symptoms. Therefore, the wisdom of employing a "routine" radiographic metastatic bone series is open to serious question.[59] On the other hand, the value of routine screening with radionuclide *bone scans* has not been properly evaluated, and there is reason to believe that these studies are more valuable than radiographs in detecting early bone involvement. This is because radiologic examination of bony structures will not demonstrate primary or metastatic lesions unless the localized mineral content of the bone has been reduced by 50 per cent or more. The radionuclide bone scan, on the other hand, is a measure of reparative bone activity, which may be considerable even in the presence of an early metastatic bone lesion.

To summarize, we do not recommend routine radiographic metastatic bone surveys *in the absence of bone symptoms.* In the presence of localized skeletal symptoms, however, multiple radiographic views of the suspected bone(s) should be obtained. *If* these prove to be negative, a bone scan should probably be performed. The reason for recommending this order of examinations is that bone scans, while apparently sensitive for metastatic tumor involvement, are certainly not specific and may appear to be "positive" in many *inflammatory* conditions as well. The radiographic examination of *clinically suspicious* bones is therefore still important in the early evaluation for metastatic disease. The place of radionuclide bone scans in screening for subclinical bone lesions remains to be determined, but there is good reason to believe that they will be helpful.

Text continued on page 30

Figure 2–1   *A,* Massive right hilar lymph node enlargement is present in this patient with disseminated lymphoma. *B,* On the lateral projection, the hilar node mass is again seen.

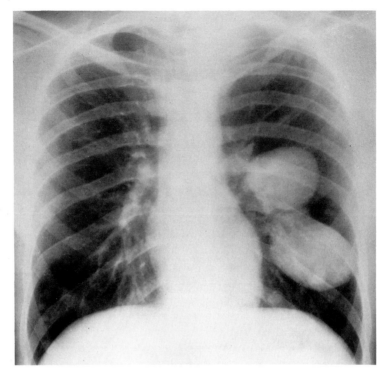

Figure 2–2   Massive circumscribed lung masses are present in this patient with disseminated, non-Hodgkin's lymphoma (see text).

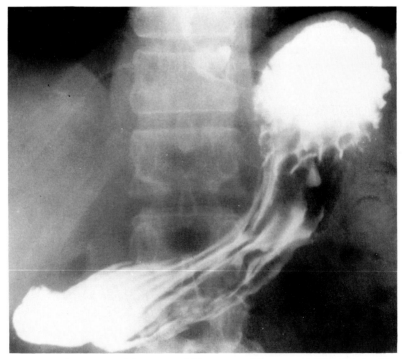

Figure 2–3   General enlargement of the gastric folds is caused by tumor infiltration in this patient with disseminated lymphoma. A triangular ulcer is also evident in the proximal body of the stomach.

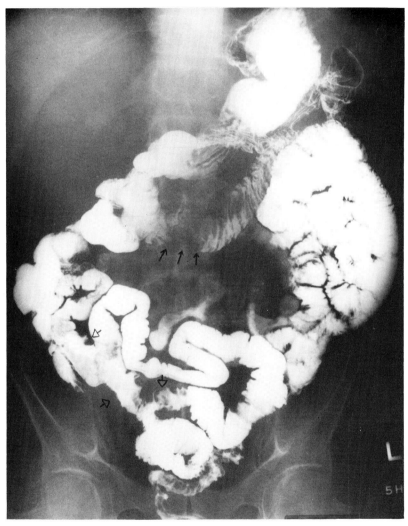

Figure 2–4 In this patient with gastrointestinal lymphoma, there is infiltration of the small bowel wall in several locations (arrowheads). Enlarged lymph nodes at the root of the small bowel mesentery partially efface the mucosal pattern of the third portion of the duodenum (vertical arrows).

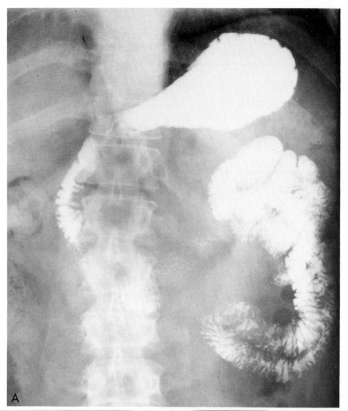

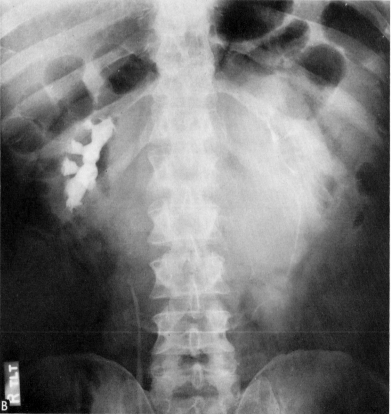

Figure 2–5 *A,* Enlargement of the duodenal loop is caused by massive retroperitoneal adenopathy in the upper para-aortic region. *B,* In the same patient, the intravenous pyelogram demonstrates lateral displacement of both kidneys and proximal ureters (together with rotation of the kidneys on their long axes) by the massively enlarged retroperitoneal lymph nodes.

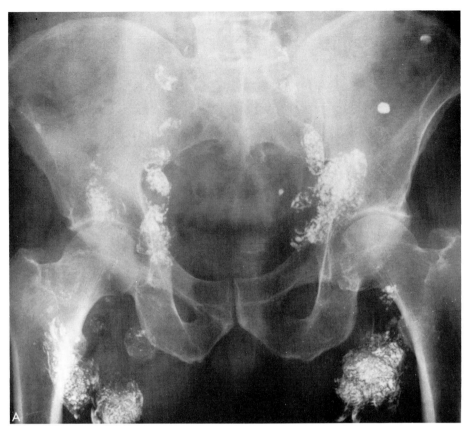

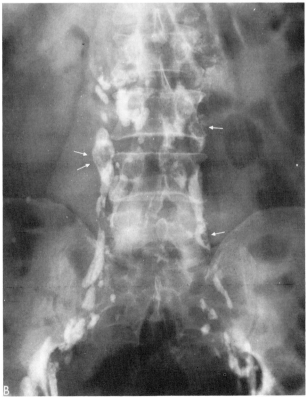

Figure 2–6 *A,* Diffuse, "bubbly" enlargement of the pelvic lymph nodes on this lymphangiogram is the "typical" appearance of aggressive non-Hodgkin's lymphomas. On the other hand, either discrete nodal filling defects (arrows; also, see text) *or* the bubbly pattern seen in non-Hodgkin's lymphoma may occur in Hodgkin's disease *(B).*

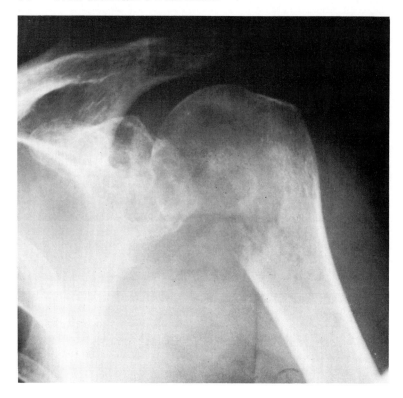

Figure 2–7 There is gross destruction of the proximal humeral epiphysis and metaphysis, with a scalloped and irregular margin, in this patient with metastatic lymphomatous involvement of bone. The tumor has also broken through the cortex inferiorly.

Metastatic non-Hodgkin's lymphoma often presents radiologically as a lytic lesion in the bone, sometimes with minimal new bone formation at the periphery of the lesion.[46] The bone metastasis, while occupying the medullary cavity, often causes scalloping of the inner surface of the cortex as well (Fig. 2–7). This contrasts with metastatic bone lesions in Hodgkin's disease: the latter quite often are mixed osteoblastic *and* osteolytic lesions and may even have a predominantly sclerotic component.[60] In Burkitt's lymphoma (see earlier section on presenting signs), osteolytic lesions in both the mandible and maxilla are common.[61] These may cause destruction of the lamina dura and displacement of the teeth, and pathologic jaw fractures may also occur.

Finally, the occurrence of paraplegia or paraparesis may be the first indication of extradural involvement by non-Hodgkin's lymphoma in the cervical, thoracic, or lumbar spine.[62] In these cases, radiologically visible tumor involvement of the adjacent vertebral bodies or accessory elements, such as the pedicles, signifies a much poorer chance for recovery of neural function following appropriate treatment. An emergency myelogram must be performed by lumbar

or cisternal puncture in these cases, and extradural tumor masses, with or without complete subarachnoid block, may be demonstrated. Immediate institution of local radiation therapy, with or without surgical decompression, should follow the radiologic demonstration of metastatic tumor and the level of involvement.

Differential Diagnosis

The differential diagnostic approach to non-Hodgkin's lymphoma is similar to that which already has been discussed for Hodgkin's disease (Chapter 1). Radiologic studies can never make an *absolute* distinction between the many diagnostic possibilities that may be present in an individual case.[63] Some of the problems in differential diagnosis have already been alluded to in earlier sections of this chapter. An intravenous pyelogram, and even a subsequent selective renal angiogram, may demonstrate the *presence* of diffuse infiltration or of a mass lesion in the kidney, without defining its specific cause. Similarly, plain film demonstrations of hepatosplenomegaly may only be confirmatory of an equivocal clinical finding, without lending further assistance in the differential diagnosis.

Some radiologic features of bone metastases secondary to non-Hodgkin's lymphoma, as compared with Hodgkin's disease, were discussed earlier, but these also lack absolute specificity. In the case of pulmonary lesions, lymphoma is decidedly the "great mimicker"; pulmonary infiltrates from a superinfection may simulate lymphomatous involvement of the lung parenchyma, or vice versa. Pleural effusions similarly may be caused by tumor involvement, or they may be secondary to hemorrhage or empyema. There is nothing specific in the radiologic appearance that will lend support to either etiology, in the absence of further discriminatory data from biopsy, clinical findings, or cytologic examination. Similarly, a perihilar interstitial infiltrate may represent lymphoma spreading from mediastinal nodes into the lungs, or alternatively, it may be the first radiologic sign of viral pneumonia or of *Pneumocystis carinii* infection.

As mentioned, even the lymphangiogram has certain important limitations. Immunologic deficiency syndromes, as well as hyperimmune states (such as "immunoblastic lymphadenopathy" or lupus erythematosus), may cause node enlargement on the lymphangiogram that simulates tumor involvement, particularly to the inexperienced observer. In defense of lymphangiography, however, it can be stated that massive and ubiquitous foamy enlargement of pelvic and periaortic nodes, often seen on lymphangiograms in patients with non-Hodgkin's lymphoma, is quite *specific* for lymphomatous involvement of these nodes (Fig. 2–6A).[37]

Finally, a word should be said for the use of radiologic techniques as "screening" studies in the differential workup of elusive symptoms such as a fever of unknown origin, unexplained weight loss, or persistent back pain. Here, even the intravenous pyelogram may have differential diagnostic value despite its relative insensitivity, as with the demonstration of lateral deviation of the mid-portions of the ureters that may accompany massive periaortic lymphadenopathy. The intravenous pyelogram is easy to perform, and it is a relatively innocuous and inexpensive means for pursuing the diagnosis in these difficult situations. On the other hand, the use of a lymphangiogram as a differential diagnostic tool should be approached with greater trepidation in the case of a patient with unexplained fever or back pain. This is because of the acknowledged risk of pulmonary oil embolization in some patients, the poorly investigated effects of long-term retention of foreign materials such as lymphangiographic contrast medium in retroperitoneal lymph nodes, and the possible effects (in the form of oil granulomata) of the lymphangiogram on subsequent diagnostic histopathologic examinations of the retroperitoneal lymph nodes. A simple "screening" posteroanterior and lateral chest radiographic examination is a minimum requirement when pursuing these difficult clinical diagnostic problems: The presence of poorly delineated but definitely enlarged hilar lymph nodes, possibly with associated mediastinal lymphadenopathy, may point strongly toward lymphomatous disease when a large list of other differential diagnoses are being considered on clinical grounds.

Localization and Staging

In view of related discussions elsewhere in this chapter and in Chapter 1, only a sequential listing of recommended radiologic examinations that should be performed for the proper anatomic *staging* of non-Hodgkin's lymphoma will be presented here.[64,65] This list should also be construed as indicating the approximate *chronologic* order of the performance of radiologic examinations, in staging a new patient who presents with known (or highly suspected) non-Hodgkin's lymphoma. These radiologic studies, of course, must be preceded by or interspersed with appropriate laboratory examinations, including a complete blood count and urinalysis, liver and renal function studies, and bone marrow biopsy. In our opinion, the chain of radiologic staging procedures proposed here, performed in order of ascending complexity or discomfort for the patient, *should be terminated* if and when disseminated (stage IV) disease has been demonstrated. This is based upon the premise that proved localized and regional lymph node involvement might be treated effectively with intensive radiation therapy, with or without adjunctive chemotherapy; on the other hand, disseminated (stage IV) disease, with discontinuous tumor infiltrations or masses in parenchymatous organs, necessitates chemotherapy as the primary modality of treatment. Dogmatic determination of the exact extent of disease, once the decision has been made that stage IV disease is present, becomes an academic matter in most cases.

As stated previously, all cases of *primary* extranodal non-Hodgkin's lymphoma, as opposed to Hodgkin's disease in extranodal sites, should be staged vigorously. This is because there is a high rate of definitive control (using radiotherapy) in this form of disease, when the lymphoma is confined to the extranodal primary site or to the primary site and regional lymph nodes only.[37]

Our recommended list of sequential radiologic examinations, in ascending order of their complexity, is:

1. Standard chest radiographs.
2. Lung and mediastinal tomography, only if equivocal findings are noted on the plain chest films. *Lateral* tomography may be helpful in delineating paramediastinal lung lesions.[59]
3. Radiographic bone studies in areas with specific symptoms (followed by radionuclide bone scans for detailed correlation with symptoms and with radiographic studies).
4. Inferior cavography, with excretory urography performed as part of the same study.
5. Bipedal lymphangiography (if not medically contraindicated).
6. Selective angiography for specified indications (i.e., renal masses or kidney enlargement; hepatic enlargement; defects on liver scan; laboratory liver function abnormalities).

If the patient reaches the last level in this series of radiologic examinations and if all studies, including bone marrow aspiration and percutaneous liver biopsy, also remain negative, laparotomy with open bone marrow biopsy and segmental liver biopsy should at least be *considered*.[54, 66, 67] Extensive sampling of mesenteric lymph nodes, open liver biopsy, and splenectomy are necessary components of this procedure, when properly performed.

Usually in cases of non-Hodgkin's lymphoma, however, the preceding radiologic and other noninvasive studies performed preoperatively will obviate the need for a laparotomy. Surgical staging should not be undertaken lightly in non-Hodgkin's lymphoma, a disease known to be disseminated widely at first presentation in a majority of cases.[68]

Radiologic Follow-up

This topic has also been mentioned in earlier sections, and the specifications for continued radiologic follow-up of treated patients with Hodgkin's disease (Chapter 1) apply equally to those with treated non-Hodgkin's lymphoma. Certainly, a chest radiograph at clinical follow-up visits is a minimum requirement, and serial abdominal films performed on outpatient follow-up examinations are equally important in patients who have had lymphangiograms within the past two years.[69] As with Hodgkin's disease, changes in the configuration or the position of even poorly opacified periaortic or pelvic nodes may have great significance in detecting an early recurrence (see Fig. 1–8). For this reason, as with Hodgkin's disease, follow-up abdominal radiographs performed in the months after lymphangiography are as important as the original lymphangiogram itself.

The same strictures that apply to radiologic studies of suspected bone lesions in the pretreatment workup of the patient apply equally to the patient being followed after therapy. In our opinion, "routine" metastatic bone series, performed in the absence of symptoms, are not indicated in the continued follow-up of patients with treated disease. On the other hand, it is important to maintain radiologic surveillance of treated metastatic bone lesions to assure continued healing or to detect early recurrences. As with Hodgkin's disease, non-Hodgkin's lymphoma in bone often develops into a sclerotic "island" in otherwise normal surrounding bone following successful local treatment. Radiation necrosis of bone is an unfortunate, if rare, sequel to intensive therapy. This development might be heralded by recurrence of pain, demineralization of the bone, or pathologic fracture. Needless to say, clinical and radiologic differentiation between this complication and recurrent tumor may be extremely difficult. Percutaneous needle biopsy under fluoroscopic control may provide a solution in these situations.

As with Hodgkin's disease in the post-treatment period, the development of radiologic infiltrates in the lung may herald: (1) a pulmonary infection in an immunologically deficient host; (2) radiation pneumonitis in an area of lung that was subjected to intensive irradiation (often in the lung apex or the paramediastinal regions); *or* (3) metastatic lymphoma. Only in conjunction with detailed knowledge of the clinical findings and signs can the development of radiologic infiltrates in the post-treatment period be evaluated properly. At times, fluoroscopically controlled transthoracic needle biopsy of infiltrates or apparent "masses" in the lungs may preclude the need for an open thoracotomy. In other cases, a radiologically controlled transbronchial brush biopsy of a parenchymal lung lesion may yield cytologic or bacteriologic material that will be helpful in the previously treated patient with non-Hodgkin's lymphoma. These radiologic "special procedures" should be performed when the patient is hospitalized and under close observation, whenever possible.

SUMMARY

Non-Hodgkin's lymphoma, unlike Hodgkin's disease, tends to disseminate early and to involve many lymph node regions as well as parenchymal organs, including the lungs, liver, and bone marrow. Occasionally, however, localized nodal disease can be delineated with the assistance of radiologic techniques; in other cases, primary extranodal lymphoma (relatively unusual in Hodgkin's disease) may be established by radiologic and other means, and these cases have a relatively good prognosis when involvement can be shown to be limited to the primary site and regional lymph nodes. As with Hodgkin's disease, radiologic studies have much to offer in the detection and differential diagnosis of these disorders. In view of the frequent dissemination of non-Hodgkin's lymphoma when first seen, however, the authors have suggested a careful sequence of radiologic examinations. These are to be performed in order of their increasing complexity and discomfort to the patient, with the aim of avoiding unnecessary and uncomfortable procedures whenever possible (particularly, an unnecessary exploratory laparotomy). As with Hodgkin's disease, the importance of radiologic assistance in following the *treated* patient with non-Hodgkin's lymphoma is emphasized.

References

1. Schein, P. S., Chabner, B. A., Cannellos, G. P., et al.: Potential for prolonged disease-free survival following combination chemotherapy of non-Hodgkin's lymphoma. Blood, 43:181–189, 1974.
2. Dawson, P. J., and Harrison, C. V.: A clinicopathological study of benign Hodgkin's disease. J. Clin. Pathol., 14:219–231, 1961.
3. Lukes, R. J.: Relationship of histologic features to clinical stages in Hodgkin's disease. Am. J. Roentgenol. Radium Ther. Nucl. Med., 90:944–955, 1963.
4. Peters, M., and Middlemiss, K. C.: A study of Hodgkin's disease treated by irradiation. Am. J. Roentgenol. Radium Ther. Nucl. Med., 79:114–121, 1958.
5. Freedman, S. I., Kagan, A. R., and Friedman, N. B.: Bilaterality in primary lymphosarcoma of the breast. Am. J. Clin. Pathol., 55:82–87, 1971.
6. Hamlin, J. A., Kagan, A. R., and Friedman, N. B.: Lymphomas of the testicle. Cancer, 29:1352–1356, 1972.
7. Gordon, J. D., and Paley, D. H.: Primary malignant tumors of the spleen. Statistical review and report of a case of lymphosarcoma. Surgery, 29:907–913, 1951.
8. Long, J. C., and Aisenberg, A. C.: Malignant lymphoma diagnosed at splenectomy and idiopathic splenomegaly. Cancer, 33:1054–1061, 1974.
9. Dargeon, H. W.: Lymphosarcoma in childhood. Am. J. Roentgenol. Radium Ther. Nucl. Med., 85:729–732, 1961.
10. Webster, R.: Lymphosarcoma of the thymus: Its relation to acute lymphatic leukemia. Med. J. Aust., 48:582–586, 1961.
11. Fu, Y. F., and Perzin, K. H.: Lymphosarcoma of the small intestine. Cancer, 29:645–659, 1972.
12. Whittaker, L. R.: Burkitt's lymphoma. Clin. Radiol., 24:339–346, 1973.
13. O'Conor, G. T.: Malignant lymphoma in African children. II. A pathological entity. Cancer, 14:270–283, 1961.
14. O'Conor, G. T.: Significant aspects of childhood

lymphoma in Africa. Cancer Res., *23*:1514–1518, 1963.

15. Brannan, D.: Chloroma; recent literature. Bull. Johns Hopkins Hosp., *38*:189–216, 1926.

16. Hinkamp, J. F., and Szanto, P. B.: Chloroma of the ovary. Am. J. Obstet. Gynecol., *78*:812–816, 1959.

17. Kandel, E. V.: Chloroma. A review of the literature from 1926 to 1936 and report of three cases. Arch. Intern. Med., *59*:691–704, 1937.

18. Ross, R. R.: Chloroma and chloroleukemia. Am. J. Med., *18*:671–676, 1955.

19. Leonard, B. J., Israels, M. C., and Wilkinson, J. F.: Myelosclerosis. A clinicopathological study. Q. J. Med., *26*:131–147, 1957.

20. Chievitz, E., and Thiede, T.: Complications and causes of death in polycythemia vera. Acta Med. Scand., *172*:513–523, 1962.

21. Bluefarb, S. M.: Is mycosis fungoides an entity? Arch. Dermatol., *71*:293–302, 1955.

22. Rauschkolb, R. R.: Mycosis fungoides, discussion and clinical experience at Cleveland Metropolitan General Hospital. Arch. Dermatol., *83*: 217–223, 1961.

23. Saltzstein, S. L., and Ackerman, L. V.: Lymphoadenopathy induced by anticonvulsant drugs and mimicking clinically and pathologically malignant lymphomas. Cancer, *12*:164–182, 1959.

24. Castleman, B., Iverson, L., and Pardo Menendez, V.: Localized mediastinal lymph node hyperplasia resembling thymoma. Cancer, *9*:822–830, 1956.

25. Cohen, H.: Tumor-like proliferations of lymphoid tissue. Occurrence in deltoid muscle and mediastinum. J. Mt. Sinai Hosp., *24*:750–760, 1957.

26. Lattes, R., and Pachter, M. R.: Benign lymphoid masses of probable hamartomatous nature, analysis of 12 cases. Cancer, *15*:197–214, 1962.

27. Jamplis, R. W., North, F. S., and Johnson, W. D.: Benign interlobar hyperplastic lymph node resembling thymoma. Arch. Surg., *83*:894–897, 1961.

28. Evans, N.: Lymphadenitis of secondary syphilis. Its resemblance to giant follicular lymphoadenopathy. Arch. Pathol., *37*:175–179, 1944.

29. Motulsky, A. G., Weinberg, S., Saphir, O., and Rosenberg, E.: Lymph nodes in rheumatoid arthritis. Arch. Intern. Med., *90*:660–676, 1952.

30. Zettergren, L.: Probably neoplastic proliferation of lymphoid tissue (follicular lympho-reticuloma). Reports of four cases with a survey of literature. Acta Pathol. Microbiol. Scand., *51*:113–126, 1961.

31. Kagan, A. R.: Toward an understanding of human error in the "lymphomas." Am. J. Med. Sci., *268*:271–275, 1974.

32. Banfi, A., Bonadonna, G., Carnevali, G., et al.: Malignant lymphomas. Further studies on their preferential sites of involvement and possible mode of spread. Lymphology, *2*:130–138, 1969.

33. Freeman, C., Berg, J. W., and Cutler, S. J.: Occurrence and prognosis of extranodal lymphomas. Cancer, *29*:252–260, 1972.

34. Banfi, A., Bonadonna, G., Ricci, S. B., et al.: Malignant lymphomas of Waldeyer's ring. Natural history and survival after radiotherapy. Br. Med. J., *3*:140–143, 1972.

35. Gilbert, H. A., Kagan, A. R., and Langdon, E. A.: Prognostic factors and the importance of radiation therapy in infradiaphragmatic non-Hodgkin's lymphoma. Radiology, *107*:201–205, 1973.

36. Kim, H., and Dorfman, R.: Morphologic studies of 84 untreated patients subjected to laparotomy for the staging of non-Hodgkin's lymphomas. Cancer, *33*:657–674, 1974.

37. Aisenberg, A. C.: Malignant lymphoma. N. Engl. J. Med., *288*:883–890 and 935–941, 1973.

38. Band, P. R., Silverberg, D. S., Henderson, J. F., et al.: Xanthine nephropathy in a patient with lymphosarcoma treated with allopurinol. N. Engl. J. Med., *283*:354, 1970.

39. Cox, F., and Hughes, W. T.: Disseminated histoplasmosis and childhood leukemia. Cancer, *33*: 1127–1133, 1974.

40. Ragab, A. H., Frech, R. S., and Vietti, T. J.: Osteoporotic fractures secondary to methotrexate therapy of acute leukemia in remission. Cancer, *25*:580–585, 1970.

41. Rogoff, E. E., Deck, M. D. F., and D'Angio, G.: The second sac: A complicating factor in regimens based on intrathecal medications. Radiology, *120*:568–572, 1974.

42. Veronesi, J.: The value of staging in non-Hodgkin's lymphoma (with emphasis on the histiocytic type). Cancer, *33*:446–459, 1974.

43. Olumide, A. A., Osunkoya, B. O., and Ngu, V. A.: Superior mediastinal compression: A report of five cases caused by malignant lymphoma. Cancer, *27*:193–202, 1971.

44. Salzstein, S. L.: Pulmonary malignant lymphomas and pseudolymphomas: Classification, therapy, and prognosis. Cancer, *16*:928–955, 1963.

45. Cupps, R. E., Hodgson, J. R., Dockerty, M. B., et al.: Primary lymphoma in the small intestine: Problems of roentgenologic diagnosis. Radiology, *92*:1355–1362, 1969.

46. Cremin, B. J.: The radiological appearance and incidence of lymphoma. S. Afr. Med. J., *45*: 1360–1363, 1971.

47. Wolf, B. S., and Marshak, R. H.: Roentgen features of diffuse lymphosarcoma of colon. Radiology, *75*:733–740, 1960.

48. Lusted, L. B., Besse, B. E., Jr., and Fritz, R.: Intravenous urogram in acute leukemia. Am. J. Roentgenol. Radium Ther. Nucl. Med., *80*: 608, 1958.

49. Richmond, J., Sherman, R. S., Diamond, H. D., et al.: Renal lesions associated with malignant lymphomas. Am. J. Med., *32*:184–207, 1962.

50. Lalli, A. F.: Lymphoma and the urinary tract. Radiology, *93*:1051, 1969.

51. Lee, B. J., Nelson, J. H., and Schworz, G.: Evaluation of lymphangiography, inferior venacavography and intravenous pyelography in the clinical staging and management of Hodgkin's disease and lymphosarcoma. N. Engl. J. Med., *271*: 327–337, 1964.

52. Kyaw, M., and Koehler, P. R.: Renal and perirenal lymphoma: Arteriographic findings. Radiology, *93*:1055, 1969.

53. Seltzer, R. A., and Wenlund, D. E.: Renal lymphoma. Arteriographic studies. Am. J. Roentgenol. Radium Ther. Nucl. Med., *101*:692, 1967.

54. Goffinet, D. R., Castellino, R. A., Kim, H., et al.: Staging laparotomies in unselected previously untreated patients with non-Hodgkin's lymphomas. Cancer, *32*:672–681, 1973.

55. Schwarz, G., Lee, B. J., and Nelson, J. H.: Lymphog-

raphy, cavography, and urography in the evaluation of malignant lymphomas. Acta Radiol. (Diagn.), 3:138–144, 1965.

56. Shellinger, D., Miller, W. E., Harrison, E. G., Jr., et al.: Lymphographic patterns of the subtypes of malignant lymphoma, including Hodgkin's disease. Radiology, 111:257–266, 1974.

57. Parker, B. R., Blank, N., and Castellino, R. A.: Lymphographic appearance of benign conditions simulating lymphoma. Radiology, 111: 267–274, 1974.

58. Sayoc, A. S., and Howland, W. J.: Lymphangiographic findings of mesantoin-induced pseudolymphoma. Radiology, 111:578–580, 1974.

59. Castellino, R. A., Goffinet, D. R., et al.: The role of radiography in the staging of a non-Hodgkin's lymphoma with laparotomy correlation. Radiology, 110:329–338, 1974.

60. Vieta, J. W., Friedell, H. L., and Craven, L. F.: A survey of Hodgkin's disease and lymphosarcoma in bone. Radiology, 39:1–15, 1942.

61. Whittaker, L. R.: The radiological appearance of Burkitt's tumor involving bone. Australas. Radiol., 13:307–310, 1969.

62. Mullins, G. M., Flynn, J. P., El-Mahdi, A. M., et al.: Malignant lymphoma of the spinal epidural space. Ann. Intern. Med., 74:416–423, 1971.

63. Ngan, H., and James, K. W.: Clinical Radiology of Lymphomas. Toronto, Butterworth, 1973.

64. Davidson, J. W., and Clarke, E. A.: Influence of modern radiological techniques on clinical staging of malignant lymphomas. Can. Med. Assoc. J., 99:1196–1204, 1968.

65. Johnson, R. E.: Radiotherapeutic implications of prospective staging in non-Hodgkin's lymphomas. Radiology, 110:655–657, 1974.

66. Hass, A. C., Brunk, S. F., Gulessevian, H. P., et al.: The value of exploratory laparotomy in malignant lymphoma. Radiology, 101:157–165, 1971.

67. Groth, C. G., Hellstrom, K., Hofvendahl, S., et al.: Diagnosis of malignant lymphoma at laparotomy disclosing intrahepatic cholestasis. Acta Chir. Scand., 138:186–189, 1972.

68. Desser, R. K., Moran, E. M., and Ultmann, J. E.: Staging of Hodgkin's disease and lymphoma. Diagnostic procedures including staging laparotomy and splenectomy. Med. Clin. North Am., 57:479–498, 1973.

69. Juttner, H. U., Miller, W. E., Kiely, J. M., et al.: Influence of lymphography in determining extent of disease in patients with lymphoma. Mayo Clin. Proc., 48:249–254, 1973.

Chapter Three

LUNGS AND MEDIASTINUM

Reginald F. Greene, M.D.

GENERAL CONSIDERATIONS

Primary Lung Cancer

Primary lung cancer is a common disease, and radiology plays a central role in its detection, diagnosis, and management. Primary malignancy of the lung has become the most common cause of cancer deaths among men in the United States.[1-3] However, its occurrence in females is rapidly increasing.* Ionizing radiation, asbestos, various atmospheric carcinogens, and especially cigarette smoking have been implicated as etiologic factors.[4-7] The risk of developing epidermoid carcinoma, for example, is greatly increased in smokers over nonsmokers (25:1 in males, and 12:1 in females).[3, 8] Similarly, for smokers the increased risk of developing small cell undifferentiated carcinoma is 20:1 for males and 7:1 for females.[8] No strong statistical association exists, however, between smoking and the other major histologic types of lung cancer (adenocarcinoma and large cell undifferentiated carcinoma). The chance of developing lung cancer may be increased sevenfold by exposure to asbestos.[9, 10] Six to 7 per cent of patients with lung cancer ultimately develop a second primary carcinoma of the lung.[11] A single cancer of the upper air and food passages also predisposes to a second cancer.[12] In 6 per cent of heavy

smokers, carcinoma *in situ* of the bronchus is found incidentally at autopsy.[13]

The presentation, extent, and prognosis of lung cancer vary with the histologic type.[14] All but a small percentage are of one of four major histologic types: epidermoid, adenocarcinoma, small cell undifferentiated, or large cell undifferentiated.

Epidermoid carcinoma is the most common histologic type of lung cancer, accounting for nearly one half of the total cases. It also has the most favorable prognosis (Table 3–1).[15] Epidermoid carcinoma appears to develop in heavy cigarette smokers via earlier reactive epithelial hyperplasia, squamous metaplasia, and carcinoma *in situ*.[12] These tumors tend to arise centrally in the surface epithelium of lobar, segmental, or subsegmental bronchi, accounting for the occurrence of symptoms and their earlier clinical detection. Roentgen detection, however, is often delayed until there is associated pneumonia, atelectasis, or air-trapping distal to the tumor (Figs. 3–1 and 3–2). Close surveillance of high-risk subjects (i.e., heavy smokers) using cytologic sputum examination methods has led to the discovery of epidermoid carcinomas that are radiographically occult.[16] Extension of tumor generally occurs along and through the bronchus to regional lymph nodes. The relatively favorable survival statistics for patients with epidermoid carcinoma are attributed to the lower incidence of regional lymph node and distant metastases at the time of diagnosis than in other histologic types.[14, 17, 18]

Adenocarcinoma accounts for about one

---

*Cancer deaths in 1972: male—lung 55,600, prostate 17,600, colon 16,900; female—breast 32,000, colon 19,600, lung 13,000.[1]

Table 3–1   Incidence and Survival Rates for Major Types of Lung Cancer*

Type	Overall Incidence No.	Overall Incidence %	Stage I INCIDENCE (%)	Stage I FIVE-YEAR SURVIVAL (%)	Stage II INCIDENCE (%)	Stage II FIVE-YEAR SURVIVAL (%)	Stage III INCIDENCE (%)	Stage III FIVE-YEAR SURVIVAL (%)
Epidermoid carcinoma	921	47	36	38	7	15	57	9
Adenocarcinoma	513	26	29	31	5	6	65	3
Small cell undifferentiated carcinoma	360	18	11	3†	6	4†	84	1†
Large cell undifferentiated carcinoma	181	9	34	30	9	6	57	5
TOTAL	1975	100	29		7		64	

*Adapted from a publication of the American Joint Committee for Cancer Staging and End Results Reporting, 1974.

†Two year survival.

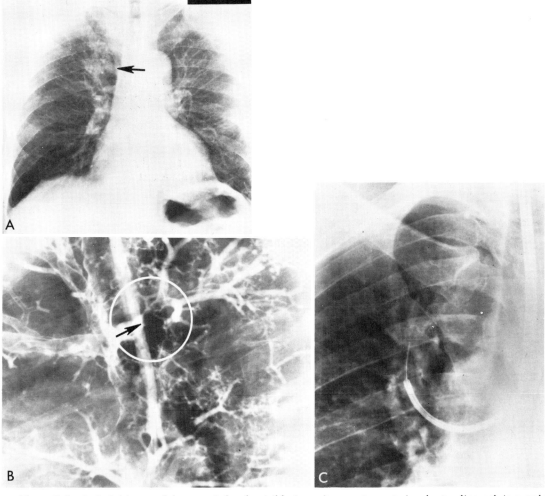

Figure 3–1   *A*, A right upper lobe mass is barely visible (arrow) on posteroanterior chest radiograph in a male smoker with hemoptysis. *B*, Bronchogram demonstrates a central endobronchial lesion (arrow) in the posterior segment of the right upper lobe. *C*, A transnasal brush biopsy of the posterior segment of the right upper lobe under fluoroscopic control was diagnostic of epidermoid carcinoma.

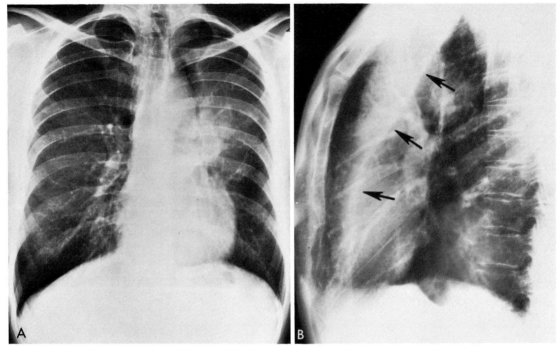

Figure 3–2 *A,* Non-productive cough, left chest discomfort, and shortness of breath were the presenting symptoms in this patient with central epidermoid carcinoma of the left upper lobe bronchus. A left perihilar density is the combined result of the tumor mass and left upper lobe atelectasis. *B,* A lateral radiograph demonstrates the airless (atelectatic) left upper lobe that is anterior to the anteriorly displaced major fissure (arrows).

quarter of all primary lung cancers (Table 3–1). In contrast to epidermoid carcinoma, these tumors tend to occur in the lung periphery, and often develop in *non-smokers.*[1, 2, 19] Because adenocarcinoma tends to extend submucosally in the bronchus and its cells cohere more tightly, exfoliation occurs less frequently than with other histologic types. In patients with the localized form (stage I), five-year survival statistics are almost as good as in those with the epidermoid variety. *Bronchoalveolar carcinoma* occurs as sheets of highly differentiated columnar cells that grow in the airspaces of the lung,* using the alveolar walls as scaffolding. This tumor frequently produces mucin and occurs in the lung periphery, especially in the vicinity of scars.[20] It has been suggested that "scar carcinoma" occurs as the result of a progression of atypical epithelial proliferation to metaplasia and finally to adenocarcinoma.[21, 22] Submucosal, endobronchial, endolymphatic, and hemato-

genous spread are common. This form of cancer may present in the form of solitary peripheral nodules, lung "consolidations," or "miliary" nodules (Figs. 3–3 and 3–18).

Small cell undifferentiated (oat cell) carcinoma is the third most common histologic type of primary lung cancer, accounting for almost one fifth of lung cancers. It is strongly linked with cigarette smoking, as well as (rarely) with occupational exposure to ionizing radiation (Table 3–1).[3] Its origin has been attributed to malignant transformation of argentaffin cells in the basal layers of bronchial epithelium. Polypeptide hormones, normally secreted by argentaffin ectodermal precursor cells, are frequently elaborated by these tumors, and cause ectopic hormonal syndromes.[23] Small cell undifferentiated carcinoma is similar to lymphoma in its histologic appearance, as well as in its associated lymphadenopathy, early systemic involvement, and relative radiosensitivity (Fig. 3–4). Submucosal, lymphatic, and vascular invasion are common. Because widespread dissemination is generally present at the time of diagno-

---

*Accordingly, this tumor has also been referred to as *bronchiolo-alveolar carcinoma* in the literature. Ed.

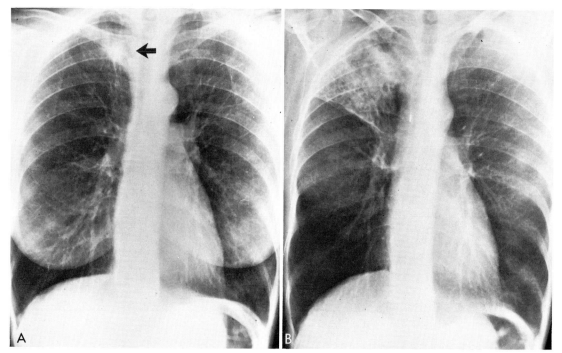

Figure 3–3 *A,* Right upper lobe opacity (arrow) in a middle-aged female with a family history of tuberculosis, a positive tuberculin skin test, and a non-productive cough. The lesion was ascribed to pulmonary tuberculosis, although no organisms were discovered in the sputum or gastric washings. *B,* A frontal radiograph after five months of antituberculous treatment shows an extension of the abnormality. There is loss in volume as well as consolidation of the right upper lobe. The lesion proved to be bronchoalveolar cell carcinoma (by mediastinal biopsy). (See also Figure 3–18.)

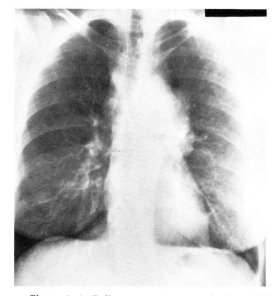

Figure 3–4 Bulky *metastatic* paratracheal and left hilar masses in a patient with small cell undifferentiated carcinoma faithfully simulate the findings of mediastinal lymphoma. The small peripheral primary lung lesion is not apparent in this study.

sis, survival is poor regardless of apparent stage with this tumor (Table 3–1).

Large cell undifferentiated carcinoma, the fourth most common type of primary lung cancer (almost one tenth of the total cases), has many similarities to adenocarcinoma (Table 3–1). Both histologic cell types have similar ultrastructures and tend to occur in the lung periphery (Fig. 3–5).[23, 24] Survival statistics by stage are similar to those for adenocarcinoma.

In addition to the four major histologic types of lung cancer, there are many less common varieties of malignancy that involve the lung parenchyma. *Bronchial carcinoids,* which account for about 5 per cent of all primary lung neoplasms, are thought to arise from the same argentaffin cells as small cell undifferentiated carcinoma (see earlier discussion). These somewhat vascular tumors tend to occur in young adults of both sexes, growing in the walls of the trachea or major bronchi. They often cause hemoptysis, bronchial occlusion, or both

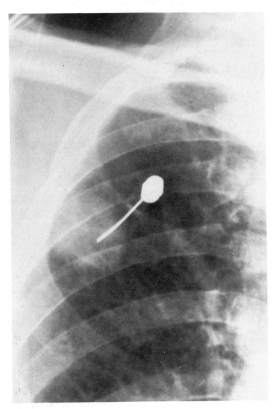

Figure 3–5 Despite the high likelihood that this newly developed nodule was malignant, a preoperative diagnosis was sought because of medical contraindications to immediate surgery in this patient. A transthoracic needle aspiration biopsy was diagnostic of large cell undifferentiated carcinoma.

(Fig. 3–6).[25] Regional metastases are common, but distant dissemination is uncommon. The carcinoid syndrome, which results from tumor secretion of 5-hydroxytryptamine, does occur rarely in bronchial carcinoids and in oat cell carcinomas.[26, 27] Other varieties of primary pulmonary malignancy are very rare and will not be considered here.

Primary Pleural Malignancy

Malignant mesothelioma, which is closely linked to asbestos dust exposure (especially the crocidolite variety), is by far the most important of the uncommon primary pleural malignancies (Fig. 3–7).[6] There is generally a forty-year latent period between exposure to asbestos and the development of a tumor. Survival data are similar to those for advanced lung cancer, and no effective treatment is known.

Primary Mediastinal Malignancy

The mediastinum is involved more commonly by secondary than by primary malignancies. The majority of primary mediastinal malignancies are lymphomas, thymomas, germinal tumors, or tracheal and esophageal carcinomas. Malignant neurogenic tumors (e.g., neuroblastoma) occur in the posterior mediastinum, particularly in children. Other primary mediastinal malignancies are very uncommon.

Lymphoma, including Hodgkin's disease, commonly arises in the mediastinal compartments and frequently coexists with more extensive disease in the neck and retroperitoneum. This group of tumors is extensively discussed in Chapters 1 and 2 and will be dealt with here only in relation to the differential diagnosis.

Thymoma is a common tumor of the anterior mediastinal compartment (Fig. 3–8). Lymphoid, mixed lymphoid, and epithelial types of thymoma are often associated with myasthenia gravis; conversely, only 15 per cent of patients with myasthenia gravis have thymoma.[28–30] The spindle cell variety of thymoma is often associated with hematologic abnormalities, such as red blood cell aplasia. Cushing's syndrome and hyperthyroidism are also known to occur in patients with thymoma.[31, 32] The ten-year survival rate is approximately 90 per cent when a thymoma is not associated with either myasthenia gravis or gross tumor invasion into adjacent structures. The ten-year survival rate drops to about 50 per cent when one of the above factors is present, and further decreases to near zero when both are present.[33] The degree of malignancy of this tumor is correlated more closely with its clinical behavior and gross morphology than with its histologic characteristics.

Germinal tumors occur with about the same frequency as thymomas. Most of the malignant varieties of germ cell origin are teratomas, but primary seminomas and choriocarcinomas of the mediastinum also occur (Fig. 3–9).

Tracheal malignancies are rare, accounting for less than 0.1 per cent of all cancers.[34] The most common tracheal malignancy is squamous cell carcinoma, followed by adenoid cystic carcinoma (cylindroma), which occasionally originates in the major bronchi (Fig. 3–10).[35] Like carcinoids, adenoid cystic

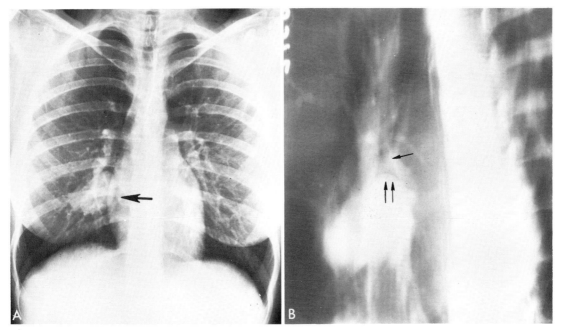

Figure 3–6 *A,* Right lower lobe opacity (arrow) in a 20-year-old female with hemoptysis. *B,* A tomogram shows an egg-shaped, endobronchial mass that occludes the right lower lobe bronchus (double arrows). The superior segmental bronchus is seen end-on and is patent (single arrow). A presumptive diagnosis of bronchial carcinoid was made and confirmed at thoracotomy. No preoperative endobronchial biopsy was obtained, for fear of causing uncontrollable hemorrhage.

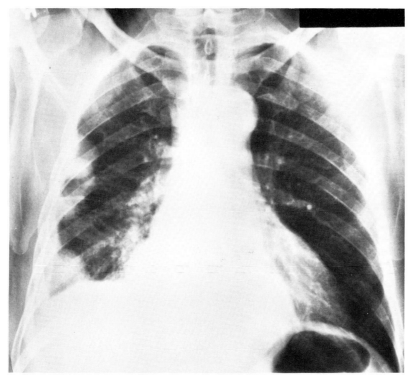

Figure 3–7 Hemispherical, lobulated masses are present along the right lateral chest wall in this 60-year-old former shipyard worker who complained of severe pleuritic chest pain. These pleural masses proved to be malignant mesothelioma.

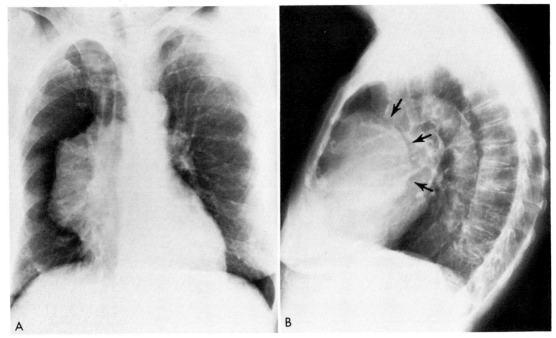

Figure 3–8 *A* and *B*, The lobulated anterior mediastinal mass (arrows) that projects into the right lung from the cardiac silhouette proved to be a malignant thymoma. This middle-aged female also had myasthenia gravis.

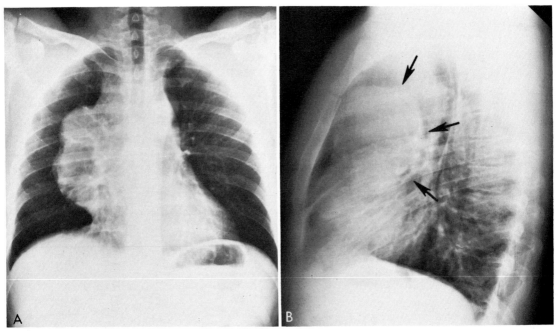

Figure 3–9 *A* and *B*, The large, lobulated, anterior mediastinal mass (arrows) that projects into the right lung of this young adult male is almost indistinguishable from the mass shown in Figure 3–8. In this case the mass is a malignant teratoma. The patient complained of a non-productive cough and dull chest discomfort.

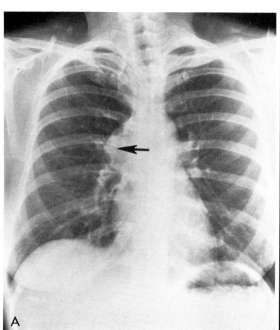 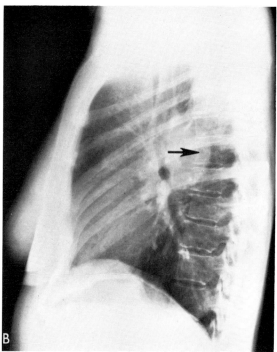

Figure 3–10 *A* and *B*, A smoothly outlined mediastinal mass projects to the right of and posterior to the trachea (arrow). The patient complained of stridor and shortness of breath. The mass proved to be an adenoid cystic carcinoma of the trachea, with a bulky extraluminal component.

carcinomas grow slowly and are locally aggressive, but only very rarely do they disseminate widely.[36] Death frequently results from tracheal obstruction or local extension into adjacent vascular structures. Long-term cures can be obtained if total excision of these localized lesions is possible. Mixed cell and mucoepidermoid carcinomas, although very uncommon, are more aggressive varieties of carcinoma that involve the trachea and major bronchi.[37] Primary cartilaginous malignancies (chondrosarcoma) also involve the trachea rarely.

Esophageal carcinoma may be of the squamous cell, adenocarcinoma, or the bulky carcinosarcoma type. These tumors are discussed in detail in Chapter 6 and will be dealt with here only in relation to the differential diagnosis.

CLINICAL CONSIDERATIONS

Presenting Signs and Symptoms

Primary mediastinal malignancies are often discovered incidentally (on chest radiographs), but only a small minority of patients with primary lung cancer (about 10 per cent) are *asymptomatic* at the time of diagnosis.[38] The largest group of asymptomatic patients have peripheral adenocarcinomas that are discovered incidentally by chest radiography. Regardless of treatment, five-year survival rates are greatest in lung cancer patients who either are asymptomatic when diagnosed, or who have had symptoms for longer than six months prior to diagnosis (18 per cent and 16 per cent respectively).[38] Survival for five years is much less frequent in patients with (1) symptoms of less than six months duration, (2) nonspecific systemic symptoms, or (3) focal metastatic symptoms (6 per cent, 9 per cent, and 0 per cent, respectively).

Local symptoms in primary lung carcinoma are usually related to their endobronchial location (Fig. 3–11): cough (75 per cent) and hemoptysis (50 per cent) are the most common symptoms present at the time of diagnosis.[39] Abundant sputum sometimes occurs in bronchoalveolar cell carcinoma. Cough or choking that occurs when eating may indicate the presence of a tracheoesophageal fistula or involvement of glossopharyngeal fibers of the recurrent laryngeal

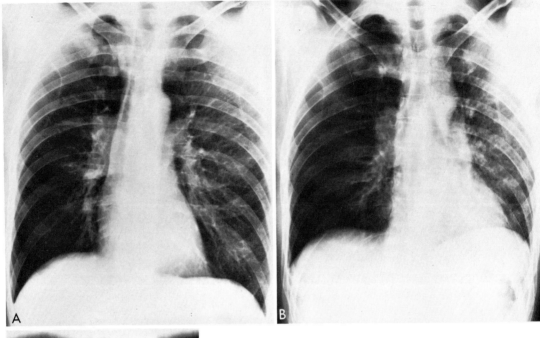

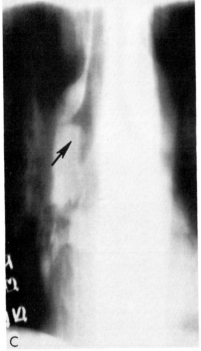

Figure 3–11 *A,* There is slight fullness of the upper margin of the right hilus and the suggestion of hypovascularity of the right lung, in a patient with shortness of breath. Symptoms were more severe than the radiographic appearance would indicate. *B,* An expiration view demonstrates trapped air in the right lung, with shift of the mediastinum to the left. *C,* A tomogram shows an endobronchial mass projecting into the right mainstem bronchus (arrow). Bronchial biopsy was diagnostic of poorly differentiated adenocarcinoma.

nerve. Fever may be part of a paramalignant syndrome or may result from pneumonitis distal to an obstructing bronchial cancer. Chest pain generally indicates involvement of some part of the chest cage (ribs, intercostal nerves, pleura, or diaphragm). Involvement of the brachial plexus by apical epidermoid lung carcinoma (Pancoast's tumor) is often associated with severe shoulder pain (Fig. 3–12). Pleural pain is a frequent accompaniment of malignant pleural mesothelioma. Shortness of breath, wheezing, and stridor often result from compromise of major airways, but they may also result from a regional ventilation/perfusion imbalance or pleural effusion. A localized expiratory wheeze can often be detected over the tumor area. Rapid enlargement of undifferentiated lung cancers, lymphomas, or teratomas may compress the trachea and cause severe stridor that will require urgent treatment.

The presence of tumor in the mediastinum can cause a large variety of symptoms in addition to those already mentioned. Hoarseness may result from direct extension of the tumor into the recurrent laryngeal nerve, or from metastatic involvement of the adjacent ductus arteriosus lymph node group. Abnormal swallowing mechanics, including aspiration and dysphagia, frequently coexist with hoarseness, since the recurrent laryngeal nerve also carries glossopharyngeal fibers. Dysphagia or odynophagia also may result from a primary esophageal tumor, or from esophageal compression by an adjacent mass in the lung or mediastinum. Compression or invasion of the superior vena cava by a primary carcinoma of the right upper lobe, metastatic paratracheal lymph nodes, or primary mediastinal cancers can result in a superior vena cava syndrome. Involvement of the stellate ganglion can cause Horner's syndrome (ptosis, meiosis, enophthalmos, and unilateral absence of sweating). Cardiorespiratory

embarrassment that cannot be explained otherwise may be the result of malignant cardiac tamponade.

Extrapulmonary Symptoms. Occasionally, a primary lung cancer is first discovered not because of local signs or symptoms, but from its extrapulmonary manifestations. Fever, malaise, weakness, and loss of weight occur frequently in lung cancer and are not always directly attributable to local or metastatic effects of the tumor. These "paramalignant" conditions, which also include finger clubbing and endocrine metabolic disorders, have been reported in 20 to 30 per cent of patients with primary lung cancers.[40] Hypertrophic pulmonary osteoarthropathy (clubbing, subperiosteal osteitis, and bone and joint pain) occurs in about 4 per cent of patients with lung cancer, but is infrequently found with the small cell undifferentiated type.[41] Symptoms produced by ectopic hormonal syndromes or pulmonary osteoarthropathy may be relieved by resection or control of the tumor. Of the cancer-related hormonal syndromes, hypercalcemia from ectopic parathormone production is probably the most common, occurring in about 10 per cent of patients with lung cancer (especially of the epidermoid type).[42, 43] The symptoms of hypercalcemia (weakness, drowsiness, nausea,

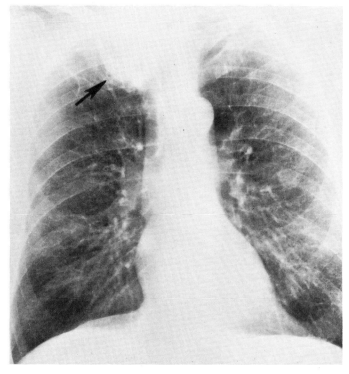

Figure 3–12 Severe, unremitting right shoulder pain was the presenting symptom of a bulky epidermoid carcinoma in the superior sulcus ("Pancoast tumor") of the right lung (arrow). Diagnosis was made by aspiration needle biopsy, under fluoroscopic control.

constipation, polyuria, and polydipsia) may occur in the absence of any clinical or radiologic evidence of bone metastases. Ectopic adrenal corticotrophic hormone, which is not uncommonly produced by small cell undifferentiated lung tumors, can cause a fulminant Cushing's syndrome (with hypokalemia, hypertension, and impaired glucose tolerance).[44, 45] Hyponatremia and decreased serum osmolarity, as a result of *inappropriate antidiuretic hormone* secretion, occur in 1 to 2 per cent of lung cancers and can be reversed with successful treatment of the tumor.[42] Gynecomastia, hyperthyroidism, various neuromyopathies, and the carcinoid syndrome (see earlier discussion) can all be produced by bronchial carcinoids as well as by small cell undifferentiated carcinomas.[27]

The initial presenting symptoms or signs may reflect the presence of extrathoracic metastases in about one fourth of patients.[3] Symptomatic bone metastases (bone pain or tenderness) often are present at the time of diagnosis. Almost one half of patients with small cell carcinoma of the lung, and a smaller percentage of those with other types, have cytologically positive bone marrow examinations at the time of diagnosis.[18] Eighteen to 39 per cent of patients with bronchogenic carcinoma have clinical evidence of brain metastases at diagnosis.[3] The highest percentage of brain metastases occur with small cell and large cell undifferentiated carcinomas. As many as 15 per cent of patients with lung cancer have been found to have surgical evidence of metastases at abdominal exploration.[46]

Differential Diagnosis

Establishing a specific diagnosis in the asymptomatic patient with a roentgenographically demonstrated pulmonary nodule generally requires a radiologically controlled or open surgical biopsy procedure. On the other hand, sputum cytology carries no risk to the patient and should be pursued with care and perseverance in all cases, although only 20 to 30 per cent of malignant solitary pulmonary nodules will be diagnosed unequivocally in this way.[47] Bronchoscopy and "blind" scalene lymph node biopsy are recognized as extremely low-yield endeavors in the differential diagnosis of pulmonary nodules. Mediastinoscopy will be diagnostic only with a minority of solitary lung nodules (about 20 per cent), but its role and that of bronchoscopy in the *staging* of known cancers is very important.[48]

Most of the local symptoms of lung cancer (fever, cough, hemoptysis, chest pain) are nonspecific and are common to a number of benign cardiorespiratory disorders. Occasionally, the presenting constellation of clinical findings allows a firm diagnosis, but often pneumonia or thromboembolism cannot be differentiated clinically from lung cancer. Chronic obstructive pulmonary disease is so common in patients with lung cancer that it serves to confuse further the clinical presentation. A "new" cough may herald a cancer, but its differentiation from pneumonia or recurrent tracheobronchitis may be difficult. An acute onset with clinical evidence of sepsis, the presence of neutrophils and pathogenic organisms in the sputum, and peripheral neutrophilia may help to make the diagnosis of pneumonia, but pneumonia and cancer often coexist. Recurrent pneumonia or incomplete clearing of an infiltrate may indicate the need for sputum cytology, endoscopy, or further radiologic studies (Fig. 3–13).

The evaluation of patients with hemoptysis presents many frustrations, and the precise site of bleeding often is not found. Excluding primary bleeding abnormalities, the major causes of hemoptysis are bronchitis, pneumonitis, bronchiectasis, and tumor. The upper air and food passages must also be excluded as bleeding sources by a thorough examination of the nose, throat, and larynx. Bronchoscopic localization is often complicated by the presence of blood throughout the tracheobronchial tree during active hemoptysis, but the site of a large localized blood clot may indicate the source of bleeding. Plain radiographs, tomography, and fluoroscopy frequently provide further clues to the site and cause of bleeding.

Clinical error may occur when a diagnosis is made in the absence of specific findings, as when patients are treated for pneumonia or pulmonary embolism in the absence of a demonstrated pathogen or vascular occlusion, respectively (Fig. 3–3). Shoulder pain from Pancoast's tumor is often treated as "bursitis" for long periods, before the tumor is recognized (Figure 3–12).

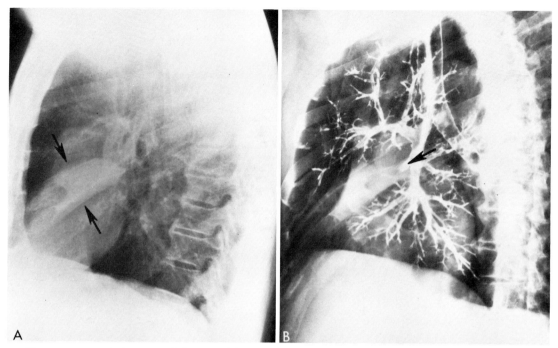

Figure 3–13 *A,* A three-month history of fever and cough accompanied persistent atelectasis and infiltration in the right middle lobe (arrows) depicted on lateral view. Two bronchial endoscopic examinations demonstrated a "normal right middle lobe orifice." Bronchial washings from the right middle lobe were negative cytologically. *B,* An oblique view during bronchography demonstrates an abrupt occlusion of the right middle lobe bronchus just distal to its origin by an epidermoid carcinoma (arrow).

Complete radiographic studies of the shoulder, neck, and lung apices may preclude this error.

Rheumatologists often see patients with lung cancer whose primary complaints are "arthritic," secondary to hypertrophic pulmonary osteoarthropathy. Pulmonary osteoarthropathy, of course, also occurs with lung sepsis, tuberculosis, and fungal infection, and in patients with congenital heart disease. Ectopic hormonal syndromes with lung cancer must be differentiated from primary endocrine tumors and hyperplasias.

Hoarseness may result directly from vocal cord tumors or inflammation, as well as from involvement of the recurrent laryngeal nerve by lung cancer. One should not *assume* that the source of abnormal cells in a sputum specimen is the lung until a thorough evaluation of the upper food and air passages has also been carried out (see Chapter 6).

Dysphagia has many causes, both benign and malignant; these in turn may be intrinsic or extrinsic to the esophagus. There is no substitute for a careful barium esophagram under fluoroscopic control to identify many of the causes of dysphagia.

Superior vena cava obstruction syndromes are most often caused by malignancies in the mediastinum, but they can also result from mediastinal fibrosis or inflammation, intrathoracic goiters, or inflammatory pericardial disease. Although Horner's syndrome is most often caused by a malignant mediastinal tumor, it very rarely may result from a benign process.

Inflammatory pleural disease, as may occur in tuberculosis, is best differentiated from pleural malignancy by thoracentesis or pleural biopsy. The histologic diagnosis of mesothelioma by means of closed (needle) pleural biopsy is difficult, and a definite diagnosis must often await open pleural biopsy or postmortem examination. The presence of hyaluronic acid in bloody pleural fluid supports the diagnosis of malignant mesothelioma.

Localization and Staging

A clinical staging classification has been adopted for lung cancer by the American Joint Committee for Cancer Staging and End Results Reporting.[15] This staging system (TNM) facilitates the exchange of information, as well helps to indicate the most appropriate mode of treatment and the individual prognosis. Survival in a patient with lung cancer not only depends on tumor histology but also on the TNM characteristics: the local extent of tumor (T), the presence of lymph node metastases (N), and the presence of distant metastases (M). Only in small cell undifferentiated carcinoma are the survival data independent of clinical staging (see Table 3–1).

Clinical TNM staging is carried out at the time of diagnosis and treatment; it should take into account the patient's history, physical examination, laboratory studies, radiologic examinations, and bronchoscopic findings. When appropriate, it should also take into consideration the results of thoracentesis, mediastinoscopy, and knowledge derived from various cytologic/histologic biopsy procedures. *Surgical* staging includes all of the above, as well as information based on direct observations and diagnostic procedures carried out at thoracotomy. *Post-surgical* staging includes the information obtained after a complete examination of the resected specimen.

We are primarily concerned here with *clinical staging*. The TNM system for lung cancer is shown in Table 3–2, and the definition of each clinical stage is shown in Table 3–3.[15]

The mucosal extent of *central* endobronchial cancers (T) generally is best determined by endoscopy. The extent of *peripheral* lung cancer, on the other hand, must be determined radiologically. The evaluation of secondary mediastinal involvement occupies a key position in staging lung cancer and in determining the likelihood of cure by resection. The mediastinum can be involved in primary lung cancer either by direct extension (T3), or by lymph node metastases (N2). Either of these circumstances relegate the disease to stage III (Table 3–3). The uniformly unfavorable survival statistics in these circumstances should encourage a conservative therapeutic course. Symptoms and signs may also indicate the presence of

Table 3–2 TNM Categories for Lung Cancer*

Primary Tumor (T)

T0   No evidence of primary tumor.

TX   Tumor proven by malignant cells in bronchopulmonary secretions; not visualized roentgenographically or bronchoscopically.

T1   Tumor 3.0 cm or less in greatest diameter, surrounded by lung or visceral pleura, without evidence of invasion proximal to lobar bronchus.

T2   Tumor more than 3.0 cm in greatest diameter, or any size that, with its associated atelectasis or obstructive pneumonitis, extends to the hilar region. Proximal extent of demonstrable tumor at least 2.0 cm distal to the carina. Associated atelectasis or obstructive pneumonitis involves less than entire lung; no pleural effusion.

T3   Tumor of any size, with direct extension into adjacent structures such as chest wall, diaphragm, mediastinum, or with proximal extent of tumor less than 2.0 cm distal to carina, or with associated atelectasis or obstructive pneumonitis of entire lung, or with pleural effusion.

Regional Lymph Nodes (N)

N0   No demonstrable metastasis to regional lymph nodes.

N1   Metastasis to ipsilateral hilar lymph nodes.

N2   Metastasis to lymph nodes in the mediastinum.

Distant Metastasis (M)

M0   No distant metastasis.

M1   Distant metastasis.

*Adapted from the American Joint Committee for Cancer Staging and End Results Reporting, 1973.

Table 3–3 Stages of Lung Cancer*

Occult	TX N0 M0
Stage I†	T1 N0 M0
	T1 N1 M0
	T2 N0 M0
Stage II	T2 N1 M0
Stage III	T3 and any N or M
	N2 and any T or M
	M1 and any T or N

*Adapted from the American Joint Committee for Cancer Staging and End Results Reporting, 1973.

†Note that Stage I includes T2 lesions that have no evidence of lymph node metastasis, and T1 lesions with metastasis to the ipsilateral nodes within the lung.

mediastinal disease (hoarseness, dysphagia, and superior vena cava or Horner's syndromes). Palpable cervical adenopathy is not very common in lung cancer, but when present it indicates concurrent mediastinal disease. Beyond these clinical considerations, the evaluation of the mediastinum must rely upon radiologic and surgical methods.

Mediastinoscopy, which has now largely supplanted scalene lymph node biopsy as a staging procedure, yields carcinomatous lymph nodes in 35 per cent of lung cancers.[48] This is of great importance, since a negative mediastinoscopy provides 90 per cent assurance that the tumor is at least resectable.[17] The incidence of positive mediastinal lymph nodes is greatest with the undifferentiated tumors.[49] The *distribution* of mediastinal lymph node involvement from lung cancer parallels normal lymph drainage patterns (Table 3–4).[50] Lymph nodes in the left tracheobronchial angle are not easily reached with mediastinoscopy, and in the case of left upper lobe cancers mediastinoscopy is often negative even when mediastinal metastases are present. Therefore, anterior transcostal explorations of the left tracheobronchial lymph nodes are often used to reach these relatively inaccessible lymph nodes. It has been reported that the findings at mediastinoscopy can be successfully predicted by mediastinal tomography.[51]

Special mediastinal biopsy procedures may be useful for diagnosing primary middle mediastinal malignancies (e.g., lymphoma). However, primary lesions of the anterior mediastinum (thymoma and teratoma) are not accessible via mediastinoscopy, and in any event primary resection is generally preferred to biopsy followed by resection in these patients.

Distant lung cancer metastases to bone, brain, and liver are often present at the time of diagnosis, and thorough preoperative evaluation for disseminated disease (M1) is therefore advisable. Clinical evidence of brain metastases has been reported in 20 per cent of epidermoid cancers, and in 39 per cent of small cell undifferentiated cancers.[3] These figures justify a noninvasive preoperative search for brain metastases with radionuclide scans or computerized axial tomography. Intraosseous metastases can be found by marrow biopsy in up to 40 per cent of patients with small cell undifferentiated carcinoma. Radionuclide bone scans are much more sensitive than the elevation of serum alkaline phosphatase or bone radiography in the detection of asymptomatic osseous metastases. Transdiaphragmatic exploration of the liver has demonstrated hepatic metastases in 8 per cent of lung adenocarcinomas and in 25 per cent of large cell undifferentiated carcinomas.[3] The diagnostic yield from liver scans in the absence of other clinical evidence of hepatic metastases has been questioned, however.[52] In summary, an orderly program of clinical evaluation to detect evidence of intrathoracic tumor extension or distant metastases is essential, prior to deciding on the mode of treatment, for the patient with lung cancer.

Clinical Follow-up

The major clinical problems that occur during or after treatment of lung cancer relate to: (1) persistence or recurrence of the primary tumor; (2) regional lymph node metastases; (3) disseminated tumor; (4) complications of treatment; and (5) intercurrent (nonmalignant) disease.

Recurrent tumor at the bronchial stump is often heralded by hemoptysis and can generally be seen bronchoscopically or demonstrated radiographically. Hemoptysis after treatment for lung carcinoma also requires a complete clinical evaluation of the upper food and air passages as well as of the remaining portions of the lung,

Table 3–4   Positive Mediastinal Biopsies by Location of Tumor*

Cancer Location	Right Paratracheal (%)	Left Paratracheal (%)	Subcarinal (%)
Right upper lobe	64	4	32
Right lower lobe	42	12	46
Left upper lobe	16	42	42
Left lower lobe	21	29	50

*Data from Carlens, F.: Appraisal of choice and results of treatment for bronchogenic carcinoma. Chest, 65:443, 1974.

since multiple primary carcinomas often occur. Recurrence of the primary tumor after irradiation often heralds simultaneous widespread tumor dissemination (Fig. 3–14).

The development of bulky periesophageal lymph node metastases is often signaled by dysphagia. Choking during eating or drinking further suggests the presence of a tracheoesophageal fistula.

Malaise, weight loss, fever, or cough in a patient after treatment for lung cancer may be the result of tumor recurrence or extension, radiation- or chemotherapy-induced pneumonitis, postoperative infection, disseminated tumor, or intercurrent disease. Associated symptoms often are helpful in making this critical differentiation. Bone pain suggests the development of disseminated tumor or chest wall tumor extension. Symptoms of pneumonia that occur within several months of completing radiotherapy suggest the presence of radiation pneumonitis or of intercurrent infection (Fig. 3–25). Pericarditis or effusion may occur as a result of mediastinal irradiation and must be differentiated from malignant pericardial effusion. Benign intercurrent disease is common in lung cancer patients and is often mistakenly ascribed to the malignancy itself. Certain chemotherapeutic

agents (e.g., busulfan, bleomycin, and Cytoxan) are recognized as causative agents of reactive pneumonitis that must be differentiated from tumor dissemination or intercurrent infection.[53]

The functional effects of lung cancer often become a major clinical problem. Regional abnormalities of gas exchange are often present when there is associated atelectasis or consolidation. A veno-arterial shunt effect is often reversed when the airless lung distal to an obstructing tumor becomes re-expanded in the course of palliative treatment. On the other hand, the most common functional effect of intensive lung irradiation is a parallel reduction in both ventilation and perfusion in the treated lung.

RADIOLOGIC CONSIDERATIONS

Presenting Radiographic Signs

The radiologic appearance of primary lung cancer is closely linked to the cell type (Table 3–4). Adenocarcinomas, for example, characteristically occur as solitary peripheral

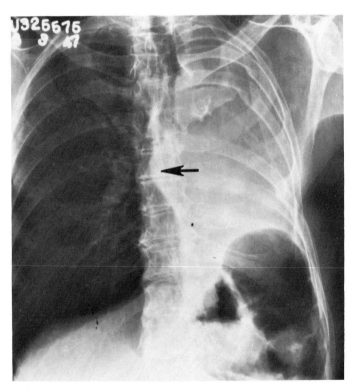

Figure 3–14 The development of periesophageal lymph node metastases six months after a left pneumonectomy for epidermoid carcinoma causes a bulge of the mediastinal pleura (arrow). This is best demonstrated on an overexposed film.

lesions, while undifferentiated carcinomas often present as multiple, centrally located radiographic densities.

Radiologically Occult Carcinomas. Although the vast majority of lung cancers are discovered only after they have become symptomatic, there is great interest now in detecting asymptomatic lung cancers, since the prognosis in "early" carcinomas is more favorable than in symptomatic cancers (about 45 per cent five-year survival).[54] The results of early detection efforts with screening radiography, however, have been disappointing to date. About one patient with cancer can be found in 5,000 asymptomatic males over 45 years old undergoing screening chest radiographs.[55] Only 20 per cent of the 121 "new" lung cancers found in a photofluorographic survey of 6,027 males from 1951 to 1961 were detected within six months of a previously negative roentgenogram.[56] Of all the patients with lung cancers discovered through this screening survey, only 8 per cent survived five years. Therefore, it appears that screening radiographs can indeed detect asymptomatic lung cancers but that overall mortality is not subsequently affected by the currently employed treatment methods. In spite of the disappointing results of screening radiography for lung cancer in the general population, interest in screening persons at high risk for lung cancer is growing. The U.S. Department of Health, Education, and Welfare in fact recommends that screening for cardiopulmonary disease be carried out only in high-risk groups, rather than in general populations, and that standard radiographic methods rather than photofluorography be used.[57]

Intensive sputum cytologic evaluation of patients who are at high risk for developing lung carcinoma has resulted in an increased detection of radiologically occult carcinomas.[16] The Mayo Clinic Lung Project, for instance, has found 15 cases over a 15-month period while using triennial chest radiography with pooled sputum cytologic testing in male smokers over 45 years of age. Although there is evidence that the prompt excision of occult carcinomas identified by endobronchial biopsy will result in prolonged survival, patients undergoing this procedure also have a high incidence of multiple lung carcinomas (about 20 per cent).[16, 58–60] Sputum-positive, radiographically occult lung carcinomas are often centrally located, endobronchial squamous cell carcinomas that are best localized by bronchoscopy. True radiologically occult carcinomas are very uncommon and should be differentiated from carcinomas that are missed because of inadequate radiologic examination or observer error (Fig. 3–1 and Table 3–5).[19, 24, 61, 62]

Solitary Pulmonary Nodules. Radiographic abnormalities are present in the vast majority (about 99 per cent) of patients with lung cancer (Table 3–5). A significant percentage (about 30 per cent) are first detected roentgenologically as solitary pulmonary nodules; more than 50 per cent of adenocarcinomas present in this way. Peripheral lung carcinomas are favorably situated for radiographic detection, but they are not usually perceived until they reach about 1 cm in diameter. Clinical chest radiography can actually resolve nodules less than 1 mm in diameter, but the contrast offered between a small cancer and the air-filled normal lung is ordinarily not sufficient for initial detection until the lesion is much larger. The likelihood of early radiographic detection of an asymptomatic peripheral lung cancer depends not only on the density produced by the tumor mass and its location, but also on the rate of growth of the individual tumor. Assuming that the tumor starts as a single malignant cell, a mass 1 cm in diameter is actually the result of 20 cell generations, which may occur over varying periods of time. Therefore, a cancer nodule 1 cm in diameter may not be so much an "early" as a "small" cancer. Aggressive lung cancers grow so rapidly that the period during which they are both small *and* asymptomatic is very short. There may be little chance, therefore, for their "early" detection. On the other hand, less aggressive lung cancers grow more slowly, so that the time span during which they are both small and asymptomatic is longer and the actual chance of their "early" detection by periodic screening examinations is greater.

Malignant pulmonary nodules may be smooth or irregular in outline, and they may be solid or cavitated. The majority of the 10 per cent of primary lung cancers that do cavitate are epidermoid carcinomas.[61] Cavitation almost never occurs in small cell undifferentiated carcinomas.[62] Malignant pulmonary nodules can present at any size. About two thirds of adenocarcinomas and small cell undifferentiated carcinomas, and one third of

Table 3–5   Radiographic Findings in Lung Cancer

Radiographic Finding	163 Squamous Cell Carcinomas† %	126 Adeno-carcinomas‡ %	114 Small Cell Undifferentiated Carcinomas§ %	97 Large Cell Undifferentiated Carcinomas# %
Peripheral lesion	31	74	32	65
Atelectasis	37	10	18	13
Consolidation	20	15	24	25
Hilar/perihilar abnormality	40	18	78	32
Mediastinal abnormality	2	3	13	10
Pleural effusion	4	5	5	2
No abnormality	3	1	0	0
Single abnormality	64	70	38	58

†Data from Byrd, R. B., Miller, W. E., and Carr, D. T., et al.: The roentgenographic appearance of squamous cell carcinoma of the bronchus. Mayo Clin. Proc., 43:327, 1968.

‡Data from Lehar, T. J., Carr., D. T., Miller, W. E., et al.: Roentgenographic appearance of bronchogenic adeno-carcinoma. Am. Rev. Resp. Dis., 96:245, 1967.

§Data from Byrd, R. B., Miller, W. E., Carr, D. T., et al.: The roentgenographic appearance of small cell carcinoma of the bronchus. Mayo Clin. Proc., 43:337, 1968.

#Data from Byrd, R. B., Miller, W. E., Carr, D. T., et al.: The roentgenographic appearance of large cell carcinoma of the bronchus. Mayo Clin. Proc., 43:333, 1968.

epidermoid and large cell undifferentiated carcinomas, are less than 4 cm in diameter when first seen.[19, 24, 61, 62]

Atelectasis and Consolidation.   Almost one half of all patients with lung cancer show roentgenologic evidence of atelectasis, consolidation, or both at the time of diagnosis (Table 3–5). As might be expected, this presentation is especially common in patients with centrally located, endobronchial epidermoid carcinomas. When the lesion is located within lobar or mainstem bronchi and is totally occlusive, atelectasis is the frequent result (Fig. 3–2). Lobar endobronchial lesions can cause expiratory air-trapping in the affected lung, or peripheral pneumonitis (Fig. 3–11). Tumors that are located peripheral to the lobar bronchi do not often cause atelectasis, because collateral ventilation between lung alveoli can maintain normal gas volumes in the distal lung. Bronchogenic lobar spread of bronchoalveolar cell carcinoma can often cause the roentgenographic appearance of lobar consolidation (Fig. 3–3); in these cases, the tumor itself actually causes the lobar density.

In lung primaries, *hilar and mediastinal* enlargement are most often found with undifferentiated tumors and in association with other radiographic abnormalities (Fig. 3–4).

Primary mediastinal malignancies occur in characteristic locations. For roentgenographic diagnostic purposes it is convenient to divide the mediastinum into anterior, middle, and posterior compartments.

The common primary malignancies of the *anterior mediastinum* (germinal tumors including teratomas, thymomas, and lymphomas) are sometimes perceived only on lateral radiographs (Fig. 3–15). When these tumors attain sufficient size, they also project into the lungs on the frontal chest view (Fig. 3–8). Rarely, mediastinal malignancies also occur superiorly within intrathoracic thyroid, parathyroid, neurogenic, and mesenchymal tissues. The majority of malignancies in the *middle mediastinum* are caused by primary (lymphomatous) and metastatic tumors in lymph nodes and by central tracheobronchial lung cancers. Efficient radiologic detection and delineation of these tumor masses will depend upon well-penetrated frontal and lateral views (Fig. 3–10). Strategically located mediastinal masses can displace, compress, or invade the trachea, esophagus, great vessels, and nerves. Phrenic palsy with diaphragmatic elevation can also occasionally be detected roentgenographically. Malignant masses of the *posterior mediastinum* are caused primarily by large cancers of the esophagus and of the lymph nodes, as well as occasional malignant neurogenic tumors; they present roentgenographically as mass lesions adjacent to the aorta and the spine (Fig. 3–16).

Chest wall, pleural, and diaphragmatic abnormalities are observed roentgenographically in a minority of lung cancers. Chest wall involvement may result from peripheral lung cancers occurring in the superior sulcus or along the lateral chest wall (Fig. 3–12). Rib or vertebral destruction may be evident in these cases. Pleural effusion, alone or in combination with other findings, is detected in only about 10 per cent of lung cancers and generally indicates direct pleural involvement by tumor. Pleural effusion and lobulated pleural/extrapleural masses are characteristic of mesothelioma and of advanced lung cancers (Fig. 3–7). *Extra*pulmonary radiographic or clinical abnormalities such as hypertrophic pulmonary osteoarthropathy or bone metastases often provide the first evidence of a lung cancer.

Differential Diagnosis

"Normal" Chest Film. Many patients with primary lung cancers first present with extrapulmonary symptoms, and unfortunately the ititial chest radiograph is often suboptimal. As a result, the chest lesion may be overlooked until much later. To avoid lengthy and misdirected searches for a primary tumor, the physician should obtain good quality erect chest roentgenograms before excluding the lung as the source for a malignancy. Often multiple chest views, fluoroscopy, or tomography are needed to detect or rule out a primary lung cancer.

Solitary Pulmonary Nodules. In about 30 per cent of patients with primary lung cancers, the only radiographic abnormality is a solitary pulmonary nodule; not all solitary nodules, however, are malignant. Solitary metastatic renal cell and colon carcinomas occur and are difficult to differentiate from primary pulmonary adenocarcinomas. There is a wide range in the reported incidence of malignancy within resected solitary lung nodules (10 to 78 per cent), possibly resulting from variations in the definition of "nodule" and in the criteria used for resection, as well as from geographic differences in the incidence of benign granulomatous infections.[63–67] The recommendation frequently voiced by surgeons that all asymptomatic solitary pulmonary nodules. should be re-

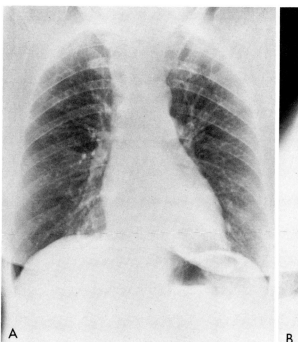 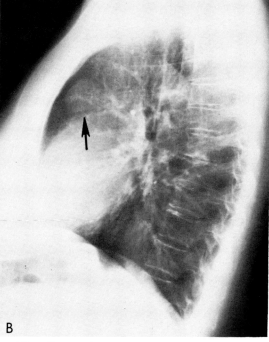

A   B

Figure 3–15 The standard radiograph (*A*) in a patient with malignant thymoma failed, even in retrospect, to reveal the anterior mediastinal mass (arrow) that is easily seen on the lateral view (*B*). (See also Figure 3–8.)

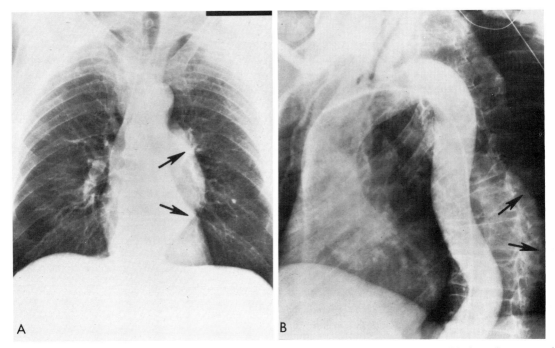

Figure 3–16 *A,* The large mass that displaces the mediastinal pleura (arrows) is inseparable from the aorta and simulates an aortic aneurysm. *B,* A thoracic aortogram showed the mass to be *non*vascular (arrows). The diagnosis was lymphoma in the posterior mediastinum.

sected is based on the belief that about 50 per cent are malignant and that the five-year cure rate for resected asymptomatic malignant nodules is excellent (30 to 45 per cent).[68–71]

Other physicians take the opposite view, arguing that the actual incidence of carcinoma in asymptomatic solitary pulmonary nodules is so low (0.25 to 16 per cent) that most surgery proves to have been unnecessary.[72–74] The truth probably lies between these extreme viewpoints. By integrating the clinical and the radiologic features and by employing modern biopsy techniques, one can identify those lung nodules that are very likely to be malignant, very unlikely to be malignant, or indeterminate.

There are two dependable radiographic findings that indicate the benignity of pulmonary nodules: the long-term absence of growth, and the presence within the nodule of benign calcification(s).

Absence of Growth. Malignancies in the lung generally double their volumes in 1 to 16 months.[75–77] There are, however, significant exceptions to this rule. Some aggressive malignancies, such as metastatic choriocar-

cinoma, are known to be capable of doubling their volumes in less than 1 month. "Scar" carcinomas, on the other hand, are frequently indolent and may take more than 16 months to double their volumes.[21] A solitary pulmonary nodule that shows *absolutely* no growth on chest roentgenograms for 2 or more years can safely be assumed to be benign.[78] Using this "rule," a number of benign nodules will be resected but only very rarely will malignancies be regarded as benign. The common benign lung lesions such as hamartomas and infectious granulomas are known occasionally to grow and to simulate lung cancer. Great care must be taken in making radiographic measurements, since small changes in lesional diameters signify much larger changes in their *volumes.* Technical variations in the roentgenograms can also cause artifactual diameter variations.

Benign Calcifications. Central, stippled, or laminated calcifications are dependable signs of benignity when they are identified centrally within pulmonary nodules (Fig. 3–17). Curvilinear ("popcorn") calcification often occurs in benign hamartomas. Neither soft tissue nodules with small eccentric calcifications nor those that develop in areas of pre-existing lung calcifications can safely be regarded as benign, however. The error of characterizing end-on vessels or calcifications that are near but not actually within nodules as "benign" calcifications, may be avoided with multiple fluoroscopic spot films or *tomography*. Histologic calcification is often present in lung cancer but is not detectable roentgenographically.[79]

The following characteristics of pulmonary nodules are *not* regarded as dependable roentgenographic signs for differentiating benign from malignant lesions: (1) type of margination (smooth, *versus* irregular or umbilicated); (2) size; (3) presence or absence of satellite lesions; (4) cavitation; (5) extensions to the pleura; and (6) homogeneity or inhomogeneity in density. The intuitive belief that cancers are irregular and that benign lesions are smooth is *not* supported by experience. Umbilication or notching occurs in granulomas and hamartomas, as well as in primary lung cancers. Satellite lesions, cavitation, and linear extension to the pleura can

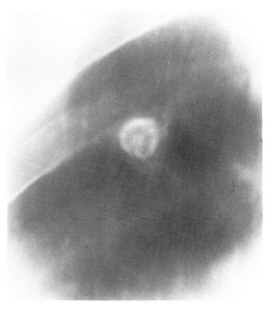

Figure 3–17 A tomographic study demonstrates the "target calcification" of a benign granuloma. This is one form of calcification in pulmonary nodules that is a dependable indicator of benignity.

occur both in cancers and in granulomas. Cancers may be homogeneously dense; alternatively, they may be associated with true air bronchograms or focal emphysema. Similarly, chronic pneumonitis may exhibit inhomogeneities as a result of cholesterol deposits, focal emphysema, or irregular consolidation.

There are three commonly encountered clinical circumstances that require further decisions to be made about the management of solitary lung nodules:

A nodule identified roentgenographically possesses one of the indicators of benignity. If indeed benign calcification *or* two-year size stability is present, the lesion can safely be assumed to be benign.

An uncalcified nodule of unknown growth history is identified. In this circumstance, certain clinical features may help to reduce the likelihood of malignancy. In patients below 35 years of age, solitary nodules rarely are malignant. The chance of having a primary lung malignancy is reduced in the patient who has never smoked. On the other hand, if the patient is a smoker over 35 years of age and is in good general health, resection of the nodule is a wise course, since there may be a significant lung cancer risk and the operative risk itself is low. If the cancer risk seems relatively low (as in the nonsmoking patient under 35 years of age) *or* if the risk of thoracotomy is significant (as in the elderly patient in poor general health), it is wise to make a considerable effort to obtain a diagnosis *before* thoracotomy is undertaken. For this purpose, percutaneous needle aspiration or bronchial brush biopsy of lung lesions under radiologic control are useful methods. About 90 per cent of lung cancers can be diagnosed by needle aspiration, and 70 per cent by bronchial brushing.[80–82]

There is a nodule with ambiguous roentgenographic calcification or an uncertain growth history. Resection is still probably the best choice in these circumstances, when cancer risk is not low and general health factors are satisfactory. When cancer risk is low or general health is unsatisfactory, needle aspiration or bronchial brushing is probably preferable to primary resection or to roentgenographic observation as a first step. The choice between resection, observation, and radiologic biopsy in a given patient will depend on the relative cancer and operative risks, and of course the patient's preferences.

Atelectasis and Consolidation. Because atelectasis or consolidation are frequent roentgenographic manifestations of lung cancer or of simple pneumonia, differentiation may be difficult. An inappropriate therapeutic response to adequate treatment for pneumonia, and the persistence or recurrence of consolidation or atelectasis, should lead the physician to perform further studies (Fig. 3–13). In these situations, detailed radiographic examination to determine the patency of the proximal bronchi can be obtained using high-penetration grid films, fluoroscopic spot films, tomography, or contrast bronchography. Bronchography can demonstrate the presence of an endobronchial lesion but cannot always differentiate between cancers and benign lesions. Bronchography may have an adverse effect on some noncancerous acute inflammatory lung diseases and its use should be deferred until the patient is afebrile. The bronchographic demonstration of an endobronchial lesion should lead to direct biopsy either by endoscopy or by a radiologically controlled method. When cavitation occurs it is often difficult to differentiate tissue necrosis distal to a lung carcinoma from a simple lung abscess. Lobar consolidation resulting from bronchoalveolar cell carcinoma is often indistinguishable roentgenographically from pneumonitis (Fig. 3–18).

Hilar Enlargement. Hilar enlargement occurs in benign as well as in malignant conditions. A major problem when hilar enlargement is observed is to differentiate roentgenographically between vascular and solid masses. The lung hilar vessels often become enlarged in chronic obstructive pulmonary disease, pulmonary arterial hypertension from any cause, pulmonary embolism, congestive heart failure, and mitral stenosis, and they can simulate lymph node enlargement. Fluoroscopic demonstration of intrinsic (vascular) pulsations or a change in hilar size with Valsalva's maneuver can often establish the correct diagnosis. True hilar lymph node enlargement can also usually be differentiated from vascular structures with tomography; only in rare circumstances is pulmonary arteriography needed to differentiate vascular from solid hilar abnormalities. Unilateral hilar lymph node enlargement usually is the result of a malignancy, but occasionally it will occur in sarcoidosis or in mycobacterial, bacterial, or mycotic infections.

Bilateral, symmetrical, and smooth hilar

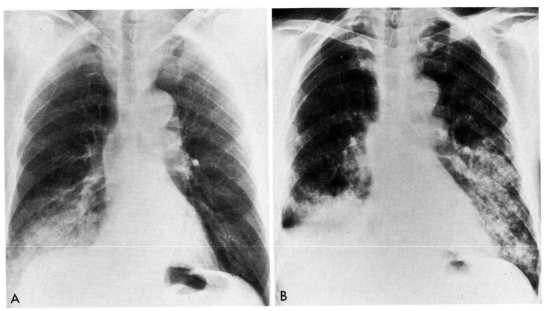

Figure 3–18 *A,* The nonhomogeneous opacification in the right lower lobe is indistinguishable from a pneumonia, in this patient with bronchoalveolar cell carcinoma. The patient complained of shortness of breath and a cough productive of abundant whitish sputum. (See also Figure 3–3.) *B,* Six months after diagnostic resection of the right lower lobe, there was evidence of tumor in the remainder of the right lung as well as spread to the left lung.

lymph node enlargement often is the result of sarcoidosis (see Fig. 1–4 in Chapter 1), but when it is associated with massive mediastinal adenopathy, lymphoma (including Hodgkin's) or small cell lung carcinoma is often the cause (Fig. 3–4; see also Fig. 1–1 in Chapter 1). Occasionally, metastases from a distant primary tumor such as renal cell carcinoma can cause symmetrical, bilateral hilar lymphadenopathy simulating sarcoidosis or lymphoma. Because there is no absolutely specific radiologic sign that can differentiate malignant from benign hilar lymph node enlargement, biopsy is often required for a diagnosis.

Mediastinal Enlargement. The roentgenologic differential diagnostic considerations with mediastinal masses are particularly complex; this is not only because benign and malignant solid masses must be differentiated from each other, but solid lesions must also be separated from vascular structures. Almost 10 per cent of patients with primary mediastinal tumors are considered at first to have a vascular lesion such as an aneurysm.[83]

The anterior mediastinal compartment may be encroached upon by various vascular or related structures (such as a dilated pericardium or right ventricle, an ascending aortic aneurysm, or dilated internal mammary arteries). Ultrasound study can usually identify pericardial effusions. A "mass" in the middle mediastinum may be the result of a pericardial effusion or enlargement of the great vessels. A dilated superior vena cava or azygos vein can often be identified by its decrease in size with Valsalva's maneuver. Radionuclide blood pool scans can often identify large vascular lesions. Aneurysm of the descending aorta, the primary vascular cause of an enlargement in the posterior mediastinum, may sometimes be difficult to distinguish from a solid tumor without performing angiography (Fig. 3–16). Some solid tumors can be differentiated from vascular lesions by their ability to concentrate radionuclides.[84] Goiters can often be identified by their ability to concentrate labeled pertechnetate or iodides.[13] A "negative" iodide scan, however, does not *exclude* goiter as the cause of an anterior mediastinal mass. Pneumoperitoneum may occasionally be diagnostic in evaluating a mediastinal mass that is suspected of being a diaphragmatic hernia (and that does not contain stomach or bowel).

The roentgenographic evaluation of mediastinal masses should begin with the review of all available earlier chest examinations, together with multiple current chest views (posteroanterior, lateral, and both obliques). Fluoroscopy with barium swallow may also aid in the localization and identification of mediastinal lesions. Tomography can help in defining a mass and identifying calcifications within the lesion. When vascular lesions have been excluded the differentiation of benign and malignant masses is the principal task.

In the *anterior mediastinal compartment* the common malignant tumors (lymphoma, malignant thymoma, germinal malignancies) must be differentiated from the common benign lesions (intrathoracic goiter, benign thymic or bronchogenic cysts, dermoid, and benign vascular enlargements). When observed fluoroscopically, goiters almost invariably move cranially during the act of swallowing; in addition, they often contain calcium and they frequently displace the trachea up to the level of the larynx. Rapid enlargement of a benign goiter from internal hemorrhage can simulate the rapid growth of a malignant mass. In children, thymic enlargement may be caused by simple thymic hyperplasia, but lymphomas originating in the thymus may have a similar roentgenographic appearance. Benign cysts that cannot be differentiated from solid malignant lesions require removal for positive identification. Occasionally, large amounts of mediastinal fat that accumulate in patients with endogenous (as in Cushing's syndrome) or exogenous obesity may simulate malignant masses. The fat generally extends symmetrically through all of the mediastinal compartments. Parathyroid tumors rarely become large enough to produce roentgenologic mediastinal masses; they are generally associated with clinical and roentgenographic osseous signs of hyperparathyroidism.

Masses in the anterior mediastinum that also involve the middle mediastinum usually are lymphomas or represent metastatic lymph nodes. Lung tumors in the anterior segments of the upper lobes may be juxtamediastinal and may simulate small mediastinal tumors that project into the lung. These primary lung cancers can usually be differentiated from mediastinal masses by fluoroscopic demonstration of their excursion with the lung on deep breathing, or by tomography.

Malignancies confined to the *middle mediastinum* are more apt to be secondary than primary. It is generally known that lung cancers often metastasize to the mediastinum, but it may be forgotten that extrathoracic malignancies also commonly metastasize to the mediastinum (Fig. 3–19). It is not uncommon for cancers of the breast, kidney, thyroid, prostate, or other malignancies, to metastasize to hilar or mediastinal lymph nodes. Inflammatory mediastinal adenopathy is usually, but not always, associated with pulmonary consolidations.

The major primary malignant tumors of the *posterior mediastinum* (neurogenic, esophageal, and lymph nodes) must be differentiated from benign lesions. Smooth benign cysts of the neurenteric, bronchogenic, or duplication variety are sometimes identified by their characteristic roentgenographic appearances. Other benign lesions of the posterior mediastinum include neurogenic tumors and paraspinal infections. Intrathoracic meningoceles, sometimes occurring in neurofibromatosis, can be identified by their expansion with coughing. Esophageal carcinoma masses are readily confirmed with barium studies.

Pleura, Chest Wall, and Diaphragmatic Abnormalities. Pleural effusion must be differentiated from solid pleural masses and from pulmonary abnormalities. Demonstration of free fluid movement with decubitus views or fluoroscopy is diagnostic. Pleural effusion is rare as an isolated finding in lung cancer, but is not uncommon with tuberculosis and other infections. Bilateral effusions and cardiac enlargement are usually associated with congestive heart failure. However, in combination with multiple pulmonary lesions, bilateral effusions are often indicative of a disseminated malignancy. Extrapleural mass lesions with rib destruction can be caused by fungal or tuberculous infection, as well as by multiple myeloma or by metastatic or primary lung cancer. Pleural biopsy and thoracentesis, often under fluoroscopic control, can provide material for histologic (or cytologic) and cultural studies.

Extrathoracic Radiographic Findings. True hypertrophic pulmonary osteoarthropathy occurs in lung cancer but may also be caused by bronchiectasis or benign lung infections and can be simulated by the periosteal reaction of postphlebitic syndrome. Bone metastases from lung cancer are usually osteolytic, but in small cell undifferentiated carcinoma and in carcinoid tumors they occasionally may be osteosclerotic.

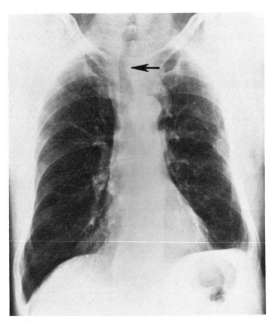

Figure 3–19 The trachea is displaced locally by a left superior mediastinal metastasis from a renal cell carcinoma (arrow).

Localization and Staging

The process of radiologic localization and staging of lung cancer often must precede the determination of a precise cytologic or histologic diagnosis. Once a pulmonary lesion is detected and a *presumptive* diagnosis of lung cancer is made, more detailed radiologic examination is required: tumor localization, exclusion of artifactual densities, determination of benign or malignant roentgenographic characteristics, and presumptive tumor staging are in fact often carried out simultaneously. The combined radiologic diagnosis and staging procedure follows the clinical TNM system and must answer the following questions:[15]

(1) How long has the lesion been present?

(2) Has the lesion increased in size during the observation period?

The first two questions are best answered by reviewing and comparing all available previous radiographs. Reviewing reports on earlier studies is not an adequate substitute for examining the radiographs themselves.

(3) Is the "lesion" an artifact such as a button, skin mole, nipple, or hair braid?

(4) Is the location of the lesion intrathoracic but extrapulmonary, such as a benign bone island in the rib or a traumatic extrapleural hematoma?

(5) Is the lesion mediastinal, or is it juxtamediastinal (that is, intrapulmonary) in location?

(6) In what bronchopulmonary segment is the lung lesion located?

(7) Is the lesion solitary?

Fluoroscopic observation of the mass during rotation and stereoscopic or multiple views can easily discern the extrathoracic nature of moles, nipples, and braids, as well as the parenchymal location of deep pulmonary nodules. Pulmonary lesions that are adjacent to the rib cage or mediastinum are best identified fluoroscopically by their movement relative to the ribs or the mediastinal structures during deep breathing.

(8) What are the detailed morphologic characteristics of the lesion?

(9) Does the lung lesion contain benign calcifications?

(10) Is the lesion surrounded by lung and contained within the visceral pleura (T1)?

(11) What is the proximal extent of the lesion in the bronchus (T1 versus T2 or T3)?

Multiple radiographic views and tomograms can provide more detailed information about the lung mass. Overlying vessels seen end-on or calcifications in the adjacent lung can be differentiated from true calcific nodules with these methods. The proximal extent of a tumor can sometimes be inferred from its dynamic effects; for instance, obstructive left upper lobe atelectasis indicates the presence of tumor in or around the major left upper lobe bronchus. The additional finding of air-trapping in the left lower lobe (hyperlucency of the lobe during expiration) would imply that the tumor had extended into the left lower lobe or the left mainstem bronchus, as well. Endobronchial tumor that causes only fractional narrowing of the bronchus may not cause visible expiratory airtrapping, but it may still cause transient mediastinal shift with respiration, only recog-

nizable at fluoroscopy. There has been considerable interest in the functional effects of lung cancers before and after treatment, but the clinical role of radionuclide ventilation and perfusion scans is yet to be established.

(12) Is there ipsilateral hilar (N1) or mediastinal (N2) adenopathy?

Detailed radiologic inspection of the lung hila is needed to detect adenopathy. Lymph node metastases, when present, occur in predictable locations (Figs. 3–4 and 3–14). Films of the esophagus during maximum distension with barium can demonstrate subcarinal or paraesophageal adenopathy. Oblique views without barium and tomography may also be useful for this determination (Fig. 3–20). Negative results using mediastinal tomography closely correlate (in 95 per cent of cases) with negative mediastinoscopy.[51] Therefore, tomography may help to select suitable candidates for mediastinoscopy.

(13) Does the lung lesion extend to the chest wall or the mediastinum (T3)?

Extension of tumor to the mediastinum may also be inferred by finding abnormalities attributable to mediastinal nerve invasion. Recurrent nerve or phrenic nerve palsies can be determined by roentgenologic observations of vocal cord or diaphragmatic movement. Tomography and high-penetration grid films are also useful in detecting mediastinal adenopathy.

Angiograms are often necessary to exclude direct involvement of the heart and great vessels by centrally located tumors (Fig 3–21). The following are considered to be angiographic signs of inoperability:[85]

1. Occlusion of the superior vena cava
2. Occlusion or concentric narrowing of the left main pulmonary artery
3. Complete or partial occlusion of the right pulmonary artery or its bifurcation
4. Occlusion of the right ascending pulmonary artery branch, plus abnormality of the superior vena cava
5. Occlusion of the pulmonary veins
6. Any vascular abnormality contralateral to the lung tumor

Intraosseous or selective catheter azygography can be used to demonstrate azygos vein obstruction, which generally indicates inoperability.[86] Detail spot films or tomography may be necessary to detect involvement of the chest wall by a lung tumor.

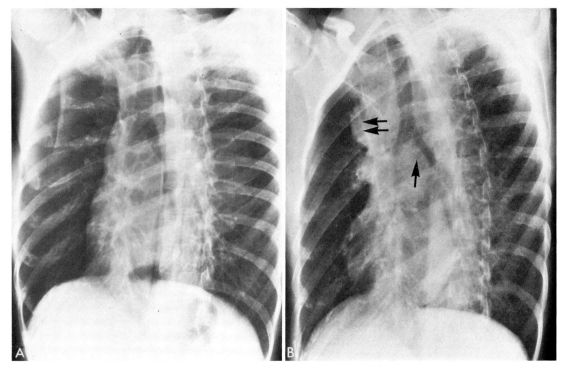

Figure 3–20   Oblique views are often of great value in detecting hilar and mediastinal adenopathy. In comparison with a left anterior oblique view in a *normal* patient (*A*), the paratracheal (double arrows) and subcarinal (single arrow) adenopathy is easily detected in a patient with small cell undifferentiated carcinoma of the lung (*B*).

(14) Is there a pleural effusion (T3)?

It should be noted that fairly large effusions can occupy a subpulmonic location and be difficult to recognize without decubitus views.

(15) Is there evidence of distant metastatic disease (M1)?

Brain and bone scans are sensitive indicators of metastatic disease. Bone metastases may also be evident when radiographs are obtained specifically of symptomatic sites. However, the radionuclide bone scan is generally more sensitive (but less specific) than radiography in the detection of early metastatic disease. Osseous hyperemia caused by a nearby tumor, as well as many "benign" abnormalities, may result in a positive bone scan.

lesions, but many studies are indeterminate when the radiographic findings alone are considered. For indeterminate lesions, additional clinical and specialized radiologic studies are warranted. Lung lesions that are centrally located can often be studied adequately by bronchoscopy or by sputum examination. More peripherally located lung cancers sometimes may be diagnosed, short of thoracotomy, only by radiologically controlled needle or bronchial brush biopsy procedures. The biopsy of an otherwise inaccessible peripheral lung or chest wall lesion under radiologic control has greatly influenced the modern management of pulmonary lesions. The discussion that follows is concerned with technical considerations, clinical applications, results, and complications of these procedures.

Radiologically Controlled Biopsy Procedures

Standard radiographic examinations will themselves allow differentiation between some benign and malignant lung

TRANSTHORACIC (PERCUTANEOUS) NEEDLE ASPIRATION BIOPSY

Percutaneous needle aspiration biopsy antedates the development of modern radiologic image intensifiers and was employed in the diagnosis of tumors and infections of the lung prior to 1940.[87] Extensive application of this technique, however, did not occur until the availability of modern radiologic imaging systems allowed the precise localization of small lesions within the thorax. The smallest lesion that can be biopsied by this method is about 5 mm in diameter.

The transthoracic biopsy technique requires precise three-dimensional localization. Using local anesthesia and fluoroscopic image intensifier control, a fine needle (18 to 20 gauge) containing a stylet is directed through an intercostal space toward the lung lesion, while the patient is breathing quietly. A double-needle technique developed at the Massachusetts General Hospital allows the operator to obtain multiple samples through a single pleural puncture and minimizes the amount of potential tracking of material from

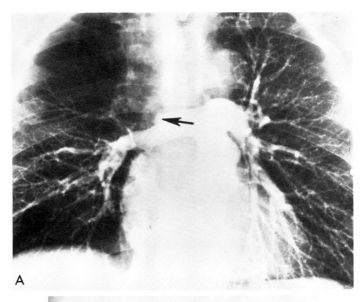

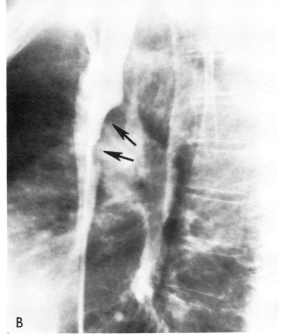

Figure 3–21 *A,* An angiographic study (pulmonary arteriogram) in a patient with carcinoma of the right upper lobe shows occlusion of the ascending ramus of the right pulmonary artery (arrow). *B,* Lateral view of a superior vena cava contrast study in the same patient also demonstrates medial and posterior encroachment (double arrows) on the vena cava by tumor. The combination of findings shown in *A* and *B* indicates inoperability.

the lesion through the lung and chest wall. With this modification, an 18 gauge needle is inserted into the lung just short of the lesion. Its stylet is removed and a longer 22 gauge needle with its own stylet is inserted through the 18 gauge needle. The inner needle is then inserted under radiologic control directly into the lesion, and as many samples as needed are obtained. Samples are obtained by removing the stylet of the 22 gauge needle and attaching a 6 ml syringe, with which suction is applied to the inner needle during withdrawal. After all of the bacteriologic and cytologic samples have been obtained, blood drawn from the patient's antecubital vein is injected via the outer needle during its removal. This maneuver helps to reduce the incidence of pneumothorax. If multiplane or biplane fluoroscopic image amplification is not available, then the patient must be rotated carefully during the needle placement to assure accurate localization. Microbiologic samples must be carefully handled and cytology specimens are rapidly fixed in preparation for staining.

The most common complication of this procedure is pneumothorax, which occurs in about 25 per cent of cases.[80] However, the pneumothoraces are generally small and require only clinical and radiographic observation. In less than 10 per cent of cases, pneumothorax following needle biopsy requires aspiration or a chest tube. Other complications are rare. Hemoptysis, which occurs in about 2 per cent of cases, is usually transient and mild. However, careful evaluation of bleeding and clotting factors (hemogram, platelet count, prothrombin time, and partial thromboplastin time) is an essential part of patient evaluation prior to performing this procedure. In contrast to large-core percutaneous biopsy procedures, deaths reported from fine needle aspiration biopsy are exceedingly rare. One death from fine needle biopsy of the lung, recently reported, resulted from fatal intrapulmonary bleeding in a patient with a uremic clotting defect.[88] The following should be considered relative (or in some cases absolute) contraindications to the procedure: a bleeding or clotting defect, pulmonary arterial hypertension, respiratory insufficiency, or local bullous lung disease.

The primary value of needle aspiration biopsy of the lung is its high diagnostic yield, as well as its safety. The yield of specific diagnoses of benign disease from needle aspiration biopsy is very low, but the overwhelming majority of cancers can be identified.[80, 81] At the Massachusetts General Hospital, negative needle aspiration biopsies have been obtained in only 5 per cent of proven lung cancers. The continued use of the double-needle technique, and the resulting higher volumes of bacteriologic and cytologic material obtained safely with this approach, may lead to an increased diagnostic yield in benign lung lesions as well. Because more than nine out of ten lung cancers can reliably be identified by the transthoracic needle aspiration technique, this method has application in patients in whom the risk of other diagnostic modalities, particularly thoracotomy, is high or in whom the presumed risk of cancer is low.

The primary clinical applications of needle aspiration biopsy include the diagnosis of (1) solitary pulmonary nodules (Figure 3–5), (2) chest wall lesions, (3) superior sulcus (Pancoast's) tumors (Fig. 3–12), and (4) multiple pulmonary nodules. This technique has also been used in the diagnosis of thick-walled cavities (Fig. 3–22) and pulmonary consolidations, although bronchial brushing is generally preferred in these circumstances. The potential risk of seeding tumor cells along the needle track is a theoretical possibility, but, in spite of the extensive use of needle aspiration biopsy, seeding has not been demonstrated clinically. Tumor cell seeding has been reported, however, with large-bore needle techniques.[89]

BRONCHIAL BRUSH BIOPSY

The clinical use of endobronchial brush biopsy, like needle aspiration biopsy, was linked to the development of high-resolution radiologic image intensification.[90] Bronchoscopists often employ brush biopsy without radiologic control, but their efforts are generally limited to the more centrally located lesions. Using three-dimensional radiologic localization methods and fully manipulable catheters, even peripheral lung lesions can regularly be entered via the endobronchial route. After administering atropine to dry the mucous membranes, a catheter is passed transnasally into the trachea to serve as a conduit. A special manipulable catheter is then passed through the conduit catheter

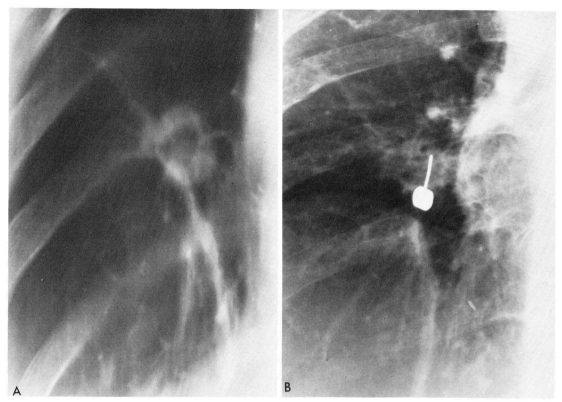

Figure 3–22   *A,* A tomographic section through a cavitary adenocarcinoma of the right lower lobe shows the lesion to have a thick wall. *B,* Anteroposterior localization film from a diagnostic transthoracic needle aspiration biopsy shows the needle in the wall of the cavity (also confirmed on a lateral film).

and directed under the image amplifier toward the lesion to be examined. When the lesion is reached, a polythene-sheathed nylon brush is passed through the manipulable catheter; cytologic or bacteriologic samples are obtained when the brush is advanced beyond its sheath into the lesion. Reciprocating movements are used to scrape the lesion with the brush, and the brush is then retracted into its sheath and withdrawn.

The primary indications for bronchial brush biopsy include: (1) non-resolving pulmonary consolidations (Fig. 3–23), and (2) cavitary lesions (Fig. 3–24). A brush biopsy also may be made of pulmonary nodules, but percutaneous needle biopsy is usually employed for this kind of lesion. About 70 per cent of lung cancers can be diagnosed with bronchial brushing.[82] In keeping with this experience, negative results have been obtained at the Massachusetts General Hos-

pital in 30 per cent of proven carcinomas. Complications are exceedingly rare. Unlike fiberoptic bronchial endoscopy, tubings with very small cross sections are used in radiologic bronchial brush biopsy and problems with ventilation are negligible. As with needle aspiration and other biopsy procedures, careful anticipatory studies of the bleeding and clotting factors must be done. Pneumothorax is a very rare complication of brush biopsy. In terms of safety and low morbidity, this method is probably superior to all other lung biopsy procedures. Therefore, it is often the specialized diagnostic method first used.

Radiologic Follow-up

The proper use of radiologic studies in the follow-up of patients with lung cancer

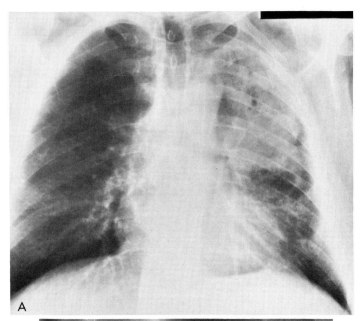

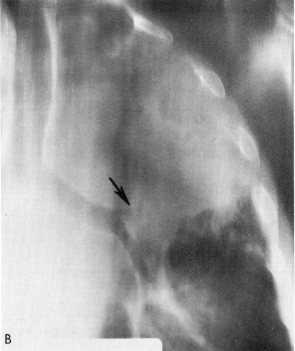

Figure 3–23 *A,* Sputum cytology, mediastinoscopy, supraclavicular biopsy, and bronchoscopy on two occasions were not diagnostic in a patient with a poorly differentiated epidermoid carcinoma. The patient had fever and hemoptysis. There is opacification of the left upper lobe. Cavitation is manifested by "bubbles" of gas in the middle of the opacified lobe. *B,* A tomographic section demonstrates occlusion of the left upper lobe bronchus at its origin (arrow)

requires an appreciation of the major clinical problems that can occur.

Persistent or Recurrent Local Tumor. Careful plain film chest radiography or tomography immediately *prior* to the initiation of radiation therapy for lung cancer is essential as a baseline to monitor tumor treatment response. Undifferentiated small cell tumors often show a rapid "lymphoma-like" response to irradiation or chemotherapy. Lobar atelectasis will often clear quickly after irradiation of the compromised bronchus. Unfortunately, however, recurrence of these undifferentiated tumors is not uncommon, and distant spread is the rule.

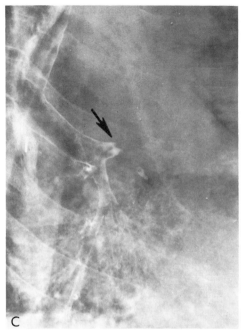

C

Figure 3-23 *Continued C,* A bronchographic study in this patient verifies the presence of an occluded left upper lobe bronchus (arrow), but adds no new information. *D,* A localization film is shown from a bronchial brush biopsy, which provided the final diagnosis.

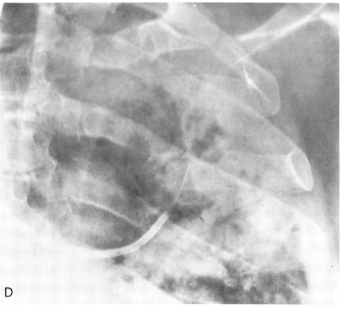

D

Recurrence of tumor in the bronchial stump can usually be recognized on plain films, tomograms, or bronchography in patients who experience hemoptysis after lung resections for cancer. Recognition of recurrence at the resection line aids in the differentiation between a second primary lung cancer and recurrent disease. Occasionally, in cases that are difficult to evaluate, radiologically visible separation of surgical clips at the resection site aids in the detection of a tumor recurrence.

Regional Lymph Node Metastases. Metastatic enlargement of mediastinal lymph nodes in lung cancer often occurs after successful local treatment of the primary lesion (Fig. 3–14). Tumor involvement of the subcarinal nodes or recurrent cancer in a mainstem bronchus may invade locally into the adjacent mediastinal tissues and result in a

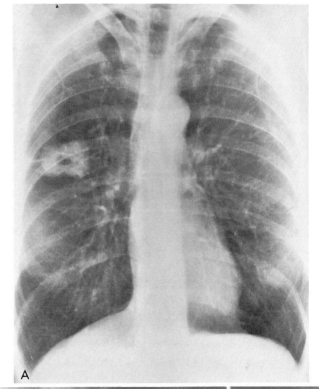

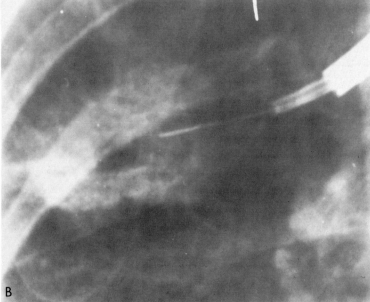

Figure 3–24 *A,* This thick-walled cavity in the right upper lobe is an epidermoid carcinoma in a patient with hemoptysis. *B,* A localization film from a diagnostic bronchial brush biopsy shows the brush within the wall of the small cavity.

tracheoesophageal fistula or disastrous vascular communication.

Disseminated Disease. A disappointingly large number of patients with lung cancer who are thought to be cured of local disease develop clinical or radiologic evidence of distant dissemination. Radiologic evidence of dissemination is most often found in the bone or brain. Multiple intrapulmonary metastases, as a late development in disseminated lung cancer, are also common.

Complications of Treatment. Empyema and bronchopleural fistula from leaks at the bronchial resection line may occur as complications of lobectomy or pneumonectomy. *Persistent* roentgenographic air-fluid levels in the chest following a lung resection often herald an empyema. Late empyemas that develop a year or more after surgery are difficult to recognize radiologically, unless air enters the space through a bronchopleural or pleurocutaneous communication. The mediastinum becomes relatively fixed postoperatively, so that no further contralateral mediastinal shift may be recognizable even with large empyema collections.

Intensive lung irradiation often causes radiation pneumonitis. It can be recognized (1) by its geographic distribution, defined by the margins of the radiation portals, and (2) by the temporal relationship to radiation therapy. The earliest radiologic sign of radiation pneumonitis is consolidation in the irradiated segment(s), which may coincide with or follow shortly the termination of treatment (Fig. 3–25). Later in its course, radiation pneumonitis becomes more cicatricial, causing contraction of the affected lung. Radiation osteitis (in the ribs), myelitis,

or pericarditis may also occur, rarely, when the time elapsed since treatment is greater than 18 months.

Chemotherapy used as the primary treatment in small cell undifferentiated carcinoma may occasionally injure the lung directly, or it may so depress the bone marrow that opportunistic infections occur. Radiologic biopsy procedures frequently play a central role in the diagnosis of these opportunistic infections. Chemotherapeutic agents (e.g., actinomycin D) used in combination with radiation therapy may act synergistically to produce injury in the irradiated lung.

Intercurrent Disease. Symptoms and signs of benign disease such as pulmonary embolism, myocardial infarction, stroke, or pneumonia are often mistakenly ascribed to a previously diagnosed lung cancer. The proper use of radiologic studies such as pulmonary arteriography, radionuclide scans, bronchial brushing, or needle aspiration biopsy in these circumstances depends on a high index of clinical suspicion of intercurrent disease.

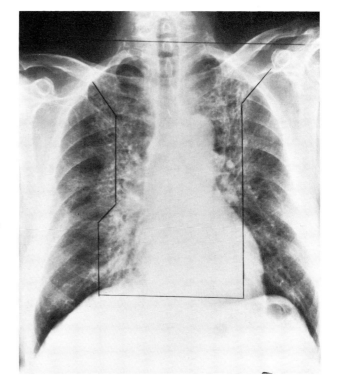

Figure 3–25 Progressive shortness of breath, fever, and cough developed in this patient near the end of a course of lung irradiation for small cell undifferentiated carcinoma. The opacities in the central regions of the lungs correspond to the margins of the treatment portals, which are shown by the black lines. This proved clinically to be acute radiation pneumonitis.

References

1. Silverberg, E., and Holleb, A. I.: Cancer statistics, 1972. Cancer, 22:2, 1972.
2. Cutler, S. J.: End Results in Cancer. U. S. Department of Health, Education, and Welfare, Public Health Service. (Report No. 3). Washington, D. C., Government Printing Office, 1968.
3. Selawry, O. S., and Hansen, H. H.: Lung cancer. In Holland, J. F., and Frei, E. (eds.), Cancer Medicine. Philadelphia, Lea & Febiger, 1973.
4. United States Department of Health, Education, and Welfare, Public Health Service: Smoking and Health: Report of the Advisory Committee to the Surgeon General of the Public Health Service. (Publication No. 1103.) Washington, D. C., Government Printing Office, 1964.
5. Wagoner, J. K., Archer, V. E., Lundin, F. E., et al.: Radiation as the cause of lung cancer among uranium miners. N. Engl. J. Med., 273:181, 1965.
6. Wagner, J. C.: Asbestos cancer. J. Natl. Cancer Inst., 46:5, 1971.
7. Buell, P., Dunn, J., and Breslow, L.: Cancer of the lung and Los Angeles-type air pollution. Cancer, 20:2139, 1967.
8. Kreyberg, L.: Histological Typing of Lung Tumours. Geneva, World Health Organization, 1967.
9. Selikoff, I. J., Hammon, E. C., and Churg, J.: Mortality experiences of asbestos insulation workers 1943–1968. In Shapiro, H. A. (ed.), Conference on Pneumoconiosis, Johannesburg, April 23–May 2, 1969. London, Oxford Univ. Press, 1970, pp. 180–186.
10. Auerbach, O., Stout, A. P., Hammond, E. C., et al.: Changes in bronchial epithelium in relation to sex, age, residence, smoking and pneumonia. N. Engl. J. Med., 267:111, 1962.
11. Smith, R. A.: Development and treatment of fresh lung carcinoma after successful lobectomy. Thorax, 21:1, 1966.
12. Epstein, S. S., Payne, P. M., and Shaw, H. J.: Multiple primary malignant neoplasms in the air and upper food passages. Cancer, 13:137, 1966.
13. Auerbach, O., Stout, A. P., Hammond, E. C., et al.: Bronchial epithelium in former smokers. N. Engl. J. Med., 267:119, 1962.
14. Feinstein, A. R., Gelfman, N. A., and Yesner, R.: The diverse effect of histopathology on manifestations and outcome of lung cancer. Chest, 66:225, 1974.
15. The American Joint Committee for Cancer Staging and End Results Reporting: Clinical staging system for carcinoma of the lung. Ca, 24:87, 1974.
16. Sanderson, D. R., Fontana, R. S., Woolner, L. B., et al.: Bronchoscopic localization of radiographically occult lung cancer. Chest, 65:608, 1974.
17. Sarin, C. L., and Nohl-Oser, H. C.: Mediastinoscopy: A clinical evaluation of 400 consecutive cases. Thorax, 24:585, 1969.
18. Hansen, H. H., and Muggia, F. M.: Staging of inoperable patients with bronchogenic carcinoma with special reference to bone marrow examination and peritoneoscopy. Cancer, 30:1395, 1972.
19. Lehar, T. J., Carr, D. T., Miller, W. E., et al.: Roentgenographic appearance of bronchogenic adenocarcinoma. Am. Rev. Resp. Dis., 96:245, 1967.
20. Campobasso, O.: The characteristics of peripheral lung tumours that suggest their bronchioloalveolar origin. Br. J. Cancer, 22:655, 1968.
21. Ripstein, C. B., Spain, D. M., and Bluth, I.: Scar cancer of the lung. J. Thorac. Cardiovasc. Surg. 56:362, 1968.
22. Meyer, E. C., and Liebow, A. A.: Relationship of interstitial pneumonia honeycombing and atypical epithelial proliferation to cancer of the lung. Cancer, 18:322, 1965.
23. Razzuk, M. A., Race, G. J., Lynn, J. A., et al.: Observations on ultrastructural morphology of bronchogenic carcinoma. J. Thorac. Cardiovasc. Surg., 59:581, 1970.
24. Byrd, R. B., Miller, W. E., Carr, D. T., et al.: The roentgenographic appearance of large cell carcinoma of the bronchus. Mayo Clin. Proc., 43:333, 1968.
25. Moersch, H. J., and McDonald, J. R.: Bronchial adenoma. J.A.M.A., 142:299, 1950.
26. Gowenlock, A. H., Plat, D. S., Campbell, A.C.P., et al.: Oat cell carcinoma of the bronchus secreting 5-hydroxytryptophan. Lancet, 1:304, 1964.
27. Sandler, M., Scheuer, P. J., and Watt, P. J.: 5-hydroxytryptophan secreting bronchial carcinoid tumour. Lancet, 2:1067, 1961.
28. Jamplis, R. W., and Cressman, R. L.: Current concepts of thymomas. Am. J. Surg., 98:202, 1959.
29. Joseph, W. L., Murray, J. F., and Mulder, D. G.: Mediastinal tumors—problems in diagnosis and treatment. Chest, 50:150, 1966.
30. Seybold, W. D., McDonald, J. R., Clagett, O. T., et al.: Tumors of the thymus. J. Thorac. Cardiovasc. Surg., 20:195, 1950.
31. Scholz, D. A., and Bahn, R. C.: Thymic tumors associated with Cushing's syndrome: Review of three cases. Mayo Clin. Proc., 34:433, 1959.
32. Franken, E. A., Jr.: Radiologic evidence of thymus enlargment in Grave's disease. Radiology, 91:20, 1968.
33. Wilkins, E. W., Edmunds, L. H., and Castleman, B.: Cases of thymoma at the Massachusetts General Hospital. J. Thorac. Cardiovasc. Surg., 52:322, 1966.
34. Houston, H. E., Payne, W. S., Harrison, E. J., Jr., et al.: Primary cancer of the trachea. Arch. Surg., 99:132, 1969.
35. Janower, M. L., Grillo, H. C., MacMillan, A. S., Jr., et al.: The radiological appearance of carcinoma of the trachea. Radiology, 96:39, 1970.
36. Grillo, H. C.: Benign and malignant diseases of the chest. In Shields, T. W. (ed.), General Thoracic Surgery. Philadelphia, Lea & Febiger, 1972, pp. 555–575.
37. Sniffen, R. C., Soutter, L., and Robbings, L. L.: Mucoepidermoid tumors of the bronchus arising from surface epithelium. Am. J. Pathol., 34:671, 1958.
38. Gupta, A. K., Pryce, D. M., and Blenkinsopp, W. K.: Pre-operative length of history and tumour size in central and peripheral bronchial carcinomata. Thorax, 20:398, 1965.
39. Cohen, S., and Hossain, M.S.A.: Primary carcinoma of the lung: A review of 417 histologically proved cases. Chest, 49:67, 1966.

40. Rassan, J. W., and Anderson, G.: Incidence of paramaligant disorders in bronchogenic carcinoma. Thorax, *30*:86, 1975.
41. Yacoub, M. H.: Relation between the histology of bronchial carcinoma and hypertrophic pulmonary osteoarthropathy. Thorax, *20*:537, 1965.
42. Azzopardi, J. G., Freeman, E., and Poule, G.: Endocrine and metabolic disorders in bronchial carcinoma. Br. Med. J., *4*:528, 1970.
43. Azzopardi, J. G., and Whittaker, R. S.: Bronchial carcinoma and hypercalcaemia. J. Clin. Pathol., *22*:718, 1969.
44. Rees, L. H.: Hormone production by lung tumors. Tubercle (Suppl.), *3*:49, 1973.
45. Liddle, G. W., Island, D. P., Ney, R. L., et al.: Nonpituitary neoplasms and Cushing's syndrome: Ectopic "adrenocorticotropin" produced by nonpituitary neoplasms as a cause of Cushing's syndrome. Arch. Intern, Med., *111*:471, 1963.
46. Bell, J. W.: Abdominal exploration in one hundred lung carcinoma suspects prior to thoracotomy. Ann. Surg., *167*:199, 1968.
47. Lillington, G. A.: The solitary pulmonary nodule— 1974. Am. Rev. Resp. Dis., *10*:699, 1974.
48. Pearson, F. G.: An evaluation of mediastinoscopy in the management of presumably operable bronchial carcinoma. J. Thorac. Cardiovasc. Surg., *55*:22, 1968.
49. Marchand, P.: Mediastinoscopy. S. Afr. Med. J., *46*:285, 1972.
50. Carlens, F.: Appraisal of choice and results of treatment for bronchogenic carcinoma. Chest, *65*:443, 1974.
51. James, E. C., and Ellwood, R. A.: Mediastinoscopy and mediastinal roentgenology. Ann. Thorac. Surg., *18*:531, 1974.
52. Rosenthal, S., and Kaufman, S.: Liver scan in metastatic disease. Arch. Surg., *106*:656, 1973.
53. Rosenow, E. C.: The spectrum of drug-induced pulmonary disease. Ann. Intern. Med., *77*:977, 1972.
54. Woolner, L. B., Fontana, R. S., and Bernatz, P. E.: Early bronchogenic carcinoma: Problems in detection, localization and treatment. Surg. Clin. North Am., *53*:761, 1970.
55. Gilbertson, V. A.: X-ray examination of the chest: An unsatisfactory method of detection of early lung cancer in asymptomatic individuals. J.A.M.A., *188*:130, 1964.
56. Weiss, W., Boucot, K. R., and Cooper, D. A.: The survival of men with measurable proved lung cancer in relation to growth rate. Am. J. Roentgenol. Radium Ther. Nucl. Med., *98*:404, 1966.
57. United States Department of Health, Education, and Welfare, Public Health Service: The chest x-ray as a screening procedure for cardiopulmonary disease. (Publication No. 8036.) Washington, D.C., Government Printing Office, 1973.
58. Woolner, L. B., David, E., and Fontana, R. S.: In situ and early invasive bronchogenic carcinoma: Report of 28 cases with postoperative survival data. J. Thorac. Cardiovasc. Surg., *60*:275, 1970.
59. Melamed, M. R.: The cytological presentation of malignant lymphomas and related diseases in effusions. Cancer, *16*:413, 1963.
60. Grzybowski, S., and Coy, P.: Early diagnosis of carcinoma of the lung. Simultaneous screening with chest x-ray and sputum cytology. Cancer, *25*:113, 1970.
61. Byrd, R. B., Miller, W. E., Carr, D. T., et al.: The roentgenographic appearance of squamous cell carcinoma of the bronchus. Mayo Clin. Proc., *43*:327, 1968.
62. Byrd, R. B., Miller, W. E., Carr, D. T., et al.: The roentgenographic appearance of small cell carcinoma of the bronchus. Mayo Clin. Proc., *43*:337, 1968.
63. Gracey, D. R., Byrd, R. B., and Cugell, D. W.: The dilemma of the asymptomatic pulmonary nodule in the young and not-so-young adult. Chest, *60*:479, 1971.
64. Edwards, W. M., Cox, R. S., and Garland, L. H.: The solitary nodule (coin lesion) of the lung: An analysis of 52 consecutive cases treated by thoracotomy and a study of preoperative diagnostic accuracy. Am. J. Roentgenol. Radium Ther. Nucl. Med., *88*:1020, 1962.
65. Nolin, S. M., Dwork, R. E., and Glaser, S.: Solitary pulmonary nodules found in a community-wide chest roentgenographic survey. Am. Rev. Tuberc., *79*:427, 1959.
66. McClure, C. D., Boucot, K. R., Shipman, G. A., et al.: The solitary pulmonary nodule and primary lung malignancy. Arch. Environ. Health, *3*:127, 1961.
67. Comstock, G. W., Vaughan, R. H., and Montgomery, G.: Outcome of solitary pulmonary nodules discovered in an x-ray screening program. N. Engl. J. Med., *254*:1018, 1956.
68. Katz, S., Peabody, J. W., Jr., and Davis, E. W.: The solitary pulmonary nodule. D. M., April, 1961.
69. Steele, J. D., Kleitsch, W. P., Dunn, J. E., et al.: Survival in males with bronchogenic carcinomas resected as asymptomatic solitary pulmonary nodules. Ann. Thorac. Surg., *2*:368, 1966.
70. Jackman, R. J., Good, C. A., Clagett, O. T., et al.: Survival rates in peripheral bronchogenic carcinomas up to four centimeters in diameter presenting as solitary pulmonary nodules. J. Thorac. Cardiovasc. Surg., *57*:1, 1969.
71. Seybold, W. D.: Solitary or "coin" lesions of the lung. Postgrad. Med., *36*:424, 1964.
72. Trunk, G., Gracey, D. R., and Byrd, R. B.: The management and evaluation of the solitary pulmonary nodule. Chest, *66*:236, 1974.
73. Jones, R. C., and Cleve, E. A.: Solitary circumscribed lesions of the lung: Selection of cases for diagnostic thoracotomy. Arch. Intern. Med., *93*:842, 1954.
74. Nathan, M. H.: Management of solitary pulmonary nodules: An organized approach based on growth rate and statistics. J.A.M.A., *227*:1141, 1974.
75. Weiss, W., Seidman, H., and Boucot, K. R.: The Philadelphia pulmonary neoplasm research project. Am. Rev. Resp. Dis., *111*:289, 1975.
76. Garland, L. H., Coulson, W., and Wollin, E.: The rate of growth and apparent duration of untreated primary bronchial carcinoma. Cancer, *16*:694, 1963.
77. Wolff, G.: Die Bedeutung der verdoppelungszeit fur die Differentialdiagnose von Runderherden.

(The significance of the growth doubling time for the differential diagnosis of coin lesions.) Fortschr. Rontgenstr., *101*:366, 1964.

78. Good, C. A.: Roentgenologic appraisal of solitary pulmonary nodules. Minn. Med., *45*:157, 1962.

79. Salzman, E.: Lung Calcifications in X-ray Diagnosis. Springfield, Ill., Charles C Thomas, 1968.

80. Nordenstrom, B.: Transthoracic needle biopsy. N. Engl. J. Med., *276*:1081, 1967.

81. Sinner, W. N.: Transthoracic needle biopsy of small peripheral malignant lung lesions. Invest. Rad., *8*:305. 1973.

82. Bibbo, M., Fennessy, J. J., Chien-Tai, L., et al.: Bronchial brushing technique for the cytologic diagnosis of peripheral lung lesions: A review of 693 cases. Acta Cytol., *17*:245, 1973.

83. Oldham, H. N., and Sabiston, D. C.: Primary tumors and cysts of the mediastinum. Arch. Surg., *96*: 71, 1968.

84. Ito, Y., Okuyama, S., Awano, T., et al.: Diagnostic evaluation of ^{67}Ga scanning of lung cancer and other diseases. Radiology, *101*:255, 1971.

85. Abrams, H. L.: Angiography. Boston, Little, Brown, 1971.

86. Skinner, D. B., Dreyfuss, J. R., and Nardi, G. L.: Azyography in the evaluation of operability of pulmonary carcinoma. N. Engl. J. Med., *267*:232, 1962.

87. Sappington, S. W., and Favorite, G. O.: Lung puncture in lobar pneumonia. Am. Rev. Med. Sci., *191*:225, 1936.

88. Pearce, J. G., and Patt, N. L.: Fatal pulmonary hemorrhage after percutaneous aspiration lung biopsy. Am. Rev. Resp. Dis., *110*:346, 1974.

89. Wolinsky, H., and Lischner, M. W.: Needle track implantation of tumor after percutaneous lung biopsy. Ann. Intern. Med., *71*:359, 1969.

90. Hattori, S., Matsuda, M., Sugiyama, T., et al.: Cytologic diagnosis of early lung cancer; brushing method under x-ray television fluoroscopy. Chest, *45*:129, 1964.

Chapter Four

JAWS AND ALVEOLAR RIDGES

NEAL W. FREY, D.D.S., M.Sc.D.,
STUART C. WHITE, D.D.S., PH.D., AND
HENRY M. CHERRICK, D.D.S., M.S.D.

CLINICAL CONSIDERATIONS

Presenting Signs and Symptoms

Various types of primary and metastatic tumors affect the jaws and surrounding soft tissues. *Squamous cell carcinoma* (epidermoid carcinoma) is the most common primary malignancy and originates in the soft tissues (mucosa).[1-4] Depending upon its location, squamous cell carcinoma in the oral region exhibits one of three distinct growth patterns: ulcerative, exophytic, or verrucous. The ulcerative form is the most common and appears as a craterlike defect with rolled mucosal margins. Palpation of the surrounding tissue suggests induration and infiltration.

Small lesions (under 1 cm) are usually asymptomatic and are generally discovered on routine dental examination. As the lesion increases in size, pain is often the first symptom. When the carcinoma is in close proximity to the teeth, exfoliation or loosening of the dentition is a common finding. Advanced lesions invade the underlying osseous structures, but pathologic fractures are rare. In edentulous patients wearing a dental prosthesis, large soft tissue lesions may impinge on the appliance, causing pain or dislodgment. When carcinoma occurs on the maxillary alveolar ridges or gingivae, involvement of the maxillary sinus is com-

mon. When the antrum is involved, symptoms may include pain, headache, facial asymmetry, and nasal discharge.

Metastatic carcinoma in the jaws is not a common tumor, but because metastases produce early clinical signs and symptoms they may offer the first clinical indication of an undiscovered primary carcinoma at a distant site (for instance, the lung). The posterior body of the mandible is the most common site. The usual clinical symptoms are discomfort or pain followed by paresthesia or anesthesia of the lip or chin secondary to mandibular nerve involvement. Teeth in the affected area may become extruded and exfoliated, or roots may be resorbed. A definite swelling or expansion of the bone is almost always found, and occasionally erythema is noted in the overlying mucosa. Metastases from the lower portion of the body (prostate, gastrointestinal tract, kidney) to the jaws, without involvement of the lungs, are difficult to explain, but the possible importance of the vertebral venous plexus as a route for metastasis has been discussed at length.[5]

Sarcomas are rare primary malignancies of the jaws. The most common are fibrosarcoma, osteosarcoma, chondrosarcoma, and Ewing's sarcoma. As a group, sarcomas are more likely to occur in younger patients than are carcinomas. Clinically, most sarcomas of the jaws exhibit a rapid growth rate, and often the initial clinical sign is facial asymmetry. They are fleshy-appearing tumors and ulcerate the oral mucosa only after attaining considerable size. Pain is a late symptom and generally occurs only after secondary infection or nerve involvement. Teeth are displaced and frequently exfoliated.

The *malignant lymphomas,* although not rare tumors, are uncommon primary lesions of the jaws. Lymphosarcoma (including the Burkitt's variety) and reticulum cell sarcoma are the most common lymphomas to affect the jaws. The clinical signs and symptoms are discussed in Chapter 2.

Differential Diagnosis

SQUAMOUS CELL CARCINOMA

Squamous cell carcinoma must be differentiated from leukoplakia, papillomas, erosions, and specific as well as nonspecific white patches on the oral mucosa. Approximately 17 per cent of white patches represent premalignant lesions or already invasive carcinomas. Definitive diagnosis is made only by incisional or excisional biopsy. Papillomas are exophytic growths that are often difficult to differentiate from verrucous carcinomas. Diagnosis is made by biopsy, but obtaining an adequate specimen for biopsy may be difficult particularly when the lesion is small. Repeated biopsies may be necessary. Erosions and nonspecific ulcers generally heal uneventfully following removal of the etiologic factor. When these lesions do not respond favorably within two weeks, biopsy is indicated. Specific ulcers such as mycotic and bacterial infections may simulate carcinomas clinically, and diagnosis is sometimes established only with specially stained smears, fluorescent microscopy, cultures, biopsies, or a combination of these techniques.

METASTATIC CARCINOMA

All benign and malignant tumors within the jaws may cause pain and swelling, but the pain caused by diseases of the temporomandibular joint, caries, and trigeminal neuralgia can simulate the pain of malignancy. Patients who present with peripheral nerve deficiencies (i.e., facial anesthesia or paresthesia) as well as swelling of the jaws are generally considered to have a malignant disease, inasmuch as benign lesions of the jaws rarely, if ever, cause both these symptoms. Definitive diagnosis of metastatic carcinoma in the jaw is made by history, physical examination, appropriate radiologic studies including standard skeletal and long bone surveys, and biopsy. Occasionally, metastases are multiple within the jaws, and this helps to differentiate them from other lesions. If the primary tumor has not been localized by other means, classifying it histologically may also be difficult because the metastasis is often poorly differentiated.

SARCOMA

Sarcomas of the jaws must be differentiated from odontogenic tumors, benign expansile lesions, and reactive and inflammatory processes. Odontogenic tumors and expansile lesions have a capacity for aggressive growth; they often simulate sarcomas clinically because of their size and resulting deformity, but direct correlation of their radiographic appearances helps to differentiate these lesions. Reactive and inflammatory lesions can resemble osteosarcoma or chondrosarcoma clinically as well as radiographically. Eliminating the instigating factors for an inflammatory process in the mouth often helps to make the definitive diagnosis. Reactive and proliferative osseous lesions can appear similar to sarcomas microscopically, and a generous biopsy is necessary to establish the diagnosis.

LYMPHOMAS

Diagnosis of lymphoma in the jaws is made primarily by biopsy and by correlation with clinical symptoms. Microscopically, difficulty may arise in differentiating the lymphomas from reactive and proliferative lymphoid disease (such as benign lymphoid hyperplasia, Sjögren's disease, and Mikulicz's disease) and inflammatory lesions. When a diagnosis of lymphoma of the jaws or the overlying mucosa is made, a complete systemic evaluation of the patient is necessary to rule out the possibility that the lesion may have metastasized from another site.

Therapeutic Decisions and Staging

SQUAMOUS CELL CARCINOMA

The prognosis and the treatment plan for patients with oral carcinoma depend on the degree of differentiation of the tumor, the size of the primary lesion, its location, and whether metastasis has already occurred.[6, 7] The finding with the gravest effect on prognosis is the presence of metastatic adenopathy; however, destruction of underlying bone (mandible or maxilla) indicates that the primary tumor is biologically aggressive. Surgery should play a major role in treating those oral carcinomas that destroy bone. Table 4–1 contains a modification of the TNM classification that applies to the oral cavity only.

A major clinical consideration when squamous cell carcinoma occurs in the oral cavity is whether the osseous structures or the enveloping periosteum is involved. When the malignancy has invaded the periosteum or bone, the generally accepted procedure is to do a wide local resection with a

Table 4–1 TNM Classification for Oral Malignancies

Primary Tumor (T)
TIS	Carcinoma in situ
T1	Tumor 2 cm or less in size
T2	Tumor 2–4 cm
T3	Tumor greater than 4 cm

Regional Lymph Nodes (N)
N0	No palpable nodes
N1	Movable homolateral nodes
N2	Movable contralateral or bilateral nodes
N3	Fixed nodes

Distant Metastasis (M)
M0	No distant metastases
M1	Distant metastases present

Stages
Stage I	T1	N0	M0
Stage II	T2	N0	M0
Stage III	T1 to T3	N1	M0
Stage IV	T1 to T3	N2, N3	M1

tumor-free margin of 2 to 3 cm. Whenever possible, the mandibular condyle is preserved for future reconstructive purposes. Occasionally, the outer table or lower half of the mandible can be saved to allow fixation of a dental appliance.

METASTATIC CARCINOMA

Metastasis to the jaws and surrounding tissues generally occurs late in the course of disease. The identification of these and other concurrent sites of metastasis is accomplished by physical, radionuclide, and radiographic examinations. Palliative therapy generally consists of chemotherapy or local irradiation.

SARCOMAS AND LYMPHOMAS

Primary sarcomas of the jaws have traditionally been treated with surgery. The possibility of distant metastasis must be ruled out before therapy is initiated. Chest radiographs, liver and bone scans, palpation of the cervical lymph nodes, and careful general physical examination are essential in determining whether metastasis has taken place ("staging"). Lymphomas limited to the jaws and oral cavity occur rarely. Appropriate therapy should be determined by the local or regional extent of tumor.

BENIGN TUMORS

Many benign expansile central lesions in the jaws, mainly the odontogenic tumors (such as ameloblastoma, ameloblastic fibroma, and odontogenic fibroma), are initially treated by conservative therapy. Unfortunately, because of the high recurrence rate of these tumors, a second or even a third procedure is often necessary. Ameloblastomas of the maxilla generally require more aggressive surgery than those of the mandible. When recurrences do occur, careful radiographic examination of the margins of the tumor is most important. It is generally recognized that the surgical tumor-free margins should be a minimum of 1 cm.

Clinical Follow-up

SQUAMOUS CELL CARCINOMA

Clinical follow-up is vital in patients treated for squamous cell carcinoma of the jaws. Erosions, ulcers, and additional areas of leukoplakia and erythroplakia should be regarded with a high level of suspicion. Enlarged or tender cervical lymph nodes may be the first signs of metastasis.

Patients who have undergone irradiation should be followed closely for the occurrence of osteoradionecrosis of the jaws. Early detection is important for the successful treatment of this condition. Establishment of excellent oral hygiene and the use of topical fluoride treatments on the teeth have reduced radiation caries significantly in patients whose salivary glands were in the field of irradiation.

SARCOMAS AND LYMPHOMAS

The clinical follow-up of patients treated for sarcomas and lymphomas consists of careful examinations of the local tissues and cervical lymph nodes. Blood-borne metastasis is not uncommon, and chest radiographs should be taken periodically.

RADIOLOGIC CONSIDERATIONS

RADIOGRAPHIC PROJECTIONS OF THE JAWS

Numerous radiographic projections of the maxilla and mandible are available for depicting bone lesions. It is desirable to see the entire lesion in three dimensions, with demonstration of all its borders. Curved surface tomography (Panorex, Orthopantomograph, and Panelipse) gives a broad, generally useful panoramic view of the teeth and supporting structures of the jaws from the facial aspect (Fig. 4–1). Supplemental radiographs are usually taken for greater definition. This requirement may be fulfilled by the use of intraoral periapical, lateral jaw, and lateral skull views, or a combination of these projections. Mediolateral and anteroposterior relationships of jaw tumors may be visualized in the body of the mandible by a combination of intraoral periapical, occlusal, and lateral jaw films. The region of the angle and ramus of the mandible will usually require a lateral jaw radiograph, in combination with posteroanterior skull and reverse Towne projection radiographs to provide adequate coverage. The region of the condyle is best covered with lateral laminographic views and other special views as required. Multiple hypocycloidal or circular tomographic projections in several planes may be required to localize tumors in the jaws effectively, particularly lesions in the maxilla. Bone destruction in the palate and in other areas within the maxilla is difficult to see on conventional radiographs because of superimposition of complex bony structures and the relative thinness of the bony palate. The radiologist who is expert in dental or head and neck radiology is the best judge of the appropriate views needed in a given situation.

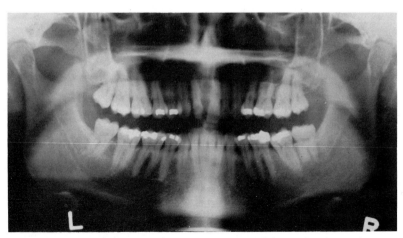

Figure 4–1 A panoramic radiograph provides broad coverage of the teeth, jaws, and contiguous structures of the orofacial region. This type of film is frequently used for initial screening purposes.

Presenting Radiographic Signs

The malignant lesions considered in this discussion are primary as well as secondary tumors involving the gingival, palatal, and alveolar ridge areas of the maxilla, in addition to the gingival, alveolar ridge, and vertical ramus areas of the mandible.

In general, malignancies affecting the mandible or maxilla tend to exhibit ragged, irregular, noncorticated, or poorly delineated borders radiographically. More slowly growing benign tumors tend to exhibit smooth, regular, corticated borders that may expand the affected bone (see also Chapter 14, on sarcomas). A malignant lesion of the jaws may be osteolytic, osteoblastic, or a combination of the two, resulting radiographically in a radiolucent, sclerotic, or "mixed" appearance, respectively.

Primary mucosal carcinomas that originate within the oral cavity and affect the jaws are usually of soft tissue origin and spread by local extension into the alveolar bone, causing osteolysis. These lesions do not produce new bone within the tumor, under the periosteum, or in adjacent bone. Sclerosing osteitis may occur in the adjacent bone secondarily, however, if the tumor becomes ulcerated and infected. New periosteal bone formation or bone production within the tumor may be associated with a primary sarcoma, and the radiographic appearance is variable. Metastatic carcinoma in the jaws may produce bone within the lesion, but this occurs rarely.

Malignant tumors do not usually cause resorption of adjacent tooth roots, although it has been noted in some patients. On the other hand, a rapidly invading tumor destroys supporting periodontal bone to the extent that teeth may become loosened and be retained only by surrounding soft tissue, or they may be exfoliated. Benign tumors, cysts, and infections are more frequently associated with actual resorption of tooth roots.

A slight increase in soft tissue opacity located outside the periphery of tumor-involved bone may be indicative of an associated soft tissue mass. Frequently, a clear-cut soft tissue mass is delineated radiographically near an area of bone destruction, thereby indicating the presence of a malignant growth.

Multiple areas of bone destruction in a jaw, or, rarely, in both jaws are suggestive of a metastatic origin. Areas of irregular central or cortical bone destruction, without radiographic signs of soft tissue swelling or a visible or palpable growth in the oral cavity, also point toward possible jaw metastases. The posterior body of the mandible is the most frequent site of metastases. While a primary locally invasive carcinoma tends to destroy the jaw as it advances, metastatic carcinoma tends to infiltrate and to leave ragged pieces of separated bone within the tumor mass.

In general, all destructive jaw lesions presenting a radiographic appearance consistent with a tumor should be biopsied. In addition, apparent periapical infections that do not respond to therapy should also be biopsied. Whenever tissue is submitted to the pathologist for histologic examination from intraosseous lesions it should always be accompanied by multiple radiographic views of the area.

SQUAMOUS CELL CARCINOMA

The most common malignant bone involvement is local invasion of squamous cell carcinoma (epidermoid carcinoma) from adjacent mucosa into the premolar and molar area of the mandible, although osseous involvement in other areas of both jaws may occur.[8] A radiolucent "dished-out" or **U**-shaped osseous excavation occurring along the superior alveolar border and extending down into medullary bone is the typical appearance (Fig. 4–2). The superficial bone destruction may have a clearcut margin, indicating "erosion" caused by the pressure of an overlying gingival tumor growth. In other patients an irregular, ragged margin indicates actual "invasion" of the alveolar bone.[9] No evidence of periosteal reaction or new bone formation within the tumor is seen. The accompanying shadow of a soft tissue growth may frequently be seen. However, mucosal carcinoma invading from the gingiva into the buccal or lingual surfaces of the alveolar bone may not be apparent radiographically. On occasion, the appearance of such invasive lesions can also simulate that of a primary central (medullary) bone lesion on a conventional radiograph. Invasion and destruction of bone in the hard palate and the maxil-

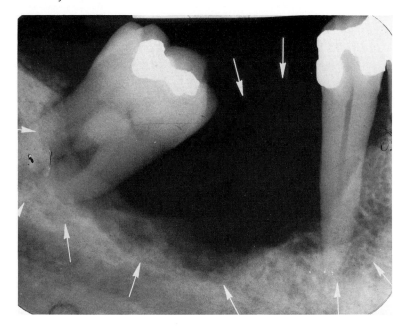

Figure 4–2 A periapical projection in the molar region of the mandible of a 50-year-old male. The irregular loss of bone is characteristic of an infiltrating carcinoma from the overlying mucosa. Note that the border of the lesion is ill-defined, the molar tooth is undermined, and there is no evidence of root resorption. A soft tissue mass adjacent to the lesion could be seen on the original radiograph. The inferior alveolar nerve canal is immediately subjacent to the lesion.

lary alveolar ridge by carcinoma of the overlying oral mucosa may occasionally be seen. Ultimately, the maxillary sinus and nasal fossa may also become involved.

CENTRAL SQUAMOUS CELL CARCINOMA

A rare primary carcinoma of bone that develops most often within the mandible, but may also appear in the maxilla, is the central squamous cell carcinoma. The tumor is lytic, producing a single, central radiolucent area in the bone; it is thought to be derived from odontogenic epithelium or from epithelial cells trapped embryologically within the jaws.[10, 11] The bone margins surrounding this lesion are ragged, indicating an invasive tumor, and the lesion may eventually erupt through the cortical plate. While new bone is not produced inside the lesion, irregular opacities may be seen radiographically within the lesion, which represent pieces of bone left in the wake of the advancing tumor. This lesion must be differentiated from metastases to the jaws (by histologic examination), from locally-invading extraosseous mucosal tumors (by clinical examination), and from antral carcinomas spreading into the maxillary alveolar bone (by careful radiographic examination of the antrum). Shear reports

a more frequent occurrence of central carcinoma of the jaws in older males.[10]

OSTEOSARCOMA

The most common type of primary sarcoma arising in the jaws is osteosarcoma (osteogenic sarcoma). In addition, the jaws are involved metastatically in 6.5 per cent of other sarcomas,[12] the mandible usually being affected. Primary osteosarcomas of the jaws have a somewhat better prognosis than osteosarcomas in other bones. Advanced cases of primary osteosarcoma of the jaws present a varied appearance radiographically: lytic, sclerotic, or a combination of the two ("mixed"). Garrington and coworkers reported approximately equal distribution of the three types in a series of 56 cases analyzed.[12] The tumor is usually unicentric, and it typically exhibits irregular borders highly suggestive (or diagnostic) of malignancy. Expansion of bone may be observed radiographically in the sclerotic type of sarcoma, which may grow more slowly, whereas the lytic type destroys bone rapidly as it advances. The cortical plates may also be destroyed, predisposing to pathologic fracture of the jaw. Periosteal new bone formation in these tumors varies from none, to increasing amounts of irregular, layered, or right-angled spicules of bone ("sun-ray" effect) at the bone surface (Fig. 4–3). A very early radiographic sign of osteosarcoma in the jaw may be a widened periodontal membrane space, or a radiolucency around one or more teeth. The mean age of patients with occurrence in the jaws is about 33 years, and there is a greater incidence in males.[13]

A few patients who have had benign lesions subjected to therapeutic irradiation have been reported subsequently to develop jaw sarcomas.

CHONDROSARCOMA

The mandibular alveolar ridges and ramus or the maxillary alveolar ridges and palate may become involved by a primary chondrosarcoma. The radiographic appearances are similar to those manifested by osteosarcoma: lytic, sclerotic, or mixed. The tumor may show a single radiolucent area of irregular bone destruction, multiple loculations, or radiolucencies with sclerotic densities inside the destructive lesions. Frequent bone expansion at the labial, buccal, and lingual margins occurs.[14] In some cases, a sun-ray periosteal reaction similar to that produced by some osteosarcomas is seen peripherally. A ground-glass appearance within the area of bone destruction may be evident in other patients. Teeth in close re-

lation to the tumor may be resorbed, loosened, or exfoliated. When the lesion is small, widening of the periodontal membrane space may be noted, as in early osteosarcoma.[15] Peak incidence is in the fourth and fifth decades of life, with a male to female ratio of 2 to 1. Clinically, chondrosarcomas behave differently from osteosarcomas of the jaws: they usually occur at a later age, are slower growing, and are slower to produce metastases.[8] Differentiation from a benign chondroma is crucial, and the roentgenograms can provide evidence of malignancy (biologic aggressiveness) when a diagnosis based on tissue sections is in doubt.

FIBROSARCOMA

Fibrosarcoma may arise centrally within the jaws or in the periosteum of the mandible or maxilla.[13, 16] Radiographically, the appearance of central fibrosarcoma resembles that of osteosarcoma. Dahlin and Ivins describe a case presenting as an ill-defined central radiolucency in the bone, with subsequent cortical perforation and periosteal reaction.[16] Periosteal fibrosarcoma of the jaws is rare; there may be no radiographic evidence of bone loss or simply a smooth excavation along the bone border.[8] Fibrosarcoma is most common before age 50 but

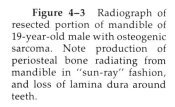

Figure 4–3 Radiograph of resected portion of mandible of 19-year-old male with osteogenic sarcoma. Note production of periosteal bone radiating from mandible in "sun-ray" fashion, and loss of lamina dura around teeth.

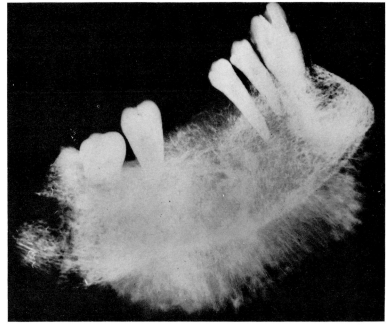

may occur at any age, including in young children.

EWING'S SARCOMA

Ewing's sarcoma is an uncommon primary malignant tumor in the jaws; it occurs occasionally in the maxilla but more often in the mandible. The lesion may assume a variety of radiologic appearances, including irregular bone destruction or lysis, sclerosis, multiple distinct loculations, and periosteal new bone formation.[17] In most cases a radiolucency confined to the central portion or medulla of the bone is noted, with indistinct margins, but some tumors may cause bone expansion. Areas of sclerosis may be seen within or around the radiolucency. A finding that is often associated with Ewing's sarcoma is periosteal new bone formation, producing a laminated or onionskin effect along the bone surface.[17] This may consist of a single layer or multiple layers of new bone parallel to the cortical surface. In addition, some cases have motheaten cortical margins, with right angle spicules of periosteal new bone entering the soft tissues and giving a sun-ray effect. Teeth may be loosened and lost. Ewing's sarcoma occurs mainly in children and young adults, usually under 25 years of age,[18] with males affected twice as often as females.

RETICULUM CELL SARCOMA OF BONE

Reticulum cell sarcoma of bone is regarded as belonging to the malignant lymphoma group ("histiocytic lymphoma"). This lesion does not occur commonly in the jaws, but when found it is most often in the mandible. The tumor is destructive and exhibits poorly defined, invasive margins highly suggestive of malignancy. A sclerotic bone reaction may be evident overlying or surrounding the area of radiolucency.[8] The alveolar crest or mandibular ramus may be involved, with undermining and loss of teeth. Generally, there is no sign of periosteal new bone formation. In the maxilla, the tumor sometimes extends into the nasal cavity. It usually occurs in patients under 40 years of age, but this sarcoma sometimes may affect a younger age group (under 20 years). Men are affected more often

than women, in a ratio of about 2 to 1. Hodgkin's disease and lymphocytic lymphoma occur even less frequently in the jaws. When observed radiographically, the lesions are usually lytic or destructive; occasional osteoblastic activity may also be evident, however.

BURKITT'S TUMOR

Burkitt's tumor (African jaw lymphoma) often affects the premolar and molar regions of the jaws. This lesion is osteolytic, and the early radiographic findings are loss of lamina dura around the erupted teeth, enlargement of a developing tooth crypt, and small focal areas of radiolucency within the bone.[19, 20] Later, the jaw radiolucencies coalesce into larger areas of bone loss that may be multilocular in appearance. Teeth become resorbed or undermined and are shed as the mass increases in size. Subperiosteal new bone formation may be seen radiating into the adjacent soft tissues. This tumor also has the potential to expand the jaws greatly.[21] Peak age incidence is in children between 3 years and 8 years of age, and this tumor is rare in patients over 15 years of age.[20] Occurrence is mainly in central eastern Africa, but cases have now been reported from many areas of the world, including the United States. (See also Chapter 2.)

MULTIPLE MYELOMA

Multiple myeloma frequently involves the jaws bilaterally, usually in the premolar, molar, angle, and ramus areas of the mandible. The lesion is lytic and may present radiographically as numerous, well-defined, circular or oval radiolucencies that are small and initially appear distinct (Fig. 4–4). Later, these punched-out areas of destruction may become confluent and form large areas of bone destruction. No apparent bone reaction occurs around each tumor, but the inside of the cortical plate may become scalloped or rarely may even be penetrated, with the development of a pathologic fracture. Solitary lesions or generalized osteoporosis may be the modes of presentation in other patients. Cranial bone lesions are common in this disease, and supplemental radiographs of the skull are indicated. Men are affected more often than women,

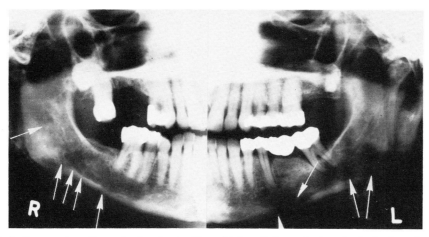

Figure 4–4   Panoramic radiograph of patient with multiple radiolucent lesions in the body and ramus of mandible, demonstrated to be deposits of multiple myeloma. In addition, internal aspect of the cortical plate along the inferior border of the mandible demonstrates bilateral resorption, particularly on the left.

in a ratio of 4 to 1. It is most common in patients between 40 and 70 years of age, but occurrence in younger individuals has been recorded.

METASTATIC CARCINOMA

Metastatic carcinoma is the most common malignant tumor in bones, but the jaws are rarely affected. Metastatic tumor in the jaws may point to an occult malignancy located at another primary site, or the jaw lesion may be the first indication

of metastatic spread from a known tumor. Usually, only one jaw is affected. The molar region of the mandible is more often a site of metastasis than the maxilla (Fig. 4–5). Lesions in the jaw may be single or multiple, and are of variable size. The radiographic appearance often is one of bone destruction with ill-defined, infiltrating margins, similar to primary malignant bone tumors. Small residual fragments of bone may be observed within the radiolucency, or on occasion there may be sclerosis in metastatic lesions from carcinoma of the prostate, breast, or even the lung. Periodontal bone including

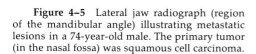

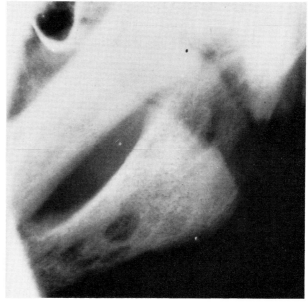

Figure 4–5   Lateral jaw radiograph (region of the mandibular angle) illustrating metastatic lesions in a 74-year-old male. The primary tumor (in the nasal fossa) was squamous cell carcinoma.

lamina dura may be lost, leading to mobility and loss of teeth, and penetration of cortical bone with pathologic fracture may develop eventually. Tumors in many sites are capable of metastasizing to the jaws; in descending order of frequency, these locations include the breast, lung, prostate, thyroid, kidney, stomach, and colon.[22] A complete medical history is extremely important when the possibility of a metastatic tumor arises.

OTHER MALIGNANT JAW LESIONS

Other malignant neoplasms also occur rarely as primary lesions in the jaws or as secondary deposits. Among these are non-Burkitt's lymphoma,[23] malignant tumor of salivary gland origin,[24, 25] solitary plasma cell myeloma, malignant melanoma, hemangioendothelioma, hemangiopericytoma, malignant schwannoma, and neuroblastoma.[26, 27]

Differential Diagnosis

The *periapical* abscess, granuloma, and cyst are peculiar to the jaws and are the direct result of infection within the tooth pulp. Radiographically, periapical involvement characteristically causes widening of the periodontal membrane space, a break in the lamina dura, or a varying amount of periapical bone destruction. When bone destruction occurs in these conditions, a radiolucency is seen that may have either well-corticated or ill-defined borders and is usually confined to the vicinity of the tooth apex. A sclerotic reaction may also be evident in surrounding bone, and root resorption may be present.

The evenly widened periodontal membrane space around one or several teeth, and periapical bone destruction resulting from pulpal infection, must be differentiated from similar radiographic signs that may indicate early osteosarcoma or chondrosarcoma, as well as scleroderma, early periapical cemental dysplasia, benign cementoblastoma, or osteomyelitis.

Localized or diffuse bone loss may also be evident around one or several teeth as the result of periodontitis, histiocytosis X, or ameloblastoma. The jaw lesions of

histiocytosis X are osteolytic and may give the appearance of "teeth floating in space," while some ameloblastomas have irregular borders suggestive of a malignant bone neoplasm infiltrating around the teeth. In addition, local destruction of supporting bone around the molar and incisor teeth is found in periodontosis and in the Papillon-Lefevre syndrome.

The radiographic appearances of central squamous cell carcinoma and of lytic metastases to the jaws may also be confused with osteomyelitis or osteoradionecrosis. Active osteomyelitis is lytic, has irregular, moth-eaten borders, may destroy cortical margins, and often contains residual pieces of devitalized bone (sequestra), as do central squamous cell carcinoma or metastatic carcinoma. Periosteal new bone formation may also be evident with osteomyelitis.

Other radiolucent bone lesions that occur centrally in the jaws are fissural cysts, follicular cysts, cysts and brown tumors of hyperparathyroidism, central giant cell granulomas, hemangiomas, multiple myeloma lesions, and sarcomas. Except for sarcomas and hemangiomas, these lesions usually have discrete or well-defined borders. They may or may not occur in close relation to the roots of teeth.

The osteoblastic type of metastatic carcinoma (usually breast or prostate), as well as primary osteosarcoma, fibrosarcoma, and chondrosarcoma, may also manifest as radiolucency in the jaw mixed with radiopacity, resembling the osteoblastic phase of Paget's disease, fibrous dysplasia, chronic sclerosing osteomyelitis, or the osteomata of Gardner's syndrome. In addition, the calcifying epithelial odontogenic cyst (Gorlin's cyst), periapical cemental dysplasia, and calcifying epithelial odontogenic tumor (Pindborg tumor) may also present a mixed osteoblastic and osteolytic appearance, with the borders becoming less defined as the lesions become more calcified. In some patients, chondrosarcoma, Paget's disease, fibrous dysplasia, or hyperparathyroidism may exhibit a diffuse, ground-glass radiographic appearance within areas of bone destruction.

Several jaw lesions tend to stimulate new bone formation under the periosteum. Garre's sclerosing osteomyelitis with proliferative periostitis is found in relation to a chronically infected lower molar in children or young adults. The periosteal reaction is observed along the lateral and inferior borders of the mandible adjacent to the infected tooth. Other benign and malignant lesions that may stimulate periosteal new bone are central hemangioma,[28] suppurative osteomyelitis, infantile cortical hyperostosis (Caffey's disease), osteosarcoma, fibrosarcoma, chondrosarcoma, Ewing's sarcoma, and Burkitt's tumor.

The punched-out radiolucencies associated with multiple myeloma must also be differentiated from the small, purely lucent lesions of active hyperparathyroidism or eosinophilic granuloma (histiocytosis X) that can occur in the mandible. Generalized osteoporosis and loss of the lamina dura are the principal findings in some cases of multiple myeloma, hyperparathyroidism, rickets, or osteomalacia, but these conditions may simply be related to aging.

MALIGNANT TRANSFORMATION

Malignant tumors rarely evolve from benign jaw lesions; of those that do, a significant number develop from benign lesions exposed to therapeutic radiation, suggesting a possible etiologic factor. On rare occasions, mucoepidermoid carcinoma, squamous cell carcinoma, and malignant pleomorphic adenoma (mixed tumor) have been reported to develop in the walls of odontogenic cysts (radicular, follicular, and residual cysts.[2, 6, 29, 30] Malignant transformation that develops in the wall of a previously benign cyst with a well-defined margin produces a radiographic irregularity in the otherwise smooth cyst margin. The malignant lesion may occur in relation to the crown or the root of an unerupted tooth. In addition, carcinoma may arise rarely within an ameloblastoma (ameloblastic carcinoma).

Spontaneous and postirradiation sarcomatous degeneration (to osteosarcoma or to fibrosarcoma) has been reported rarely within jaw lesions of monostotic or polyostotic fibrous dysplasia.[31] The malignant lesions appear radiographically as enlarging, poorly defined areas of radiolucency that may penetrate the cortex and may produce new bone within the tumor mass. Other benign jaw tumors, including central giant cell granuloma, chondroma, myxoma, and fibroma have rarely shown evidence of

malignant degeneration after irradiation. Fortunately, radiation therapy no longer is being used for benign disease. Development of osteosarcoma in a jaw affected by Paget's disease is not an uncommon complication of this condition.[13]

Localization and Staging

Careful oral radiography is important in determining the presence and extent of local invasion into the adjacent bone by primary mucosal cancers in the mouth. The extent and the location of osseous involvement are very important when the treatment plan is being formulated. When the lesion is found to extend into bone from the overlying mucosa, the treatment of choice almost always is surgery. Usually, when resection is performed, a neck dissection with the creation of a wide margin around the lesion is indicated.

Injudicious radiotherapy to such lesions carries the risk of osteoradionecrosis, with its associated pain and difficulty in management. On the other hand, when oral mucosal lesions do not involve bone they are often properly treated with radiotherapy. Carcinomas of the maxillary alveolar ridge are usually treated surgically because of their proximity to underlying bone. Bone and chest radiography are essential for the detection of metastasis (other than to cervical lymph nodes) and for appropriate assignment within the TNM system (see the earlier section on clinical staging). Conversely, metastatic deposits detected radiologically in the maxillary or mandibular arches may be the first sign of a primary lesion elsewhere in the body; they may also provide the first indication of spread from a known distant tumor.

Radiologic Follow-up

Radiography plays a role in the surveillance of the jaws after orofacial surgery, and occasionally after treatment of primary lesions elsewhere in the body. The jaws should be included in full skeletal surveys for metastatic disease, especially when bone symptoms are present and there is a high index of suspicion clinically.

When radiation therapy or chemotherapy or both are central to the treatment regimen, cessation of tumor growth, shrinkage of the tumor mass, or actual filling-in of jaw radiolucencies may be visualized radiographically. Demonstration of trabecular and cortical bone remodeling, and the reappearance of destroyed crypt walls around developing teeth and of the lamina dura adjacent to tooth roots, are indications of cessation of tumor growth and bone repair. In some cases of primary jaw carcinoma treated by radiation therapy, however, the tumor mass may be replaced by fibrous tissue without radiographic evidence of reossification.[8] Areas of persistent tumor growth may sometimes be evident alongside areas of bone repair.

Over a period of months to years following a course of intensive radiotherapy in the orofacial region, the jaws may develop radiographic signs of osteoradionecrosis. The usual clinical indications for radiographic examination in these situations are pain and pathologic fracture. Necrotic jaw lesions usually require at least six months to a year following therapy to become evident. In the absence of recurrent tumor or infection, there may be no radiographic evidence of bone necrosis. In the presence of infection, usually from an exposed root canal of a tooth or from loss in the continuity of the oral mucous membrane, there is a tendency for the necrotic bone lesion to become manifest. Localized jaw infections are usually of dental origin, and extensive osteomyelitis with osteoradionecrosis may appear as a diffuse radiolucency associated with small bony sequestra. These lesions usually progress slowly, show little subperiosteal new bone formation, and are prone to cause jaw fractures. Subsequently, the pathologic fractures may show nonunion.

The radiographic differentiation between osteoradionecrosis of the jaw with infection, and tumor persistence or recurrence is often difficult. The radiographic appearances of recurrent jaw tumor, tumor plus infection, or osteoradionecrosis plus infection may be indistinguishable, and biopsy may be necessary. Radiographs taken before, during and immediately after treatment may serve as a valuable baseline for comparison. The presence of recurrent tumor is suggested when, in later films, the destructive bone lesion is seen to be progressing concentrically from a single focus, in the region of the original tumor. The presence of osteomyelitis or necrosis is suggested by linear extension of the radiolucent lesion along the axis of the jaw, by long areas of sclerosis, and by evidence of sequestration of devitalized bone. Osteoradionecrosis is seen much more frequently in the mandible than in the maxilla.

Postoperative radiographs are also valuable for evaluation of positioning, healing, and maintenance of fabricated prosthetic and biological implants that have been inserted into the jaw.

References

1. Dorn, H. R., and Cutler, S. J.: Morbidity from cancer in the United States. Public Health Monograph No. 56. Washington, D.C., U.S. Government Printing Office, 1959, p. 186.
2. Pindborg, J. J.: Oral cancer from an international point of view. J. Can. Dent. Assoc., 31:219–226, 1965.
3. United States Surgeon General, Advisory Committee: Smoking and Health: Report of the Advisory Committee to the Surgeon General of the Public Health Service, U.S. Department of Health, Education, and Welfare. Princeton, N.J., D. Van Nostrand, 1964.
4. Vogler, W. R., Lloyd, J. W., Milmore, B. K.: A retrospective study of etiologic factors in cancer of the mouth, pharynx and larynx. Cancer, 15:246–258, 1962.
5. Stockdale, C. R.: Metastatic carcinoma of the jaws secondary to primary carcinoma of the breast. Oral Surg., 12:1095, 1959.
6. Fries, R., Grabner, H., Langer, H., Jr. et al.: Comparative investigation on the classification of carcinoma of the oral cavity. J. Maxillofac. Surg., 1:222–235, 1973.
7. Arthur, J., and Fenner, M.: Influences of grading on prognosis in carcinoma of the tongue: computer analysis of 299 cases. Clin. Radiol., 17:384–396, 1966.
8. Worth, H. M.: Principles and Practice of Oral Radiologic Interpretation. Chicago, Year Book Medical Publishers, 1972.
9. Swearingen, A. G., McGraw, J. R., and Palumbo, V. D.: Roentgenographic pathologic correlation of carcinoma of the gingiva involving the mandible. Amer. J. Roentgenol., 96:15–18, January 1966.
10. Shear, M.: Primary intra-alveolar epidermoid carcinoma of the jaw. J. Pathol., 97:645–651, 1969.
11. Morrison, R., and Deeley, T. J.: Intra-alveolar carcinoma of the jaw, treatment by supervoltage radiotherapy. Br. Dent. J. 35:321–326, 1962.

12. Garrington, G. E., Scofield, H. H., Cornyn, J., et al.: Osteosarcoma of the jaws. Cancer, 20:377–391, 1967.
13. Shafer, W. G., Hine, M. K., and Levy, B. M.: A Textbook of Oral Pathology. 3rd ed. Philadelphia, W. B. Saunders, 1974.
14. Chaudry, A. P., Robinovitch, M. R., Mitchell, D. F., et al.: Chondrogenic tumors of the jaws. Am. J. Surg., 102:403–411, 1961.
15. Waldron, C. A.: Non-odontogenic neoplasms, cysts, and allied conditions of the jaws. Semin. Roentgenol. 6:414–425, 1971.
16. Dahlin, D. C., and Ivins, J. C.: Fibrosarcoma of bone. Cancer, 5:85–99, 1952.
17. McCormack, L. J., Dockerty, M. B., and Chromley, R. K.: Ewing's sarcoma. Cancer, 5:85–99, 1952.
18. Carl, W., Schaaf, N. G., Gaeta, J., et al.: Ewing's sarcoma. Oral Surg., 31:472–478, 1971.
19. Adatia, A. K.: Radiology of Burkitt's tumour in the jaws. East Afr. Med. J., 43:290–297, 1966.
20. Adatia, A. K.: Radiology of Burkitt's tumour in the jaws. Br. Dent. J., 120:315–326, 1966.
21. O'Connor, G. T.: Malignant lymphoma in African children. Cancer, 14:270–283, 1961.
22. Clausen, F., and Poulsen, H.: Metastatic carcinoma to the jaws. Acta Pathol. Microbiol. Scand., 57:361, 1963.
23. Eversole, L. R., and Rovin, S.: Differential radiographic diagnosis of lesions of the jawbones. Radiology, 105:277–284, 1972.
24. Butt, W. P., Hollender, L., and Stener, I.: Mandibular erosion in tumours of the major salivary glands. Acta Radiol., 8:235–240, 1969.
25. Smith, R. L., Dahlin, D. C., and Waite, D. E.: Mucoepidermoid carcinomas of the jawbones. J. Oral Surg., 26:387–393, 1968.
26. Bradley, P. F., and Rowe, N. L.: Mandibular metastasis of a neuroblastoma: Report of case. J. Oral Surg., 28:781–784, 1970.
27. De Leon, E. L., Finney, R. A., Ruth, A., et al.: Neuroblastoma with metastasis to maxilla and mandible: Review of literature and report of case. J. Oral Surg., 28:773–780, 1970.
28. Sherman, R. S., and Wilner, D.: The roentgen diagnosis of hemangioma of bone. Am. J. Roentgenol., 86:1146–1159, 1961.
29. Gardner, A. F.: The odontogenic cyst as a potential carcinoma: A clinicopathologic appraisal. J. Am. Dent. Assoc., 78:746–755, 1969.
30. Breitenecker, G., and Wepner, F.: A pleomorphic adenoma (so-called mixed tumor) in the wall of a dentigerous cyst. J. Oral Surg., 36:63–71, 1973.
31. Slow, I. N., Stern, D., and Friedman, E. W.: Osteogenic sarcoma arising in a pre-existing fibrous dysplasia: report of a case. J. Oral Surg., 29: 126–129, 1971.

Chapter Five

HEAD AND NECK

Robert L. Scanlan, M.D.

CLINICAL CONSIDERATIONS

General Correlations

Carcinoma of the ear, nose, and throat has its highest incidence in elderly patients, particularly those with mucosal irritation caused by heavy smoking and drinking. Persons with poor dental care are also more likely to have cancer in the head or neck. The clinician and radiologist should be alert to the high incidence of multiple (either simultaneous or sequential) carcinomas in this area. A tumor of the head or neck may itself be a distant metastasis from another primary, which might be reflected in the chest radiograph. This situation most commonly involves metastases to the sinuses and to the lymph nodes of the neck and mandible. Melanoma and adenocarcinoma of the kidney can also metastasize to the base of tongue or buccal mucosa.

Interdisciplinary cooperation is time consuming but indispensable. Any suspicious sign or symptom of serious disease, such as an otherwise innocent radiographic skull lesion, an opacified sinus, dysphagia, pain in the ear, or diplopia, calls for a serious effort on the part of all the physicians concerned to disprove the presence of cancer.

Patients, particularly those in the high-risk groups, must also be made aware of warning symptoms (including lumps, hoarseness, nasal or aural discharge, persistent sore in the mouth, or an unexplained loose tooth) and seek early advice. Dentists should be alert to the possibility of cancer, and should examine the entire oral cavity as closely as they do the teeth (see Chapter 4). They should warn patients with persistent mucosal irritations of the potential hazard and consider biopsy of any "white patches." General physicians should not be complacent because they encounter these diseases infrequently, and they should seek the help of a specialist promptly when they suspect the presence of a malignant neoplasm and when either direct or indirect endoscopy is the only means of visualizing the suspicious area.[3]

Requests for radiologic consultations should contain sufficient history and findings to delineate the clinical problem that is being explored. For optimal results, the radiographs should be viewed by the radiologist while the patient is still present in the department, to see if the clinical question has been answered. Sinus films showing "minimal evidence of disease, probably inflammatory," but accompanied by a history of epistaxis or facial pain, will prompt the radiologist to look at the films much more carefully; he may suggest further specialized studies, which could reveal an extensive tumor barely visible on the plain films. Special equipment such as polydirectional tomography must therefore be accessible.

Radiology is gross pathology, and "histologic" diagnoses should not be made by the radiologist. The fact that an isolated polypoid lesion in the antrum is usually a retention cyst does not mean that a similar lesion may not be a malignant tumor in a patient of any age. Again, clinical correlation is essential. Earlier radiographs are invaluable for making comparisons that will help to determine the presence or absence of a significant lesion. A major radiologic necessity is a series of postoperative or post-radiotherapy baseline radiographs of the treated primary tumor area, for use in future comparative studies.

The otolaryngologist often must see many patients in a short period of time. Review of every study with the radiologist, while highly desirable, is often not possible. However, any inconsistencies or major differences of opinion should be reconciled by close consultation and additional studies, if indicated.

The pathologist should have adequate information about the *source* of biopsy specimens as well as pertinent radiologic studies of the area. For example, esthesioneuroblastoma growing intracranially and into the nose may be called an adenocarcinoma if the only information available to the pathologist is that the patient has a "tumor of the nose." A meningioma growing into the middle ear histologically may resemble a chemodectoma, or a chemodectoma presenting in the posterior fossa may simulate a vascular meningioma.

The radiation therapist must insist upon a detailed knowledge of the limits of a tumor so that the entire tumor will be encompassed in the field of therapy. This might well require cerebral angiography or other contrast studies with their attendant risk, discomfort, and expense. As mentioned, consideration should be given to repeating certain studies following treatment, first to establish a baseline and then at intervals to assess tumor response or the possibility of local recurrence.[4, 5]

Presenting Signs and Symptoms

Loosening of teeth can be an early symptom of a gingival carcinoma, but it is also a late symptom in maxillary sinus carcinoma and intranasal carcinoma. Trismus is a late finding in all cancers of the tonsillar region and maxillary sinus. Persistent "sinusitis," nasal discharge, and headache are early symptoms of carcinoma of the sinuses and nasopharynx. Most patients with sphenoid carcinoma had been treated for "headache" for at least 6 to 12 months before a definitive diagnosis was reached. Otitis media occurring in an adult Chinese as a *new* finding signifies carcinoma of the nasopharynx until proven otherwise. Exophthalmos is a late finding in cancer of the sinuses, except in the rare primary lesions occurring high in the maxillary sinus and destroying the roof of the antrum early. Invasion of the cavernous sinus (involving cranial nerves III, IV, V, or VI, and the ophthalmic vein) is a late finding in cancer of the sinuses or nasopharynx.

Intranasal tumors cause unilateral nasal discharge (commonly bloody). A visible external deformity almost always connotes contiguous bone erosion. Exophthalmos, diplopia, or paresthesia of the cheek (infraorbital nerve involvement) all mean extension beyond the nasal cavity (or, in the case of primary sinus tumors, beyond the maxillary or the ethmoid sinus).

Carcinomas of the external ear or parotid gland that extend into the external ear canal can cause a conductive hearing loss. The facial nerve can be compromised by tumor extension either within the temporal bone or after it exits from the stylomastoid foramen. A tumor of the salivary gland that causes facial (seventh) nerve paralysis is malignant by definition. This clinical finding occurs in a minority of patients, however; over 70 per cent of malignancies of the parotid gland occur superficial to the seventh nerve and do not cause a neurologic deficit. Most benign tumors also occur in this so-called superficial parotid lobe. *Painful* swelling usually points toward sialoadenitis, and if both parotids or lacrimal glands are enlarged, inflammatory disease is also much more likely than a tumor. Xerostomia or dryness of the conjunctiva may be associated symptoms in these patients.

The actual extent of bulky exophytic or infiltrating tumors of the laryngopharynx often cannot be determined by indirect laryngoscopy. Much information on tumor staging can be gained from carefully selected radiographic procedures performed in conjunction with direct laryngoscopy and multiple biopsies (see section on radiologic considerations). Most lesions in the laryngopharyngeal region only become symptomatic relatively late in their course, except when the vocal cords are involved primarily.

Enlarged metastatic lymph nodes at the base of the skull or in the lower third of the neck (especially the supraclavicular region) indicate a poor prognosis, but nodes elsewhere in the neck, even when fixed to the carotid, may merit specialized radiographic studies to demonstrate or to rule out carotid invasion, as well as to determine the adequacy of collateral blood flow through the circle of Willis at the base of the brain (thereby influencing the approach to a possible en bloc carotid resection). At present, over half these patients may sustain postoperative hemiplegia despite careful surgery.

All lesions of the laryngopharynx that are exophytic, poorly differentiated, or small, and that do not interfere with cord movement, should be considered for irradiation. Any lesion, regardless of its *apparent* size, must be regarded as extensive if it is associated with otalgia, dysphagia, odynophagia, hemilaryngeal paralysis, or problems with chewing or articulation. The rate of treatment success is related to tumor *size* in supraglottic and laryngeal "ridge" lesions (epiglottis, aryepiglottic and pharyngo-epiglottic folds), is less dependent on size in lesions of the pharyngeal walls, and is not dependent on size in lesions of the pyriform sinus.[6] Finally, it should be emphasized that the clinical finding most critical in determining prognosis is the presence or absence of histologically positive lymph nodes in the neck.

Medullary and undifferentiated thyroid carcinomas can affect deglutition by contiguous invasion of the cervical esophagus. Esophageal invasion has not been observed, as a rule, with papillary or follicular thyroid carcinomas. Lymphosarcoma involving the thyroid is usually associated with generalized (systemic) disease. Hoarseness (when caused by local pressure, not nerve invasion) or deviation of the trachea can be associated with a thyroid carcinoma, but also may occur with benign goiter or bleeding into the gland (the latter is usually associated with pain). With thyroid cancer, these findings are not necessarily poor prognostic signs.

Medullary carcinomas of the thyroid can now be diagnosed with the help of an immunoassay for serum calcitonin. The diagnosis can also be suspected when there is associated hypertension (pheochromocytoma), hypercalcemia (parathyroid ade-

noma), diarrhea, a familial incidence of medullary carcinoma or multiple mucosal neuromas.[7]

Parathyroid adenomas can become clinically manifest by tracheal compression (rarely), renal lithiasis (calcium oxalate or phosphate calculi), duodenal ulcer, weakness, or an insidious personality change (hypercalcemia). The diagnosis can now be confirmed with serum parathormone immunoassay.[8] Associated radiographic bone changes can simulate those found in multiple myeloma, carcinomatous metastases, Paget's disease, hypervitaminosis D, or chronic renal failure.

Differential Diagnosis

Squamous cell carcinoma is the most common malignant tumor of the head and neck region, with different patterns of histologic differentiation and clinical presentation at various anatomic sites. Adenocarcinomas (including salivary gland tumors) and lymphomas are somewhat less common. Metastatic lesions and primary sarcomas are rare. Examples of tumors originating elsewhere that metastasize or extend to the upper respiratory and digestive tracts (primarily involving the paranasal sinuses) are chordomas, pituitary tumors, meningiomas, melanomas, and lesions of the kidney, colon, and lung.

Mucoceles of the ethmoid, frontal, or maxillary sinuses can mimic carcinomas by destroying bone and, in turn, causing exophthalmos and extraocular paresis. Benign lesions (mucocele, osteoma, fibroma, papilloma) are in fact much more common than cancers in the ethmoid, frontal, and sphenoid sinuses; this is probably one of the reasons that carcinomas in the sinuses are often diagnosed late.

Tumors of the intranasal, nasopharyngeal, and ethmoid regions are relatively unusual. In addition to the ordinary epithelial cancers, gliomas, encephaloceles, olfactory esthesioneuroblastomas, malignant schwannomas, plasmacytomas, lymphomas, and melanomas can occur here. Papillomas can behave in a malignant fashion even when they look benign histologically; on the other hand, they can sometimes evolve histologically into a malignant tumor. Often, a small needle or punch biopsy specimen will yield a true diagnosis of squamous cell carcinoma with minimal difficulty, but the problems of making a firm diagnosis with rare tumors or with Wegener's granulomatosis utilizing a small biopsy specimen may be monumental, especially with crushed tissue.

Metastatic masses in the neck from an unknown primary tumor can provide a serious problem in differential diagnosis. The primary site of adenocarcinoma that metastasizes to the cervical lymph nodes usually is the thyroid or salivary gland (rarely the base of tongue or pharyngeal wall). The most common primary site of adenocarcinoma that metastasizes to the lower neck, however, is the thorax or abdominal cavity. Other "masses" include thyroglossal duct cysts that are situated commonly over the thyrohyoid membrane, or a lingual thyroid that can fill the entire vallecula and thereby also simulate a malignant tumor. A dermoid cyst originating in the floor of the mouth can be confused with a thyroglossal duct cyst *or* a tumor of the pyramidal lobe of the thyroid. Laryngoceles, branchial cleft cysts, esophageal diverticula, and carotid aneurysms are usually situated more laterally in the neck. Neurofibromas, lipomas, cervical adenitis, and benign carotid body tumors also may occur in these locations. Large scirrhous masses that invade the cervical vessels and the brachial plexus have been caused, on occasion, by fibromatosis.

Therapeutic Decisions and Staging

Patients with primary head and neck lesions that are large (T3 or T4) or undifferentiated, as well as those with fixed metastatic cervical nodes and localized or regional lymphomas, should be considered for irradiation for at least part of the therapeutic program. Patients with very large lesions (T4), and those with head and neck cancers causing invasion of bone or functional impairment (stridor, dyspnea, trismus), are for all practical purposes *not* candidates for irradiation alone. The treatment of ipsilateral neck nodes should be elective with most lesions of the oral cavity (especially T3 and T4 lesions; treatment of T1 and T2

lesions must be individualized). This is true in general also for non-midline lesions of the oropharynx and laryngopharynx, except for very localized vocal cord carcinomas.

Despite these generalizations, it is our opinion that in squamous cell carcinomas of the respiratory and digestive tracts, few existing statistical data can be applied effectively to the individual patient. Clinical decisions must depend on a detailed knowledge of the contiguous structures involved and the location of the primary lesion, whether leukoplakia is present, whether the patient is an alcoholic, and, most important, the presence of clinically positive nodes.

If a portion of the mandible can be saved in a patient with carcinoma of the anterior tongue or floor of mouth who has undergone partial mandibular resection in continuity with the primary lesion, the functional results are excellent. In sinus surgery, the orbit must always be sacrificed if it is involved by tumor extension. Invasion of the prevertebral fascia is a poor prognostic sign in patients with oropharyngeal cancer. Radiation portals should be carefully altered if the base of skull is shown by careful roentgenologic examination to be involved by a cancer of the nasopharynx. The hard palate should be suspected at least of harboring tumor extension in a patient who has a lesion of the floor of the nasal cavity.

Temporal bone resections are worthwhile only if an ear lesion can be demonstrated to be confined to the external ear canal. These tumors sometimes extend into the middle ear via the annular ligament, leaving a normal tympanic membrane; involvement of the middle ear or inner ear is a very poor prognostic sign. If necessary, dura can be replaced and venous sinus bleeding controlled during the operation, but the position of the carotid artery within the petrous bone restricts the medial, anterior, and inferior margins of any attempted excision. Cylindromas of the parotid gland are also capable of extending into the petrous bone via the seventh nerve canal.

In carcinomas of the maxilla, extension into the pterygoid plates, cribriform plate, posterior ethmoid cells, sphenoid sinus, or retro-orbital space connotes a poor prognosis with *any* treatment. Clinical involvement of the infraorbital nerve (extension through the anterior maxillary wall) means that the skin of the cheek must also be removed. If the

frontal sinus, nasal septum or anterior ethmoid cells are involved, the standard surgical procedure will also have to be modified. The infratemporal space is a particularly difficult area to evaluate for tumor
extension before surgical exploration.

With supraglottic laryngeal primaries,
the decision to perform a limited (supraglottic) laryngectomy should be modified if it
can be demonstrated that:[9-13]

1. There is 2 cm or more invasion of the
   base of tongue, or there is extension
   into the suprahyoid region.
2. Involvement of the pharyngeal mucosa is 180° or greater.
3. Invasion of the arytenoids or inter-
   arytenoid space is present.
4. Tumor is in the laryngeal ventricle,
   or below the surface of the false cord
   or anterior commissure.
5. There is extension to the inferior
   aspect of the pyriform sinus.
6. Cartilage invasion has occurred.

The limited supraglottic operation is best
suited for lesions of the laryngeal epiglottis,
since they are often confined to the supraglottic larynx and spare the vocal cords.

Similarly, the decision to attempt a
hemi-laryngectomy rather than a total
laryngectomy in unilateral vocal cord lesions
should be reconsidered if:[12, 14, 15]

1. Subglottic extension is greater than
   1 cm.
2. The false vocal cord is involved.
3. There is involvement of the anterior
   third of contralateral vocal cord.
4. The thyroid cartilage is invaded.

Preoperative pulmonary function must
always be evaluated carefully before laryngeal surgery is undertaken, and chest radiography is therefore required for correlative
purposes, as well as to rule out metastases.

Clinical Follow-up

Following primary treatment, adenocystic
carcinomas (cylindromas) of the salivary
glands are known to be capable of metastasizing quite late, especially to the lungs.
Follicular thyroid cancers may metastasize
to the lungs, bone, or brain. Tumors of the
oral cavity can recur within the mandible,
presumably through a previously unrecog-

nized extension along the mandibular nerve.
New (second) primaries in the upper or
lower respiratory and digestive tracts are
especially common, and recurrences at
points of surgical pharyngeal anastomoses
can also occur. However, it should be remembered that post-treatment dysphagia
could also reflect the occurrence of an entirely new lesion in the cervical esophagus.
Respiratory difficulties in the post-treatment
period may be caused by pneumothorax or
aspiration pneumonia, as well as by a new
primary in the lung. Differentiating between
post-treatment laryngeal edema, radiation
necrosis of the larynx or mandible, or tumor
recurrence can be extremely difficult.[16]

RADIOLOGIC CONSIDERATIONS

Tomography

Body section radiography, called *tomography* (from the Greek *tomo,* "to cut"), came
into being in the 1930s with the work of
Vallebona and Ziedes des Plantes.[17] It has
allowed major advances to be made in radiology of the head and neck region. As linear
tomography of good quality provides more
information than even the highest quality
stereoscopic conventional films, so does
polydirectional tomography greatly exceed
linear tomography, with a capability of
placing approximately a 1 mm thick section
of tissue in sharp focus. Lesions can be
revealed by polydirectional tomography
when there is little or no indication of their
presence on conventional roentgenograms
(Fig. 5–1). This modality is therefore indis-
pensible in studies of the head and neck
region, particularly the temporal bones.

Computerized tomography has revolutionized the radiology of the orbit and brain.
(See also Chapter 17.) Because of the low fat
density of the orbital contents, it is easy to
demonstrate the bulb of the eye and its lens,
as well as the optic nerve. Frequently, the
ocular musculature is also seen. Because
non-fatty tumors contrast sharply with the
fat of the orbit, they are readily demonstrated and localized. Intracranial extension
of orbital tumor, or intraorbital extension of
intracranial tumor, is often demonstrable by
computerized tomography (Fig. 5–2).

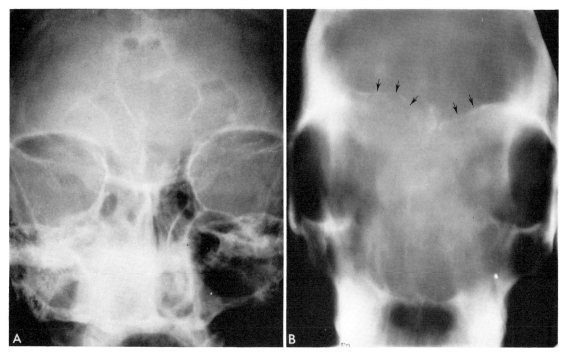

Figure 5–1 Extensive carcinoma of nasal accessory sinuses. *A,* Standard Caldwell (anterior) projection shows opacification of frontal, ethmoid, and maxillary sinuses, as well as the nasal fossa, on the reader's left. *B,* A single polytomographic "cut" in the same patient, showing extensive facial bone destruction by the soft-tissue mass, with invasion of the floor of the frontal cranial fossa (arrows). The extent of bone involvement could not have been inferred from the plain films without tomography.

Figure 5–2 Computerized tomography (EMI scan) in neurofibromatosis showing developmental defect in posterior wall of right orbit (small arrow), posterior orbital tumor (large arrow), and resulting exophthalmos. Globe is shown by X.

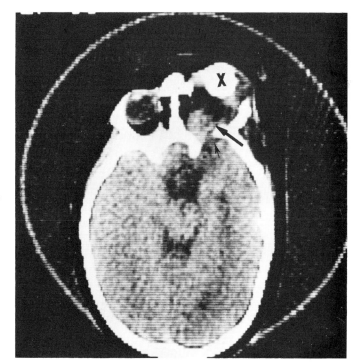

Radiation Exposure

The theoretical or actual hazard of x-rays in medical dosages has been heralded and often exaggerated in the lay press. This may be a source of undue concern not only to patients undergoing diagnostic studies, but also to those who have had or are about to have therapeutic irradiation. The potential hazard has tended to overshadow the dramatic contribution of radiation in the diagnosis and treatment of cancer of the ear, nose, and throat.

In head and neck cancer patients, the gonads are sufficiently remote from the area being examined to eliminate even a theoretical genetic concern. For the same reason, potential irradiation of a fetus is not a matter of concern in pregnant women. An exception is the use of femoral arterial catheterization for angiography of the head and neck. Here, fluoroscopy of the pelvis may produce significant amounts of local irradiation. Radiation is most dangerous to the fetus in the first 6 weeks of development when the embryo and its organ systems are being formed.[18-20] If pregnancy is a possibility and angiography is essential, some route other than the femoral can be employed for introducing a vascular catheter.

Fluoroscopy and cine radiography are the only quantitatively significant sources of somatic radiation in radiologic diagnosis. The increasing use of videotape recording of the fluoroscopic image has eliminated the added radiation of the conventional cinefluorogram. In a procedure such as laryngography, the patient could receive from 25 to 75 rads, but the exposure is localized to the larynx alone.

Naturally occurring "background" radiation is usually stated to be 0.1 rad per year (*whole body*). A chest radiograph is 0.01 rad, and a skull radiograph is 0.05 rad. In tomography, the dose to the patient is equivalent to the exposure from conventional radiographs.[21] To produce an erythema or epilation of the skin at diagnostic x-ray kilovoltages requires approximately 300 rads, which is equal to the dosage of 6,000 skull radiographs. Obviously, even the most complete tomographic and angiographic studies fall far below this. The rare radiation-related thyroid cancer would require at least 4 times the *maximum* dose received from radiologic examination of the head and neck.[22, 23] Similarly, the diagnostic dose is well below the leukemogenic dose range.

The lens of the eye has been reported as being at risk from extensive head and neck tomography. Merriam and Focht have studied radiation cataracts and their dose relationships; they found no cataracts in patients receiving less than 175 rads.[25-28] One cataract was found following 200 rads given in a single dose. With radiation therapy fractionated in the usual manner, the *minimum* dose required to produce an opacification of the lens was 400 rads. However, many patients receiving up to 6900 rads did not develop cataracts. Prior animal work has been misleading, since the rabbit lens is particularly sensitive to radiation and there is also legitimate debate as to how much lens opacity constitutes a "cataract."

In summary, patients should be reassured that with medical radiation everything is done to lower the dose to that level which is absolutely necessary for proper diagnosis and treatment, and exposure at this level does not carry significant genetic or somatic risk.

Skin and External Ear

In skin cancer, radiologic studies rarely show direct bony invasion that is not clinically evident. However, Dodd and associates have demonstrated invasion of the osseous cranial nerve canals from carcinomas of the lip, nose, face, and ear.[29] Cancer may traverse the infraorbital canal from a lesion of the lower eyelid, or may traverse the mental foramen or mandibular canal from a lesion of the lip or gingiva. Lesions may then extend intracranially to the gasserian ganglion. Similar extension may be demonstrated radiologically and clinically with the seventh nerve. Enlargement or destruction of the basal skull canals can be shown by plain film radiographs as well as by tomography. These neurovascular extensions are of the utmost import to therapy and prognosis.

Malignant tumors of the external auditory canal and middle ear usually arise in a chronically infected ear and most commonly are squamous cell carcinomas. However, adenocystic carcinomas, which apparently arise from metaplasia of the lining epithelium of the eustachian tube, will occasionally invade the ear or the temporal bone. These are difficult to diagnose clinically as well as radiographically. The bony canal of the external ear is rarely examined radiographically with the same thoroughness as the middle and inner ear, unless the radiologist is alerted by the clinician and does a special study with this area in mind. Rhabdomyosarcomas may arise in the external ear canal in children (usually less than 6 years of age) and are extremely malignant. Local recurrence is frequent, along with distant metastases, particularly to the lungs.[30] Polydirectional tomography in basal, anteroposterior, and lateral projections, with "slices" 1 mm apart, should depict the soft tissue mass and, most important, the bone destruction, which in turn will suggest the diagnosis.

Orbits

Roentgenographic study of the orbits is being revolutionized by computerized tomography (see previous discussion). Many tumors are readily perceived against the orbital fat, so that not only the presence or absence of tumor, but also very precise localization is possible. Orbital extension of tumor from the cranial cavity or from the nasal accessory sinuses is readily appreciated, as are even minute amounts of tumoral calcium (see below).

In general, radiologic study of the orbits has been underutilized despite the major contributions of Pfeiffer and Dandy.[31-33] Hanafee has shown the value of orbital venography and selective internal carotid arteriography, particularly with subtraction, in the depiction of orbital tumors.[34-36]

With tumors in the orbit, radiography (without contrast materials) and conventional tomography may show only an increased soft tissue density in the orbit (or slight enlargement of the orbit, in patients with long-standing, increased intraorbital pressure). Pressure erosion of the osseous margins is seen with lacrimal gland tumors; actual bone invasion may occur with carcinomas. The bone involvement may either be osteolytic *or* osteoblastic, with primary or metastatic lesions in the orbit.

Pressure changes may be observed radiographically, with contiguous erosion of the inferior orbital fissure (for example, with juvenile angiofibroma of the nasopharynx extending into the orbit), or there may be actual bone destruction as with the very extensive perineural invasion seen in tumors of the nasal accessory sinuses. In fact, contiguous bone invasion of the orbit from lesions of the nasal accessory sinuses, including mucoceles as well as carcinomas, is very common. A combination of intracranial and orbital extension was found in 80 per cent of the cases reported by Dandy.[33] The most pronounced hyperostic (new bone formation) changes are seen with meningiomas of the sphenoid wing. Osteo- and chondrosarcomas also occur in the orbit rarely. They may arise in patients with pre-existing Paget's disease or osteochondromas.

Careful study of the bony optic canal is highly informative and is best accomplished in the basal projection with conventional tomography, as demonstrated by Harwood-Nash with optic gliomas in children.[37] In addition, computerized tomography will beautifully display extension of a tumor through the canal, from the orbit into the cranial cavity or vice versa.

Soft tissue calcification within the orbit is of the utmost importance,[38] and in a child *may* be indicative of a retinoblastoma. Reese found that almost every retinoblastoma contains calcium, 75 per cent of these being dense enough to be demonstrated radiographically.[39] One third of the tumors were bilateral. The majority of calcified orbital tumors in adults are benign lesions such as meningiomas. In addition, radiologic calcification may be seen with atretic globes (following destruction of the eye, as with infection), and cataracts also may calcify.

Since the advent of computerized tomography, the need for contrast studies of the orbit has been altered. Angiography still will be required for the differential diagnosis of vascular lesions such as aneurysm, arteriovenous fistula (i.e., a carotid-cavernous fistula), and venous thromboses, but negative (air injection) and positive contrast orbitography has been superseded by computerized tomography. Orbital venography, which, before the development of computerized tomography, was considered by many to be the safest and most reliable contrast study, will probably continue to be used, but in a much more limited role.

Salivary Glands

Salivary gland tumors provide a special challenge to diagnostic radiology.[40] Is a tumor in the region of the salivary gland within the gland, or external to it? If within the gland, is it growing in an expansile or an invasive manner? Is a "salivary gland tumor" in reality (1) a hard, fixed lymph node, (2) a prolonged cervical transverse process, or (3) a styloid process? Are there lung metastases? If so, are they from an unknown primary with a *metastasis* to the salivary gland, or are they from a primary in the salivary gland? Is the salivary gland mass solid or cystic? The answers to these questions are often made more difficult because there may be lymph nodes within the gland that themselves may contain metastatic cancer or a primary lymphoma.

Sialography (injection of radiologic contrast material into the salivary gland duct, using topical anesthesia) has been of considerable value in determining whether a palpable tumor is actually within the salivary gland (Fig. 5–3). Its benign or malignant nature can also be assessed with some accuracy. *Benign* tumors will grow in an expansile manner, displacing the salivary ducts circumferentially. As visualized radiographically, all the ducts will fill normally and extend to the periphery of the gland. The filling defect of a benign tumor in the gland is sharply delimited (Fig. 5–3). A *malignant* tumor will grow in an irregular manner, producing an irregular filling defect within the gland. The ducts are absent or distorted, with irregular lumina and distribution, and contrast material may extravasate into the periductal tissues.

It is most advisable for the radiologist to examine the patient carefully himself, so that he can accurately delineate for the clinician the relationship between the palpable salivary gland tumor and the radiographic findings. Use of metal (i.e., radiopaque) skin markers about the periphery of the palpable tumor may also be helpful.

The technique of contrast sialography is relatively simple. However, at times ducts within the mouth cannot be cannulated because of an unusually small orifice or because there are multiple orifices. This technique is detailed elsewhere.[41, 42] The procedure is well tolerated by patients, and discomfort is relatively minor. Complications are infrequent and consist of local swelling and discomfort of short duration. Acute infection in the gland is a contraindication to a contrast study, as is allergy to the contrast.

In the differential diagnosis of enlargement of the salivary gland, a prime concern of the radiologist is to exclude calculus in a duct, with obstruction of the gland. The calculi are radiopaque, and in the sublingual area they are readily demonstrated by an intraoral film without contrast injection. For the parotid duct, a lateral projection with the mouth open and the tongue depressed by a tongue blade, and a posteroanterior soft-tissue film with the cheeks puffed out, similarly may show a calcification in the duct. Using contrast sialography, an enlarged, infected gland with diffuse sialectasis and no focal lesion is readily distinguished from a tumor. Inflammatory salivary gland changes frequently are bilateral. Occasionally, a deep parotid tumor may deform the air column as outlined by the pharyngeal soft tissues in the submentovertex (basal) skull radiograph.[43]

Ultrasound scanning clearly distinguishes between solid and cystic salivary gland tumors. Although experience is still limited, there is evidence to suggest a distinction in patterns between malignant and benign tumors.[44] Radionuclides such as technetium are secreted by the salivary glands, thereby providing an outline of the glands. However, the use of scintiscanning of the salivary glands has not become widespread, perhaps because of its limited spatial resolution.

Nose

Regrettably, these carcinomas tend to be less localized than simple clinical examination would indicate. Biopsy of the remaining tissue margins at the time of definitive surgery commonly shows residual tumor. The hard palate and anterior upper alveolar ridge can also be invaded by a tumor in the mucosa of the nasal vestibule. As a result of these factors, tumors within the nose initially are often treated inadequately.

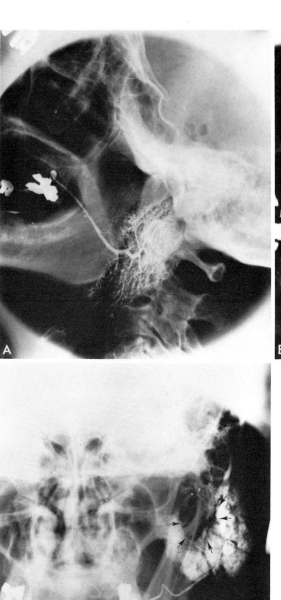

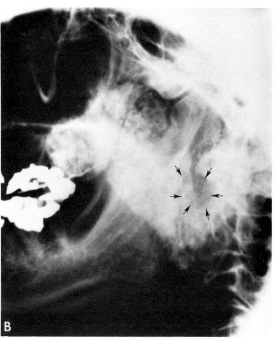

Figure 5–3   *A,* Lateral view from a normal parotid sialogram. Note the extensive, delicate arborizations. *B,* Abnormal study (lateral view). Mixed tumor within the parotid gland displaces the opacified ducts and lobules (arrows). *C,* Anterior view from sialogram (arrows depict tumor within gland); same patient as in *B.*

Diagnostic radiology may be particularly helpful in nasal tumors arising at a level above the middle turbinate, in order to rule out invasion of the antrum or of the frontal or ethmoid sinuses. Tumors at the apex of the nasal cavity may show evidence only of decreased aeration on conventional films, even with invasion of the adjacent sinuses. However, destruction of the bony margin between the nasal cavity and the cranial cavity may sometimes be demonstrated with polydirectional tomography.

Differential considerations in tumors occurring at the cranionasal junction are legion. For example, esthesioneuroblastomas are believed to arise in the olfactory mucous membrane and to extend both intracranially and into the nose and the nasal accessory sinuses simultaneously.[45, 46] Primary granular myoblastomas and melanomas have also been encountered in this area; they grow in an expansile, noninvasive manner and are enormously vascular. Meningiomas have been reported to arise within the nose,[47] but most of these have originated intracranially in the olfactory groove and the primary extension remains intracranial. However, these tumors can extend rarely into the sinuses, orbits, nasal cavity or nasopharynx. In these patients, carotid angiography is most helpful in delimiting preoperatively the intra- and extracranial extent of the tumor, as well as the details of its blood supply.

Meningoencephaloceles can extend through the foramen cecum and the cribriform plate into the nasal cavity and may simulate a tumor, particularly in infancy. However, they are usually associated with gross midline anomalies such as cleft palate and hypertelorism.[48]

Nasal Accessory Sinuses

Carcinoma of the nasal accessory sinuses may be very difficult to identify radiographically; in particular, plain film changes may be minimal. Destruction of the bony sinus margins is the key radiographic finding. Unfortunately, the presence of cancer is often not suspected and is diagnosed late. Paulus and Dodd quote Wille's series of 220 patients, 131 of whom were treated symptomatically for 2 to 6 months, and 47 for 6 to 26 months before the correct diagnosis was made and proper treatment instituted.[49, 50]

Radiologic masses within the nasal accessory sinuses usually are benign and represent a blocked mucous gland or a submucosal accumulation of fluid (the "gravitational cyst"). Much less frequently seen is a mucocele, which is caused by major blockage of the osteum of the sinus. The latter entity can be markedly expansile, occasionally with roentgenologic destruction of the bony sinus margins.

Inflammatory sinus disease can also mimic a malignant tumor.[51] However, more than one sinus is usually involved and the symptomatology facilitates the correct diagnosis. With a single sinus involved, as for example with an empyema, an acute loss of the bony sinus margin or osteosclerosis caused by osteomyelitis in the wall can be confused with a tumor radiographically; again, the clinical picture should point to the actual diagnosis. Allergic polypoid mucous membrane changes are usually diffuse, involving all the sinuses and the nasal cavity and producing a homogeneous "ground-glass" appearance on the plain films. Localized polyposis and papillomatosis may be more bewildering.[52] For example, the condition known as inverted papilloma produces a radiographic picture identical to that of carcinoma, but with a predominantly benign histologic appearance. However, some of these lesions actually do contain areas of carcinoma. Nasal and sinus granulomata, either specific as in leprosy or nonspecific as in Wegener's, and mucormycosis as seen with diabetes, can mimic the appearance of carcinoma radiographically. In addition to primary benign tumors such as osteomas, neurinomas and nasopharyngeal angiofibromas can extend into the sinuses.

Fastidious radiographic technique and an experienced radiologist are essential in examining the nasal sinuses. Polydirectional tomography has proved invaluable in demonstrating abnormal contents of nasal accessory sinuses and invasion of the bony margins, changes which may not be evident on ordinary linear tomography because of blurring from dense "companion shadows" (densities cast by out-of-focus structures). Bony invasion by one of these tumors usually is osteolytic, but it can also stimulate sclerotic changes. Therefore, one should not assume that a sclerotic or "blastic" radiographic reaction in a sinus margin is *necessarily* indicative of low-grade chronic inflammatory disease. In the presence of tumor accompanied by infection and blocked sinuses, it is difficult (or impossible) to distinguish the radiographic findings caused by the primary tumor from those of secondary infection.

With the addition of polydirectional tomography, the sinus margins and the potential routes of tumor spread are depicted.[29, 53] For example, enlargement or destruction of the infraorbital neural foramen anteriorly, or of the foramen ovale or rotundum or of the superior orbital fissure posteriorly, may be identified. Perineural tumor extension is common and in fact has been encountered at neurosurgical procedures for the control of local pain.[54]

Radiologically demonstrated invasion of the pterygoid plates or extension into the cranial cavity is usually accepted as a sign of inoperability. However, in sinus or nasal tumors extending to the region of the cribiform plate, Ketcham and associates have used a combined surgical approach, adding a frontal craniotomy through a separate incision to the transfacial approach.[55] Careful preoperative evaluation again is essential. Polydirectional tomography of the nasal sinuses is traditionally performed at 0.5 cm intervals in the anteroposterior projection. Tomographic "cuts" of 0.5 cm are also obtained in the lateral projection, and the submentovertex (basal) projection may be exceptionally informative with some lesions (particularly in evaluating the sphenoid sinus, optic canals, and pterygo-maxillary recess). Basal tomography yields a superb anatomic display of tumor extent; its major drawback is that the position is difficult for many of these patients to maintain.[56]

Catheter carotid angiography with selective internal and external carotid injections has not been useful in most patients, since these lesions are usually squamous cell carcinomas and are relatively avascular. However, in tumors of the sphenoid and the pituitary, where the transphenoidal surgical approach is increasingly being used, it is important to determine the exact position of the carotids preoperatively and whether or not they are invaded.[57] The demonstration of displacement of meningeal vessels, indicating intracranial (epidural) extension, would be highly useful information prior to treatment. Occasionally, a vascular tumor is encountered in this area, and charting the feeding vessels as well the tumor vasculature could also be useful. It is possible in certain cases, through selective catheterization, to inject thrombogenic material into a supplying blood vessel and infarct a tumor preoperatively, thus lessening the surgical blood loss.

Caution should be exercised in differentiating between actual tumor extension into a sinus cavity, and roentgenologic opacity due to a blocked sinus osteum. Mucoceles are a continuing source of surprise in the differential diagnosis of "masses" within the sinuses. Pressure erosion and expansion of the bony sinus margins with these lesions are not always easily distinguished from neoplasm.

Finally, a complete radiographic baseline study of the affected region is mandatory following the subsidence of surgical and radiation reactions, to assist in interpreting changes at a later date when tumor recurrence is suspected.

Nasopharynx

Tumors of the nasopharynx, while relatively infrequent, can be insidious and vicious. They are often diagnosed as late as one to two years after the onset of symptoms. Malignant tumors within the small nasopharyngeal space can spread readily into the sinuses, orbits, and base of the skull, penetrating through the neurovascular foramina into the cranial cavity and blocking the eustachian tube without reaching a large size.

Unexplained serous otitis media in an adult with a recent hearing loss is one of the earlier clinical manifestations. If the middle ear is not drained, infection may spread to the mastoid bone, and extension to the cranial cavity from this site may occur.[58] Tumor invasion of the bones of the skull base and its nerves may result in severe pain, diplopia, and facial numbness.[59] Epistaxis, nasal obstruction, or "nasal speech" may also occur, but all too often the first evidence of a nasopharyngeal tumor is spread to the regional lymphatics, as evidenced by a neck mass.

Careful radiologic examination can help to direct attention to the proper diagnosis.[60] The nasopharynx should be examined carefully on *all* radiographs of the skull, sinuses, or orbits. Conversely, all mastoid radiographs should also include lateral and basal views of the nasopharynx.

In children and adolescents, one expects normally to see excessive soft tissue ("adenoids") in the posterior portion of the nasopharynx. An actual tumor mass in the nasopharynx usually will be convex anteriorly, may extend inferiorly into the oropharynx, or superiorly (with sclerosis or destruction) into the skull base or into the sphenoid sinus. Squamous cell carcinomas in this area may occur even in childhood, as do rhabdomyosarcomas. *Nonmalignant lesions that may be detectable on the lateral study of the nasopharynx include congenital fibromyxolipomas and other polypoid lesions which may obstruct the airway. Herniation of the cerebral third ventricle into the nasopharynx (encephalocele) through the embryonic nasocranial duct is encountered infrequently, usually in patients with other midline anomalies such as cleft palate and hypertelorism.[61] The radiologist and clinician must always maintain a high index of suspicion, even if the typical nasopharyngeal "mass" turns out subsequently to be lymphoid hyperplasia or a Tornwaldt's cyst. The infrequency of significant nasopharyngeal lesions at any age should not encourage complacency or a fear of "crying wolf."

In addition to a mass, another sign of a nasopharyngeal tumor on the lateral view is displacement of the eustachian tube orifice,[62] and anterior displacement of the soft palate by the soft-tissue mass is often apparent as well (Fig. 5–4). The antrum, ethmoid, and sphenoid sinuses should also be carefully inspected for evidence of invasion. The base (submentovertex or axial) projection of the skull is invaluable in the radiologic delineation of this region. This radiographic view will help to demonstrate soft-tissue abnormalities of the nasopharynx, invasion of the skull base with osteolytic or sclerotic reaction, and impaired aeration of one or both mastoids.[63, 64]

Unfortunately, the correlation between radiologic and clinical findings in the nasopharynx may sometimes be poor. Radiologic changes are often subtle and easily overlooked. The area of clinical suspicion may initially direct the radiologist's attention away from the primary lesion as, for example, with a serous otitis media secondary to a nasopharyngeal cancer. On the other hand, the clinician's view of the nasopharynx,

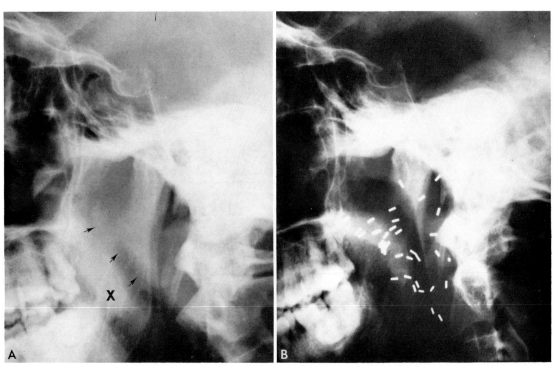

Figure 5–4   *A,* Lateral view shows large soft-tissue tumor in the roof of the nasopharynx (arrows) pushing the uvula (X) and soft palate anteriorly. *B,* Following radiation therapy, the tissues of the nasopharynx, soft palate, and airway are more normal in appearance. Opacities are interstitial radon seeds.

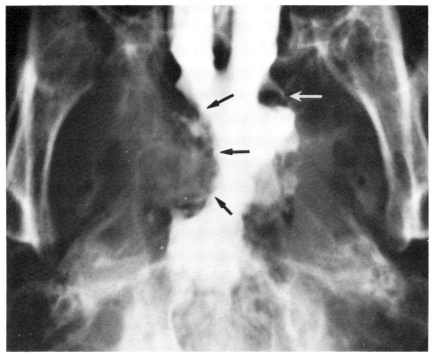

Figure 5–5 Nasopharyngogram (basal view) demonstrating a bulky nasopharyngeal tumor on the reader's left (black arrows), with obliteration of the eustachian tube. Normal tube is well-filled with contrast material on the opposite side (white arrow).

using a mirror or an endoscope, may be deceiving as to the depth of the nasopharynx, so that the actual extent of submucosal spread of a nasopharyngeal carcinoma, or of an extramucosal tumor such as a chordoma or myeloma, is not readily appreciated. The larger ulcerative or tumefactive lesions are readily defined, but infiltrative ones or those arising within the eustachian tube may not be visualized directly. As stated, if either the radiologist or the clinician suspects a tumor, together they should make a major effort to affirm or to deny its presence; the consequences of a missed or late diagnosis may be grievous.

Among the special radiologic investigations, *polydirectional tomography* in various projections has been extremely rewarding. This will demonstrate invasion of the sinuses, orbits, and foramina in the base of the skull (Fig. 5–1), as well as lytic and sclerotic bone changes in the skull base and pterygoid fossa. Tomography also gives a better appraisal of temporal bone involvement with the attendant risks of infection, meningitis, or venous sinus thrombosis.

In addition to anteroposterior and basal projections, lateral tomograms are of prime importance in showing not only the soft-tissue mass of the primary tumor, but also invasion of the clivus and of the ethmoid and sphenoid sinuses. These special examinations are long and tedious for the patient and require very exacting study by the radiologist for changes which are often very minimal. However, the knowledge gained is essential to rational treatment planning.[65]

Nasopharyngography using positive contrast material details the soft-tissue anatomy of the nasopharynx and the eustachian tubes and is quite useful in detecting early lesions and in determining the extent of known tumors (Fig. 5–5).[62] The examination is simple and well tolerated. With the patient supine and the head extended, 10 to 20 cc of a contrast substance such as colloidal barium or Dionosil is instilled into the nostrils. Lateral and submentovertex (basal) radiographic views are obtained. Fluoroscopy is then performed and "spot" films are taken in several projections, using various maneuvers.

Carotid angiography is also useful, on

occasion. It is employed primarily whenever an angiofibroma (see below) or a meningioma, which may extend into this region and exactly simulate a carcinoma of the nasopharynx, is suspected. A carotid aneurysm may also penetrate into the sphenoid sinus and then into the nasopharynx, simulating a malignant tumor (Fig. 5–6).

Pneumoencephalography may occasionally be necessary, if it is suspected that an encephalocele extends into the roof of the nasopharynx. In such cases, the air-filled third ventricle can be identified in the nasopharynx with the use of this special study.[48]

Neurinomas can produce a soft-tissue mass in the nasopharynx and neurologic impairment simulating a carcinoma.[69] However, among benign lesions of the nasopharynx, the most distinctive is the juvenile angiofibroma. This is usually a tumor of teenage males, but it has been seen in females and we have seen one patient with symptoms beginning in the fourth decade. Plain films and tomography demonstrate

an expansile mass in the pterygomaxillary fossa that pushes the posterior wall of the maxillary sinus anteriorly and the pterygoid plate posteriorly.[66] These tumors also frequently expand into the superior and inferior orbital fissures and erode into the basisphenoid bone and the sphenoid sinus. The usual symptoms are nasal obstruction and epistaxis, and there may be considerable deformity of the face. As mentioned, when this condition is suspected carotid angiography is highly desirable.[67, 68] The demonstration of an extremely vascular tumor in this area would dictate that any biopsy be performed under carefully controlled conditions, in the hospital. Some groups feel that the clinico-radiologic findings are so characteristic that biopsy is *not* essential. A case has been reported of 2,000 cc of blood loss within a very short period after biopsy. Angiographic identification of the exact feeding vessel, which can sometimes be tied off or embolized preoperatively, can be a decided advantage in reducing blood

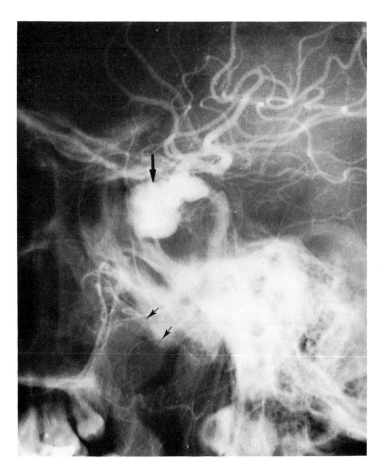

Figure 5–6 Lateral film from carotid arteriogram shows post-traumatic carotid aneurysm eroding into the sphenoid sinus and the nasopharynx, causing a soft-tissue mass in the nasopharynx (small arrows). Large arrow points to the remaining lumen of the aneurysm; most of this large aneurysm is filled with clot and therefore does not opacify.

loss at surgery. In many of these patients who have undergone operations previously, with incomplete tumor removal or a recurrence, it is well to study the vertebral as well as the carotid circulations so that all potential feeder vessels are mapped out.

Laryngopharynx

Radiologic examinations in this area may depict tumor extent with considerable precision.[62, 70-72] However, it is important to note that *edema* following an endoscopic biopsy procedure can cause changes identical to those of tumor, for periods of up to two weeks following biopsy. Subglottic tumor extension may be difficult or impossible to appreciate clinically; if shown to be present by radiologic means, subglottic extension is an unfavorable prognostic factor (Fig. 5–7). Involvement of the anterior commissure of the vocal cords or penetration of the thyroid cartilage may indicate that a surgical procedure is preferable to radiation therapy. Fluoroscopic study of the *movement* of the larynx, best recorded on videotape or by cinefluoroscopy,[73] is valuable both pre- and postoperatively. The rapid laryngeal movements can then be viewed repeatedly and in slow motion, without additional irradiation or discomfort to the patient. For example, vocal cord movement (or the lack of it) is important in staging a laryngeal tumor, and a failure of approximation of the hyoid bone and thyroid cartilage during Valsalva's maneuver may indicate tumor invasion or a neurologic deficit.[74] A serious impairment of normal laryngeal movement indicates the need for a surgical procedure as the primary therapy.[75]

Conventional lateral radiographs of the neck to show the airway, cartilage, and soft tissue may be invaluable.[72] Newer techniques derived from mammography have also been helpful, including low-dose single emulsion film-screen combinations and *xeroradiography*. The display of soft tissue planes on these studies is superb (see also Chapters 13 and 14). The use of very high kilovoltage technique* blurs out the bones and does for the anterior view of the neck

what xeroradiography has done for the lateral view (Fig. 5–7).

Tomography of the larynx in the anteroposterior projection will also blur out interfering shadows from the cervical spine. One series of "cuts" is obtained with the patient phonating "E" during expiration, and another series is performed during quiet respiration. Minimal changes in the mucosal surfaces of the endolarynx are not optimally shown, but gross structures are well demonstrated.

Barium studies of the oral cavity, pharynx, and proximal esophagus can be of great value for elucidating lesions in this area.[76-80] The base of tongue, valleculae, pyriform sinuses, and proximal esophagus are well shown; this should be combined with the "bugler" technique (expiration against pinched nose and pursed lips) in frontal, lateral, and oblique projections to distend the pyriform sinuses maximally. In addition to "spot films," cine studies or videotaping provide a good permanent record. In particular, when positive contrast *laryngography* (see below) is not possible, the combination of tomography and barium studies is useful.

One problem in the diagnosis of lesions in the proximal esophagus is the presence of an inconstant venous plexus occurring anteriorly in the postcricoid region over an area 2 cm in length. This may produce a rather bulky, slightly irregular defect, with the region otherwise appearing normal.[81] The patient experiencing an acute episode of dysphagia caused by the presence of a foreign body (such as a piece of food lodged at the cricoid level) should undergo a barium contrast examination after the foreign body is removed to be certain that a partially obstructing neoplasm was not the precipitating cause. On occasion, a thyroid carcinoma can extend into the space between the trachea and esophagus and simulate a primary tumor of the esophagus or a laryngeal neoplasm.

Contrast laryngography has been the special radiologic study of greatest diagnostic value.[82] Premedication with atropine is required; thus glaucoma and asthma are contraindications. Severe respiratory insufficiency is also a major contraindication, since the patient necessarily aspirates a considerable amount of the contrast substance (oily Dionosil), which is a local irritant capable of lowering pulmonary ventilation

---

*The author has employed the 350 kilovolt Hewlett-Packard Chest Unit with 0.25 cm copper filtration.

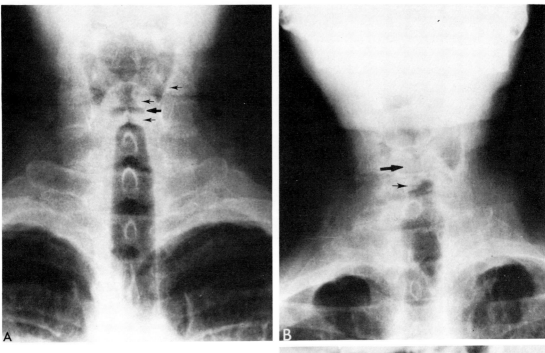

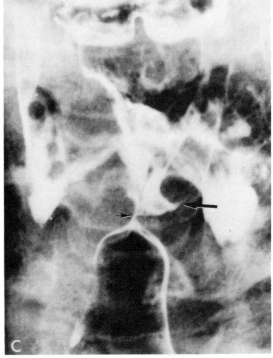

Figure 5–7 *A,* Normal larynx during phonation, showing true vocal cords (lowest small arrow), laryngeal ventricles (large arrow), false cords (middle small arrow), and pyriform sinuses (upper small arrow). Obscuring bone shadows are minimized with the use of special 350 kilovolt technique (Hewlett Packard 350 KV Field Emission Chest Unit, with 0.25 mm Cu filter). *B,* Large laryngeal tumor (large arrow) in another case, showing subglottic extension into trachea on reader's left (small arrow). *C,* Positive contrast laryngogram on same patient showing thickening of the right cord (on reader's left) with obliteration of the laryngeal ventricle (small arrow), as result of the carcinoma. Normal left ventricle of patient is shown by large arrow.

and perfusion. Local anesthesia is employed, either topically or by local nerve blocks (or by a combination of both), so hypersensitivity to these substances or to iodine-containing contrast materials is another contra-

indication. Laryngography should not be performed soon after multiple biopsies, because of the edema and hypercontractility of the affected region.

Laryngography is a stressful examination to the patient as well to the examiner. It has been dubbed by some radiologic technicians as the "larynGAGogram" and should not be regarded as trivial. When properly performed, the study is not hazardous but it is uncomfortable. Some examiners sedate the patient, but this is usually not necessary and adds another source of potential complications. Once the patient is locally anesthetized and relaxed, a substance such as oily Dionosil or a special colloidal barium (a substance that has not yet been approved by the Food and Drug Administration in this country) is introduced under fluoroscopic control to coat the posterior and lateral walls of the pharynx and the valleculae, epiglottis, larynx, and proximal trachea. Cine, videotape, or spot film studies are then obtained under fluoroscopy in multiple projections, with and without Valsalva's maneuver or phonation. It is wise to fluoroscope carefully during the laryngogram to spot suspicious areas of immobility or inflexibility, as well as to maintain proper coating with the contrast material.

Tumors may be purely tumefactive, ulcerative, or infiltrative, or they may present a combination of these patterns (Fig. 5–8). The plain films and the contrast studies should be carefully studied together to reveal cartilaginous invasion, involvement of the anterior commissure of the vocal cords, or subglottic extension, each of which profoundly affects the choice of therapy and the expected morbidity and mortality rates.

Since an appreciable amount of aspirated contrast material ends up in the lung bases, it is important at the end of the examination to have the patient attempt to empty as much as possible of the material out of the lungs, using postural drainage with the head of the table slightly down. He should also be cautioned about eating or drinking for an hour or two, while the local anesthetic is still effective.

Skull Base

In addition to the tumors previously discussed, such as esthesioneuroblastoma and meningioma, other primary tumors may originate in the skull base (see also Chapter 15). Adenocarcinoma of the pituitary rarely is seen and represents malignant degeneration of a pre-existing adenoma. This condition is associated particularly with Nelson's syndrome,[83] in which pituitary neoplasms (often malignant) are noted following bilateral adrenalectomy for Cushing's syndrome.

Chordomas are locally malignant tumors arising in the midline of the clivus or in the vertebrae from notochordal rests.[84] They are highly malignant locally, but only rarely cause distant metastases. There is marked bone destruction and local extension into the cranial cavity or spinal canal, with resultant neurologic deficits. In the skull base, these tumors are thought to arise from the spheno-occipital synchondrosis. Often, calcific debris or neoplastic calcification is seen in and about the lesion. Heffelfinger and associates have studied 55 patients with chordomas of the skull clivus. Twenty-two had chondroid elements that were classified as chondroid chordomas. The average age of the patients was 38, 10 years younger than chordomas elsewhere in the neuraxis; more females than males were affected, unlike the rates for other chordomas.[85]

There has been considerable confusion about the differential diagnosis of chordoma and chondrosarcoma in the skull base.[86] Chondrosarcomas more characteristically arise lateral to the midline, and roentgenologic calcification is extremely common. Some have erroneously been classified as chordomas. Chondrosarcomas are also highly destructive and are locally malignant.

An osteogenic sarcoma may arise *de novo* in the skull, facial bones, or cervical spine, or it may be secondary to Paget's disease. Postirradiation osteogenic sarcomas also occur, as with individuals who have been treated at an early age for a retinoblastoma.

Chemodectomas (Non-chromaffin Paragangliomas)

These highly vascular tumors, which are infrequent but not rare, require angiography for a complete assessment of their size and extent, their blood supply, and their relationship to major vessels. This is particularly true of the *carotid body* and *intravagus glomus tumors*.[87] Biopsy of these le-

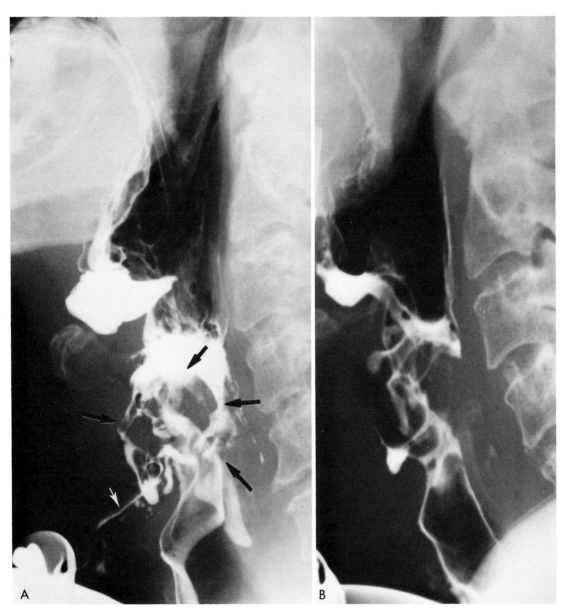

Figure 5–8 *A,* Lateral view from positive contrast study (laryngogram) showing huge tumefactive and ulcerative carcinoma of the larynx distorting the regional anatomy (black arrows). Note the anterior soft-tissue fistula (white arrow).

B, Improvement following radiation therapy.

sions may be accompanied by severe hemorrhage. Symptoms include hearing loss, pulsating tinnitus, and cranial nerve involvement (particularly IX, X, and XI); occasionally, a vascular mass is seen through the eardrum.[88-92, 96]

It seems reasonable that any neck tumor noted clinically to be fixed to the carotid artery should be studied angiographically before an attempted biopsy. The relationship of the tumor to the carotid and the presence of tumor vascularity are useful information, and an aneurysm must be excluded. The collateral blood supply to the brain can also be assessed before an attempt at surgical removal is made, with the attendant threat of a severe postoperative neurologic deficit (see earlier clinical discussion). The extension of *glomus jugulare* tumors into the jugular vein can also be well demonstrated angiographically, as well as alternate routes of venous drainage from the brain if the jugular vein must be resected at surgery (see below).

Glomus tumors within the temporal bone include the *glomus tympanicum,* which is confined to the tympanic cavity. Tomography of the temporal bone is indicated. I have collected (not personally viewed) 24 patients with an unusual anomaly: the internal carotid artery passed through the middle ear and presented as a red, pulsatile mass simulating a glomus tympanicum tumor.[93] In these cases, attempts at surgical removal led to severe hemorrhage and to temporary or permanent neurologic deficits. This anomaly is readily recognized by tomography and may be confirmed by angiography. Other confusing anomalies in the temporal bone are absence of the bony plate over the jugular bulb or over the intra-osseous portion of the carotid, the latter giving an anterior pulsatile mass.[87] I have seen one instance in which a glomus tympanicum tumor was accompanied by dehiscence of the jugular plate, an anomaly recognized subsequently on tomography. In this patient, the tympanic membrane was incised inferiorly into the jugular bulb, resulting in severe hemorrhage unrelated to the tumor. Obviously, in patients with suspected vascular tumors, careful preoperative evaluation of this area and special radiologic studies as indicated are a necessity.

Glomus jugulare tumors arise in the wall of the jugular bulb at the base of the skull and may extend into the temporal bone. In one of our patients, the tumor extended within the jugular vein as far as the angle of the mandible. The capability for extension of this type of tumor was not recognized until relatively recently; therefore, inapparent tumor extension often was not included in the radiation treatment fields, perhaps accounting for inadequate results with radiation therapy in some centers when it has been used as a palliative measure for these tumors. Within the cranium, glomus jugulare tumors also may invade the middle ear cavity, the petrous bone apex, the posterior cranial fossa, and the condyles of the foramen magnum.

Conventional radiography, particularly the exaggerated Waters projection with the mouth open, portrays the jugular fossa to good advantage. Tomography may be extremely useful in delineating the extent of glomus jugulare tumors. If it can be obtained, tomography in the submentovertex (basal) projection is most informative, but anteroposterior and lateral tomographic projections are also helpful. Carotid angiography may serve to demonstrate tumor vessels and a filling defect in the jugular bulb (if the jugular vein is still patent). If the jugular is not patent at the base of the skull, retrograde injection of contrast material through a catheter in the jugular vein will show the lesion. Posterior fossa myeloencephalography (by introduction of contrast material through a lumbar puncture) has shown that intracranial extension of these tumors is quite common.

Chemodectomas in all locations tend to be familial and are more common in females. They are bilateral in 6 to 10 per cent of patients. Within the temporal bone, they are notoriously more extensive than first surmised and are therefore much more prone to recur than at other sites. It is again emphasized that biopsies may result in severe hemorrhage and should not be performed except under carefully controlled (hospital) conditions. These lesions are slowly growing and usually are not immediately life-threatening. Surgical removal is the treatment of choice, whenever possible; however, radiation therapy has been effective in palliating some chemodectomas.[94, 95] Because of the delayed effects of radiation, one must wait 6 to 12 months before making a final decision about the efficacy of treatment. Excellent *symptomatic* relief may be obtained with irradiation in some patients, even before "objective" changes in the tumor can be appreciated, and this may last for years.

Metastases in the Head and Neck

Skull and cervical spine metastases frequently come to the attention of the diagnostic radiologist. Myeloma bone lesions tend to be diffuse and to involve the mandible, whereas skull metastases from breast carcinomas are infrequently associated with mandibular lesions; when present, the latter may consist of one or two isolated defects in the mandible. Other common sources of metastases to the head and neck region are the genitourinary tract and lung. Melanoma is commonly metastatic to the brain but infrequently to bone; metastases may occur within the nasal accessory sinuses and orbits, as well as in the parotid gland and cervical lymph glands.

In the differential diagnosis of suspected metastases in the skull, one must also consider inflammatory lesions, such as syphilitic gummata, which are now infrequent and tend to present a mixed osteolytic and osteoblastic appearance on roentgenograms. Tuberculosis may occur in the nasopharynx and be indistinguishable from carcinoma; in the skull, tuberculous lesions are usually osteolytic. Histiocytosis, particularly those forms known as eosinophilic granuloma and Hand-Schüller-Christian disease, can also cause lytic defects in the skull and other bones that are indistinguishable from metastases.[96-100] It is therefore important for the radiologist, in consultation with the clinician, at least to consider inflammatory disease in the differential diagnosis; otherwise, special cultures may be omitted at an initial biopsy or operative procedure.

In the differential diagnosis of a lateral neck mass, radiologic studies may be of exceptional value.[101, 102] Ultrasound will distinguish quite accurately between a cystic mass and a solid tumor. A cystic mass is probably a branchial cleft cyst and there may be no need for an extensive cancer survey. In other patients, plain radiographs of the neck may demonstrate that a "hard fixed node" in the superior lateral neck is actually a prolonged second cervical trans-

verse process or a prominent styloid process.

Given a new clinical finding of a solid tumor in the upper or mid-neck, which is consistent with a metastatic node, careful roentgenographic study of the nasal accessory sinuses, nasopharynx, and chest are in order.[103] If negative, tomography of the sinuses and nasopharynx and contrast studies of the nasopharynx and pharynx might be considered. The pyriform sinuses are also a common site for an asymptomatic primary tumor. Metastatic nodes presenting in the left supraclavicular area and lower third of the neck ("Virchow nodes") require careful investigation of the chest and abdomen for an occult primary.

As discussed earlier, angiography is of particular value when neck tumors are fixed to the carotid, in order to determine the presence of vessel invasion, an aneurysm (Fig. 5–9) or chemodectoma, as well as to determine the collateral supply to the brain and the potential for neurologic damage if the carotid must be sacrificed. While conventional radiographs of a hemangioma may show phleboliths or finer calcifications in the soft tissues, angiography is often disappointing in assisting in the differential diagnosis of this entity. However, arteriovenous malformations may be readily shown, and direct embolization through a radiologic catheter of arteries feeding a hemangioma or arteriovenous anomaly, to initiate a thrombotic process and to reduce their bulk, has been useful in selected patients.

Thyroid and Parathyroid Tumors

Malignant thyroid tumors include the relatively benign papillary and follicular types, diffuse anaplastic thyroid carcinoma, and medullary thyroid carcinoma (MTC).[104] MTC is characterized by an intermediate grade of malignancy between the favorable papillary and follicular types, and the highly malignant anaplastic carcinoma of the thyroid; it is associated with a high incidence of early regional lymph node metastases. A familial variety of MTC has been described, and multiglandular tumors involving the thyroid, parathyroid, or adrenals (pheochromocytoma) may occur in the patient with MTC or may be present in

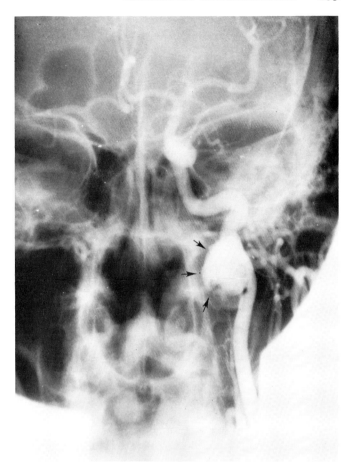

Figure 5–9 Deep upper cervical neck "mass" was shown to be an aneurysm (post-traumatic) by carotid angiography (arrows). Anterior view is shown.

family members (or have been present in ancestors). Thyrocalcitonin is secreted by medullary thyroid carcinomas, and high levels may be found in the primary tumor itself as well as in metastatic deposits. This hormone, which suppresses the resorption of bone and the release of calcium, is antagonistic to parathormone.

Thyroid tumors, when benign, may displace the trachea laterally and compress it. When the trachea is displaced anteriorly on lateral neck roentgenograms by a posterior extension of a thyroid mass, it is almost always malignant. I have seen one exceptional case in which a colloid cyst of the thyroid ruptured and set up a violent reaction in the retrotracheal soft tissues, thus simulating tumor extension.

In addition to the mass and possible tracheal deformity, roentgenologic calcification may occur in thyroid tumors.[105] Dense circumferential calcification denotes a thyroid adenoma. However, innumerable very small psammomatous calcifications may be

evident in some malignant carcinomas of the thyroid, and they may require special roentgenologic techniques (similar to those used in mammography) and oblique projections to demonstrate. It must be remembered also that thyroid tissue may occur in atypical locations. For example, the thyroid isthmus may extend high in the neck. Hill and associates have depicted a calcified thyroid cancer within a lingual thyroid, occupying most of the tongue.[106] Thyroglossal duct cysts may also encroach upon the vallecula.

In the study of the thyroid and its function, radionuclide examinations are of critical importance. In addition to depicting thyroid gland anatomy and uptake, distant metastases may be identifiable if function is present (i.e., in the more well-differentiated malignancies). The lingual thyroid is also best depicted in this manner. Ultrasound (echography), with the advent of the newer gray-scale techniques, has been a very useful adjunct to radionuclide studies, particularly in elucidating the "cold" thyroid nodule.[107-109] Echography will distinguish clearly between solid and cystic masses. Cystic masses in the thyroid may occasionally be malignant but they are usually benign, and the depiction of gross pathology within the gland by ultrasound is surprisingly good.

Thermography can occasionally be of assistance in diagnosing thyroid or parathyroid lesions, if performed after cooling the skin of the neck by applying alcohol. Malignant tumors may register as isolated "hot" areas because of their increased metabolic activity, but this method is not specific and its diagnostic sensitivity is not yet known.

Parathyroid tumors may present as very difficult clinical problems.[110] Patients with this entity may have passed repeated ureteral calculi, and have normal blood calcium and phosphorus levels and normal skeletal radiographs, but nevertheless will prove to have an elevated parathormone level indicating hyperparathyroidism. Hyperparathyroidism may present as a "brown tumor" of any bone or of a nasal accessory sinus, mimicking other primary tumors or metabolic disorders. In the *typical* case of hyperparathyroidism presenting with bone demineralization, subperiosteal resorption of bone, renal calculi, and cysts or "brown tumors" of bone, however, the radiologist is on more familiar ground.

Special diagnostic radiologic studies may be helpful in two ways: (1) selective arterial catheterization (arteriography) may lead to the demonstration of a vascular stain from a parathyroid tumor in the neck or mediastinum;[111] (2) selective venous sampling for parathormone can compare the venous drainage of the parathyroids bilaterally. The latter method apparently is satisfactory for lateralizing a tumor, but not for achieving exact localization. On occasion, angiography may also be helpful in demonstrating the effects of large *thyroid* tumors on the major vessels of the neck preoperatively.[57]

References

1. Knudson, R. J., Hatch, H. B., Ochsner, A., et al.: Multiple carcinomas of the lung and upper respiratory tract. Chest, *48*:140, 1965.

2. Stefani, S. and Eells, R. W.: Carcinoma of the hypopharynx: A study of distant metastases, treatment failures and multiple primary cancers in 215 male patients. Laryngoscope, *81*:1491, 1971.

3. MacComb, W. S., and Fletcher, G. H.: Cancer of the Head and Neck. Baltimore, Williams & Wilkins, 1967.

4. Lederman, M.: The classification and staging of cancer of the larynx. Br. J. Radiol., *25*:462, 1952.

5. Lederman, M.: Radiotherapy of cancer of the larynx. J. Laryngol. Otol., *84*:867, 1970.

6. Lalanne, C. M., Cachin, Y., Juillard, G., et al.: Telecobalt therapy for carcinoma of laryngopharynx. Am. J. Roentgenol. Radium Ther. Nucl. Med., *111*:78, 1971.

7. Weichert, R. F.: The neural ectodermal origin of the peptide secreting endocrine glands: A unifying concept for the etiology and multiple endocrine adenomatosis and the inappropriate secretion of peptide hormones by nonendocrine tumors. Am. J. Med., *49*:232–241, 1970.

8. Samaan, N. A., Hickey, R. C., Hill, C. S., et al.: Parathyroid tumors: Preoperative localization and association with other tumors. Cancer, *33*:933–939, 1974.

9. Norris, C. M.: Causes of failure in surgical treatment of malignant tumors of the larynx. Ann. Otol. Rhinol. Laryngol., *68*:487, 1959.

10. Som, M. L.: Conservation surgery for carcinoma of the supraglottis. J. Laryngol. Otol., *84*:655, 1970.

11. Delahunty, J. E., and Nassar, V. H.: Application of total organ laryngeal section. Arch. Otolaryngol. *90*:342, 1969.

12. Kirchner, J. A.: One hundred laryngeal cancers studied by serial section. Ann. Otol., Rhinol. Laryngol., *78*:689, 1969.

13. Kirchner, J. A., and Som, M. L.: Clinical and histological observations on supraglottic cancer. Ann. Otol. Rhinol. Laryngol., *80*:638, 1971.

14. Harrison, D. F. N.: The pathology and management of subglottic cancer. Ann. Otol. Rhinol. Laryngol., *80*:6, 1971.

15. Kirchner, J. A., and Som, M. L.: Clinical significance of fixed vocal cord. Laryngoscope, *81*:1029, 1971.

16. Kagan, A. R., Calcaterra, T., Ward, P., et al.: Significance of edema of the endolarynx following curative irradiation for carcinoma. Am. J. Roentgenol. Radium Ther. Nucl. Med., *20*:169, 1974.

17. Westra, D.: History of tomography. *In* Berrett, A., Brunner, S., and Valvassori, G. (eds), Modern Thin Section Tomography. Springfield, Ill., Charles C Thomas, 1973, pp. 3–17.

18. Rugh, R.: Radiology and the human embryo and fetus. *In* Dalrymple, G. V., Gaulden, M. E., Kollmorgen, G. M., et al., Medical Radiation Biology. Philadelphia, W. B. Saunders, 1973. pp. 83–96.

19. Oppenheim, B. E., Griem, M. L., and Meier, P.: Effects of low-dose prenatal irradiation in humans: Analysis of Chicago lying-in data and comparison with other studies. Radiat. Res., *57*:508–44, 1974.

20. Gaulden, M. E.: Possible effects of diagnostic x-rays on the human embryo and fetus. J. Arkansas Med. Soc., 70:424–35, 1974.

21. Swingle, L. P., and Kelsey, P. A.: Radiation Dose in Body Section Roentgenography. In Berrett, A., Brunner, S., and Valvassori, G. (eds.), Modern Thin Section Tomography. Springfield, Ill., Charles C Thomas, 1973, pp. 312–315.

22. Simpson, P. L., and Hempelmann, L. H.: Association of tumors and roentgen-ray treatment of thorax in infancy. Cancer, 10:42–56, 1957.

23. Latourette, H. B., and Hodges, F. J.: Incidence of neoplasia after irradiation of thymic region. Am. J. Roentgenol. Radium Ther. Nucl. Med., 82:667–671, 1959.

24. Chin, F. K., Anderson, U. B., and Gilbertson, J. B.: Radiation dose to critical organs during petrous tomography. Radiology, 94:623–627, 1970.

25. Teske, H. J., Schmitt, G., and Ewen, K.: Measurements on the radiation exposure of the eye in skull radiology. Radiology, 12:420–424, 1972.

26. Quisling, R. G., Seeger, J. F., Gabrielson, T. O., et al.: Radiation dose to eye lens and gonads during transfemoral cerebral angiography. Radiology, 112:715–717, 1974.

27. Van Elegem, P., Kleiner, S., and Hotton, F.: L'irradiation du patient Lors De Latomographie Du Rocher. Ann. Radiol. (Paris), 17:33–35, 1974.

28. Merriam, G. R., and Focht, E. F.: Radiation cataracts and relation to dose. Am. J. Roentgenol. Radium Ther. Nucl. Med., 77:759–785, 1957.

29. Dodd, G. D., Dolan, P. A., Ballantyne, A. J., et al.: The dissemination of tumors of the head and neck by cranial nerves. Radiol. Clin. North Am., 8:445–461, 1970.

30. Linthicum, F. H., and Schwartzman, J. A.: An Atlas of Micropathology of the Temporal Bone. Philadelphia, W. B. Saunders, 1974.

31. Pfeiffer, R. L.: Roentgenography of exopthalmos, with notes on the roentgen ray in opthalmology. Am. J. Ophthalmol., 26:724–741, 816–833, 901–911, 1943.

32. Pfeiffer, R. L.: A new technique for roentgenography of the optic canals. Am. J. Roentgenol. Radium Ther. Nucl. Med., 29:410–415, 1933.

33. Dandy, W. E.: Orbital Tumors. New York, Oskar Piest, 1941.

34. Hanafee, W. N., and Dayton, G. O.: The roentgen diagnosis of orbital tumors. Radiol. Clin. North Am., 12:403–412, 1970.

35. Hanafee, W. N., Shiu, P., and Dayton, G. O.: Orbital venography. Am. J. Roentgenol. Radium Ther. Nucl. Med., 104:1828, 1968.

36. Hanafee, W. N., and Shinno, J.: Second order subtraction with simultaneous bilateral carotid injections. Radiology, 86:334–342, 1966.

37. Harwood–Nash, D. C.: Axial tomography of the optic canals in children. Radiology, 96:367–374, 1970.

38. Zismor, J., and Raskind, R. H.: Orbital calcifications. In Newton, T. H., and Potts, D. G. (eds.), Radiology of the Skull and Brain, Vol. 2. St. Louis, C. V. Mosby, 1971, pp. 525–540.

39. Reese, A. B.: Tumors of the Eye. New York, Harper & Row (Hoeber), 1951.

40. Blady, J. V., and Hocker, A. F.: Sialography: Its technique and application in the roentgen study of neoplasm of the parotid gland. Surg. Gynecol. Obstet., 67:777–787, 1938.

41. Potter, G. D.: Sialography and the salivary glands. Otolaryngol. Clin North Am., 6:509–522, 1973.

42. Meine F. J., and Woloshin, H. J.: Radiologic diagnosis of salivary gland tumors. Radiol. Clin. North Am., 8:475–485, 1970.

43. Becker, W. (ed.): Atlas of Otorhinolaryngology and Bronchoesophagology. Philadelphia, W. B. Saunders, 1969.

44. Sample, F.: Personal communication.

45. Singer, L.: Ear, nose, and throat. In Minckler, J. (ed.), Pathology of the Nervous System, vol. 1. New York, McGraw-Hill, 1968, pp. 679–696.

46. Obert, G. J., Devine, K. D., and McDonald, J. R.: Olfactory neuroblastoma. Cancer, 13:205–215, 1960.

47. Kjeldsberg, C. R., and Minckler, J.: Meningiomas presenting as nasal polyps. Cancer, 29:153–156, 1972.

48. Pollack, J. A., Newton, T. H., and Hoyt, W. F.: Transphenoidal and transethmoidal encephaloceles: A review of clinical and roentgen features in 8 cases. Radiology, 90:442–453, 1968.

49. Paulus, D. D., Jr., and Dodd, G. D.: The roentgen diagnosis of tumors of the nasal cavity and accessory paranasal sinuses. Radiol. Clin. North Am., 8:343–360, 1970.

50. Wille, C.: Malignant tumors in the nose and its accessory sinuses. Otolaryngology, (Suppl.), 1947.

51. Zizmor, J., Noyek, A. M.: Inflammatory diseases of the paranasal sinuses. Otolaryngol. Clin. North Am., 6:459–472, 1973.

52. Becker, W. (ed.): Atlas of Otorhinolaryngology and Bronchoesophagology. Philadelphia, W. B. Saunders, 1969.

53. Dodd, G. D., Collins, L. C., Eagen, R. L., et al.: Systematic use of tomography in the diagnosis of carcinoma of the paranasal sinuses. Radiology, 72:379–393, 1959.

54. Leavens, M. E., and Barrash, J. M.: Sensory rhizotomy (cranial and spinal) and gasserian ganglionectomy in pain of the head and neck resulting from cancer. In Anderson Hospital & Tumor Institute, Neoplasia of the Head and Neck. Chicago, Year Book Medical Publishers, 1974, 261–279.

55. Ketcham, A. S., Chietien, P. B., Schour, L., et al.: Surgical treatment of patients with advanced cancer of the paranasal sinuses. In Anderson Hospital & Tumor Institute, Neoplasia of the Head and Neck. Chicago, Year Book Medical Publishers, 1974, pp. 187–209.

56. Hanafee, W., and Gussen, R.: Correlation of basal projection tomography in clinical problems. Radiol. Clin. North Am., 12:419–430, 1974.

57. Medellin, H., and Wallace, S.: Angiography and neoplasms of the head and neck. Radiol. Clin. North Am., 8:307–321, 1970.

58. Singer, L.: Ear, Nose, and Throat. Pathology of the Nervous System, Vol. 1. In Minckler, J. (ed.), New York, McGraw-Hill, 1968, pp. 679–696.

59. Ho, A. K. T.: Primary carcinoma of the nasopharynx. Laryngoscope, 72:1351–1378, 1962.

60. Jing, B. S.: Tumors of the nasopharynx. Radiol. Clin. North Am., 8:323–342, 1970.

61. Pollack, J. A., and Newton, T. H.: Encephalocele and Cranium Bifidum. In Newton, T. H., and Potts, D. G. (eds.), Radiology of the Skull and Brain, Vol. I. St. Louis, C. V. Mosby, 1971, pp. 634–647.

62. Fletcher, G. H., and Jing, B. S.: The head and neck. In Hodes, P. J. (ed.), Atlas of Tumor Radiology. Chicago, Year Book Medical Publishers, 1968, 1–367.

63. Ho, H. C.: Radiological diagnosis of nasopharyngeal carcinomas — Special reference to its spread to the base of the skull. In Muir, C., and Shanmugaratnam, K. (eds.), Cancers of Nasopharynx Symposium. Flushing, N.Y., International Union against Cancer, 1967.

64. Rizzuti, R. J., and Whalen, J. P.: Nasopharynx. In Newton, T. H., and Potts, D. G. (eds.), Radiology of the Skull and Brain, vol. 1. St. Louis, C. V. Mosby, 1971, pp. 241–259.

65. Fletcher, G. H.: The place of roentgen diagnosis in treatment planning for cancers of the nasopharynx, paranasal sinus, and laryngopharynx. Radiol. Clin. North Am., 8:293–305, 1970.

66. Holman, C. B., and Miller, W. E.: Juvenile nasopharyngeal fibroma: Roentgenologic characteristics. Am. J. Roentgenol. Radium Ther. Nucl. Med., 94:292–298, 1969.

67. Rosen, L., Hanafee, W. N., and Naham, A.: Nasopharyngeal angiofibroma and angiographic evaluation. Radiology, 86:103–107, 1966.

68. Wilson, G. H., and Hanafee, W. N.: Angiographic findings in 16 patients with juvenile nasopharyngeal angiofibroma. Radiology, 92:279–284, 1969.

69. Fee, E., Epsy, C. D., and Konrad, H. R.: Trigeminal neurinomas. Laryngoscope, 80:371–376, 1975.

70. Seaman, W. B.: Contrast radiography in neoplastic disease of the larynx and pharynx. Semin. Roentgenol., 9:301–309, 1974.

71. Hill, B. J.: Radiology of the larynx. Otolaryngol. Clin. North Am., 6:549–561, 1973.

72. Baclesse, F.: Tumeurs Malignes du Pharynx et du Larynx. Paris, et Cie, 1960.

73. Landman, G. H.: Laryngography and Cinelaryngography. Assen Netherlands, Royal Van Gorcum Ltd., 1970.

74. Ardran, G. N., Kemp, F. H., and Marland, P. M.: Laryngeal palsy. Br. J. Radiol., 27:201–209, 1954.

75. Gilbert, H. A., and Kagan, A. R.: Recurrence patterns in squamous cell carcinoma of the oral cavity, pharynx, and larynx. J. Surg. Oncol., 6:357–379, 1974.

76. Seaman, W. B.: Examination of the pharynx. In Margulis, A. R., and Burhenne, H. J. (eds.), Alimentary Tract Roentgenology, St. Louis, C. V. Mosby, 1973, pp. 299–336.

77. Donner, M. W.: Swallowing mechanism and neuromuscular disorders. Semin. Roentgenol., 9:273–282, 1974.

78. Kirchner, J. A.: Problems in the diagnosis of pharyngeal paralyses. Laryngoscope, 68:1641, 1958.

79. Ramsey, G. H., Watson, J. S., Gramiak, R., et al.: Cine-fluorographic analysis of the mechanism of swallowing. Radiology, 64:498, 1955.

80. Templeton, F. E., and Kredel, R. A.: The cricopharyngeal sphincter. Laryngoscope, 53:1–12, 1943.

81. Pittman, R. G., and Fraser, G. M.: The post-cricoid impression on the esophagus, Clin. Radiol., 16:34, 1965.

82. Powers, W. E., McGee, H. H., and Seaman, W. B.: Contrast examination of the larynx and pharynx. Radiology, 68:169–178, 1957.

83. Rovitt, R. L., and Berry, R.: Cushing's syndrome and the hypohysis: A re-evaluation of pituitary tumors and hyperadrenalism. J. Neurosurg., 23:270–295, 1965.

84. Dahlin, D. C.: Bone Tumors. Springfield, Ill., Charles C Thomas, 1967.

85. Heffelfinger, M. J., Dahlin, D. C., MacCarty, P. S., et al.: Chordomas and cartilaginous tumors at the skull base. Cancer, 32:410–420, 1973.

86. Di Chiro, G., and Anderson, W. B.: Clivus. Clin. Radiol., 16:211–223, 1965.

87. Wallace, S., and Medellin, H.: The value of angiography in head and neck tumors. In Anderson Hospital & Tumor Institute, Neoplasia of the Head and Neck. Chicago, Year Book Medical Publishers, 1974, pp. 159–174.

88. Britton, B. H.: Glomus tympanicum and glomus jugulare tumors. Radiol. Clin. North Am., 12:543–551, 1974.

89. Alford, B. R., and Guilford, F. R.: A comprehensive study of tumors of the glomus jugulare. Laryngoscope, 72:766–787, 1962.

90. Capps, F. C.: Tumors of the glomus jugulare or tympanic body. J. Fac. Radiol., 8:312–324, 1957.

91. Riemenschneider, P. A.: Roentgenographic diagnosis of the glomus jugulare. Am. J. Roentgenol. Radium Ther. Nucl. Med., 69:59–65, 1953.

92. Guild, S. R.: Glomus jugulare in man. Ann. Otol. Rhinol. Laryngol., 62:1045–1071, 1953.

93. Scanlan, R. L., Britton, B. H., Rumbaugh, C. L., et al.: Anomalous course of the internal carotid artery through the middle ear. Presented at Radiological Society of North America Meeting in Chicago, 1967. To be published.

94. Williams, J. G.: Radiotherapy of tumors of the glomus jugulare. J. Fac. Radiol., 8:335, 1957.

95. Simonton, K. M.: Paraganglioma (chemodectoma) of the middle ear and mastoid. J.A.M.A., 206:1531–1534, 1968.

96. Terry, R., and Johnson, L. C.: Syllabus and bibliography, from course on Bone Diseases at the International Academy of Pathology.

97. Lichtenstein, L.: Integration of eosinophilic granuloma of bone, Letterer-Siwe disease and Schüller-Christian disease as related manifestations of a single nosological entity. Arch. Pathol., 56:84–102, 1953.

98. Fisher, R. H.: Multiple lesions of bone in Letterer-Siwe disease: Report of a case with culture of paracolon arizena bacilli from bone lesions and blood, followed by response to therapy. J. Bone Joint Surg., 35A:445, 1953.

99. Bouchard, J.: Radiation Therapy of Tumors and Diseases of the Nervous System. Philadelphia, Lea & Febiger, 1966, p. 202.

100. Holmes, G. W., and Schultz, M. D.: Therapeutic Radiology. Philadelphia, Lea & Febiger, 1950.

101. McIrath, D. G., ReMine, W. H., Devine, K. D. et al.: Tumors of the parapharyngeal region. Surg. Gynecol. Obstet., *116*:88–94, 1963.

102. Perez, C. A., Jesse, R. H., and Fletcher, G. H.: Metastatic carcinoma and cervical lymph nodes unknown primary site. *In* Anderson Hospital & Tumor Institute, Neoplasia of the Head and Neck. Chicago, Year Book Medical Publishers, 1974.

103. Dodd, G. D., and Jing, B. S.: The place of diagnostic radiology in diagnoses and treatment for head and neck cancer. *In* Anderson Hospital & Tumor Institute, Neoplasia of the Head and Neck. Chicago, Year Book Medical Publishers, 1974, pp. 175–186.

104. Hill, Stratton C., Jr.: Malignant thyroid tumors: Their manifestations. *In* Endocrine and Nonendocrine Hormone-Producing Tumors. Chicago Year Book Medical Publishers, 1973, pp. 323–338.

105. Freeman, D., and Lindsay, S.: Medullary carcinoma of the thyroid gland. Arch. Pathol., *80*:575–582, 1963.

106. Wallace, S., Hill, C. S, Paulus, D. D., Jr., et al.: The radiologic aspects of medullary (solid)

107. thyroid carcinoma. Radiol. Clin. North Am., *8*:463–475, 1970.

108. Rosen, I., Walfish, P. G., and Miskin, M.: The use of B mode ultrasonography in changing indications for thyroid operations. Surg. Gynecol. Obstet., *139*:193–197, 1974.

108. Taylor, K. J. W., Carpenter, B. E., and Barrett, M. R.: Gray scale ultrasonography in the diagnosis of thyroid swellings. J. Clin. Ultrasound, *2*: 327–330, 1973.

109. Crocker, E. F., McLaughlin, A. F., Kossoff, M. E., et al.: The gray scale echographic appearance of thyroid malignancy. J. Clin. Ultrasound, *2*: 305–307, 1973.

110. Deftos, L. J., Keutmann, H. T., Niall, H. D., et al.: Parathyroid hormones and parathyroid neoplasms. *In* Anderson Hospital, Endocrine and and Nonendocrine Hormone-Producing Tumors, Chicago, Year Book Medical Publishers, 1973, pp. 297–308.

111. Doppman, J. L., Mallette, L. D., Marx, S. J., et al.: The localization of abnormal mediastinal parathyroid glands. Radiology, *115*:31–36, 1975.

Chapter Six

ESOPHAGUS

Harvey M. Goldstein, M.D.

CLINICAL CONSIDERATIONS

Presenting Signs and Symptoms

Difficulty in swallowing is the most frequent complaint of patients with esophageal carcinoma. This is *not* an early finding.[1] The onset of painful swallowing usually denotes full thickness involvement of the wall of the esophagus with proximal dilatation. Weight loss is an earlier symptom of esophageal carcinoma than difficulty in swallowing. A medical examination for weight loss ordinarily does not include a barium esophagram, however, unless symptoms of a deglutition disorder are present. The cancer can extend to involve the recurrent laryngeal nerve, which causes hoarseness; the trachea or bronchus, resulting in cough after eating; or the investments of the heart, which can cause pericardial effusion.

The common sites of esophageal carcinoma are associated with the locations of the natural anatomic constrictions of the esophagus: the cricopharyngeal area (upper third of the esophagus), the left bronchus (middle third), and the diaphragmatic opening (lower third). To be more specific, the upper third of the esophagus encompasses the hypopharynx or region of the pharyngoesophageal constrictor muscles, the cervical esophagus, and the mediastinal esophagus above the arch of the aorta. The middle third extends from the upper border of the aortic arch to the left primary bronchus. The lower third includes the re-

mainder of the esophagus to the diaphragmatic hiatus, which in turn includes the cardioesophageal junction. Most esophageal carcinomas are found in the middle and lower thirds. However, a relatively great incidence of cancer in the upper third of the esophagus has been reported in South Africa.[2] Worldwide, cervical esophageal carcinomas are reported rarely (10 per cent in most series), and often careful indirect laryngoscopy reveals that a retrocricoid carcinoma is actually invading the cervical esophagus secondarily.

Tylosis palmaris and plantaris is sometimes associated with carcinoma of the esophagus.[3]

Differential Diagnosis

Benign manifestations such as congenital short esophagus, diverticulum, peptic esophagitis with inflammatory stenosis, lye stricture, achalasia, diaphragmatic hernia, esophageal web, and Plummer-Vinson syndrome can all give symptoms identical to those of cancer.[4] The issue of differential diagnosis may become even more confusing, because cancer has been associated occasionally with these benign conditions; this is usually explained on the basis of the repeated injury and subsequent repair to the epithelial surfaces that may occur with each of them.

Benign tumors of the esophagus are usually small and asymptomatic.[5] When symptomatic, they may cause difficulty in

110

swallowing; however, hemorrhage denotes malignancy. The common benign tumors occur mainly in the lower third of the esophagus and are usually leiomyomas, polyps, or cysts. Duplications or foregut cysts occasionally occur in the middle third as well.

Very large polypoid masses within the esophagus indicate a soft tissue sarcoma or a so-called carcinosarcoma.[6, 7] Sarcomas of the esophagus, notably leiomyosarcomas, seem to have a low rate of metastasis, but extensive data for these generalizations are lacking.

Adenocarcinomas and adenocanthomas of the esophagus occur but are exceedingly rare.[8] A common error is to confuse them with adenocarcinomas of the esophagogastric junction, which actually arise from the cardia of the stomach. Subsequent contiguous spread of tumor into the esophagus from the cardia of the stomach can produce an ulcerative lesion resembling primary cancer of the esophagus. Mucous and chief-like cells remain at the proximal and distal ends of the normal esophagus, and consequently adenocystic carcinomas (salivary gland–type carcinomas) have been reported.

Metastases to the esophageal wall are rare, despite the frequency of metastases to the mediastinal and hilar lymph nodes. Breast carcinoma is the most common tumor to metastasize to the esophagus, but intramural deposits from melanomas and carcinomas of the lung, kidney, thyroid, and testicle have all been reported.

Practically all the problems of differential diagnosis of benign esophageal lesions and esophageal carcinoma can now be resolved by esophagoscopy. A trans-esophagoscopic biopsy is false-negative in one of ten patients because of luminal narrowing so severe that the lesion is missed by the biopsy forceps. If this anatomic situation is foreseen in advance, cytologic brushing alone may be diagnostic. Bronchoscopy to rule out a primary lung carcinoma or tracheobronchial extension from an esophageal primary tumor (carinal invasion; extrabronchial compression) is also important.

Therapeutic Decisions and Staging

No known correlation exists between the degree of histologic differentiation of a tumor and its gross appearance or prognosis. Treatment failure is related to local tumor extension and is only secondarily attributable to associated regional lymph node metastases, distant metastases, or both.[9, 10] The subepithelial extension of the tumor along the esophagus cannot be appraised well by routine radiologic techniques. However, the greatest single problem in the staging of this disease, at present, is that there is no reliable means of demonstrating transmural spread into the surrounding mediastinal tissues. Autopsy studies have shown that almost one third of patients with esophageal cancer die of local disease, without bulky regional or distant metastases.

It has been estimated via autopsy and surgical specimens that a five-year cure rate of 20 per cent (including a 14 per cent postoperative mortality rate) is possible for resectable lesions.[11] However, only 50 per cent of patients have lesions that are deemed resectable at the time of diagnosis. Most of these resectable lesions are 6 cm or less in length on esophagrams. A 10 per cent five-year cure rate, or less, is usually reported. The failure to cure epithelial cancer of the esophagus may be attributable to the fact that the esophagus is very thin at the levels where carcinomas typically develop. Local extension occurs early, and cervical and abdominal lymph node metastases are not uncommon.

Clinical Follow-up

Despite treatment, death often results from local effects of the tumor, actually leading to starvation. The proponents of vigorous treatment of carcinoma of the esophagus advocate a combination of surgery and irradiation.[12, 13] The use of surgery or irradiation alone also has ardent supporters.[14, 15] All other procedures, whether for recurrence or initial palliation, are even less satisfactory than surgery or irradiation. Gastrostomy (for alimentation), surgery for the creation of a pharyngeal fistula (for salivary diversion), or insertion of tubes (to aid swallowing) typically yields little success. Hemorrhage, erosion, fistula formation, or prosthesis migration and obstruction often occur with indwelling tubes.

Postoperative mortality (at a rate of 15 to 20 per cent) is usually attributable to pneumonia, pulmonary embolism, wound infection, or dehiscence of esophagogastrostomy anastomoses accompanied by mediastinitis and empyema. Patients who develop a postoperative leak at the esophagogastric anastomosis usually die. Irradiation of a gastroesophageal anastomosis within the thoracic cavity (because of recurrence or residual disease) is not without risk.

Postirradiation strictures and fistulae can simulate mucosal and paraesophageal recurrences. Radiation pneumonitis or myelitis may also occur. It is of interest to note that 20 per cent of the patients who survive tumors of the upper respiratory and digestive tracts (head and neck) eventually develop another primary carcinoma in the lung or in the upper respiratory or digestive tract (including the esophagus).[16]

RADIOLOGIC CONSIDERATIONS

Presenting Radiographic Signs

EXAMINATION TECHNIQUE

Meticulous examination technique is essential to the accurate roentgenographic assessment of esophageal neoplasms. Because a tumor may develop in any portion of the esophagus, and because dysphagia is often poorly localized by the patient, roentgenologic examination must include the entire esophagus. The optimal examination includes fluoroscopic observation of the esophageal circumference, as well as filming of at least two complementary anatomic projections. Additional radiographs are then obtained in any position necessary to characterize a suspected lesion. Radiographs of the distended, barium-filled esophagus, as well as collapsed mucosal pattern views, may be obtained. Occasionally, double contrast studies of the esophagus are indispensable to visualize a small lesion protruding into the lumen or a minimal amount of mucosal irregularity.[17] Repetitive viewing with cineradiography may provide motility information important to the diagnosis of a suspected lesion.[18]

Cineradiography and rapid-sequence "photospots" are also particularly helpful for evaluation of the cervical esophagus, because of the rapid passage of barium in this region. For complete radiographic evaluation of an esophageal neoplasm, it is advisable also to examine the remainder of the upper gastrointestinal tract. This procedure is particularly advisable with tumors involving the distal esophagus, inasmuch as they frequently originate in the gastric cardia or fundus and represent secondary extension to the esophagus (see the preceding discussion of differential diagnosis).

CRITERIA OF MALIGNANCY

Virtually all esophageal malignancies produce some degree of luminal narrowing. The narrowed area is usually irregular and nodular, and ulceration of the tumor is common. At fluoroscopy, a malignant narrowing is unchanging and rigid, with no distensibility despite continuous ingestion of barium. Demonstration of mucosal destruction in the narrowed area is also critical to the radiologic diagnosis of esophageal cancer. An abrupt transition in diameter at the junction of the tumor with the normal esophagus, resulting in an overhanging edge or "shelf" formation, is an additional reliable feature of malignancy.

PATTERNS OF MALIGNANCY

The radiologic manifestations of esophageal malignancies may be subdivided into four patterns (Fig. 6–1): annular constricting, polypoid (or fungating), infiltrative (or stenosing), and ulcerative.[19-24] In many cases features of more than one pattern may be present.

The annular constricting type of esophageal cancer is the most common and is similar in appearance to the "apple-core" carcinoma of the colon. Prominent overhanging margins at the proximal and distal extremes of the gross tumor are characteristic (Fig. 6–2). The constricted portion of the esophageal lumen is typically irregular and ulcerated. If obstruction by the tumor is marked, sufficient barium will not traverse the constricted area, and the inferior margin

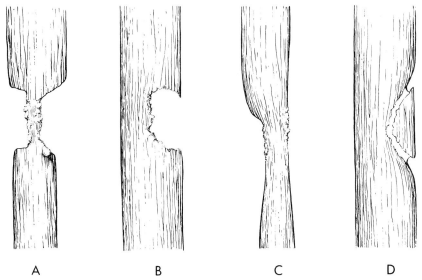

Figure 6–1 Schematic representation of the four basic radiographic patterns of esophageal carcinoma. *A,* annular constricting; *B,* polypoidal; *C,* infiltrative; *D,* primary ulcerative.

of the lesion may not be adequately visualized.

Some variation in the polypoidal pattern also occurs quite frequently. When limited to only one wall, this type of tumor presents as an abrupt, irregular, marginal filling defect with some luminal encroachment (Fig. 6–3). Eventually, the tumor may encircle the entire esophageal circumference, which results in an annular appearance, or it may continue its intraluminal growth and cause obstruction in this manner. When multiple polypoidal tumor components are present, the appearance of esophageal varices may be mimicked (Fig. 6–4).[25]

The infiltrative type of carcinoma is the most difficult to diagnose confidently. It is characterized by a gradual, tapered narrowing without overhanging edges. Since most of the growth of this tumor occurs in the submucosa, there is relative sparing of the overlying mucosa, with resulting close resemblance to a benign stricture (Fig. 6–5). Asymmetry of the tapered contours and the presence of small marginal irregularities in the narrowed area may provide clues to the correct diagnosis. This appearance is also commonly seen in the distal esophagus when it is secondarily infiltrated by a gastric neoplasm.

Although some ulceration is frequently noted within esophageal malignancies of any type, the primary ulcerative variety is the most unusual. When visualized in profile, the ulcer is characteristically meniscoid in shape and occurs within a relatively flat tumor mass that is protruding into the esophageal lumen (Fig. 6–6). It is critical to visualize this type of tumor in profile, in order to appreciate fully the type of ulceration. This appearance is analogous to the more familiar tumor of the stomach, where a prominent ulceration may occur within a malignant mass.

HISTOLOGIC VARIETIES

Although the vast majority of malignant esophageal tumors are squamous cell in origin, several other malignant neoplasms occur occasionally and may be encountered on radiologic examination. These include adenocarcinoma, carcinosarcoma, sarcoma, lymphoma, and metastases to the esophagus. Adenocarcinoma usually involves the distal esophagus and almost always represents extension from the gastric cardia or fundus, even if the gastric component is small (Fig. 6–7). True primary adenocarcinoma of the esophagus is rare and probably arises from heterotopic gastric mucosa or a columnar-lined esophagus.[8, 26] Carcinosarcoma, consisting of both malignant squamous epithelial and stromal elements, is typically a bulky, polypoid lesion that expands the esophageal lumen (Fig. 6–8).[7, 27]

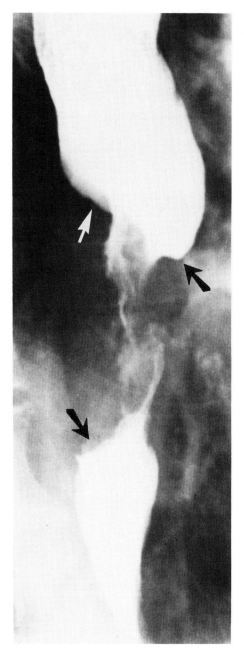

esophagus is usually from secondary spread, but rarely it can arise primarily within the esophagus (Fig. 6–9).[30, 31] The esophagus is the most uncommon portion of the gastro-intestinal tract to become involved with lymphoma. Direct extension from adjacent

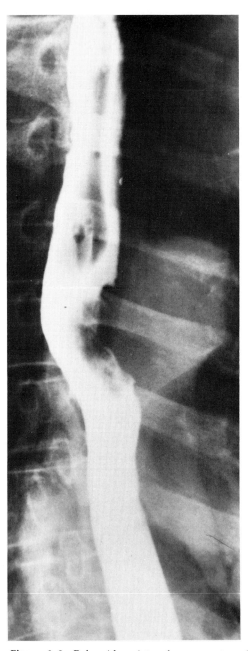

Figure 6–2 Annular constricting type of esophageal carcinoma. Esophagram demonstrates a prominent overhanging "shelf" at both ends of the lesion (arrows). The constricted area is irregular with destruction of the mucosal pattern.

Pure sarcomas are also rare and occur much less commonly than their benign stromal tumor counterparts. Their radiologic appearance is not characteristic, although a large extraluminal component may be present.[28, 29] Melanosarcoma involving the

Figure 6–3 Polypoid variety of squamous carcinoma. At the level of the aortic knob, an irregular polypoid mass arises from the esophageal mucosa and protrudes into the lumen. There is no obstruction to the flow of barium.

the earlier section on criteria of malignancy).[32, 33] Metastasis to the esophagus usually results from direct extension of an adjacent tumor and is seen most frequently with primary breast and lung tumors. When transmural invasion occurs, the radiographic

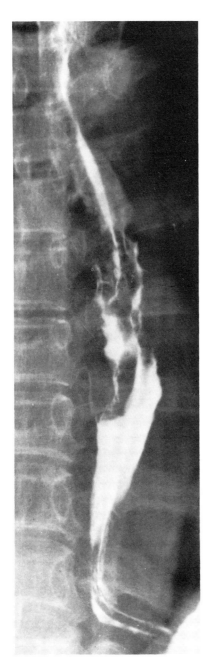

Figure 6–4 Varicoid carcinoma. Squamous cell carcinoma of the mid-esophagus with multiple varicoid defects simulating the appearance of varices. The lack of change with repeated swallowing and respiratory maneuvers suggests the diagnosis of tumor rather than of true varices.

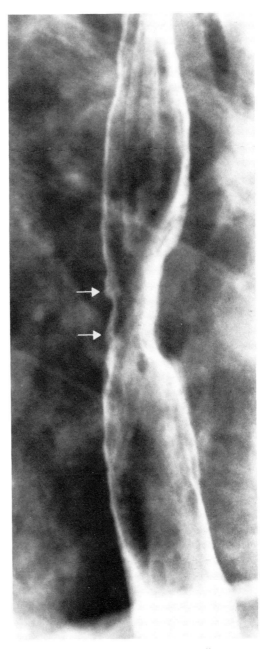

Figure 6–5 Infiltrating squamous cell carcinoma. Double contrast esophagram demonstrates a persistent asymmetrical narrowing of the distal esophagus. Several fine serrations (arrows) are present along one contour, suggesting malignancy.

lymph nodes can occur, or lymphoma may actually originate in the esophageal submucosa. Several different radiographic appearances may be present, which range from benign to typically malignant (see

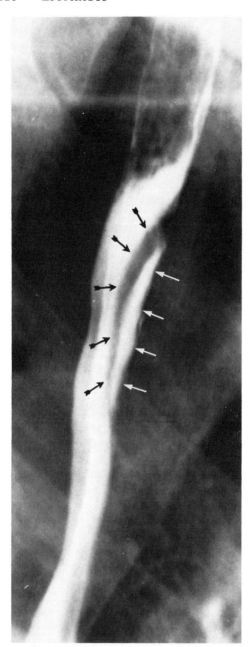

Figure 6–6 Primary ulcerative carcinoma. Barium swallow demonstrates a large meniscoid-shaped ulcer (white arrows) occurring in a flat tumor mass (black arrows).

Differential Diagnosis

Because an esophageal malignancy may demonstrate a variety of radiologic appearances, it must be differentiated from a num-

appearance may be indistinguishable from a polypoid or annular primary esophageal carcinoma. In general, with the exception of some carcinosarcomas and lymphomas, the radiographic appearance of these unusual esophageal neoplasms is indistinguishable from the usual squamous cell carcinoma.

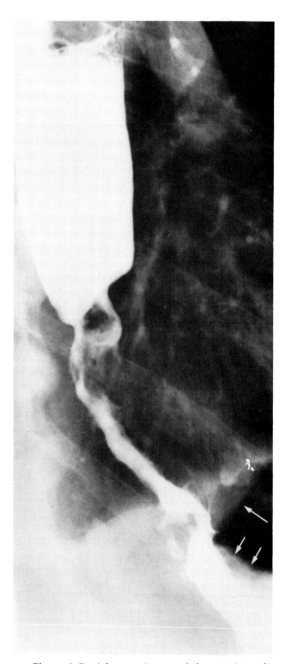

Figure 6–7 Adenocarcinoma of the gastric cardia with extensive invasion of the distal esophagus. Esophagram demonstrates tumorous constriction of the distal third of the esophagus. The largest portion of the lesion is on the esophageal side with only a small component of the tumor seen in the stomach (arrows).

techniques usually provide definitive information. On the other hand, if there is a positive or suspicious radiologic examination, a negative endoscopic examination should not be accepted without further evaluation. This situation may arise with

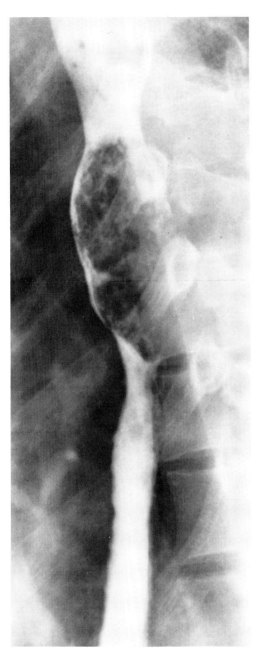

Figure 6–8 Carcinosarcoma. The bulky, intraluminal esophageal mass with expansion of the esophageal lumen is characteristic of carcinosarcoma.

ber of other possible esophageal abnormalities. Despite careful clinical assessment and optimal radiologic examination, occasionally the radiographic distinction between benign and malignant disease of the esophagus is not possible. Fortunately, modern endoscopic biopsy and cytologic

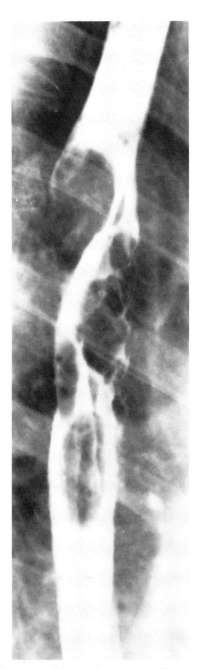

Figure 6–9 Metastatic melanoma. The esophagram shows a multilobular mass in the mid-esophagus. The proximal overhanging edge and irregularity indicate a malignant lesion.

cancers that are largely submucosal and in which superficial biopsies may be misleading, as well as in neoplasms that cause high-grade obstruction, mechanically preventing adequate visualization and biopsy.

ESOPHAGITIS

Benign causes of esophageal narrowing, such as strictures associated with peptic esophagitis or previous corrosive ingestion, provide the most common and difficult problems of radiologic differentiation. Strictures may be particularly difficult to differentiate from the infiltrating form of carcinoma (see the earlier discussion of patterns of malignancy). Benign strictures are characterized by relatively symmetrical narrowing with tapered margins, rather than the abrupt edges seen with most malignant neoplasms (Fig. 6–10 A and B). With a benign stricture, the narrowed area tends to be smoother and to retain its mucosal pattern. The length of the narrowed area is variable and is not helpful in differentiating benign from malignant processes. The presence of a hiatal hernia or unequivocal gastroesophageal reflux may favor the diagnosis of a peptic stricture, but these secondary features should not be considered more important diagnostically than the appearance of the lesion itself.

ACHALASIA

Narrowing of the distal esophageal segment associated with achalasia may also be difficult to distinguish from an obstructing neoplasm arising in the distal esophagus or proximal stomach. With either achalasia or obstructing carcinoma, considerable dilatation of the proximal esophagus may occur. Intermittent partial opening of the narrowed segment, caused by the gravitational effects of continued barium ingestion in the upright position, will often provide a clue to the correct diagnosis of achalasia. In addition, administration of methacholine chloride (Mecholyl) in conjunction with esophagography may help to differentiate these conditions by creating deep contractions in the proximal denervated esophagus of achalasia.[34]

BENIGN NEOPLASMS

Benign tumors of the esophagus are the other major potential differential diagnostic problem. The most common lesion of this group is the intramural leiomyoma.[5, 35] Unlike the polypoid variety of carcinoma, a benign intramural tumor will generally have a smooth surface with stretching, rather than destruction of the overlying mucosa. When seen in profile, rather sharp right angles may be formed at the esophageal wall at the point from which these tumors arise (Fig. 6–11).[36] Not infrequently, an extra-esophageal soft tissue component of an intramural tumor may also be visualized against the air-filled lung adjacent to the mediastinum.

FOOD MATERIAL

An intraluminal filling defect caused by impacted food is not ordinarily a diagnostic problem because of the associated history. However, it should be remembered that food bolus obstructions often occur because of an underlying esophageal lesion.

VARICES

If esophageal varices are large, they may be confused with the diffuse polypoidal variety of carcinoma, or varicoid carcinoma (Fig. 6–4).[25] Unlike the rigid filling defects of carcinoma, esophageal varices will change in size and shape with each swallow and with various respiratory maneuvers.

EXTRINSIC MASSES

When visualized in profile, extrinsic impressions on the esophagus, such as from adjacent lymphadenopathy, may cause significant narrowing. When extrinsic masses are large, the esophagus may also be displaced to some degree. Typically, the impression upon the esophagus is eccentric and smooth, with a gradual transition to the uninvolved esophagus above and below the extrinsic mass.[36]

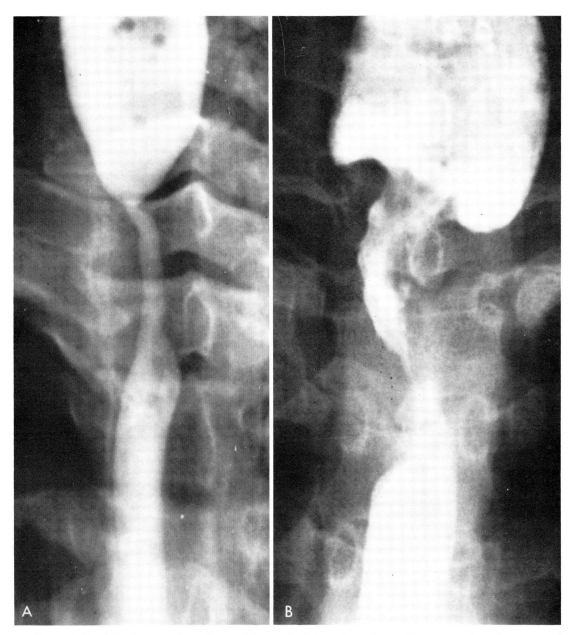

Figure 6–10   *A,* Benign corrosive stricture of the proximal thoracic esophagus. The narrowed area is smooth and the adjacent esophageal margins taper symmetrically. *B,* Squamous carcinoma of the proximal thoracic esophagus in a different patient. The narrowed area is irregular and ulcerated, and there are overhanging edges proximally (see also Fig. 6–2).

Localization and Staging

The responsibility of the radiologist in the evaluation of a suspected esophageal neoplasm has two aspects. First, he suggests the diagnosis of esophageal malignancy. Second, he makes a roentgenologic assessment of the extent of esophageal and extra-esophageal spread that is critical to clinical decisions regarding therapy.

The barium study can provide valuable information regarding the vertical extent of gross tumor involvement of the esophagus, as well as aiding in diagnosis. Radiographic documentation of the superior and inferior extent of a lesion is essential in any

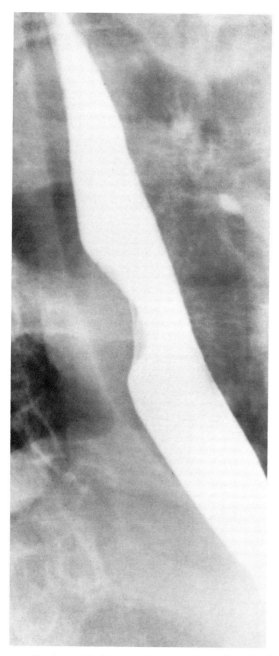

Figure 6–11 Benign leiomyoma of the distal esophagus. Barium swallow demonstrates a smooth submucosal mass arising at right angles from the esophageal wall.

treatment planning. Careful fluoroscopic or cineradiographic observation of disrupted esophageal peristalsis and the limitations of normal distensibility may yield information regarding the true vertical extent of a tumor. Use of a spasmolytic agent in conjunction with an esophagram may also

aid in the delineation of the inferior extent of a tumor by causing relaxation and improved filling of the normally expansile esophagus below the obstruction (Fig. 6–12).[37] Vertical extension from the primary lesion occurs via submucosal lymphatics, and often this lymphatic spread extends beyond the gross radiologic and pathologic margins of the tumor. Occasionally, secondary esophageal implantation sites or cancerous involvement of virtually the entire esophagus may result from submucosal infiltration (Fig. 6–13).[24]

Unfortunately, local extraesophageal tumor spread has usually occurred by the time the primary esophageal lesion is discovered. Depending upon the site of the primary lesion, lymphatic spread may involve mediastinal, supraclavicular, and subdiaphragmatic nodes. In addition, direct extension into the mediastinum, tracheobronchial tree, aorta, heart, mediastinal pleura, and lungs often occurs because of the strategic anatomic location of the esophagus and the lack of a true serosa to retard spread. The initial esophagram may also provide evidence of local mediastinal extension. For example, perforation into the mediastinum or a fistulous communication with the tracheobronchial tree may be demonstrated (Fig. 6–14). In addition, a discontinuity in the normal smooth esophageal course or in the esophageal axis, as manifested by angulation at the tumor site (Fig. 6–15) or by offsetting of the barium columns above and below the tumor, is indicative of cancerous infiltration into surrounding structures.[38]

Completion of an upper gastrointestinal series at the time of esophagography may provide information regarding extension of a distal esophageal neoplasm to the stomach or, more likely, extension of a primary gastric neoplasm into the distal esophagus. In addition, attention to the retrogastric area may reveal evidence of the frequent involvement of subdiaphragmatic lymph nodes in the celiac group.[39]

In addition to the barium study of the esophagus, other conventional radiologic examinations are frequently helpful in assessing lymph node involvement or direct mediastinal extension. Frontal and lateral chest radiographs may demonstrate adenopathy or invasion of mediastinal structures. Tomography or xeroradiography can be utilized for more definitive evaluation of suspected mediastinal abnormalities. Positive contrast tracheobronchograms are now utilized infrequently, probably because of the widespread preoperative use of tracheobronchoscopy.

Azygography (azygos vein angiograms) may be utilized to evaluate resectability of esophageal neoplasms because of the anatomic proximity of the azygos vein and the distal two thirds of the thoracic esophagus.[40] The examination is simple and may be performed via transfemoral direct catheteriza-

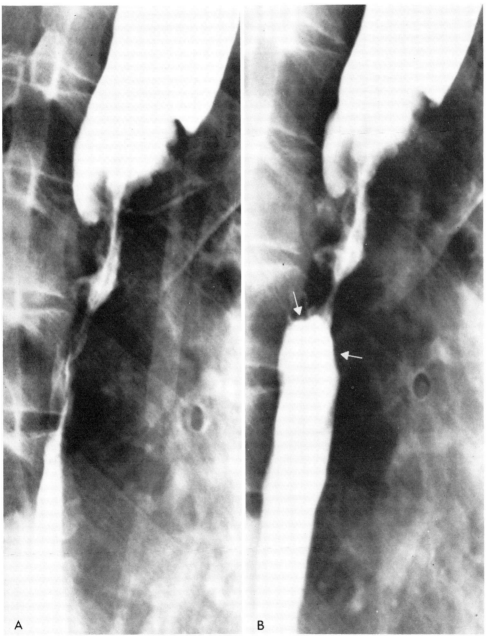

A   B

Figure 6–12 Squamous cell carcinoma of the mid-esophagus. *A,* Esophagram demonstrates an obvious lesion with proximal overhanging margins. The distal extent of the tumor cannot be determined because of poor filling as a result of the obstruction. *B,* Following 20 mg of parenteral propantheline bromide, relaxation and subsequent filling of the uninvolved esophagus below the tumor facilitate assessment of the gross distal extent (arrows).

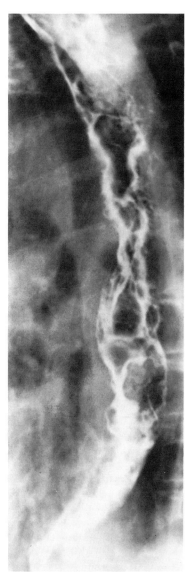

Figure 6–13 Squamous cell carcinoma with involvement of the entire thoracic esophagus. The esophagram demonstrates a nodular neoplasm involving the whole thoracic esophagus, presumably secondary to diffuse submucosal extension.

tion of the azygos vein or indirectly by intraosseous contrast material injection into a lower rib. Significant impingement or obstruction of the azygos venous system by the primary neoplasm itself or by metastatic nodes indicates unresectability (Fig. 6–16A and B).

The controlled injection of air (pneumomediastinography) into the mediastinal soft tissues, supplemented with tomography, allows radiographic outlining of the size and shape of esophageal neoplasms and provides information regarding tumorous attachments to adjacent mediastinal organs.[41, 42] In addition, visualization of enlarged metastatic nodes is also facilitated by the insufflated air. The examination may be performed in conjunction with tracheo-

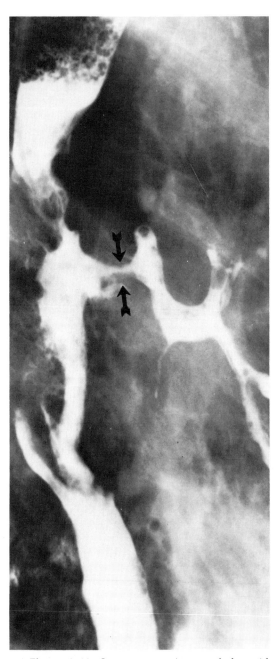

Figure 6–14 Squamous carcinoma of the mid-esophagus with a bronchial fistula. The esophagram shows an extensive tumor of the mid-esophagus with barium filling the left bronchial tree through the communicating fistula (arrows).

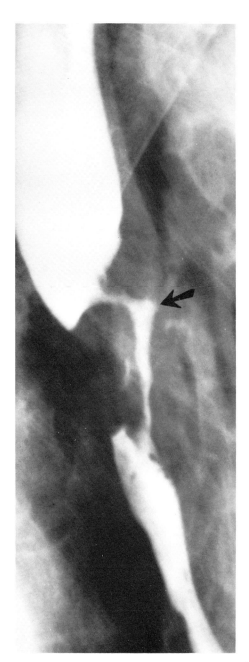

Figure 6–15 Squamous cell carcinoma of the esophagus. There is disruption of the esophageal axis as evidenced by sharp angulation (arrow) of the constricted portion of the esophagus. Distortion of the axis indicates adherence to adjacent mediastinal structures.

bronchial endoscopy (bronchoscopy) or as a separate procedure. It has not achieved widespread popularity but, from available reports, appears to be an accurate and a safe procedure when performed properly.

Prior to surgical management of an esophageal malignancy with colonic interposition in the chest, examination of the colon with barium enema and mesenteric arteriography is advisable. Preoperative barium studies of the colon will exclude any unrecognized abnormalities such as tumors, strictures, or diverticular disease that might interfere with the subsequent passage of food. Mesenteric arteriography is performed to evaluate the anatomic integrity of the colonic marginal artery. Demonstration of this blood supply is useful in selecting the optimal portion of the colon for interposition, in order to prevent a later anastomotic breakdown secondary to ischemia.

Evaluation for distant metastases must be done before deciding upon definitive treatment, and it is also dependent chiefly upon radiologic imaging techniques. Information regarding direct mediastinal spread and the presence of pulmonary metastases may be gained by routine chest radiography. Pulmonary infiltrates secondary to aspiration or tracheobronchial fistulas must sometimes be differentiated from metastases. Skeletal surveys and radionuclide bone scans are usually not performed unless focal symptoms are present. Bone metastases are most common in the axial skeleton and have been reported in the later stages of the disease in over 5 per cent of patients with esophageal cancer (Fig. 6–17).[43] Hepatic scanning provides a good screening test for liver metastases and, if indicated, may be supplemented with hepatic arteriography.

Radiologic Follow-Up

Barium study of the esophagus (or an interposed intestinal segment) is also the primary examination in the follow-up evaluation of the patient treated by surgery or radiation. As with surgical resection of any gastrointestinal tract neoplasm, early (four to six weeks) postoperative evaluation of the esophagus is essential to establish the patency and integrity of the surgical anastomosis, as well as to define any deformity that might represent residual tumor or postoperative change. After the initial baseline study, repeat esophagrams at regular inter-

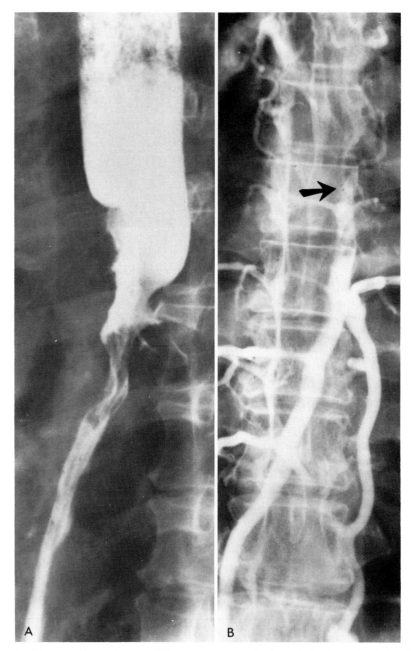

Figure 6–16 Unresectable carcinoma of the esophagus. *A*, Barium study shows the irregular, ulcerated mid-esophageal tumor. *B*, Intraosseous azygogram demonstrates complete obstruction of the azygos vein (arrow), indicating unresectability of the neoplasm.

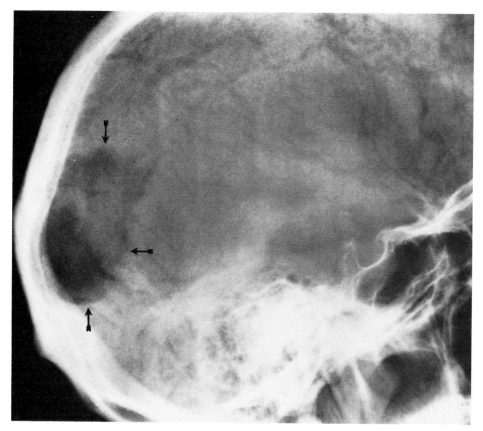

Figure 6–17   Squamous cell carcinoma of the esophagus with a bony metastasis. There is a large, irregular, lytic metastatic deposit in the occipital area of the skull (arrows).

vals should be utilized to evaluate the patient for potential local recurrence of disease.

Similarly, during and following radiotherapy, periodic esophagrams will aid in the assessment of treatment progress. Commonly, a smooth, benign-appearing narrowing of the esophagus evolves during and after treatment, from the stenosis of an irregular tumor (Fig. 6–18). In particular, if slight mucosal irregularities in the treated area persist, it may be most difficult to determine radiologically whether any residual tumor remains. Occasionally, perforation of necrotic neoplastic tissue occurs during radiotherapy, which may result in mediastinitis or communication with the tracheobronchial tree.

Regular interval chest radiographs for evaluation of the mediastinal structures and lung fields are also necessary in following the treated patient. Radiation-induced pneumonitis, usually localized to the paramediastinal portions of the lung, may occur in patients who have received high-dose mediastinal radiotherapy, and should not be confused with pulmonary metastases (Fig. 6–19). Pulmonary metastases from esophageal carcinoma usually will appear as distinct nodular densities in the lung fields, although ray-like lymphangitic tumor extension from the mediastinum into the adjacent lung may occasionally provide a difficult (and crucial) diagnostic problem.

As with the pretreatment evaluation, bone radiographic surveys and scans, liver scans, and the radiologic examination of other clinically relevant areas will complement clinical and laboratory findings in following the treated patient.

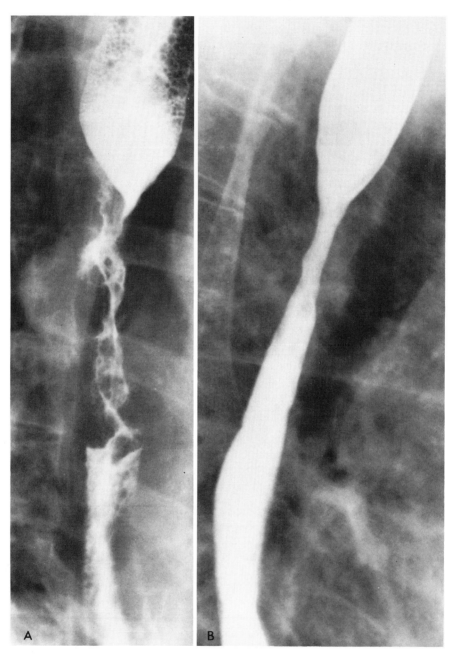

Figure 6–18   Carcinoma of the esophagus. *A*, Pre-treatment esophagram demonstrates a long irregular neoplasm. *B*, Two months following completion of radiotherapy a relatively smooth stricture is present in the same area. No gross tumor is visible now.

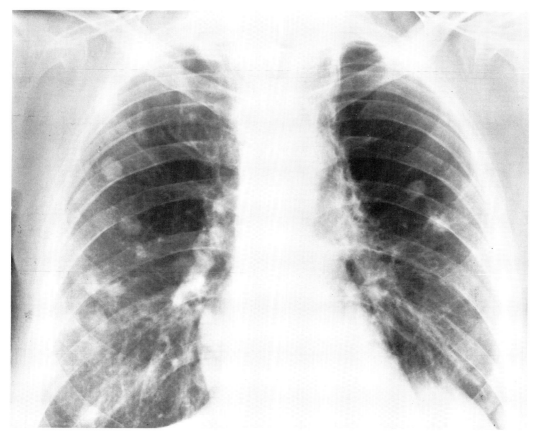

Figure 6–19 Pulmonary metastases secondary to squamous cell esophageal carcinoma. Frontal chest radiograph demonstrates bilateral multiple nodular metastases. The shaggy mediastinal margins are secondary to radiation change.

References

1. Palmer, E. D.: Carcinoma of the esophagus; survival and the fallacy of early diagnosis. U.S. Armed Forces Med. J., 8:1317, 1957.
2. Coetzee, T.: Carcinoma of the oesophagus. S. Afr. J. Surg., 4:107–122, 1966.
3. Parnell, D. D., and Johnson, S. A. M.: Tylosis palmaris et plantaris: Its occurrence with internal malignancy. Arch. Dermatol., 100:7, 1969.
4. Jacobsson, F.: The Paterson-Kelly (Plummer-Vinson) syndrome and carcinoma of the esophagus. In Tanner, N. C., and Smithers, D. W. (eds.), Neoplastic Diseases at Various Sites. Vol. R., Tumors of the Oesophagus. Edinburgh and London, E. S. Livingston, Ltd., 1961.
5. Attah, E. B., and Hajdu, S. I.: Benign and malignant tumors of the esophagus at autopsy. J. Thorac. Cardiovasc. Surg., 55:396–404, 1968.
6. Hughes, J. H., and Cruickshank, A. H.: Pseudo-sarcoma of the oesophagus. Br. J. Surg., 56:72–76, 1969.
7. Moore, T. C., Battersby, J. S., Vellios, F., et al.: Carcinosarcoma of the esophagus. J. Thorac. Cardiovasc. Surg., 45:281–288, 1963.
8. Lortat-Jacob, J.-L., Maillard, J. N., Richard, C. A., et al.: Primary esophageal adenocarcinoma: Report of 16 cases. Surgery, 64:535–543, 1968.
9. Buch, B. A., and Fletcher, W. S.: Esophageal cancer: Results of therapy in an indigent population. J. Surg. Oncol., 5:101–111, 1973.
10. Mosley, R. V.: Squamous cell carcinoma of the esophagus. Surg. Gynecol. Obstet., 126:1242, 1968.
11. Merendino, K. A., and Mark, V. H.: An analysis of one hundred cases of squamous cell carcinoma of the esophagus, part II. Surg., Gynecol., Obstet., 94:110–114, 1952.
12. Akakura, I., Nakamura, Y., Kakegawa, T., et al.: Surgery of carcinoma of esophagus with pre-operative radiation. Chest, 57:47, 1970.
13. Nakayama, K.: Statistical review of five-year survivals after surgery for carcinoma of the esophagus and cardiac portion of the stomach. Surgery, 45:883, 1959.
14. Moore, W. T., Arnold, G. E. and Day, L. H.: Surgical treatment of carcinoma of the cervical esophagus. South. Med. J., 11:1159–1163, 1967.
15. Wilson, S. E., Plested, W. G., and Carey, J. S.: Esophagogastrectomy versus radiation therapy for mid-esophageal carcinoma. J. Thorac. Surg., 10:195, 1970.
16. De la Pava, S., Pickren, J. W., Cabrera, A., et al.:

Subclinical carcinoma of the esophagus. Study of second primary carcinoma. N. Y. State J. Med., 64:524–527, 1964.

17. Suzuki, H., Kobayashi, S., Endo, M., et al.: Diagnosis of early esophageal cancer. Surgery, 71: 99–103, 1972.

18. Berridge, F. R., and Gregg, D. M.: The value of cinematography in the diagnosis of malignant strictures of the esophagus. Br. J. Radiol., 31:465–471, September, 1958.

19. Brombart, M.: In Margulis, A. R., and Burhenne, H. J. (eds.), Alimentary Tract Roentgenology, Vol. 1, 2nd ed. St. Louis, C. V. Mosby, 1973, pp. 372–380.

20. Golden, R., Cimmino, C. V., Collins, L. C., et al.: Section 5: Digestive Tract. In Robbins, L. L., (ed.), Golden's Diagnostic Radiology. Baltimore, Williams & Wilkins, 1969, pp. 101–109.

21. Marshak, R. H.: The roentgen findings of benign and malignant tumors of the esophagus. J. Mt. Sinai Hospital, 23:75–89, 1956.

22. Stein, G. N., and Finkelstein, A. K.: Tumor Atlas of the Gastrointestinal Tract: The Esophagus and Stomach. Chicago, Year Book Medical Publishers, 1973, pp. 2–83.

23. Wiot, J. W., and Felson, B.: Current concepts in cancer. I. Esophagus: Radiographic differential diagnosis. J.A.M.A., 226:1548–1552, 1973.

24. Zboralske, F. F., and Friedland, G. W.: Diseases of the esophagus: Present concepts. Calif. Med., 112:33–51, 1970.

25. Silver, T. M., and Goldstein, H. M.: Varicoid carcinoma of the esophagus. Am. J. Dig. Dis., 19: 56–58, 1974.

26. Turnbull, A. D. M., and Goodner, J. T.: Primary adenocarcinoma of the esophagus. Cancer, 22:915–918, 1968.

27. McCort, J. J.: Esophageal carcinosarcoma and pseudosarcoma. Radiology, 102:519–524, 1972.

28. Camishion, R. C., Gibbon, J. H., Jr., and Templeton, J.: Leiomyosarcoma of the esophagus. Ann. Surg., 153:951–956, 1961.

29. Goodner, J. T., Miller, T. R., and Watson, W. L.: Sarcoma of the esophagus. Am. J. Roentgenol. Radium Ther. Nucl. Med., 89:132–139, 1963.

30. Burnett, J. M., and St. John, E.: Primary melano-sarcoma of the esophagus. Radiology, 57:868–870, 1951.

31. Garfinkle, J. M., and Cahan, W. G.: Primary melanocarcinoma of the esophagus: First histologically proven case. Cancer, 5:921–926, 1952.

32. Bickel, J.: Hodgkin's disease of the esophagus. Acta Radiol., 35:371–374, 1951.

33. Caruso, R. D., and Berk, R. N.: Lymphoma of the esophagus. Radiology, 95:381–382, 1970.

34. Ennis, J. T., and Lewicki, A. M.: Mecholyl esophagography. Am. J. Roentgenol. Radium Ther. Nucl. Med., 119:241–244, 1973.

35. Glanville, J. N.: Leiomyomata of the esophagus. Clin. Radiol., 16:187–190, 1965.

36. Schatzki, R., and Hawes, L. E.: The roentgenological appearance of extramucosal tumors of the esophagus: Analysis of intramural extramucosal lesions of the gastrointestinal tract in general. Am. J. Roentgenol. Radium Ther., 48: 1–15, 1942.

37. Ghahremani, G., Heck, L. L., and Williams, J. R.: A pharmacologic aid in the radiographic diagnosis of obstructive esophageal lesions. Radiology, 103:289–293, 1972.

38. Akiyama, H., Kogure, T., and Itai, Y.: The esophageal axis and its relationship to the resectability of carcinoma of the esophagus. Ann. Surg., 176:30–36, 1972.

39. Guernsey, J. M., Doggett, R. L. S., III, Mason, G. R., et al.: Combined treatment of cancer of the esophagus. Am. J. Surg., 117:157–161, 1969.

40. Crummy, A. B., Wegner, G. P., Flaherty, T. T., et al.: Azygos venography: An aid in the evaluation of esophageal carcinoma. Ann. Thorac. Surg., 6:522–527, 1968.

41. Holub, E., and Simecek, C.: Pneumomediastinography in carcinoma of the esophagus. Thorax, 23:77–82, 1968.

42. Nordenström, B.: Paravertebral approach to the posterior mediastinum for mediastinography and needle biopsy. Acta Radiol., 12:298–304, 1972.

43. Goodner, J. T., and Turnbull, A. D. M.: Bone metastases in cancer of the esophagus. Am. J. Roentgenol. Radium Ther. Nucl. Med., 111:365–367, 1971.

Chapter Seven

STOMACH

Gerald W. Friedland, M.D.

CLINICAL CONSIDERATIONS

Presenting Signs and Symptoms

About 95 per cent of all gastric malignancies are adenocarcinomas.[1-4] Although their incidence is declining in the United States, they still rank fifth in frequency among all malignant neoplasms. Indeed, the Third National Survey of the National Cancer Institute estimates that 22,900 new cases of gastric carcinoma will occur in the United States during 1975; of these, 14,000 will occur in males and 8,900 in females, giving a male to female ratio of 1.6 to 1.[5] They usually occur in patients over the age of 65 years.[1] Adenocarcinomas at the esophagogastric junction seem to occur more often in males (male to female ratio of 7 to 1) who also have a hiatal hernia, heartburn, and a duodenal ulcer.[6]

Early or superficial gastric carcinoma (carcinoma limited to the mucosa and submucosa),[7-13] first recognized in France and the United States in the mid-1930s,[14-17] is most often diagnosed in Japan today. However, physicians in the United States are now finding this entity with increasing frequency.[18] In Hawaii, for example, Americans of Japanese descent constitute 35 per cent of the population; yet, of the five patients with early gastric carcinoma reported in a Hawaiian series, none were Japanese-American and three were Caucasian.[19]

Other gastric neoplasms comprise only 5 per cent of all gastric malignancies; nearly all are leiomyosarcomas or malignant lymphomas.[1-4, 20, 21] Malignant lymphomas involving the stomach are either of the Hodgkin's or non-Hodgkin's (histiocytic or lymphocytic) variety.[22-24] Most are diffuse in histologic type rather than nodular, and diffuse histiocytic lymphoma is the most frequent type found.[22, 23] Both lymphocytic and histiocytic lymphomas can have a fibrotic stroma, and these are referred to as "desmoplastic."[25-27] Dorfman asserts that most extranodal malignant lymphomas that were previously called Hodgkin's disease are actually examples of histiocytic lymphoma.[28] The term "malignant lymphoma" best describes *both* Hodgkin's and non-Hodgkin's lymphomas.[29] Burkitt's lymphoma involving the stomach rarely occurs in the United States.[30] Other rare primary gastric malignancies include carcinoids, leiomyoblastomas, squamous cell carcinomas, adenoacanthomas, angiosarcomas, and carcinosarcomas.[20, 31-34]

Most secondary gastric neoplasms originate in the pancreas or the colon.[35] Other secondary neoplasms in the stomach are rare; they include malignant melanoma, carcinoma of the breast, Kaposi's sarcoma, and carcinoma of the kidney.[36-41]

Early gastric carcinoma usually causes vague symptoms; as many as 23 per cent of patients have no complaint relative to the tumor.[7] When present, symptoms (in order of frequency) include epigastric pain or "hunger pain" (46 per cent), discomfort or nausea (18 per cent), anorexia (3.2 per cent), and weight loss (0.8 per cent).[7] A cooperative international study found that the most common symptoms occuring *first* were epigastric pain (37 per cent), weight loss (14 per cent), dysphagia (14 per cent), vomiting (12 per cent), anorexia (11 per cent), and weakness (5 per cent).[42]

By the time most patients in the United States consult a physician, the carcinoma has already extended beyond the gastric mucosa and submucosa. At this stage, patients may complain of pain similar to that caused by a peptic ulcer; indeed, as many as one third of patients report that a physician had treated them for an ulcer for three to six months before they underwent a gastric resection. Food and antacids may or may not relieve the pain. Later, nausea, vomiting, and finally pyloric obstruction develop. In the later stages of the disease, weight loss is almost universal. When the carcinoma arises in the region of the esophagogastric junction, the patient will experience difficulty in swallowing as the carcinoma narrows and obstructs the lumen. About one out of four patients complain of either constipation or diarrhea. Because blood continuously seeps from the surface of the neoplasm, most patients eventually become anemic, although few actually experience serious bleeding; when a patient develops serious gastrointestinal bleeding, the usual cause is hemorrhagic gastritis or a chronic peptic ulcer and not a primary or secondary gastric carcinoma.[43] Leiomyosarcomas, however, may cause deep ulcers and may bleed massively.

On physical examination, the physician may elicit abdominal tenderness or palpate an abdominal mass. Adenocarcinoma, leiomyosarcoma, and malignant lymphoma can all produce a palpable mass, but only a localized lymphoma is potentially curable at this stage. Unfortunately, as many as 50 per cent of patients in the United States with a gastric carcinoma already have evidence of metastatic disease by the time they consult their physicians. The clinician should carefully palpate the liver and the left supraclavicular area for an enlarged, hard lymph node (Virchow's node), inspect the skin and accessible mucosa for metastases, ecchymoses, or jaundice, check the skin creases for acanthosis nigricans, and examine the abdomen carefully for ascites and the rectum for adjacent metastases in the pouch of Douglas (shelf of Blumer).

Advanced leiomyosarcomas, carcinomas, and malignant melanomas can also cause free gastric perforation into the peritoneal cavity, and both gastric leiomyosarcomas and carcinomas are prone to form fistulas, particularly between the stomach and colon.[21, 44] Rarely, such fistulas can extend into the pericardial sac, producing pneumopericardium.[45]

No evidence exists to support the contention that benign gastric ulcers are premalignant lesions.[46] Polypoidal carcinomas do not arise from degeneration of adenomatous polyps.[21] However, in some quarters this remains a controversial issue; almost 4 per cent of "gastric polyps" removed by endoscopic polypectomy prove to be carcinomatous.[21, 47] Some authors have stated that as many as 40 per cent of villous adenomas are premalignant,[46] but others have found this figure much too high.[21] Numerous reports suggest that patients with chronic atrophic gastritis are more likely to develop gastric carcinoma than are patients whose gastric mucosa is normal.[48-52] In one study, for example, 363 patients with atrophic gastritis were restudied 11 to 18 years after initial biopsy and gastric secretory tests; 13 per cent of them had developed carcinoma of the stomach.[49] Good evidence exists that patients with pernicious anemia have an increased incidence of gastric carcinoma (Fig. 7–1).[53, 54] Sliding hiatal hernia seems to predispose slightly toward carcinoma at the esophagogastric junction; in one series, 35 per cent of patients with a carcinoma in this region had a hiatal hernia, whereas a hernia existed in only 6 per cent of patients with a carcinoma elsewhere in the stomach.[6] After either a partial gastrectomy or a gastroenterostomy and vagotomy for benign duodenal or gastric ulcer, some patients have developed atrophic gastritis; later, a few of these patients may present with a carcinoma, usually in the region of the stoma.[52, 55-59] Persons with blood type A have a significantly higher incidence of carcinoma (particularly lesions in the gastric antrum) than persons of other blood groups.[60] Some patients with Menetrier's disease also seem prone to develop gastric carcinoma.[61] For a long time, physicians believed that the presence of a duodenal ulcer made the stomach "immune" to gastric carcinoma; this is clearly not true.[6, 62] When patients with a duodenal ulcer do develop carcinoma, it

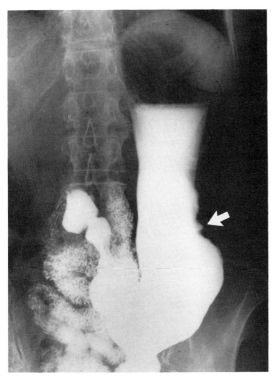

Figure 7–1 Gastric adenocarcinoma (arrow) in a patient with pernicious anemia. The long, thin, tubular stomach that lacks mucosal folds, particularly in the fundus where the folds normally are prominent, is characteristic of pernicious anemia. No metastases were found in the local nodes or the liver at surgery.

may be more likely to occur at the esophagogastric junction.[6]

Differential Diagnosis

Nearly all lesions simulating gastric malignancies are amenable to diagnosis by radiology, gastroscopy, biopsy, or some combination of these techniques.

Reports from different parts of the world give remarkably similar figures for the rate of detection of a gastric lesion of any kind (95 or 96 per cent), and for the percentages of malignancies accurately diagnosed by an upper gastrointestinal series (72 per cent, 79 per cent, 70 per cent).[18, 63, 64] If radiologists repeat equivocal examinations, they can increase the accuracy rate by 10 to 15 per cent.[64] Some physicians treat patients who have an equivocally benign gastric ulcer

with medical therapy for a period of six to eight weeks or longer to determine whether or not it will heal.[14] Unfortunately, benign gastric ulcers, particularly in the elderly, may take a long time to heal, and as many as 12 per cent of ulcerating carcinomas temporarily "heal" completely.[47]

Because they feel surgeons should know if the left hepatic artery arises anomalously from the left gastric artery, some radiologists recommend preoperative arteriography for all gastric malignancies; the surgeon then will not inadvertently sever the left gastric artery, which could infarct the left lobe of the liver.[65] Others, however, are of the opinion that preoperative arteriography adds no further information in patients with gastric carcinoma except when: (1) fundal masses (neoplasm or varices) exist; (2) patients present with gastric hemorrhage; or (3) carcinoid tumors or leiomyosarcomas are suspected.[66, 67]

Radionuclide scans can demonstrate a primary gastric malignancy. Of 27 patients studied using technetium-99m sulphur colloid, a positive gastric scintiphotograph was obtained in 6 of the 8 who had a carcinoma; there was one false-positive.[68] To increase the accuracy of this test the patient must fast, and the examination must be performed in the upright position.[68] It is still too early to determine the specificity of this technique and its practical value. Gallium-67 citrate scans are of no value in the detection of malignant lymphoma of the stomach.[69]

Most patients who have an early gastric carcinoma secrete some acid after Histalog or pentagastrin tests; only one fifth of patients with advanced carcinomas have absolute anacidity.[14, 70] One study suggests that an elevated level of lactic dehydrogenase in gastric juice correlates well with the presence or absence of gastric carcinoma; using this technique as a screening method, 1,534 individuals were examined and 7 cases of gastric carcinoma were discovered, 3 of them early.[71, 72]

Roentgen examination with barium remains the single most important technique for detecting gastric cancer. It is easy and painless to perform and to repeat. However, it cannot show the histologic nature of the lesion, and it often overlooks small lesions on the anterior and posterior walls of the stomach.[8, 73]

Using the newer fiberoptic gastroscopes, endoscopists can now see the whole stomach and can detect lesions invisible or equivocal on a barium study; the instrument also allows biopsy.[73] By spraying barium in the stomach, the endoscopist can see lesions better and take radiographs later.[74] Endoscopy is accurate in 61 to 84 per cent of all cases, with a false-positive rate of 10 to 20 per cent.[47, 75] To the endoscopist, early malignant lymphoma and early carcinoma often look alike.[75] Unfortunately, endoscopy with the new fiberoptic endoscopes and gastrocamera still carries a limited morbidity and mortality rate, as did the procedure performed with the older instruments.[76]

Guided gastrobiopsy, during which the endoscopist takes at least six "bites" of the lesion, and guided cytodiagnosis, during which the endoscopist brushes the lesion to obtain cells, have largely replaced exfoliative cytology of blind gastric washings.[18, 73] This does not mean that exfoliative cytology is a useless procedure; one series gives 81 per cent positive results with antral carcinomas and 93 per cent positive results with carcinomas at the esophagogastric junction; another claims an overall accuracy rate of 95 to 97 per cent.[18, 77-79] Non-directed gastric cytology can detect as many as 74 per cent of malignant lymphomas.[79] On the other hand, guided gastrobiopsy is accurate in 80 to 95 per cent of all cases; there are no false-positives.[47, 73, 81] Endoscopists also have the option of performing a polypectomy, for about 4 per cent of gastric polyps are carcinomatous.[47] The examination is relatively difficult to perform, however, and requires extensive training and expertise. Guided cytodiagnosis has an accuracy of 90 per cent, with 8 per cent false-positives.[18] If physicians perform both guided gastrobiopsy and guided cytodiagnosis in all patients with a known gastric lesion, they will diagnose nearly all gastric carcinomas.[47] Both Japanese and European authors recommend a *combination* of roentgen examination, endoscopy, guided gastrobiopsy, and guided cytodiagnosis for all patients with a gastric lesion.[8, 47, 73] It is important to emphasize that, even with the entire stomach as a specimen, distinguishing between a poorly differentiated adenocarcinoma, or a pseudolymphoma, and a malignant lymphoma can still be difficult.

Therapeutic Decisions and Staging

Two vital factors influence the selection of appropriate therapy: the type of gastric neoplasm and the extent of disease. Gastric carcinoma metastasizes most commonly to the liver (70 per cent), the peritoneum, omentum, and mesentery (43 per cent), the lung and pleura (33 per cent), and the bones (11 per cent).[16] A small percentage metastasize to the skin or the adrenal glands. Carcinoid tumors metastasize most frequently to the draining lymph nodes and to the liver. For reasons that remain obscure, foregut (tracheobronchial and upper gastrointestinal) carcinoid tumors more commonly give rise to osseous metastases than do those arising from midgut structures.[82] The four important places to search for metastases from a stomach tumor, therefore, are the lungs, bones, liver, and the abdominal lymph nodes. Stereo posteroanterior and lateral chest radiographs, supplemented by tomography, will help to exclude pulmonary metastases. At the present time, a technetium-99m polyphosphate bone scan of the entire skeleton is superior to clinical symptomatology, serum alkaline phosphatase determinations, and skeletal radiographs for the early detection of bone metastases.[84] Although sensitive, the bone scan method is nonspecific and false-positives are common.[84] The physician should, therefore, always correlate "positive" areas found on the scan with radiographic and clinical findings.[84]

At laparotomy, the surgeon should document the local extent of the gastric neoplasm, other abdominal extension, and particularly the presence or absence of nodal and hepatic metastases. If the liver contains metastases, if ascitic fluid positive for malignancy is present in the peritoneum, or if the surgeon can see gross implants on the serosa or in the retrouterine or rectovesical pouch, the only possible surgical benefit is palliation. The surgeon should also biopsy clinically negative nodes and liver. If lymphoma is suspected on frozen sections, the surgeon should also consider splenectomy, in addition to extensive nodal and hepatic biopsies. Radiopaque markers should be placed on all biopsied masses and nodes, regardless of whether the frozen sections are positive or negative; this will enable the radiologist to observe the position of the markers (for evidence of tumor growth) during the postoperative period, and may guide the radiotherapist as well.

The need for some kind of practical staging system becomes evident when one studies survival figures. When gastric carcinoma has spread to the regional lymph nodes, the five-year survival rate falls dramatically from 44 per cent to 6 per cent.[63] The overall five-year survival rate is 12 per cent. If the gastric cancer is truly localized when the surgeon resects it, the five-year survival rate increases to 50 per cent.[83] The International Union Against Cancer offers a clinical classification (T) as well as a histologic classification (P) for staging gastric cancer. It recommends use of the histologic classification for tissues that are removed surgically.[85] The American Joint Committee for Cancer Staging and End Results Reporting has also compiled a *TNM classification* that defines the surgical extent of gastric tumors at exploration and subsequent pathologic examination of specimens.[86] In stage IA, the tumor is confined to the mucosa (T1), without node involvement (N0) or distant metastases (M0). In stage IB, the tumor extends to, but not through, the serosa (T2), without involvement of regional lymph nodes (N0) or any remote tissues (M0). In stage IC, the tumor extends through the serosa (T3) without involving regional lymph nodes (N0) or remote tissues (M0). In stage II, there is diffuse involvement of the gastric wall (linitis plastica) (T4), without node involvement (N0) or spread to distant tissues (M0). A neoplasm also is classified as stage II if it involves the gastric wall to any degree (T1 through T4), and has extended to the regional lymph nodes (N1), but has not produced distant metastases (M0). The neoplasm is classified as stage III when it involves the wall of the stomach to any degree (T1 through T4) and has spread to abdominal lymph nodes remote from the tumor (N2), but has not yet metastasized to remote tissues or organs (M0). Any gastric cancer that has spread to distant organs (M1), regardless of the extent of the primary tumor or the status of the regional lymph nodes, is classified as stage IV.

The calculated five-year survival results for gastric carcinomas classified as T1, T2, or T3 (but N0 and M0) is 50 to 90 per cent.[86]

The prognosis for a patient with stomach cancer depends also on how deeply the neoplasm has penetrated the wall; actual size and location of the primary tumor is less important (Figs. 7–2 and 7–3).[86] Unlike the Dukes' classification for carcinoma of the colon, the staging systems for gastric cancer have not yet undergone sufficient trial to prove their clinical usefulness.

Every patient who has a malignant lymphoma should undergo bipedal lymphography. At best, gallium scans will detect gross abdominal node involvement in only 75 per cent of patients with malignant lymphoma, and hepatic uptake obscures a large fraction of the upper abdomen.[69] Gray-scale ultrasonography may occasionally reveal intra-abdominal nodes that are inaccessible to the usual diagnostic methods, but the image resolution is still inadequate. On posterior views, the spine effectively shields many of the lymph nodes, and on anterior views the nodes may be hidden by abdominal gas shadows. Perhaps computerized transverse axial tomography will solve many of these problems in the future.

If gross liver metastases are present, the physician will often discover a large liver, sometimes with a hard, nodular edge, upon palpation. About 20 per cent of patients with liver metastases, however, have no clinical evidence of spread. When gastric carcinomas have metastasized to the liver, liver function tests are altered in the following percentages of cases: serum glutamic oxalacetic transaminase (SGOT), 89 per cent; serum glutamic pyruvic transaminase (SGPT), 88 per cent; lactate dehydrogenase (LDH), 85 per cent; serum alkaline phosphatase, 76 per cent; serum gamma globulin, 62 per cent; serum alpha globulin, 61 per cent; urine urobilin, 59 per cent.[87] Liver radionuclide scintigraphy detects proved hepatic metastases in 89 per cent of cases in which the liver is palpable, and in 75 per cent in which the liver is not palpable; false-negatives occur in 16 per cent and false-positives in 6 per cent.[88] Liver scanning therefore has an accuracy rate too low for use as a routine screening method for metastases in clinically normal livers, unless it is combined with other diagnostic tests.

Newly available gray-scale ultrasonography has proved superior to liver scanning.[89, 90] One series suggests that it is diag-

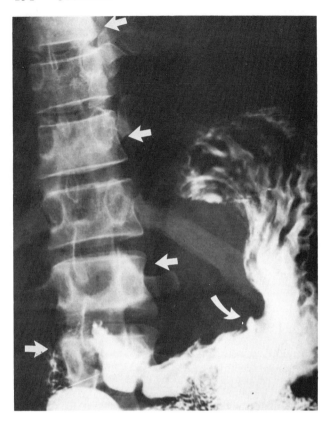

Figure 7–2 Relatively small adenocarcinomatous ulcer on the lesser curve of the stomach (curved arrow); there are already osteoblastic metastases in the vertebrae (straight arrows).

nostic in 82 per cent of all cases, contributory in 10 per cent, and spurious in only 8 per cent, giving an overall accuracy rate of 92 per cent.[89] In addition, it can show nodes in the porta hepatis and possibly may be able to distinguish between malignant lymphoma and other neoplasms.[90, 91]

In one well-controlled series, needle biopsy of the liver with metastases was positive in 45 per cent when performed by the transthoracic route, and in 49 per cent by the subcostal route. When both approaches were used, the total positive yield was increased to 58 per cent.[92]

Peritoneoscopy can help to detect superficial miliary hepatic metastases, as well as metastases between the liver and the diaphragm and serosal excrescences on the mesentery and bowel.[93, 95-97] However, it has not yet achieved a sufficient degree of flexibility to permit visualization and biopsy of all potentially affected intraperitoneal lymph nodes. It will provide the correct diagnosis in about 69 per cent of liver metastases.[96] If used for inspection and biopsy of the liver only, a peritoneoscope with an outside diameter that is considerably smaller than the fiberoptic instrument may

well prove adequate and more comfortable for the patient.[97] When a patient has clear-cut symptoms and findings that suggest the presence of the carcinoid syndrome, the liver usually contains metastases, and the urine will usually have high levels of 5-HIAA.[82] Although some authors find selective arteriography useful for showing the thickness of the stomach wall preoperatively in gastric carcinomas and for determining the presence or absence of nodal and hepatic metastases, others do not share this optimism.[65-67, 98, 99] However, it is undisputed that arteriography clearly depicts the richly vascular metastases from carcinoid tumors and leiomyosarcomas.[65, 99]

Surgery offers the only hope at present for curing gastric carcinoma. Surgeons still do not agree, however, about exactly how much of the stomach should be resected. Whether or not a total gastrectomy is a worthwhile endeavor remains unanswered. Some favor it (Fig. 7–3) for certain specific indications;[63, 100-105] others feel that surgeons will not increase survival rates by extending the scope of gastric resection.[106, 107] A compromise seems to be that if the distal stomach is involved, the surgeon should remove

80 to 90 per cent of the stomach and at least 5 cm beyond the macroscopic extent of tumor; only if the carcinoma involves the fundus, or if linitis plastica is present, should the surgeon consider removing the entire stomach together with the distal one-third of the esophagus.[101] The operative mortality rate for partial gastrectomy is 10 per cent, and for total gastrectomy 34 per cent.[63] The prognosis for localized gastric lymphoma is far superior to that of adeno-carcinoma; resection often results in long-term control, and the overall uncorrected five-year survival is 25 per cent.[108, 109] If necessary, the surgeon can treat gastric malignancy by resecting the spleen, trans-verse colon, and, less successfully, the pan-

creas (body and tail) in contiguity with the stomach. Early postoperative complications may include hemorrhage, acute pancreatitis, peritonitis, intra-abdominal abscess, duo-denal stump fistulas, gastric retention, pul-monary embolism, or pneumonia.

Some physicians treat patients with advanced gastric carcinoma with chemo-therapy and radiation therapy. Only three chemotherapeutic agents (5-fluorouracil, mitomycin, and BCNU) have exhibited clinically significant activity.[110, 111] In one study radiation therapy alone did not pro-duce an objective response; 5-fluorouracil alone, on the other hand, produced an ob-jective response in 17 per cent of treated patients.[112] When patients received both

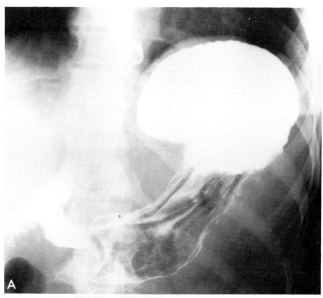

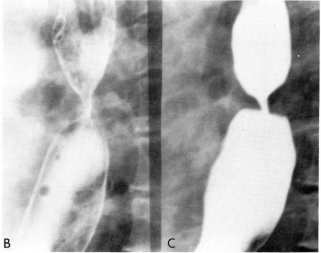

Figure 7–3 *A,* A large adenocarci-noma has produced a classic "apple-core" lesion in the pyloric antrum. The patient underwent a total gastrectomy. Eight years later, the patient developed a benign eso-phageal stricture because of tryptic eso-phagitis (*B* and *C*). There was no evidence of tumor recurrence. (Courtesy of F. R. Ber-ridge, F. R. C. P., Cambridge, England.)

5-fluorouracil and radiation therapy, the objective response rate rose to 55 per cent.[112] In another study, 5-fluorouracil plus radiation proved significantly better than a placebo plus radiation.[113] Many physicians, however, feel that the benefit of this therapy does not outweigh the adverse side effects, especially in an incurable disease, and so do not advise its use.

Recent evidence suggests that patients suffering from inoperable, recurrent, or residual adenocarcinoma of the stomach may obtain palliation from treatment with fast neutrons.[114] The tumor regresses satisfactorily, but the stomach develops dense fibrosis and contracture, with destruction of the mucosa. These patients must therefore undergo gastrectomy four to six months after treatment.[114]

Only if carcinoids of the stomach are under 2 cm in diameter should surgeons excise them locally; otherwise these tumors should be treated like an adenocarcinoma of the stomach (see preceding discussion). Adenoacanthomas require a surgical approach similar to that for adenocarcinomas of the stomach. Since leiomyosarcomas spread through the bloodstream and not by means of the lymphatics, regional lymph node dissection is unnecessary.

Clinical Follow-up

At present, most patients in the United States with gastric carcinoma have advanced disease at the time the diagnosis is made. Consequently, only 12 per cent of treated patients will survive five years.[83] Nevertheless, the physician should make every attempt to detect an early recurrence of tumor, and should re-examine the patient within one month after surgery and at regular intervals thereafter. At each follow-up visit, the physician should perform a complete history and physical examination, and request a complete blood count, posteroanterior and lateral chest radiographs, and an abdominal roentgenogram. If the measured distance between clips placed at the time of surgery increases on the abdominal roentgenogram, this almost invariably indicates tumor recurrence. Every patient should have a routine upper gastrointestinal series one month after surgery to serve as a baseline for future study. This simple precaution can prevent a considerable amount of confusion at a later date, for only by knowing what defects and deformities remain as the result of surgery will the radiologist be able to detect an early tumor recurrence. On the other hand, the physician should not place undue reliance upon the postoperative radiologic findings; all the diagnostic difficulties encountered before surgery become magnified when surgical deformities are present and when the stomach remnant empties rapidly through an enterostomy stoma. Therefore, each patient must also undergo endoscopy postoperatively, supplemented by guided gastrobiopsy and guided cytodiagnosis if the gastroscopist finds a lesion. Unfortunately, most gastric carcinomas recur on the serosal rather than the mucosal surface;[115] the chances of detecting a superficial mucosal recurrence, therefore, remain slight.

Another tool currently used for detecting a recurrent tumor is the serum carcinoembryonic antigen (CEA) determination. Recent evidence suggests that steadily rising values may possibly be helpful for following stomach cancers,[117] but daily serum levels of the antigen may fluctuate by as much as 35 per cent in a given patient.[118]

Following gastrectomy, many patients lose weight and develop diarrhea or the dumping syndrome.[116] Since the portions of the gastrointestinal tract that absorb organic iron and folic acid or produce intrinsic factor may be removed or bypassed, nearly all patients will eventually become anemic if they are not treated with inorganic iron, vitamin B_{12}, and folic acid. Because the surgeon usually resects the vagus nerves, the gallbladder may fail to empty well; the resultant bile stasis causes an increased incidence of gallstones following gastrectomy. Postoperative afferent loop syndromes and blind loop syndromes may also prove troublesome. In a Billroth II (gastrojejunal) anastomosis, food may leave the stomach and proceed down the small bowel before pancreatic and biliary secretions from the duodenal remnant can "catch up" and mix with it. Malabsorption may result; its well-known signs and symptoms include osteomalacia and bone pain. Patients who have undergone a Billroth I gastrectomy are less likely to develop nutritional and postprandial problems, but if the carcinoma arises in the gastric antrum—a frequent occurrence—the surgeon is obliged to remove the duodenum and to perform a Billroth II procedure.

When surgeons perform a total gastrectomy and remove the lower end of the esophagus, they are also excising the vestibular sphincter—the only truly effective antireflux mechanism in this area.[119, 120] Pancreatic juices can therefore gain free access to the esophagus, erode the mucosa, and cause an esophageal stricture (tryptic esophagitis) (Fig. 7–3). To prevent this, surgeons have now devised techniques to increase the distance between the esophagus and the pancreatic duct orifice.

The physician should carefully observe all patients who have potentially premalignant conditions.[121] Endoscopic polypectomy has now become a routine procedure, thereby eliminating the need to follow many gastric polyps. Physicians should continue to observe all patients who have had multiple polyps, however, because an early cancer can lurk between the polyps or develop at a later date. Because patients who have the Peutz-Jeghers syndrome or the Cronkite-Canada syndrome seem no more prone to develop gastric carcinoma than the general population, no special need exists to follow their polyps. The following groups of patients with benign disease require an annual investigation: (1) all patients who have undergone previous gastrectomy or gastroenterostomy; (2) all patients with pernicious anemia or absolute anacidity, and all members of a family with pernicious anemia; (3) all patients with Menetrier's disease.

Some surgeons advise "second-look surgery" in suspected recurrences of cancer of the stomach. The chance for prolonging survival is small, but patients may obtain relief of symptoms from a palliative procedure.[122]

RADIOLOGIC CONSIDERATIONS

Presenting Radiographic Signs

On occasion, the radiologist will diagnose a neoplastic mass projecting into the gastric fundus on an ordinary chest radiograph, or recognize a thick-walled stomach or a tumor mass on a plain abdominal radiograph.[123] Mucinoid adenocarcinomas and gastric leiomyomas may calcify and thereby become visible on non-contrast plain films.[123, 124] Very rarely, gastric carcinomas may present with pneumopericardium (see above), and gastric carcinomas, leiomyosarcomas, and metastatic melanomas in the stomach may perforate, producing pneumoperitoneum.[21, 45]

During an upper gastrointestinal series, most radiologists take multiple views of the stomach.[125] *Mucosal pattern views* with small amounts of barium may show lesions that are obscured when the stomach is filled completely with barium, but views are also taken of the *barium-filled stomach*. Many radiologists now favor dilute-barium, high-kilovoltage techniques over the previously used dense-barium low-kilovoltage techniques (which tend to obscure nodular filling defects in the filled stomach). *Air-contrast studies* of the stomach have been used by radiologists for almost 65 years,[126] and have recently undergone many refinements,[127-130, 151] especially in Japan. Some radiologists do not use this method routinely, but reserve it for second studies of difficult or equivocal lesions.[63] One-sixth grain of morphine intramuscularly will increase gastric peristalsis, enabling the radiologist to assess suspiciously rigid areas in the gastric wall.[61]

When the gastric cancer has spread in the mucosa but no deeper than the submucosa, it clearly merits the title "early," for appropriate surgery at this stage will cure 95 per cent of patients.[7, 8, 11, 13] Japanese physicians classify early gastric carcinoma into three morphologic types. Type I is called *protruded,* and includes pedunculated polyps with malignant change and polypoid cancers. Type II is termed *superficial;* there is no significant protrusion or ulceration. In type IIa the lesion is slightly elevated; a IIb lesion is flat; and a IIc lesion is slightly depressed or eroded. In type III the lesion is *ulcerated.* Japanese radiologists most commonly are able to diagnose types IIc and III. A shallow ulcer (type IIc or III) is the most common radiographic feature of early gastric cancer; frequently, this presents as an irregular erosion with deeper central ulceration. The mucosal folds adjacent to the ulcer terminate abruptly and often have clubbed ends.

Advanced malignant gastric neoplasms can become ulcerated and may also infiltrate the stomach wall (producing large polypoidal masses), may form fistulas, or can displace the stomach. Each of these gross forms produces rather characteristic radiologic findings.[61, 132] Malignant gastric ulcers have no specific characteristics with regard to their size, location, or number. They can vary in size from tiny to huge, and they can arise anywhere in the stomach. Multiple gastric ulcers, however, do suggest the presence of malignant lymphoma or metastases rather than carcinoma or leiomyosarcoma.

Radiologists always attempt to view any ulcer in at least two projections: in profile and face-on. When viewed in profile, an ulcer is seen as a constant projection from the barium-filled gastric lumen. Looking at an ulcer face-on is rather like looking down on a volcanic crater from above; the term "ulcer crater," therefore, appropriately describes its appearance. By rotating the patient on the table, the radiologist can view fluoroscopically any ulcer in the fundus or body of the stomach and in the lesser and greater curve of the antrum in profile, obliquely, and face-on. However, it is technically difficult for the radiologist to see ulcers on the anterior and posterior walls of the antrum in direct profile, even when the radiographic tube is angled cephalad or caudad.

Practically speaking, the most difficult roentgenographic problem in this area is the differentiation of benign from malignant gastric ulcers. When one examines the projection of a malignant gastric ulcer in profile, it has a rather characteristic appearance (Fig. 7–4). It appears to penetrate into a tumor mass, and hence appears as a projection from the barium-filled lumen; however, because the original tumor mass itself protrudes into the stomach, the ulcer rarely projects in profile beyond the expected contours of the lumen. Exceptions to this rule include rare, deep, penetrating malignant ulcers, as well as those cases in which an *infiltrative* gastric carcinoma has undergone peptic ulceration. Usually, the malignant ulcer does not lie exactly in the center of the tumor mass, and the floor of the ulcer is often irregular; its margins are also irregular and nodular, as opposed to a benign gastric ulcer. Although the width of a carcinomatous ulcer often exceeds its depth, the reverse is often true for ulcers in leiomyosarcomas and malignant lymphomas. Because the neoplastic mass surrounding a carcinomatous ulcer protrudes like a wart into the gastric lumen, the white intraluminal barium seen on a radiograph may cease abruptly at the

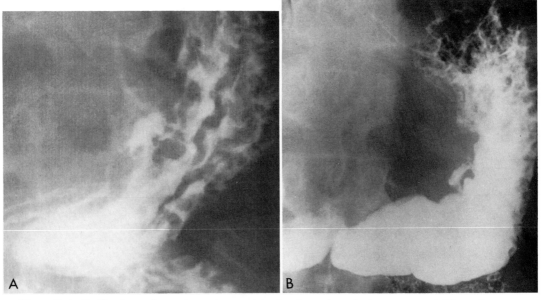

Figure 7–4 Profile views of a carcinomatous gastric ulcer located on the lesser curve. *A,* Mucosal-pattern spot film. The ulcer in the center of the film has an irregular floor, its width exceeds its depth, and irregular mucosal folds radiate towards its nodular edge. *B,* When the stomach is distended with barium, the defect in the lesser curvature of the stomach caused by the well-defined, irregular, angular neoplastic mass (within which the ulcer is embedded) becomes evident.

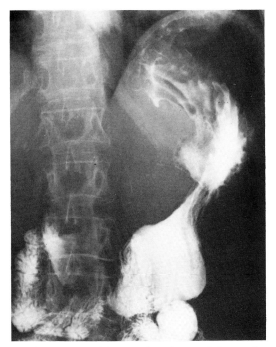

Figure 7–5 Malignant lymphoma. A huge ulcer lies within a large, rather smooth mass on the lesser curvature.

margin of the neoplasm. Although ulcerated gastric lymphomas and leiomyosarcomas can look exactly like carcinomas,[132-136] more often the tumor mass tapers smoothly toward the normal gastric wall (Figs. 7–5 and 7–6). Gastric carcinomas tend to be more angular at their margins; both lymphomas and leiomyosarcomas also often form large extramural soft tissue masses (Fig. 7–6). The radiologist can distinguish between intramural and extramural masses: defects in the gastric barium column whose centers seem to lie within or outside the projected luminal contour of the stomach are likely to be intramural or extramural masses, respectively.[135]

When viewed face-on, a malignant gastric ulcer often has an irregular, angular margin (Fig. 7–7). Stellate mucosal folds may radiate toward this margin and then terminate, but their ends usually expand to form irregular nodules. The wart-like neoplastic mass surrounding the ulcer is seen to create a well-defined, irregular, lucent rim when the radiologist compresses the stomach (Fig. 7–8). Multiple malignant ulcers are most likely to be lymphoma or

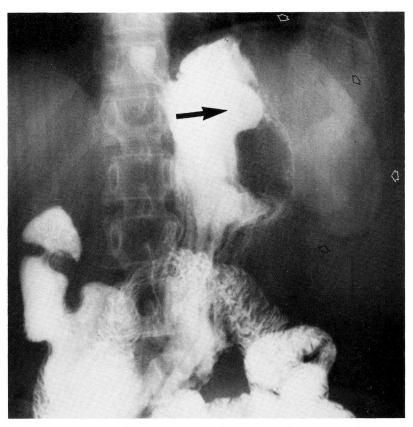

Figure 7–6 Leiomyosarcoma. A large mass projects into the gastric lumen and also extends laterally into the soft tissues (small open arrowheads). A huge ulcer lies within the mass (large straight arrow).

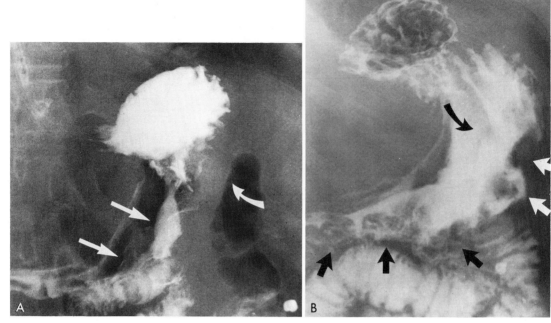

Figure 7–7 Malignant lymphoma. *A,* Supine, mucosal pattern view. An ulcer that has an irregular, angular outline is seen face-on (upper straight white arrow). Air outlines part of the irregular, barium-coated mass within which the ulcer lies (lower straight arrow). The extragastric component of the mass impresses on the air-filled colon (curved arrow). *B,* In the prone position, barium partially obscures the ulcer (curved black arrow), but multiple polypoidal filling defects come into view (straight arrows).

metastatic melanoma, and sometimes each ulcer surrounded by an equal mass of neoplasm assumes the appearance of a "bull's-eye" lesion (Fig. 7–9).[41] This bull's-eye appearance also may occur in leiomyosarcoma and in the rare carcinoid tumors and Kaposi sarcomas of the stomach.

When viewed in profile, carcinomatous

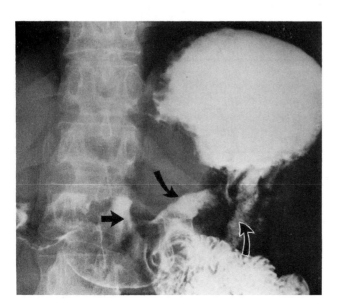

Figure 7–8 Carcinomatous ulcer (upper curved arrow). The ulcer appears angular, and a well-defined mass (straight arrow and lower curved arrow) surrounds the ulcer. The pathologist interpreted the frozen sections as indicating a benign ulcer, so a simple partial gastrectomy was performed. Subsequent permanent sections showed an adenocarcinoma.

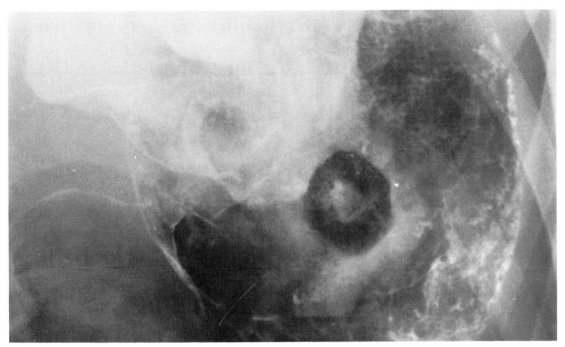

Figure 7–9   Malignant lymphoma. "Bull's-eye" lesion. (From Harell, G., Dunnick, R., and Parker, B.: Multiple bull's-eye lesion in lymphoma. Am. J. Roentgenol., in press, 1976.)

gastric ulcers may exhibit a feature known as the meniscus sign (Carman's sign). The ulcer itself assumes a meniscoid shape, the convexity of the meniscus facing the gastric wall, and its concavity facing the gastric lumen. In the antrum, however, the concavity may face the gastric wall and the convexity the lumen (Fig. 7–10).

In about 10 per cent of cases, mucus, food, blood, or necrotic tissue fills the ulcer, so that barium will not adhere to its walls. In these circumstances and when the patient is obese, the radiologist may fail to detect a small malignant ulcer.

Malignant neoplasms that infiltrate the gastric wall often elude detection. If a neoplasm contains a significant amount of fibrous tissue, it will stiffen the gastric wall and become manifest as an area of rigidity on an upper gastrointestinal series. On the other hand, if an infiltrating neoplasm is soft and pliable (like some malignant lymphomas) the radiologist may fail to detect it even if it has spread widely. The esophagogastric junction and the gastroduodenal junction do not provide barriers to neoplastic spread.[152] A gastric carcinoma, for example, may spread beneath the submucosa up the wall of the esophagus, where it may simulate a benign stricture (Fig. 7–11; see also Chapter 6).

During fluoroscopy, the radiologist observes the stomach carefully to detect areas of rigidity. Such areas can become apparent in various ways. Gastric peristalsis may skip one segment of the gastric wall; a rigid segment may also appear abnormally straight (straight outlines in the stomach, as in Figure 7–10, are abnormal until proved otherwise). The infiltrated segment may see-saw with peristaltic waves like wood floating upon the ocean.[14] If the area of rigidity completely encircles the stomach, barium may pour into the duodenum as if the stomach were a metal pipe; the more extensive the neoplasm, the more marked is this particular feature. When the neoplasm infiltrates the entire stomach (linitis plastica), the resultant rigid, small, narrow stomach is often referred to as a "leather-bottle stomach." Desmoplastic neoplasms also may narrow the luminal caliber (Fig. 7–12). When this occurs in the pylorus, the neoplasm may obstruct the gastric outlet. A rigid neoplasm that encircles part of the body of the stomach can cause a local, broad, shallow constriction; this is then referred to as an "hour-glass stomach." Softer neoplasms, on the other

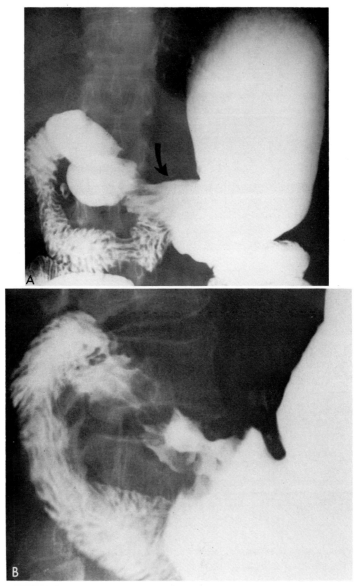

Figure 7–10   Adenocarcinoma of the pyloric antrum. *A,* Barium-filled stomach. The superior edge of the pyloric antrum appears straight (curved arrow); such appearance is always abnormal. *B,* When external compression is applied, a prepyloric ulcer with a characteristic meniscus sign (Carman's sign) appears (see text).

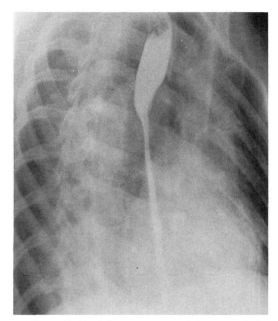

Figure 7-11 Adenocarcinoma of the stomach that has spread up the esophagus beneath the mucosa and has produced a long, smooth esophageal stricture.

hand (particularly some lymphomas), may actually widen the luminal caliber.

Malignant neoplasms usually thicken the gastric wall (Figs. 7-13, 7-14) in addition to altering its pliability. In infiltrating the stomach, they may thicken the wall, the gastric folds, or both.[61] Because the serosal and omental fat that surrounds the stomach may cast a lucent shadow on a radiograph, the radiologist can often measure the actual thickness of the gastric wall between the barium-filled lumen and the lucent serosal fat line. Until proved otherwise, the radiologist should consider that a gastric wall thicker than 1 cm results from neoplastic infiltration.[35] The area of thickening may protrude into the gastric lumen like a rigid plaque. Malignant lymphomas and carcinomas as well as some benign conditions may thicken the gastric folds. Ragged-appearing, generally thickened folds are nonspecific, but multiple, thick, intersecting, arcuate segments producing scalloped inner stomach contours are nearly always caused by a malignant lesion.[35] Although the radiologist may find that neoplastic thickened folds are less pliable than normal, malignant lymphomas may be soft in consistency and need not necessarily stiffen the folds. Characteristically, in the

presence of a neoplasm barium clings well to the enlarged folds and the stomach does not contain either excess fluid or mucus.[133]

Any malignant gastric tumor can present as one or more nodular filling defects. On mucosal pattern views with small amounts of barium, carcinomas usually cause multiple round or oval, firm filling defects. If the radiologist applies compression to the barium-filled stomach or uses the dilute-barium, high-kilovoltage technique (Fig. 7-15), the nodules again can be recognized as round or oval filling defects within the barium-filled lumen when seen face-on; when seen in profile, they produce semicircular scalloped defects in the stomach margin. On barium-air contrast studies, barium coats the nodules, which then project into, or are silhouetted in, the air-filled lumen. Polypoidal masses near the esophagogastric junction frequently invade, narrow, and finally obstruct the distal esophagus (Fig. 7-17). Often the radiologist will recognize a polypoidal defect at the esophagogastric junction when the patient takes his first

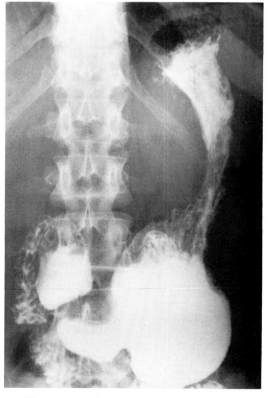

Figure 7-12 A gastric carcinoma has narrowed the lumen of the upper two thirds of the stomach.

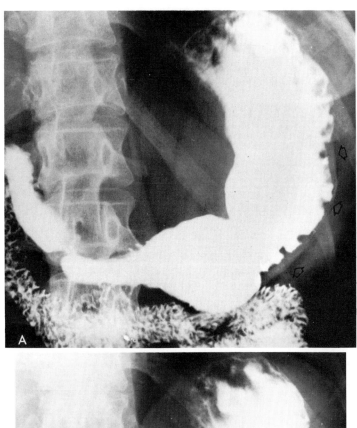

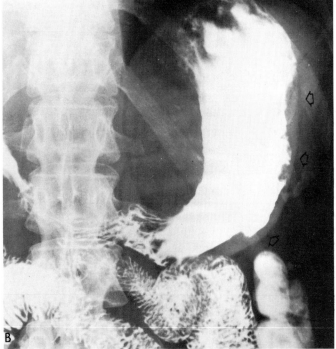

Figure 7–13   Gastric adenocarcinoma. *A,* The neoplasm has thickened the gastric wall along the greater curvature (open arrows). The radiologist did not recognize this. *B,* One year later, the gastric wall has increased considerably in thickness (open arrows), and the infiltrating neoplasm has destroyed the mucosa of the upper two thirds of the stomach, producing an irregular nodular outline.

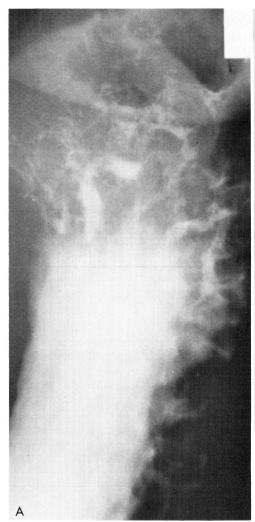

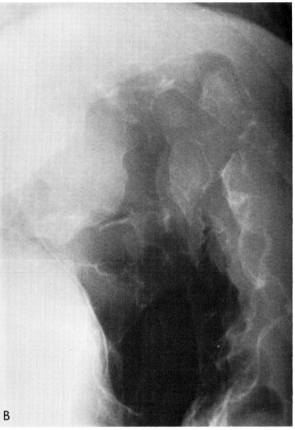

Figure 7–14 Malignant lymphoma. *A,* Initial study. The radiologist noted large, serpiginous gastric folds and recommended a repeat study after a short interval. *B,* Six months later, the folds have increased dramatically in size and have assumed a scalloped appearance. (Courtesy of George Harell, M. D., Stanford University.)

swallow of barium in the upright position: instead of pouring from the esophagus into the stomach in a smooth, steady stream, the barium splits or fragments, like water splashing on a jagged rock. If the radiologist then places the patient in the left-anterior-oblique (LAO), 30 to 60° upright position, the mass, hanging into the now *air*-filled gastric fundus, will stand out in sharp focus (Fig. 7–17).[9] Likewise, in the supine or LAO-Trendelenburg (head-down) positions, the mass projects as a filling defect into the *barium*-filled fundus (Fig. 7–18).[9] Polypoidal carcinomas of the distal stomach, like infiltrating carcinomas, may convert the pylorus into a rigid conduit that permits the barium to pour unimpeded by the pyloric sphincter mechanism into the small bowel.

On a radiograph, gastric fistulas are characterized by barium-filled tracts that extend outside the lumen. Their presence also may be deduced, for instance, when the colon fills before barium has entered the cecum. Sometimes, only a barium enema will outline a gastrocolic fistula. Gastric carcinomas, leiomyosarcomas, malignant lymphomas, metastatic melanomas, and transverse colon carcinomas spreading to the stomach can all form such fistulas.

Extraluminal malignant neoplasms can also alter the appearance of the stomach. A leiomyosarcoma in the stomach wall may remain entirely extraluminal. Both a carcinoma of the pancreas and a carcinoma of the colon can invade the stomach directly.[35] A carcinoma of the body or of the tail of the pancreas, for instance, can invade the upper posterior wall or the greater curvature

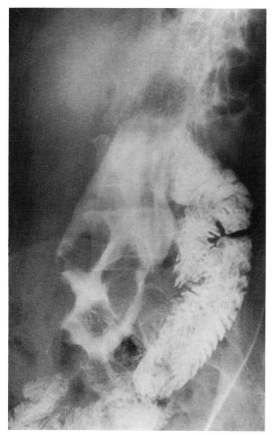

Figure 7–15 Polypoidal gastric carcinoma. Steep oblique view of the stomach using the dilute barium, high kilovoltage technique. Huge polypoidal masses within the barium-filled stomach overlie the right iliac wing and the lumbosacral spine.

cinoma of the breast develops an apparent linitis plastica, the most likely diagnosis is extensive peritoneal implantation.[35]

Differential Diagnosis

The most common problem confronting the radiologist in the diagnosis of stomach lesions is the differentiation of benign and malignant gastric ulcers.[136-139] Both the appearance of the ulcer itself and the character of the surrounding tissue differ in the two diseases (see also the preceding section). When viewed in profile, a smooth ulcer that projects beyond the gastric lumen is usually benign, although exceptions do occur. Benign ulcers frequently undermine the mucosa, and the overhanging mucosal edge is often visible as a thin, well-defined, transverse line at the mouth of the ulcer when shown in profile—the "Hampton line." When this overhanging edge is edematous, it forms a thicker collar of tissue—the ulcer collar. With rare exceptions, the presence of the Hampton line and the ulcer collar also indicates that the ulcer is benign.

When viewed face-on, the margins of

of the stomach. A carcinoma of the tail of the pancreas can deform the gastric wall and displace the stomach forward. If it invades the stomach, it will fix or tether the wall, thicken the gastric rugae, and finally ulcerate into the lumen. Carcinoma of the head of the pancreas can displace and deform the distal gastric antrum and pylorus. It can infiltrate the wall, ulcerate into the lumen and obstruct the gastric outlet.[35] Carcinoma of the splenic flexure of the colon can spread to the stomach through the gastrocolic ligament. Initially, it becomes manifest by scalloping and indenting the greater curvature. Later it, too, will frequently ulcerate into the lumen.[35]

Peritoneal implants from carcinoma of the breast may involve the stomach diffusely, or they may remain localized to the fundus or antrum. If a patient with a known car-

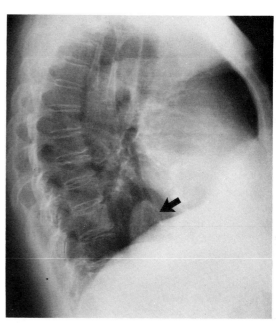

Figure 7–16 Adenocarcinoma of the stomach invading the distal esophagus. Lateral view of the chest. The superior margin of the neoplasm presents as a mediastinal mass (straight arrow).

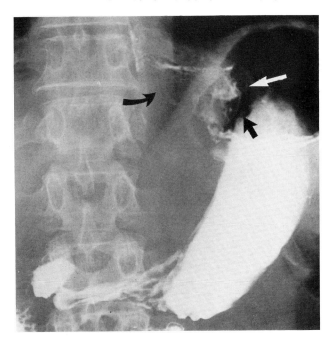

Figure 7–17 Malignant lymphoma at the esophagogastric junction. Patient is prone. A large mass, coated by barium, projects into the air-filled gastric fundus (straight arrows). The neoplasm has also invaded the distal esophagus (curved arrow). An enlarged liver has displaced and stretched the lesser curve of the stomach laterally.

benign ulcers are usually smooth and are round or oval. Malignant ulcers, by contrast, frequently have irregular, angular outlines and nodular edges.

The inflammatory thickening of the gastric wall produced by benign peptic ulcer and the intramural neoplastic protrusions associated with a malignant ulcer can be compared to two common skin lesions — a boil and a wart. An inflammatory lesion, such as a boil, merges gradually and almost imperceptibly into the surrounding normal tissue; a malignant gastric nodule, like a wart on the skin, is delineated abruptly where it joins the normal tissue. When viewed in profile, the inflammatory mass on either side of a benign gastric ulcer slopes gradually and gently and merges imper-

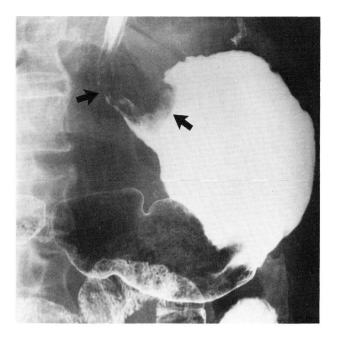

Figure 7–18   An adenocarcinoma of the esophagogastric junction which has invaded the distal esophagus, projects into the barium-filled fundus (arrow). (Courtesy of G. R. Friedland, D. M. R. E. (deceased), Pretoria, South Africa.)

ceptibly into the surrounding gastric wall; the ulcer itself is located centrally within this inflammatory or edematous mass. By contrast, neoplastic tissue projects more sharply into the lumen, and the demarcation between normal and abnormal mucosa is more distinct. Likewise, when seen face-on, the mound of inflammatory tissue around a benign ulcer blends gradually into the normal mucosa, whereas a neoplastic mass has a well-defined rim. Mucosal folds may radiate toward both benign and malignant ulcers, but, unlike the smooth, regular folds around a benign ulcer, folds radiating towards a malignant ulcer are irregular, nodular, and frequently have bulbous terminations at the edge of the tumor mass. When radiologists call an ulcer "definitely benign," they will be correct about 90 per cent of the time.[137] Aberrant pancreas and eosinophilic granuloma in the stomach can produce bull's-eye lesions that simulate those seen in malignancies.[41]

Pseudolymphomas can thicken the gastric folds and can simulate malignant lymphoma or carcinoma.[141] The term "hypertrophic hypersecretory gastropathy" refers to the radiologic, gastroscopic, and histologic hypertrophy of gastric mucosa that may accompany hypersecretion of acid and pepsin (but not necessarily of protein) in the gastric juice.[70] It may occur in patients with gastric or duodenal ulcers or with gastrinomas (the Zollinger-Ellison syndrome), as well as in apparently normal individuals.[70, 142] Patients with hypertrophic, hypersecretory gastropathy characteristically have excessive gastric secretions that make their gastric folds appear to be ill-defined. The enlarged folds themselves usually are relatively inconstant and are readily flattened by palpation.[139] Giant rugal hypertrophy, characteristic of Menetrier's disease, involves the greater curve of the stomach more than other areas.[139] Typically, these patients secrete excess protein but little or no acid in the voluminous gastric juice, although, rarely, they can have both excess protein loss and acid hypersecretion.[70] Excessive gastric mucous secretion in these patients produces characteristic, inconstant linear defects that resist coating by the barium suspension. Gastric polyposis may simulate malignant neoplastic nodules;[21, 121] if the radiologist can identify stalks, however, polyposis becomes the more likely diagnosis.

Gastric varices most often project from the esophagogastric junction, the gastric fundus, and the proximal part of the lesser curve of the stomach. Unlike neoplasms, they usually become flatter or disappear when the fundus is distended with barium or air, and the radiologist can usually demonstrate esophageal varices concurrently on an esophagram.[143, 144]

Defects from redundant mucosa and simulating neoplasms can occur occasionally at the esophagogastric junction in normal individuals, in patients with varices, or as the result of extrinsic compression from the liver or another extragastric mass.[143] Radiographs taken during a barium swallow with the patient lying prone over a bolster, radiographs exposed with the patient in different phases of respiration or lying in various positions, and radiographs taken after distending the fundus with air will usually indicate the nature of the lesion (or its absence). When large, nodular, or serpentine folds are found at the level of the esophagogastric junction extending into the fundus and upper part of the body of the stomach, the radiologist should consider subphrenic abscess or chronic pancreatitis in the differential diagnosis.[144] In pancreatitis, the duodenojejunal flexure is often depressed.[35] Pancreatitis or a pseudocyst sometimes ulcerates through the gastric wall, thereby simulating a malignant neoplasm.[35]

Rarely, Crohn's disease, tuberculosis, actinomycosis, histoplasmosis, sarcoidosis, or eosinophilic granuloma can involve the stomach and simulate a malignant neoplasm.[35, 145] A leather-bottle type stomach may occur rarely in patients with syphilis or amyloid disease,[146] or after the ingestion of large quantities of corrosive materials.

Patients with untreated pernicious anemia may develop an irregular, nodular filling defect on the greater curvature of the antrum secondary to spasm of the antral musculature. Following treatment with vitamin B_{12}, this will usually revert to normal.

Strictures of the gastric antrum following chronic peptic ulceration may simulate antral carcinoma. Benign strictures usually taper gradually and smoothly. Both malignant and benign strictures lack distensibility, but, unlike benign strictures, malignant strictures are so rigid that the lumen never closes completely when the surrounding muscle contracts.[147, 148]

Additional radiologic studies to establish the diagnosis—parietography and arteriography—have largely fallen into disrepute.* Parietography may occasionally save the patient a laparotomy: carbon dioxide (1.0 to 1.5 liters) is introduced through a needle into the peritoneal cavity, and radiographs and tomograms are then made with the stomach distended with air, in the upright position. Confusing *pseudo*-masses, such as a lobe of the liver, spleen, or left crus of the diaphragm, or an abdominal aortic aneurysm, might be elucidated in this way.

Localization and Staging

Gastric cancer can spread within the abdomen in four ways.[115] With *direct invasion,* gastric cancer spreads along the wall of the gastrointestinal tract to involve the adjacent esophagus or the first part of the duodenum, or it may involve adjacent tissues such as the pancreas, liver, and the abdominal wall directly. Frequently, it spreads directly along the greater omentum to involve the transverse colon, and a gastrocolic fistula may develop. Another mode is *lymphatic spread.* Carcinomas from the fundus and upper part of the body of the stomach tend to metastasize to the lymph nodes around the gastroesophageal junction and to lymph nodes at the hilum of the spleen; carcinomas in the lower part of the body and the pyloric antrum tend to metastasize to nodes along the lesser omentum (and from there to the porta hepatis), and to the superior mesenteric nodes. *Bloodstream dissemination* occurs via the portal vein to the liver. *Intraperitoneal seeding* depends upon the dynamics of flow of ascitic fluid: peritoneal implants occur most commonly in the pouch of Douglas, along the lower small bowel mesentery, along the superior border of the sigmoid colon, along the right paracolic gutter lateral to the cecum and ascending colon, and in the ovaries.[149] Malignant lymphomas in the stomach secondarily involve the local nodes, liver, and spleen. Leiomyosarcomas, on the other hand, rarely metastasize to the draining lymph nodes but do tend to form peritoneal implants or to spread via the bloodstream.

Posteroanterior and lateral chest radiographs and full-lung tomograms are mandatory in any patient with a malignant gastric neoplasm. Gastric carcinoma can spread from the nodes around the esophagogastric junction to the mediastinal nodes, and thence into the lungs by lymphangitic spread. Alternatively, it can spread via the portal vein to the liver, and from there through the hepatic veins and inferior vena cava to the lungs. The radiologist should, therefore, search for mediastinal and hilar nodal enlargement, pulmonary nodules, and linear interstitial changes in the perihilar regions of the lungs (lymphangitic spread).

In any patient suspected of having a gastric neoplasm, particularly near the esophagogastric junction, the radiologist should give particular attention to examining the distal esophagus. Any nodularity, irregularity, narrowing, or rigidity should be considered tumor extension until proved otherwise. All patients suspected of having a gastric malignancy on an upper gastrointestinal series must also have a full small bowel series at the same time. The radiologist should especially search for evidence of metastatic lesions indenting the duodenal sweep or the small bowel (Fig. 7–19).[149, 150] The radiographic appearance of serosal metastases is described in Chapter 8. In addition, all patients suspected of having a gastric malignancy should also have a barium enema in order to detect tumor extension, which not infrequently occurs by spread through the greater omentum or by peritoneal implants.

Although bone metastases from gastric cancer occur less frequently than metastases to other sites, a metastatic skeletal survey is essential for a complete examination of the patient. Such metastases are almost invariably osteoblastic. When a patient has a malignant lymphoma involving the stomach, bipedal lymphography should be included in the routine examination.

Hepatic angiography is not a sensitive method for detecting metastases from carcinoma of the stomach.[66] Such metastases are almost invariably less vascular than the liver, so that the radiologist must rely on displacement of arteries during the arterial

---

*Goldstein does use arteriography to embolize arteries in patients with bleeding gastric malignancies.[153]

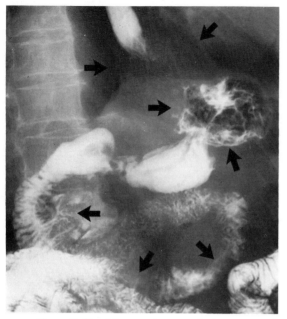

Figure 7–19 Adenocarcinoma of the proximal stomach. The neoplasm has spread into the distal esophagus (upper arrows), and secondary tumor deposits cause impressions on the duodenal sweep and jejunum (lower arrows).

phase and the possible presence of "holes" in the general whiteness of the liver during the capillary phase of the angiogram. In addition, normal hepatic parenchyma may cause defects in the hepatogram that can simulate those of metastases. Consequently, arteriography is not usually considered a routine part of the examination of a patient with gastric cancer. In the rare instances in which a leiomyosarcoma or carcinoid tumor is suspected, however, selective arteriography can be valuable because hepatic metastases from these tumors are usually richly vascularized.[65, 99]

Radiologic Follow-up

All patients should have routine post-treatment chest and abdominal radiographs, as described in the section on clinical follow-up after treatment of the tumor. On the periodic plain abdominal roentgenograms, the radiologist should pay particular attention to any increase in distance between radiopaque surgical clips. Such spreading suggests that recurrence has developed or that known residual tumor is growing.

The treating physician should refer every patient who has had gastric surgery for a gastric malignancy to the radiologist for a baseline upper gastrointestinal examination four weeks after surgery. It cannot be stressed too strongly that this simple precaution may prevent a considerable amount of confusion at a later date. The radiologist should take great care not to "flood" the stomach remnant and small bowel initially with barium, since overlapping loops may obscure the surgical anastomosis. Mucosal pattern studies with compression, and barium-air contrast studies of the anastomosis will often reveal defects that are difficult to see when large amounts of barium are given. A corollary of this is that the radiologist has to be provided with pertinent clinical information before an examination is undertaken.

The tumor may recur locally, in the regional lymph nodes, or in the adjacent viscera. The radiologic appearance will depend upon whether or not the surgeon has performed a total or a subtotal gastrectomy.[115] When the patient has undergone subtotal gastrectomy, the radiologist should search for signs of local recurrence in the gastric stump (Fig. 7–20) or in the loop of duodenum anastomosed to the stomach (the latter in Billroth I). One of the earliest signs of local recurrence is that part of the wall of the stomach becomes rigid and lacks distensibility.[115] Because the gastric stump so frequently is covered by the rib cage, the radiologist may encounter difficulty in palpating this area adequately to determine the presence or absence of gastric wall rigidity. Maximal filling with barium or air, however, may aid in demonstrating a lack of distensibility. Subsequently, nodules and ulcers may appear either in the gastric stump or in the duodenum near the anastomosis. Sometimes, local recurrence first becomes manifest through a change in size and shape of the gastroenteric stoma. As the recurring carcinoma surrounds the anastomotic stoma, it elongates and narrows it.[115] Therefore, the radiologist should consider a long, narrow, rigid stoma as local recurrence of the tumor until proved otherwise. In these instances, both the gastric stump and the esophagus often become dilated. Recurrence of tumor in the lymph nodes around the esophagogastric junction initially may produce extrinsic pressure defects in this area.[115] Subsequently, the

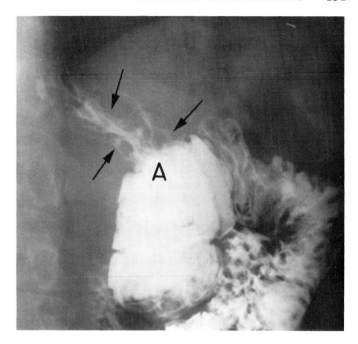

Figure 7–20 Recurrent adenocarcinoma in the gastric remnant (arrows) following Billroth II surgery. A gastrojejunal anastomosis is present (A).

tumor spreads from these nodes into the gastric remnant and may produce a narrow, rigid stomach similar to linitis plastica.[115]

As stated earlier, a tumor can spread to the small bowel and colon through peritoneal implants. A most important site to search for tumor recurrence is in the small bowel afferent loop leading to the gastroenteric anastomosis (Billroth II anastomoses). Recurrence in the afferent loop can occur from tumor within the pancreas itself or from the local lymph nodes. Therefore, the radiologist should always make a careful attempt to fill the afferent loop with contrast medium when studying the postgastrectomy stomach. Tumor recurrence can manifest itself as areas of narrowing or dilatation in the afferent loop.[115] When the pancreas is diffusely involved by tumor, the entire afferent loop may become narrowed.[115]

Enlargement of the liver usually indicates metastatic spread to that organ. Frequently, an enlarged liver will displace the lesser curve of the gastric remnant to the left or will push the stomach backward.[115]

In addition to signs of tumor recurrence, the other well-known complications of complete or partial gastrectomy can occur. These complications can be acute and occur in the early postoperative period, or they may become manifest at any time after surgery.

One example is shown in Figure 7–3, in which a patient developed tryptic esophagitis after total gastrectomy; this eventually resulted in an esophageal stricture.

References

1. Rubin, P.: Cancer of the gastrointestinal tract: Gastric cancer diagnosis. J.A.M.A., 228:883–884, 1974.
2. Palmer, W. L.: Carcinoma of the stomach. In Bockus, H. L. (ed.), Gastroenterology. 3rd ed., vol. 1. Philadelphia, W. B. Saunders, 1974, pp. 949–982.
3. Lowe, W. C.: Neoplasms of the Gastrointestinal Tract. Flushing, N.Y., Medical Examination Publishing, 1972, pp. 70–124.
4. Brandborg, L. L.: Polyps, tumors and cancer of the stomach. In Sleisenger, M. H., and Fordtran, J. S. (eds.), Gastrointestinal Disease. Philadelphia, W. B. Saunders, 1973, pp. 581–604.
5. Third National Survey of the National Cancer Institute. CA, 25:10, 1975.
6. MacDonald, W. C.: Clinical and pathologic features of adenocarcinoma of the gastric cardia. Cancer, 29:724–732, 1972.
7. Doi, H.: Radiologic diagnosis of early gastric cancer. In Radiologic and Other Biophysical Methods in Tumor Diagnosis. Chicago, Year Book, 1975, pp. 245–254.
8. Kawai, K.: Present results in early detection of stomach cancer by radiologic means. In Grundmann, E., Grunze, H., and Witte, S. (eds.), Early Gastric Cancer. New York, Springer, 1974, pp. 82–85.

9. Kobayashi, S., Yamada, A., Kawai, B., et al.: Study on early cancer of the cardiac region. X-ray findings of the surrounding area of the oesophago-gastric junction. Australas. Radiol., *16*:258–270, 1972.

10. Kobayashi, S., Kizu, M., and Kasugai, T.: Gastric acid secretion in relation to gross type of gastric cancer. Am. J. Gastroenterol., *60*:366–371, 1973.

11. Koga, M., Nakata, H., Kiyonari, H., et al.: Roentgen features of the superficial depressed type of early gastric carcinoma. Radiology, *115*:289–292, 1975.

12. Sakita, T.: Endoscopy in the diagnosis of early ulcer cancer. Clin. Gastroenterol., *2*:345–360, 1973.

13. Shirakabe, H., and Ichikawa, H.: Early gastric cancer. *In* Hodes, P. L. (ed.), Tumor Atlas of the Gastrointestinal Tract. Chicago, Year Book, 1973, pp. 277–357.

14. Gutmann, R. A.: Forty years of early diagnosis of gastric cancer. *In* Grundmann, E., Grunze, H., and Witte, S. (eds.), Early Gastric Cancer. New York, Springer, 1974, pp. 69–75.

15. Golden, R.: Diagnostic Radiology. Vol. 3. Baltimore, Williams & Wilkins, 1970.

16. Stout, A. P.: Pathology of carcinoma of the stomach. Arch. Surg., *46*:807–822, 1943.

17. Stout, A.P.: Tumors of the stomach. Armed Forces Institute of Pathology, fasc. 21. Washington, D.C., U.S. Government Printing Office, 1953.

18. Prolla, J. C., and Kirsner, J. B.: Handbook and Atlas of Gastrointestinal Exfoliative Cytology. Chicago, The University of Chicago Press, 1972. pp. 30–47.

19. Raines, D. R., Helman, R. M., and Johnson, L. F.: Early gastric carcinoma in Hawaii. An unusual experience in non-Japanese. Am. J. Gastroenterol., *61*:190–194, 1974.

20. Nelson, R. S.: Malignant tumors of the stomach other than carcinoma. *In* Bockus, H. L. (ed.), Gastroenterology. 3rd ed., vol. 1. Philadelphia, W. B. Saunders, 1974, pp. 998–1017.

21. Marshak, R. H., and Lindner, A. E.: Polypoid lesions of the stomach. Semin. Roentgenol., *6*:151–167, 1971.

22. Dorfman, R. F., and Kim, H.: Relationship of histology to site and to prognosis in Hodgkin's disease and non-Hodgkin's lymphomas. Front. Radiation Ther. Onc., *9*:196–202, 1974.

23. Jones, S. E., Fuks, Z., Bull, M., et al.: Non-Hodgkin's lymphomas. IV. Clinicopathological correlation in 405 cases. Cancer, *31*:806–823, 1973.

24. Kaplan, H. S.: Hodgkin's Disease. Cambridge, Harvard University Press, 1972, p. 169.

25. Bennett, M. D., and Millett, Y. L.: Nodular sclerosing lymphosarcoma. A possible new clinicopathological entity. Clin. Radiol., *20*:339–343, 1969.

26. Millett, Y. L., Bennett, M. H., Jelliffe, A. M., et al.: Nodular sclerotic lymphosarcoma. A further review. Br. J. Cancer, *23*:683–692, 1969.

27. Uribe, A. R., and Rappaport, H.: Malignant lymphoma, histiocytic type with sclerosis (sclerosing reticulum cell sarcoma). Cancer, *29*:946–953, 1972.

28. Dorfman, R. F.: Personal communication, 1975.

29. Lee, Y-T.N., and Spratt, J. S.: Malignant Lymphoma: Nodal and Extranodal Diseases. New York, Grune & Stratton, 1974, pp. 239–244.

30. Ferris, R. A., Hakkal, H. G., and Cigtay, O. S.: Radiological manifestations of North American Burkitt's lymphoma. Am. J. Roentgenol. Radium Ther. Nucl. Med., *123*:614–629, 1973.

31. Cope, V., and Warwick, F.: The role of radiology in the detection of endocrine tumors in the G.I. tract. Clin. Gastroenterol., *3*:621–642, 1974.

32. Lavin, P., Hajdu, S. I., and Foote, F. W., Jr.: Gastric and extragastric leiomyoblastomas: clinicopathologic study of 44 cases. Cancer, *29*:305–311, 1972.

33. Altshuler, J. H., and Shaka, J. A.: Squamous cell carcinoma of the stomach: Review of the literature and report of a case. Cancer, *19*:831–838, 1966.

34. Pack, G. T.: Unusual tumors of the stomach. Ann. N.Y. Acad. Sci., *114*:985–1011, 1964.

35. Ferrucci, J. T., and Janower, M. L.: Localized infiltrating lesions of the stomach. Semin. Roentgenol., *6*:168–181, 1971.

36. Beckly, D. E.: Alimentary tract metastases from malignant melanoma. Clin. Radiol., *25*:385–389, 1974.

37. Pomerantz, H., and Margolin, H. N.: Metastases to the gastrointestinal tract from malignant melanoma. Am. J. Roentgen. Radium Ther. Nucl. Med., *88*:112–117, 1972.

38. Appel, M. F.: Gastric metastases from breast carcinoma. Am. Surg., *40*:253–255, 1974.

39. Joffe, N.: Metastatic involvement of the stomach secondary to breast carcinoma. Am. J. Roentgenol. Radium Ther. Nucl. Med., *123*:512–521, 1975.

40. Richey, L. E., and Cooley, R. N.: Kaposi's sarcoma: The radiographic manifestations of involvement of the stomach. Gastroenterology, *44*:195–198, 1963.

41. Reeder, M. M., and Cavanagh, R. C.: "Bull's-eye" lesions. Solitary or multiple nodules in the gastrointestinal tract with large, central ulceration. J.A.M.A., *229*:825–826, 1974.

42. Lundh, G., Burn, J. I., Kolig, G., et al.: A co-operative international study of gastric cancer (under the auspices of the International Federation of Surgical Colleges). Ann. R. Coll. Surg. Engl., *54*:219–228, 1974.

43. Lightdale, C. J., Kurtz, R. C., Boyle, C. C., et al.: Cancer and upper gastrointestinal tract hemorrhage. Benign causes of bleeding demonstrated by endoscopy. J.A.M.A., *226*:139–141, 1973.

44. Smith, D. L., Dockerty, M. B., and Black, G. M.: Gastrocolic fistulas of malignant origin. Surg. Gynecol. Obstet., *134*:829–832, 1972.

45. Cramm, R. E., and Robinson, F. W.: Pneumopericardium associated with gastric cancer. Report of a case and literature review. Gastroenterology, *60*:311–314, 1971.

46. Ming, S-C.: Histogenesis and premalignant lesions. J.A.M.A., *228*:886–888, 1974.

47. Classen, M., and Rösch, W.: Gastroscopy, biopsy and cytology in early detection of stomach cancer. *In* Grundmann, E., Grunze, H., and Witte, S. (eds.), Early Gastric Cancer. New York, Springer, 1974, pp. 113–117.

48. Bock, O.A.A.: The relationship between chronic gastritis, gastric ulceration and carcinoma of

the stomach. S. Afr. Med. J., *48*:2063–2066, 1974.

49. Cheli, R., Santi, L., Ciancamerla, G., et al.: A clinical and statistical follow-up study of atrophic gastritis. Am. J. Dig. Dis., *18*:1061–1065, 1973.

50. Crespi, M., Bigotti, A., and di Matteo, S.: Pathogenesis of stomach cancer. *In* Grundman, E., Gruze, H., and Witte, S. (eds), Early Gastric Cancer. New York, Springer, 1974, p. 35.

51. Du Plessis, D. J.: The distribution of gastritis in carcinoma of the stomach. Br. J. Surg., *61*: 521–523, 1974.

52. Skinner, J. M., Heenan, P. J., and Whitehead, R.: Atrophic gastritis in gastrectomy specimens. Br. J. Surg., *62*:23–25, 1975.

53. Kaplan, H. S., and Rigler, L. G.: Pernicious anemia and carcinoma of the stomach. Am. J. Med. Sci., *209*:339–348, 1945.

54. Hoffman, N.R.: The relationship between pernicious anemia and cancer of the stomach. Geriatrics, *25*:90–95, 1970.

55. Carter, T. L., and Martel, W.: Gastric carcinoma following long-term gastroenterostomy. Report of two cases. J.A.M.A., *225*:52–53, 1973.

56. Morgenstern, L., Yamakawa, T., and Seltzer, D.: Carcinoma of the gastric stump. Am. J. Surg., *125*:29–38, 1973.

57. Nicholls, J. C.: Carcinoma of the stomach following partial gastrectomy for benign gastroduodenal lesions. Br. J. Surg., *61*:244–249, 1974.

58. Stalsberg, H., and Taksdal, S.: Stomach cancer following gastric surgery for benign conditions. Lancet, *2*:1175–1177, 1971.

59. Taksdal, S., and Stalsberg, H.: Histology of gastric carcinoma occurring after gastric surgery for benign conditions. Cancer, *32*:162–166, 1973.

60. van Wayjen, R. G., and Linschoten, H.: Distribution of ABO and rhesus blood groups in patients with gastric carcinoma, with reference to its site of origin. Gastroenterology, *65*: 877–883, 1973.

61. Stein, G. N., and Finkelstein, A. K.: The stomach. *In* Hodes, P. J. (ed.), Tumor Atlas of the Gastrointestinal Tract. Chicago, Year Book, 1973, pp. 87–275.

62. Bateson, E. M.: Cancer of the stomach and duodenal ulcer: report of two cases with a discussion of the significance of this rare association. Clin. Radiol., *23*:208–212, 1972.

63. Nielsen, S. A., Amdrup, E., Christiansen, P., et al.: Carcinoma of the stomach. An analysis of 385 cases treated—1955 to 1964. Acta. Chir. Scand., *140*:313–320, 1974.

64. Frik, W.: Early radiologic diagnostics of stomach cancer. *In* Grundmann, E., Grunze, H. and Witte, S. (eds.), Early Gastric Cancer. New York, Springer, 1974, pp. 76–81.

65. Baum, S.: Angiography of localized gastric lesions. Semin. Roentgenol., *6*:207–219, 1971.

66. Eisen, F., and Fischerman, K.: Angiography in gastric tumours. Acta Radiol. (Diagn.), (Stockh.), *15*:193–197, 1974.

67. Wenz, W.: Abdominal Angiography. New York, Springer, 1974, pp. 64, 92.

68. Marsden, D. S., Alexander, C. H., Yeung, P. K., et al.: The use of 99m Tc to detect gastric malignancy. Am. J. Gastroenterol., *59*:410–415, 1973.

69. Adler, S., Parthasarathy, K. L., Bakshi, S. P., et al.: Gallium-67-citrate scanning for the localiza-

tion and staging of lymphomas. J. Nucl. Med., *16*:255–260, 1975.

70. Baron, J. H.: The clinical applications of gastric secretion measurements. Clin. Gastroenterol., *2*:293–314, 1973.

71. Simon, L., and Figus, A. I.: Diagnostic value of determination of lactate dehydrogenase and beta-glucuronidase activity of gastric juice. Correlation with a histologic study of the gastric mucosa. Digestion, *7*:174–182, 1972.

72. Figus, A. I., and Simon, L.: Screening for gastric carcinoma by determination of lactic acid dehydrogenase activity in the gastric juice. Digestion, *7*:266–276, 1972.

73. Debray, C. H., Housett, P., Marche, C., et al.: Diagnosis of stomach cancer today. *In* Grundmann, E., Grunze, H., and Witte, S. (eds.), Early Gastric Cancer. New York, Springer, 1974, pp. 120–125.

74. Suzuki, H., Saito, S., and Nagao, F.: Barium-spray method to improve radiographic and endoscopic views of gastric and duodenal lesions. Gastrointest. Endosc., *19*:125–126, 1973.

75. Seifert, E., Ostertag, H., and Otto, P.: Incidence, localization and accuracy of endoscopy and guided biopsy. *In* Grundmann, E., Grunze, H., and Witte, S. (eds.), Early Gastric Cancer. New York, Springer, 1974, pp. 54–62.

76. Meyers, M., and Ghahremani, G. G.: Complications of fiberoptic endoscopy. Part 1. Esophagoscopy and gastroscopy. Radiology, *115*:293–300, 1975.

77. Schade, R. O. K.: Cytology in early diagnosis. J.A.M.A., *228*:890–891, 1974.

78. Vilardell, F.: Exfoliative cytology in gastric diseases. In Bockus, H. L. (ed.), Gastroenterology. 3rd ed., vol. 1. Philadelphia, W. B. Saunders, 1974, pp. 475–486.

79. Kline, T. S., and Goldstein, F.: The role of cytology in the diagnosis of gastric lymphoma. Am. J. Gastroenterol., *62*:193–198, 1974.

80. Poole, G. J.: A new roentgenographic method of measuring the retrogastric and retroduodenal spaces: statistical evaluation of reliability and diagnostic utility. Radiology, *97*:71–81, 1970.

81. Kasugai, T., and Kobayashi, S.: Evaluation of biopsy and cytology in the diagnosis of gastric cancer. Am. J. Gastroenterol., *62*:199–203, 1974.

82. Grahame-Smith, D. G.: Natural history and diagnosis of the carcinoid syndrome. Clin. Gastroenterol., *3*:575–594, 1974.

83. Axtell, L. M., Cutler, S. J., and Meyers, M. H.: End results in cancer: Report No. 4. National Cancer Institute, National Institutes of Health. Bethesda, Md., Public Health Service, 1972, pp. 47–50.

84. O'Mara, R. E.: Nuclear techniques in skeletal neoplastic disease. *In* Radiologic and Other Biophysical Methods in Tumor Diagnosis. Chicago, Year Book, 1975, pp. 153–165.

85. Committee on TNM Classification. TNM classification of malignant tumors. Geneva, International Union Against Cancer, 1968, pp. 27–29.

86. Staging System for Carcinoma of the Stomach. Chicago, American Joint Committee for Cancer Staging and End Results Reporting, 1971, pp. 1–20.

87. Cederqvist, C., and Nielsen, J.: Value of liver func-

tion tests in predicting resectability in patients with gastric cancer. Acta Chir. Scand., *139*: 656–659, 1973.

88. Watanabe, K., Kawahira, K., and Matsuura, K.: Clinical evaluation of preoperative liver scintography in gastric carcinoma patients. Am. J. Roentgenol. Radium Ther. Nucl. Med., *121*: 720–727, 1974.

89. Taylor, K. W., Carpenter, D. A., and McCready, V. R.: Comparison of ultrasound and radioisotope examination in the diagnosis of hepatobiliary disease. J. Clin. Ultrasound, *2*:264, 1974.

90. Taylor, K. J. W., Carpenter, D. A., and McCready, V. R.: Grey scale echography in the diagnosis of intrahepatic disease. J. Clin. Ultrasound, *1*:284–287, 1973.

91. Taylor, K. J. W., Carpenter, D. A., and McCready, V. R.: Ultrasound and scintigraphy in the differential diagnosis of obstructive jaundice. J. Clin. Ultrasound, 2:105–116, 1974.

92. Conn, H. O., and Yesner, R.: A re-evaluation of needle biopsy in the diagnosis of metastatic cancer of the liver. Ann. Intern. Med., *59*:63–61, 1963.

93. Berci, G., Shore, M., Danish, J., et al.: The evaluation of a new peritoneoscope as a diagnostic aid to the surgeon. Ann. Surg., *178*:37–44, 1973.

94. Dunnick, R ., Harrell, G. S., and Parker, B.: "Bull's-eye lesions" of the stomach and small bowel. To be published.

95. Sauer, R., Fahrlander, H., and Fridrich, R.: Comparison of the accuracy of liver scans and peritoneoscopy in benign and malignant primary and metastatic tumors of the liver. Scand. J. Gastroenterol., *8*:389–394, 1973.

96. Johri, J. P., and Peschile, C.: Combined peritoneoscopy and liver biopsy in the diagnosis of hepatic neoplasm. Gastroenterology, *63*: 1016–1019, 1974.

97. Ash, S. R., and Manfredi, F.: Directed biopsy using a small endoscope. Thoracoscopy and peritoneoscopy simplified. N. Engl. J. Med., *291*: 1398–1399, 1974.

98. Rösch, J.: Arteriography in the diagnosis of tumors of the liver, spleen, and pancreas. *In* Radiologic and Other Biophysical Methods in Tumor Diagnosis. Chicago, Year Book, 1975, pp. 319–334.

99. Baum, S.: Selective arteriography. *In* Hodes, P. J. (ed.), Tumor Atlas of the Gastrointestinal Tract. Chicago, Year Book, 1973, pp. 360–387.

100. Henrichsen, S., Kronborg, O., and Brenoe, E.: Total gastrectomy for cancer of the stomach. Acta Chir. Scand., *140*:147–150, 1974.

101. Menguy, R.: Surgical treatment of gastric adenocarcinoma. J.A.M.A., *228*:1286–1287, 1974.

102. McNeer, G., Bowden, L., Booner, R. J., et al.: Elective total gastrectomy for cancer of the stomach: end results. Ann. Surg., *180*:252–256, 1974.

103. Paulino, F., and Roselli, A.: Carcinoma of the stomach. With special reference to total gastrectomy. Curr. Probl. Surg., December 1973, pp. 3–72.

104. Murakami, T.: Surgical treatment of gastric carcinoma. *In* Bockus, H. L. (ed.), Gastroenterology. 3rd ed., vol. 1. Philadelphia, W. B. Saunders, 1974, pp. 983–997.

105. Zacho, A., Cederqvist, C., and Pischerman, K.: Surgical treatment of gastric malignancies: a twenty-year series comprising mainly far advanced and high-seated tumors. Ann. Surg., *179*:94–101, 1974.

106. Gilbertsen, V. A.: Results of treatment of stomach cancer: An appraisal of efforts for more extensive surgery and a report of 1,983 cases. Cancer, *23*:1305–1308, 1969.

107. Rahbar, A., Watne, A. L., and Mendoza, C. B., Jr.: Malignant diseases of the stomach. Analysis of 121 patients. Oncology, *28*:313–318, 1973.

108. Hoerr, S. O., McCormack, L. J., and Hertzer, N. R.: Prognosis in gastric lymphoma. Arch. Surg., *107*:155–158, 1973.

109. Connors, J., and Wise, L.: Management of gastric lymphomas. Am. J. Surg., *127*:102–108, 1974.

110. Camis, R. L., and Carter, S. K.: A review of chemotherapy in gastric cancer. Cancer, *34*:1576–1586, 1974.

111. Moertel, C. G.: Chemotherapy. J.A.M.A., *228*: 1290–1291, 1974.

112. Falkson, G., and Falkson, H. C.: Fluorouracil and radiotherapy in gastrointestinal cancer. Lancet, 2:1252–1253, 1969.

113. Holbrook, M. A.: Radiation therapy. J.A.M.A., *228*:1289–1290, 1974.

114. Catterall, M., Kingsley, D., Lawrence, G., et al.: The effects of fast neutrons on inoperable carcinoma of the stomach. Gut, *16*:150–156, 1975.

115. Samuel, E.: Gastric neoplasms. *In* Sutton, D. (ed.), Textbook of Radiology. 2nd ed. New York, Churchill-Livingston, 1975, pp. 735–740.

116. Welch, C. E.: Late effects of gastrectomy. J.A.M.A., *228*:1287–1289, 1974.

117. Holyoke, E. D.: Editor's interview: Present and probable uses of CEA. CA, *25*:22–26, 1975.

118. Raury, M., Moertel, C. G., Schutt, A. J., et al.: Usefulness of serum carcinoembryonic antigen (C.E.A.) determinations during anticancer therapy for long-term follow-up of gastrointestinal carcinoma. Cancer, *34*:1230–1234, 1974.

119. Friedland, G. W., Melcher, D. H., Berridge, F. R., et al.: Debatable points in the anatomy of the lower oesophagus. Thorax, *21*:487–498, 1966.

120. Berridge, F. R., Friedland, G. W., and Tagart, R. E. B.: Radiological landmarks at the oesophago-gastric junction. Thorax, *21*:499–501, 1966.

121. Yamada, T., and Ichikawa, H.: X-ray diagnosis of elevated lesions of the stomach. Radiology, *110*:79–83, 1974.

122. Ellis, H., and Jayasekara, G.: Is "second look surgery" justified in suspected recurrences of cancer of the stomach? Br. J. Surg., *62*:226–230, 1975.

123. Wolf, B. S., and Khilnani, M.: Plain film diagnosis of gastrointestinal lesions. *In* Margulis, A. R., and Burhenne, H. L. (eds.), Alimentary Tract Roentgenology. 2nd ed., vol. 1. St. Louis, C. V. Mosby Co., 1973, pp. 137–171.

124. Myo Lwin, T. O., and Soodeen, T. H.: A case report on calcified mucinous adenocarcinoma of the stomach. J. Can. Assoc. Radiol., *24*:370–373, 1973.

125. Hanelin, J.: Some technical aspects in the demon-

stration of gastric lesion . Semin. Roentgenol., 6:235–253, 1971.

126. Elisher, V. J.: Über eine Methode zur Röntgenuntersuchung das Magens. Fortsch. Röntgenst., 18:322–340, 1911.

127. Balthazar, E., and Rosenthal, N.: Calcifying mucin producing adenocarcinoma of stomach. N.Y. State J. Med., 73:1704–1706, 1973.

128. Kreel, L., Herlinger, H., and Glanville, J.: Technique of the double contrast barium meal with examples of correlation with endoscopy. Clin. Radiol., 24:307–314, 1973.

129. O'Reilly, G. V. A., and Bryan, G.: The double contrast barium meal — a simplification. Br. J. Radiol., 47:482–483, 1974.

130. Gelfand, D. W.: The double-contrast upper gastrointestinal examination in the Japanese style. An experience with 2,000 examinations. Am. J. Gastroenterol., 63:216–220, 1975.

131. Nagoyo, T., and Yokoyama, H.: Early phases and diagnostic features. J.A.M.A., 228:888–889, 1974.

132. Janower, M. D.: Diagnostic radiology. J.A.M.A., 228:892–893, 1974.

133. Ngan, H., and James, K. W.: Lymphoma of the gastrointestinal tract. In Trapnell, D. H. (ed.), Clinical Radiology of the Lymphomas. Radiology in Clinical Diagnosis Series. London, Butterworths, 1973, pp. 107–117.

134. Nelson, R. S., and Lanza, F. L.: Gastroscopic and radiologic patterns in gastric lymphoma. In Radiologic and Other Biophysical Methods in Tumor Diagnosis. Chicago, Year Book, 1975, pp. 255–260.

135. Stein, L. A., and Margulis, A.: The spheroid sign. A new sign for accurate differentiation of intramural from extramural masses. Am. J. Roentgenol. Radium Ther. Nucl. Med., 123: 420–426, 1975.

136. Ichikawa, H.: Differential diagnosis between benign and malignant ulcers of the stomach. Clin. Gastroenterol., 2:329–343, 1973.

137. Goldberg, H. I.: Roentgen diagnosis of ulcerative diseases. In Sleisenger, M. H., and Fordtran, J. S. (eds.), Gastrointestinal Disease. Philadelphia, W. B. Saunders, 1973, pp. 496–506.

138. Wolf, B. S.: Observations on roentgen features of benign and malignant gastric ulcers. Semin. Roentgenol., 6:140–150, 1971.

139. Reeder, M. M., Olmsted, W. M., and Cooper, P. H.: Large folds, local or widespread. J.A.M.A., 230:273–274, 1974.

140. Nelson, S. W.: The discovery of gastric ulcers and the differential diagnosis between benignancy and malignancy. Radiol. Clin. North Am., 7:5–25, 1969.

141. Watson, R. J., and O'Brien, M.T.: Gastric pseudolymphoma (lymphfollicular gastritis). Ann. Surg., 171:98–106, 1970.

142. Zollinger, R. M., and Takeuchi, O.: Surgical treatment of gastrinoma and WDHA syndrome. Clin. Gastroenterol., 3:685–696, 1974.

143. Kaye, J. J., and Stassa, G.: Mimicry and deception in the diagnosis of tumors of the gastric cardia. Am. J. Roentgenol. Radium Ther. Nucl. Med., 110:295–303, 1970.

144. Feinberg, S. B., and Tully, T. E.: Secondary gastric mural abnormalities simulating primary disease in isolated chronic left subphrenic abscess and isolated chronic pancreatitis. Am. J. Roentgenol. Radium Ther. Nucl. Med., 122: 413–418, 1974.

145. Gonzales, G., and Kennedy, T.: Crohn's disease of the stomach. Radiology, 113:27–29, 1974.

146. Cummack, D. H.: Gastro-intestinal X-ray Diagnosis. Edinburgh, Livingston, 1969, p. 75.

147. Berridge, F. R., and Gregg, D. M.: The value of cinematography in the diagnosis of malignant strictures of the oesophagus. Br. J. Radiol., 31:465–471, 1958.

148. Berridge, F. R.: Personal communication, 1963.

149. Meyers, M. A.: Metastatic seeding along the small bowel mesentery. Roentgen features. Am. J. Roentgen. Radium Ther. Nucl. Med., 123: 67–73, 1975.

150. Meyers, M. A., and McSweeney, J.: Secondary neoplasms of the bowel. Radiology, 105:1–11, 1972.

151. Laufer, I., Mullens, J. E., and Hamilton, J.: The diagnostic accuracy of barium studies of the stomach and duodenum — correlation with endoscopy. Radiology, 115:569–580, 1975.

152. Meyers, M. A., Katzen, B., and Alonso, D. R.: Transpyloric extension to duodenal bulb in gastric lymphoma. Radiology, 115:575–580, 1975.

153. Goldstein, H. M., Medellin, H., Ben-Menachem, Y., et al.: Transcatheter arterial embolization in the management of bleeding in the cancer patient. Radiology, 115:603–608, 1975.

Chapter Eight

SMALL BOWEL

GERALD W. FRIEDLAND, M.D.

CLINICAL CONSIDERATIONS

Presenting Signs and Symptoms

Although small bowel tumors are rare, over 90 per cent of small bowel neoplasms are malignant. The Third National Survey of the National Cancer Institute estimates the number of new cases of primary small bowel cancer at 2200 for 1975.[1-4] Because they are rare and because they produce such vague symptoms, most physicians do not consider them in the differential diagnosis when a patient presents with abdominal complaints.

The most common primary malignant small bowel neoplasms detected during life are adenocarcinoma, carcinoid tumor, malignant lymphoma, and leiomyosarcoma.[5, 6] In autopsy series, incidental carcinoids are found more commonly than adenocarcinomas or leiomyosarcomas, because carcinoids do not cause symptoms if they remain localized within the bowel wall.[5] Rare primary malignancies include fibrosarcoma, malignant schwannoma, liposarcoma, and villous adenoma.[7-9]

Malignant lymphomas involving the small bowel are either of the Hodgkin's or non-Hodgkin's (histiocytic or lymphocytic) variety.[10, 11] Only in advanced or recurrent disease does Hodgkin's lymphoma involve the small bowel.[10, 11] Statistically, diffuse rather than nodular histiocytic and lymphocytic lymphomas occur in the small bowel; diffuse histiocytic lymphoma is the most frequent type.[10, 11] Although rare, Burkitt's lymphoma does occur in the United States.[12]

Secondary neoplasms can reach the small bowel in three ways: direct invasion, intraperitoneal seeding, and hematogenous metastases.[13] Intraperitoneal seeding, the most common method, can occur from any intra-abdominal viscus, but frequent primary sites are the stomach and pancreas. True hematogenous metastases usually arise from cutaneous melanomas and carcinomas of the breast, lung, kidney, and cervix.

Common clinical presentations include obstruction, bleeding, loss of weight, palpable mass, and perforation.[2, 4, 14, 15] If these symptoms and signs have existed for a long time, the patient more likely will have a carcinoid tumor or a leiomyosarcoma than an adenocarcinoma, which typically presents with a short history.

Most commonly, malignant small bowel neoplasms produce symptoms because they obstruct the lumen. Symptoms of partial small bowel obstruction are intermittent pain, nausea, and vomiting. As the obstruction becomes complete, the patient's abdomen distends and the vomiting becomes persistent. If the neoplasm ulcerates the mucosa, mild to moderate bleeding may result; this occurs most frequently in patients with leiomyosarcoma, adenocarcinoma, and malignant lymphoma. Leiomyosarcomas also may develop deep ulcers and may bleed massively. Carcinoid tumors, by contrast, rarely bleed. Over two thirds of patients complain of weight loss when

156

first seen. This probably results from anorexia caused by chronic obstruction and ulceration.

In about 40 per cent of cases, the neoplasm is palpable upon physical examination when the patient first seeks medical aid. Sometimes an intussusception may mimic a neoplastic mass on palpation, but this complication occurs much less frequently with malignant than benign neoplasms.[2]

About one out of every ten patients presents with free perforation into the peritoneal cavity.[16] This complication develops most frequently in patients with leiomyosarcomas but can occur with malignant lymphomas and, rarely, with adenocarcinomas; carcinoid tumors, by contrast, usually do not perforate. Leiomyosarcomas perforate most frequently, because they characteristically derive their blood supply from the periphery of the tumor; as the neoplasms grow, they compress the surrounding vessels, become ischemic, undergo central necrosis, and may then perforate.[17]

A patient with a carcinoid or malignant lymphoma may show unusual signs and symptoms. Recent evidence indicates that only 4 per cent of patients with a carcinoid tumor of the small bowel actually develop the carcinoid syndrome, characterized by diarrhea, flushing, and bronchospasm, and less frequently by tricuspid insufficiency and pulmonary valve stenosis.[18, 19] Almost all patients with this syndrome will have liver metastases. Serotonin, catecholamines, prostaglandins, kallikrein, and histamines may all play a role in producing this syndrome.[20, 21] A small number of patients with carcinoid syndrome develop thrombosis of their mesenteric vessels and present with gangrene of the small bowel, a complication that is usually fatal.[22] As many as 30 per cent of patients with carcinoid tumors develop other types of neoplasms, and metastatic carcinoid tumors themselves can be familial.[23, 24]

An association exists between malignant lymphoma and the malabsorption syndrome.[25] At times a malabsorption syndrome may exist before a lymphoma develops; on other occasions, the lymphoma may precede the malabsorption syndrome, although the precise factors leading to this syndrome remain obscure. This association is uncommon, probably occurring in only 6 per cent of cases.[25] A peculiar form of malabsorption syndrome, occurring predominantly in persons of Mediterranean ancestry, is characterized by a diffuse lymphoproliferative infiltration throughout the small bowel. A few of these patients develop a lymphoma, termed Mediterranean lymphoma.[26-29] The lymphoma can develop first in the mesenteric lymph nodes or first in the small bowel.[26] Of those patients who have lymphoma, a few develop alpha-chain disease.[30, 31]

Patients initially afflicted with the Peutz-Jeghers syndrome or, more rarely, multiple intestinal polyposis, Crohn's disease, or celiac disease, may subsequently develop an adenocarcinoma of the small bowel.[32-38] Carcinomas develop in 2 to 3 per cent of patients with the Peutz-Jeghers syndrome.[32] Although an increasing number of reports are accumulating that describe patients with Crohn's disease who develop carcinoma of the bowel, this complication is rare.[33-36] Even bypassed segments are not immune.[34-35] If a patient with Crohn's disease that had been well controlled suddenly deteriorates, or develops anemia or an intestinal obstruction, the clinician should consider this diagnosis.[36, 37]

Differential Diagnosis

Because of the rarity of small bowel neoplasms, radiologists and clinicians are more likely to consider a diagnosis of Crohn's disease, vascular insufficiency, or malabsorptive disease than one of small bowel malignancy in a patient with intestinal complaints. Methods used to arrive at the correct diagnosis include radiologic investigations, biochemical studies, peroral small bowel biopsy, and, more recently, enteroscopy.

With the exception of the few patients who present with intestinal perforation or an intussusception, the physician should refer all patients suspected of having a malignant small bowel neoplasm to a radiologist for a small bowel series using a barium suspension as the contrast agent. Using this technique alone, the preoperative diagnosis is accurate in 53 per cent of cases.[14] In patients presenting with suggestive symptoms but in whom the radiologist has failed to demonstrate a lesion, a retrograde small bowel enema will increase the diagnostic yield.[40, 41] Angiography is useful in patients suspected of having a carcinoid tumor or a leiomyosarcoma;[42–44] the exact indications for this examination are discussed in detail in the section on radiologic considerations.

An isolated case report indicates that radionuclide scanning using technetium-99m sulphur colloid may demonstrate a carcinoid tumor,[45] but in two cases surgically proved at Stanford this method failed to show the lesion; its value, therefore, still remains unclear. Gallium-67 citrate scans are of no value for detecting malignant lymphoma in the small bowel.[46] Severe malabsorption, particularly in a patient of Mediterranean ancestry with jejunal masses, should encourage the physician to search for free alpha-chains in the serum and reduced levels of IgG, IgM, and albumin, which are all characteristic of heavy chain disease.[29]

When a small bowel series shows a diffuse mucosal abnormality, a peroral suction biopsy may provide sufficient tissue to enable the pathologist to distinguish malignant from nonmalignant conditions. The drawback of this method is that it is often difficult to be sure that the biopsy instrument is located in the abnormal segment when the suction is applied.

It has recently become feasible to perform enteroscopy by threading a fiberoptic endoscope over a previously swallowed string, the tip of which is located in the small bowel.[47] Unfortunately, this technique is available only in a few centers at present.

Since virtually all patients in whom these investigations suggest a malignancy undergo surgery, the actual diagnosis is made by examining histologic sections of the specimen. Laparotomy is also indicated for patients in whom the diagnosis remains equivocal or who show signs and symptoms strongly suggestive of a small bowel malignancy, even when all preoperative investigations are negative.

Therapeutic Decisions

Two vital factors influence the selection of appropriate therapy: the type of neoplasm and the extent of the disease.

Leiomyosarcomas, fibrosarcomas, and malignant schwannomas metastasize to the liver and lungs, but usually spare the regional lymph nodes.[7] All other primary small bowel neoplasms spread first to the mesenteric lymph nodes and subsequently to the para-aortic lymph nodes and liver.[7] The three important places to search for metastases, therefore, are the lungs, liver, and abdominal lymph nodes.

Stereo posteroanterior and lateral chest radiographs supplemented by tomography will help to exclude pulmonary metastases. For all practical purposes, only biopsy at laparotomy will enable the physician to determine the exact extent of microscopic tumor invasion within the abdomen — the factor that will most influence treatment and prognosis when the chest radiographs are negative.

At laparotomy, the surgeon should document the local extent of the neoplasm, non-local abdominal extension, and in particular, the presence or absence of nodal and hepatic metastases. The surgeon should also perform a biopsy of the clinically negative nodes and liver. If lymphoma is suspected on frozen sections, the surgeon should consider splenectomy in addition to selective nodal and hepatic biopsies. Radiopaque markers must be placed on all masses and nodes selected for biopsy, regardless of whether the initial frozen sections are positive or negative; this will assist the radiotherapist in placing his treatment fields, and help the diagnostic radiologist to determine whether or not the markers are separating (indicating tumor growth) during the postoperative period.

Although most currently available investigations used for detecting nodal and hepatic metastases prior to the staging laparotomy show only large lesions, many are still useful because they may direct the surgeon's attention to appropriate areas for biopsy. These investigations include bipedal lymphography, radionuclide scanning procedures, gray-scale ultrasonography, laparoscopy, arteriography, and transverse axial tomography.

Although bipedal lymphography is mandatory for every patient who has a malignant lymphoma, it has not proved useful for detecting nodal metastases from other small bowel malignancies. At best, gallium scans will detect gross nodal involvement in only 75 per cent of patients with malignant lymphoma,[46] and hepatic uptake obscures a large portion of the upper abdomen. These scans are no longer used at Stanford for detecting lesions below the diaphragm. Gray-scale ultrasonography may occasionally uncover abdominal nodes (mesenteric, suprarenal, infradiaphragmatic) inaccessible to the usual diagnostic examination,[48, 50] but, when used for this purpose, it also suffers serious limitations. The resolution is still inadequate; on posterior views, the spine effectively shields the lymph nodes, and, on anterior views, the nodes may hide behind abdominal gas shadows. Perhaps computerized axial tomography for the whole body, now under development, will solve many of these problems in the future.

Determining the best means to detect liver metastases before surgery still remains a challenge. If gross liver metastases are present, palpation by the physician will often reveal a large liver, sometimes with a hard, nodular edge. About 20 per cent of patients with metastases have no clinical evidence of metastases to the liver, however.[51] If the fractionated lactic acid dehydrogenase, serum alkaline phosphatase activity, and fractionated serum bilirubin concentration are normal, the presence of metastatic hepatic tumor is unlikely.[52] In one well-controlled series, blind needle biopsy of the liver by the transthoracic route was positive in 45 per cent of cases, and biopsy by the subcostal route was positive in 49 per cent. When both were done, the total positive yield was increased to 58 per cent.[51] When a patient has symptoms suggesting a diagnosis of carcinoid syndrome, the liver usually contains metastases, and the urine will usually have high levels of 5-HIAA.[53]

The real problem arises when one tries to detect metastases that are very small, or when few deposits exist. Routine radionuclide liver scanning (using technetium or indium) has proved disappointing. Before metastases from intra-abdominal malignancies become visible, the lesions have already attained a diameter of 2 to 3 cm.[54] A recent report gives the overall accuracy rate as 84 per cent; there were 13 per cent false-positive and 23 per cent false-negative results.[55] Only if it is used in combination with some other technique, such as peritoneoscopy, ultrasonography, or arteriography, does liver scanning provide clinically useful information.[55] When used specifically to detect lymphomatous infiltration of the liver, the diagnostic accuracy rate of gallium scans is only 48 per cent.[46]

Conventional ultrasonography seems even less accurate than radionuclide scanning in the liver; gray-scale ultrasonography, however, has proved far superior to radionuclide scanning.[56, 57] One series suggested that it was diagnostic in 82 per cent of cases, contributory in 10 per cent, and "spurious" in 8 per cent, giving an overall accuracy rate of 92 per cent.[57] In addition, it can show nodes in the porta hepatis and may possibly be able to distinguish between malignant lymphoma and other neoplasms.[56, 58]

Laparoscopy—insertion of a fiberoptic endoscope through a tiny abdominal incision—can help to detect superficial miliary hepatic metastases, as well as metastases between the liver and the diaphragm and tumor excrescences on the bowel.[59-61] However, endoscopy has not yet achieved a sufficient degree of flexibility to permit visualization and biopsy of all the affected abdominal lymph nodes. Realistically, it will provide the correct diagnosis in about 69 per cent of individuals with liver metastases.[61] If it is to be used for biopsy and endoscopy of the liver only, an endoscope with an outside diameter that is considerably smaller than the fiberoptic instrument may prove to be more comfortable for the patient.[62]

Since the richly vascular carcinoid tumors and leiomyosarcomas comprise a high proportion of primary small bowel neoplasms, angiography holds the greatest promise at present for detecting liver metastases 0.5 to 1 cm in size.[42, 43, 63-65] Although angiography may well be the most accurate method currently available,[65] it is expensive to use as a screening procedure and it is an invasive technique. For these reasons, its use still remains limited in most institutions to specific indications given in the section on localization and staging.

Since most malignant small bowel tumors cause symptoms by partially or completely obstructing the intestine, surgical excision of the tumor and the draining mesenteric nodes will usually provide at least temporary relief of symptoms.[15, 66] Radical surgery for carcinoids may be helpful even when they have metastasized to the liver.[15, 67] Leiomyosarcoma invades locally but does not metastasize to regional lymph nodes, making lymph node dissection un-necessary.[17] Common postoperative com-plications include reobstruction from edema or stenosis at the anastomosis, anastomotic leak, and postoperative adhesions. The pa-tient can expect a favorable outcome in cases of lymphoma in stages I and II[66] and in intra-mural malignant carcinoid tumors.[68] Exten-sive small bowel disease, such as can occur in infiltrative lymphoma, precludes surgical therapy; only chemotherapy and radiation therapy will then ameliorate the patient's symptoms. Radiation therapy or chemo-therapy may also be useful for metastatic carcinoid tumors.

Clinical Follow-up

No matter what form of therapy is used, the physician should carefully evaluate the patient at least one month after the start of therapy and again at the following inter-vals: in the first year, every two months; second year, every three months; third year, every four months; fourth year, every five months, fifth year, every six months; and sixth year and thereafter, annually. This schedule should of course remain flexible; the patient should feel free to consult the physician at any time should symptoms de-velop.

Examinations at these times should include at least a complete history and physi-cal examination, complete blood count, posteroanterior and lateral chest radio-graphs, and an abdominal radiograph if the patient has undergone lymphography and still has contrast medium within the nodes. The purpose of this follow-up is to determine whether or not the primary tumor has re-curred, or whether metastases have de-veloped or known metastases regressed. The patient may also develop complications at predictable intervals, resulting from the therapy used—surgery, radiation therapy, chemotherapy, or any combination of these modalities.

The patient's physician should always request a routine small bowel series one month after surgery to serve as a baseline for future study. Repeat examinations at six-month intervals (every third visit during the first year, every second visit during the second year), or sooner if clinical symptoms

warrant, may help to identify an early recur-rence. Postoperative small bowel studies will probably have the same incidence of false-negative findings (perhaps an even greater incidence, because of postoperative changes) as studies performed before surgery.

Investigations that the patient has un-dergone prior to therapy may dictate the most appropriate tests to use for follow-up. If the patient has had either a radionuclide scan of the liver or ultrasonography of the liver and retroperitoneum before surgery, the physician can use these techniques for following known liver metastases or residual large abdominal masses. Only if no other method has previously shown the lesion should the physician elect to follow a hepatic metastasis with more invasive techniques such as angiography.

Enteroscopy is such a new technique that endoscopists do not yet know whether or not it will prove effective for detecting tumor recurrences. If it does, it could super-sede other methods.

The initial enthusiasm for the use of carcinoembryonic antigen (CEA) as a diagnostic tool and as an adjunct for the de-tection of recurrent tumor has dampened.[69–71] Recent evidence suggests that rising values are helpful for following colonic cancer, questionably helpful for stomach cancers, and of no value in small bowel neoplasms.[71] Daily values may fluctuate by as much as 35 per cent in a given patient.[69]

RADIOLOGIC CONSIDERATIONS

Presenting Radiographic Signs

Since malignant small bowel tumors frequently cause partial small bowel obstruc-tion, plain abdominal radiographs may re-veal dilated loops of small bowel up to the point of obstruction. If a high-grade obstruc-tion exists, colonic gas may appear reduced or absent. In all cases of suspected obstruc-tion, the patient should also have upright and horizontal-beam lateral decubitus films. These will demonstrate fluid levels in high, arch-shaped loops. An acute onset of ob-struction, without preceding symptoms, suggests that an intussusception may have developed (Fig. 8–1).

Leiomyosarcomas, fibrosarcomas, and

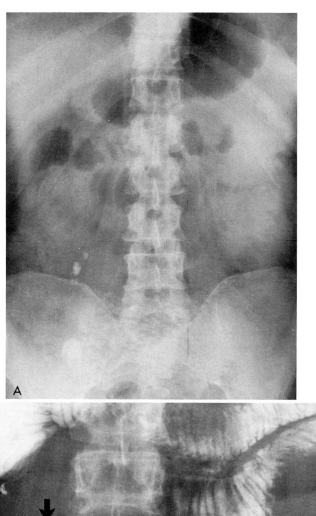

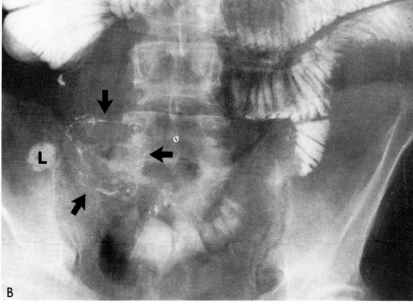

Figure 8–1   Metastatic melanoma with intussusception of the small bowel. *A,* Preliminary films show dilated, largely fluid-filled loops of small bowel; gas is absent from the colon. Note several calcified lymph nodes in the right lower quadrant. *B,* Small bowel series, using barium as the contrast agent. A small amount of barium has percolated between the intussusceptum and the intussuscipiens (arrows). A calcified abdominal lymph node is also visible (L).

malignant schwannomas of the small bowel are frequently large and may undergo central necrosis. These necrotic cavities may entrap air and produce a characteristic large, irregular gas shadow surrounded by a soft tissue mass on the plain abdominal films.[72, 73]

If a neoplastic mass involving the entire wall of the small bowel from mucosa to serosa undergoes necrosis, the intestine may perforate into the free peritoneal cavity; pneumoperitoneum results. Leiomyosarcomas, malignant lymphomas, metastatic melanomas, and carcinomas may actually present in this way.[7, 16, 72] Pneumoperitoneum is visible as free air under the diaphragm, on upright and lateral decubitus views.

A carcinoid tumor may occasionally appear as a calcified mass on a radiograph; this occurs more frequently than previously recognized.[42]

The initial radiographic diagnosis is most often made by a barium small bowel series. It is better not to do this examination at all than to do a so-called survey examination that relies entirely upon chance to demonstrate the lesion. Huge blobs of barium may hide significant lesions and give a false sense of security to the physician, while doing a gross injustice to the patient (Fig. 8–2). The difference between an uninterpretable examination and one that provides maximal information rests upon a few simple techniques. The basic principles are: (1) to fill the entire small bowel from duodenum to ileocecal valve, so that no area that could harbor the tumor is empty of barium; (2) to take steps to ensure that the transit time is rapid, so that the radiologist, patient, and technicians do not lose interest because the examination drags on for hours; and (3) to assure that every small bowel loop is adequately separated so that no lesion hides behind an overlapping loop of small bowel. These points are so important that they merit some discussion at this stage.

To assure a steady flow of barium through the small bowel, the patient should drink 16 to 20 ounces of a barium suspension, for example, Miller's mixture.[74] In the adult, no need exists to lie the patient on the right side, to add ice, or to inject physostigmine.[75] If one uses the Bradfield-Chrispin technique —that is, one thoroughly mixes 10 milliliters of Gastrografin with 20 fluid ounces of barium—one will achieve the most rapid

transit time.[75, 76] Prone overhead films are taken by a technologist every 15 minutes. If bowel loops overlap, the radiologist should place a rubber sponge beneath the prone patient, using fluoroscopic control to separate the loops before the technician takes the overhead films. Fluoroscopy plays an extremely important role in any small bowel examination; the fluoroscopist should manipulate the loops vigorously before positioning the patient for overhead films. Finally, the radiologist can display the entire length of terminal ileum using the simple technique described by Bradfield and Chrispin.[76] The tilt upside-down maneuver will frequently allow the radiologist to examine the loops of small bowel that are usually shielded from the palpating paddle or hand by the bony pelvis.[77] The Poole maneuver will demonstrate whether or not metastases have extended to the retrogastric space.[78] The amount of effort that the radiologist need expend to convert a misleading, uninterpretable examination into one that beautifully displays every segment of small bowel is so minimal that no acceptable excuse exists to produce anything but the best.

After identifying a lesion, the physician should ask certain questions: Are there changes in the lumen or in the bowel wall, or outside the wall, or in multiple anatomical sites? Is a given lesion soft and pliable, or rigid? Does the lesion invade the jejunum, the ileum, or both? Is the involved segment short or long? Are there discrete lesions? The answers to these questions will narrow the possible diagnoses to relatively few entities.

Almost all adenocarcinomas of the mesenteric small bowel are solitary lesions and are located in the jejunum, usually within 30 cm of the ligament of Treitz.[5, 6, 73] Carcinoids, implanted carcinomas from other sites, and malignant lymphomas, by contrast, almost always occur in the ileum, particularly the distal ileum.[42, 73, 79–81] They are often multiple. Exceptions to this rule include Mediterranean lymphoma and malignant lymphoma complicating celiac disease, both of which usually arise in the jejunum.[26, 38, 39]

One of the most frequent radiologic findings in small bowel neoplasms is an abnormality of luminal caliber. The observed change can consist of either narrowing or dilatation. The normal caliber of the small bowel is not more than 25 mm in the jejunum and 20 mm in the ileum. A measurement

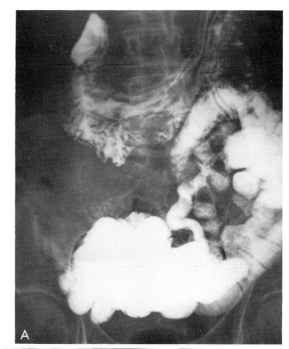

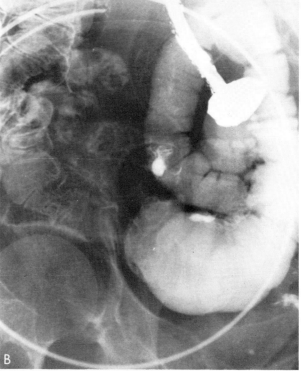

Figure 8–2 Adenocarcinoma of the distal jejunum. *A,* "Survey small bowel series," reported as normal. A large blob of barium in ileal loops overlies the distal jejunum. *B,* Antegrade "small bowel enema." Fifty ml of barium suspension was injected through the tube seen in the top right-hand corner of the figure, followed by an injection of 150 ml of 1 per cent methylcellulose solution. Only when the loops were separated by means of a balloon compression paddle (opaque ring) did a short, irregular stricture with overhanging edges between the dilated and normal caliber jejunum become apparent.

between 25 mm and 30 mm could be normal or abnormal, but any measurement greater than 30 mm is definitely abnormal.[74] Care should be taken not to measure the luminal caliber on a film either closely proximal or distal to a peristaltic wave; otherwise, false measurements will result.[74]

The most common radiologic finding caused by a small bowel neoplasm is narrowing of the bowel lumen (Figure 8–2); this is significant if it is *consistently* narrower than the normal bowel, or if it causes dilatation proximally. Adenocarcinoma (Fig. 8–2)—the most common primary small bowel malignancy detected during life—and, less frequently, a carcinoid tumor seeding along the small bowel mesentery (Fig. 8–3), a true metastatic carcinoma, or a malignant lymphoma can narrow the luminal caliber.[72, 73] All these lesions can exhibit the well-known features of a malignant stricture: it is short; it has an eccentric, irregular channel; its edges appear sharply demarcated and overhang where it joins the normal bowel; the wall is rigid, and the overlying mucosa is ulcerated.[72, 73] Although a stricture from a malignant lymphoma can exactly simulate one from an adenocarcinoma, the former often is longer and lacks the overhanging edges;[72, 73] indeed, the junction between normal and abnormal bowel in lymphoma often tapers in a uniform manner.

Increasing evidence has accumulated that both lymphocytic and histiocytic lymphomas can be desmoplastic.[82–84] Dorfman asserts that most extranodal malignant lymphomas previously called Hodgkin's disease are actually examples of histicytic lymphoma with eosinophilia.[85] For these reasons, the statement that Hodgkin's disease is often desmoplastic (i.e., the stroma is fibrotic and the neoplasm tends to form adhesions), whereas lymphosarcoma is not, is false. Moreover, it now seems that the radiologic appearance of small intestinal involvement is essentially the same for all types of malignant lymphomas.[73, 81] Peritoneal implants and malignant lymphomas often involve multiple, discontinuous bowel segments or regions.[81] Sometimes a carcinoid tumor may produce multiple, long, smooth, narrow areas of intestine by inducing smooth muscle hypertrophy.[86]

Widening of the luminal caliber extending over a long segment of bowel with a smooth or irregular featureless outline and no recognizable mucosal pattern, is the single most common finding in malignant lymphoma (Fig. 8–4).[73] Rarely, a segment of bowel involved in this manner can dilate greatly (Fig. 8–5) and assume an aneurysmal shape (aneurysmal dilatation).[87] Occasion-

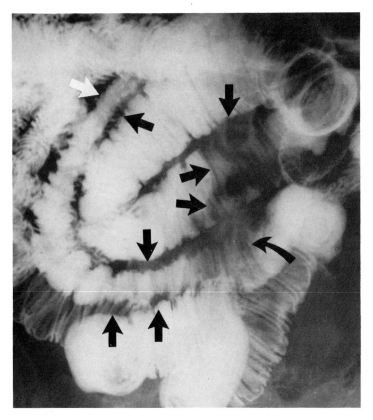

Figure 8–3 Secondary peritoneal implants from carcinoma of the pancreas. A jejunal segment between the curved arrow, lower right, and the white and the black arrows on the left remained constantly narrow and demonstrated submucosal fold thickening and "tacking" of folds. Because of diffuse mural and submucosal infiltration, the distance between this loop and adjacent loops is also increased. Multiple nodules are present as well, the most conspicuous of which are indicated by the arrows on the upper right. The two arrows at the bottom of the illustration point to defects having the characteristics of extramural masses.

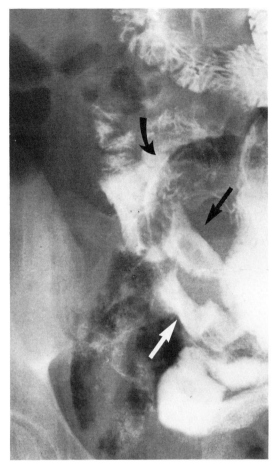

Figure 8–4 Malignant lymphoma involving the ileum. Irregular luminal outline without a mucosal pattern, because of ulceration of the mucosa (arrows). The straight arrows point to slightly deeper ulcers; the curved arrow points to a small bowel loop displaced around a large mesenteric nodal mass.

ally, diffuse submucosal lymphomatous infiltration[88] and, rarely, an infiltrative carcinoid tumor[89] can lead to a slight to moderate increase in luminal caliber involving the entire mesenteric small bowel; the folds in these patients are usually thickened (see section on fold patterns).

An intussusception may develop in association with a small bowel tumor, either before or during the radiologic examination (Fig. 8–1).[73] If barium passes through a preexisting intussusception, the appearance is that of a localized mass with luminal narrowing. Only when barium percolates between the intussusceptum and intussuscipiens does the typical so-called coil-spring pattern appear (Fig. 8–1). Both patterns will appear simultaneously if the intussusception

develops during the radiologic examination. Leiomyosarcomas, carcinoids, malignant lymphomas, and metastatic melanomas may present in this fashion.

Other important radiographic changes in malignant small bowel neoplasms involve changes in the intestinal wall. These include changes in the fold pattern as well as the occurrence of nodules, ulcers, and fistulas.

Thickening of the bowel mucosa or of the submucosa can be recognized radiologically from the fold pattern on radiographs taken with barium in the bowel.[74, 90] The normal mucosal folds appear as fine, feathery black filling defects in the white barium-filled lumen. The measured width of these folds should not normally exceed 2 mm (the folds should not be measured immediately proximal or distal to a peristaltic wave).[74] Commonly, in malignant lymphoma, the mucosa in the affected segment is completely ulcerated; the outline of the small intestinal lumen then appears smooth, or irregular and featureless, without any mucosal pattern (Figs. 8–4, 8–5).[73] Malignant lymphoma can also infiltrate the submucosa; the resulting submucosal thickening can be diagnosed when the individual folds measure greater than 2 mm in width and when they appear straightened. Nodular filling defects (described later in this chapter) also commonly accompany the submucosal thickening in malignant lymphoma (Fig. 8–6).[88]

The presence of nodules (Figs. 8–3, 8–6, 8–7) may be recognized by black, round defects within the barium-filled lumen when they are seen face-on; when seen in profile, the nodules produce semicircular, scalloped defects in the luminal margins.[74] Individual lymphoma nodules may develop a stalk and so appear as pedunculated filling defects. Multiple small nodules, usually associated with a thickened submucosal fold pattern, can occur in leukemia and carcinoid tumors as well as in lymphoma (Fig. 8–6). Leiomyosarcoma in the small intestine can present as a large, broad-based nodule, with or without a mucosal fold pattern on its surface. Large, oval, or lobulated sessile nodules most frequently represent malignant lymphoma (especially if located in the ileum) or metastases, but they can be seen rarely as an unusual manifestation of a slow-growing adenocarcinoma, usually in the jejunum.[72, 73] Whereas malignant lymphoma can some-

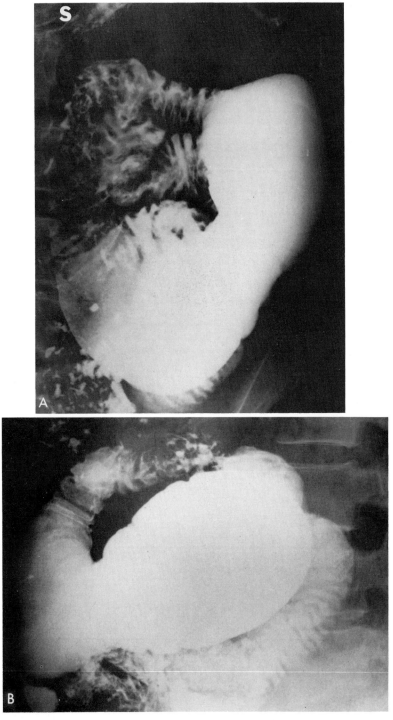

Figure 8–5   Malignant lymphoma. A jejunal loop that is involved by tumor has undergone aneurysmal dilatation. *A,* Anteroposterior view. There is residual barium in the stomach. *B,* Lateral view. Unlike Crohn's disease, there is no stricture between the dilated loop and the jejunum distal to it.

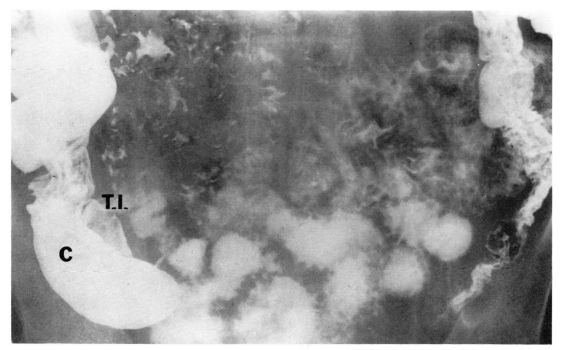

Figure 8–6   Malignant lymphoma. T. I., terminal ileum; C, cecum. The mucosal folds of the small bowel are diffusely thickened, and multiple small nodules are present between the folds.

times cause multiple small, pedunculated polyps, larger pedunculated polyps are unusual in malignant neoplasms of the small bowel; when present, they are likely to be

due to metastatic melanoma (especially if they are multiple), less often to leiomyosarcoma, and rarely to adenocarcinoma.[73]

Ulcers (Fig. 8–8) appear radiologically

Figure 8–7   Peritoneal implants from carcinoma of the pancreas. Multiple nodules with their centers projected outside the luminal contours of the bowel. The distance between the affected loops is also increased.

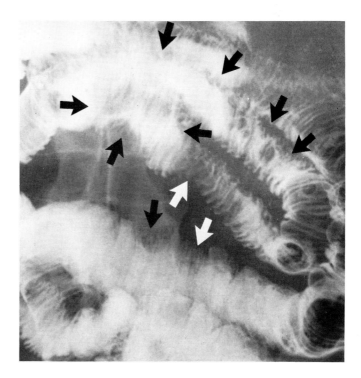

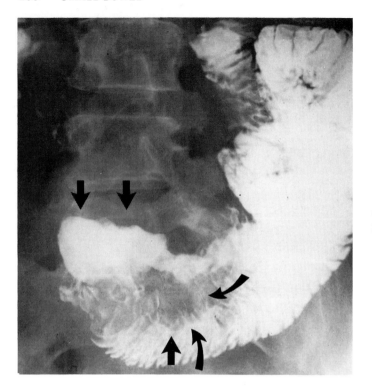

Figure 8–8 Malignant lymphoma. Large, irregular ulcer (two vertical straight arrows on left), intramural nodules (lower arrows) and mucosal "tacking" (horizontal curved arrow on right). The distance between the affected bowel loops is increased.

as protrusions from the barium-filled outline of the lumen.[71] Unlike diverticula, they do not vary in size or shape on different radiographs from the same series, or when compression is applied. Large, irregular ulcers associated with large nodules are usually secondary to leiomyosarcomas and malignant lymphomas (Fig. 8–8).[72, 73] Sizable ulcers surrounded concentrically by the rim of a tumor mass have become known as "bull's-eye lesions," because of their characteristic appearance when seen face-on during barium contrast studies.[73] These lesions occur most frequently in metastatic malignant melanomas, when they are often multiple and vary in size.[73] Less often, leiomyosarcomas, fibrosarcomas, malignant schwannomas, lymphomas, and, rarely, Kaposi's sarcomas may give rise to a similar appearance.[91]

The appearance of fistulas on a radiograph is characterized by long barium-filled tracts that extend outside the bowel lumen.[74] Their presence may sometimes be deduced when the distal colon fills before the cecum, in a patient who has not had part of the colon surgically removed (Fig. 8–9), or when there is abnormal contrast filling of the bladder or some other structure. Leiomyosarcomas,

malignant lymphomas (Fig. 8–9), and metastatic melanomas are particularly liable to form fistulas, although this phenomenon does represent an unusual complication of malignant small bowel neoplasms.[7, 72, 73]

Malignant neoplasms involving the mesentery can alter the appearance of the barium-filled small bowel loops.[74] A desmoplastic tumor can cause a persistent, sharp angulation of the bowel by shortening and thickening the mesentery. The combination of one or more small, intraluminal intestinal nodules and a sharply angulated, fixed loop of bowel, usually the terminal ileum, makes a diagnosis of carcinoid tumor almost certain.[73, 79] Mesenteric tumor implants or, less often, a desmoplastic malignant lymphoma may also kink the bowel. Any desmoplastic neoplasm in the mesentery, furthermore, may cause a radiologic feature called "tacking": the mucosal folds are pulled outside the general contours of the bowel lumen and may appear sharply angulated (Fig. 8–8).[74]

Neoplasms in the mesentery can cause widening of the distance between adjacent small bowel loops (Figs. 8–3, 8–7, 8–8). Mural thickening can also cause some separation between adjacent loops and may be difficult to distinguish from mesenteric thickening. More frequently, however, neoplastic involvement of the mesentery causes displacement of masses lying within and outside the bowel. Defects in the barium column whose estimated centers lie within or outside (Figs. 8–3, 8–4, 8–7) the projected luminal contours of the bowel are likely to be intramural or extramural masses, respectively.[92] Two thirds of leiomyosarcomas project chiefly into the peritoneal cavity, and a few of these are also pedunculated;[17, 73] a leiomyosarcoma of the small intestine, therefore, usually exhibits the radiologic features of an extramural mass. These neoplasms, furthermore, tend to seed locally by forming peritoneal implants, which make the original mass appear even larger.[17] Nodal metastases from primary small bowel neoplasms (Fig. 8–3) or peritoneal implants, usually arising from primary carcinomas elsewhere in the abdomen (Figs. 8–3, 8–7), can cause similar mesenteric or extramural mass defects. Ascites may also develop.

In summary, each small bowel malignancy has characteristic features. Most *adenocarcinomas* partially obstruct the bowel and arise in the jejunum, where they grow rapidly and usually form a short zone of constriction with an irregular, eccentric lumen and overhanging margins. Only about one third of *carcinoid* tumors are detected during life; they usually produce an almost diagnostic appearance, consisting of the combination of one or more small intramural nodules and a sharply angulated, fixed loop of bowel, usually the terminal ileum. *Leiomyosarcomas* are equally distributed throughout the mes-

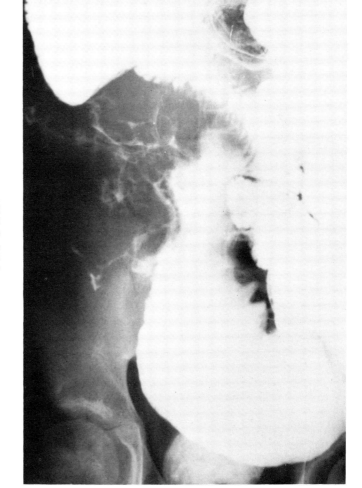

Figure 8–9 Malignant lymphoma. There is a grossly dilated loop of distal ileum (lower center). Multiple, narrow and irregular fistulae extend from this loop to the reader's left. The rectum (central, barium-filled structure beneath the dilated ileum) has filled before the cecum (by way of a fistula).

enteric small bowel; about two thirds of them project chiefly into the peritoneal cavity and exhibit the radiologic features of an extra-mural mass. Another characteristic appearance of leiomyosarcoma is that of a large, irregular ulcer within an even larger submucosal tumor nodule. *Malignant lymphomas* of the small bowel most commonly involve the terminal ileum and usually extend across the ileocecal valve to involve the cecum as well. Characteristically, malignant lymphomas involve multiple long, discontinuous segments of bowel. The luminal caliber of the involved segment is often widened and the mucosal pattern entirely obliterated because of ulceration; the bowel wall may be considerably thickened. Malignant lymphomas can, however, produce almost any roentgenologic pattern including diffuse submucosal thickening, multiple small sessile or pedunculated nodules, large irregular ulcers within larger nodules, and narrowing of the luminal caliber, with or without ulceration of the overlying mucosa. *Mesenteric tumor implants* from other primaries most often involve the terminal ileum. The involved bowel appears fixed, rigid, and angulated, and its mucosal folds appear thickened and "tacked." Characteristically, extramural masses are evident on contrast studies; the metastatic implants may subsequently grow into the bowel wall and narrow the luminal caliber. Multiple, pedunculated intraluminal nodules that vary in size and bull's-eye lesions are rather characteristic of *malignant melanoma;* the presence of a known skin primary clinches the diagnosis.

Differential Diagnosis

Common benign conditions often create difficult differential diagnostic problems. Some causes for a localized narrowing of the luminal caliber of the small bowel include Crohn's disease, vascular disease, prior surgery, extrinsic bands, radiation-induced enteritis, and, less frequently today, a time-release ("enteric-coated") potassium chloride pill.[74] In contrast to malignant bowel strictures, which usually have an eccentric lumen, most benign lesions that narrow the luminal caliber have a concentric lumen. Although benign strictures can be short, they are often longer and taper more gently into the normal bowel than do their malignant counterparts.

Several benign conditions can also cause persistent, sharp angulations of the gut and mucosal "tacking."[74] Probably the most common benign cause for this appearance in the United States is mesenteric adhesions following surgery. Previous peritonitis may cause similar adhesions. In a patient with an appropriate history who does not have either a mesenteric or an intraluminal mass, the radiologist can make a correct diagnosis of adhesions with confidence. Patients who undergo radiation therapy following surgery are particularly liable to develop radiation-induced enteritis.[93, 94] Normal small bowel is freely mobile, but adhesions from previous surgery may fix several loops in a constant anatomical pattern within the abdomen. These loops of bowel, trapped and immobilized in the field of irradiation, are more prone to develop the changes of enteritis.[93] Often, such loops become rigid and angulated, the mucosa becomes "tacked," and nodular filling defects caused by submucosal fibrosis may develop. Consequently, the radiologic appearance may *mimic* either carcinoid tumor or peritoneal tumor implants.[93] Patients with tuberculous peritonitis (a rare cause of bowel kinking), tacking, and mesenteric nodal masses almost always have simultaneous evidence of active pulmonary tuberculosis on chest radiographs.[95]

An extraluminal mass could be caused by a leiomyoma rather than a leiomyosarcoma, but it is best to regard all myomatous neoplasms as potentially malignant, especially if they exceed 7 mm in diameter.[17] A peritoneal tumor implant or a duplication cyst may rarely mimic a leiomyosarcoma roentgenographically.

A communicating abscess with regional enteritis may resemble the large ulcers seen in leiomyosarcomas, malignant lymphomas,[73] and the rare schwannomas and fibrosarcomas. However, other distinguishing roentgenologic features of regional enteritis are almost always present.

Stenotic regional enteritis, characterized by multiple areas of small bowel stenosis accompanied by proximal dilated loops with a smooth, featureless mucosal lining, may resemble malignant lymphoma. However, unlike malignant lymphoma, the loops usually contain a considerable amount of retained food and fluid secretions and show signs of chronic obstruction.[72]

Both regional enteritis and malignant

lymphomas can have thickened folds exhibiting a pattern of submucosal infiltration, an irregular bowel outline, intraluminal nodules, and extraluminal fistulas. In contrast to malignant lymphoma, however, in regional enteritis the inflammation often produces temporary spasm; characteristic linear ulcers occur, the submucosal nodules are usually regular or symmetrical, and the bowel loops are often more widely separated. Inflammatory pseudotumor may cause submucosal nodules and can even obstruct the lumen or cause an intussusception.[96]

When the radiologist has performed the best possible small bowel examination, the patient's symptoms may still suggest a small bowel lesion although the examination itself is negative. More sophisticated techniques may then enhance visualization of a lesion. These include an antegrade small bowel enema (Fig. 8–5) and a retrograde small bowel enema. An antegrade small bowel enema involves intubation of the small bowel and the controlled injection of barium followed by methylcellulose or magnesium sulfate through the tube. A retrograde small bowel enema is performed by doing an initial conventional barium enema, followed by administration of water under fluoroscopic control until reflux through the ileocecal valve results in retrograde contrast filling of the entire small bowel.[40, 41] Both methods may be extremely uncomfortable and at times painful, even when the patient has been given Valium and Demerol, but the duration of discomfort is brief and equals that of many other commonly used diagnostic procedures such as esophagoscopy and bronchoscopy.[41]

Angiography is sometimes valuable in demonstrating the primary lesion in patients with carcinoid tumors, but it seems that not until the carcinoid has invaded the mesentery and infiltrated the lymph nodes will angiography outline the lesion.[42, 43] At that stage, the branches of the distal mesenteric and intestinal arterial arcade appear stellate or irregular in the area of the lesion, the neoplasm itself "stains" slightly (that is, it takes up contrast medium and appears white), and its draining veins may be obstructed.[43] These angiographic appearances are not diagnostic.[43] Idiopathic mesenteric fibrosis or any active inflammatory or neoplastic process that causes local mesenteric infiltration and retraction can have a similar appearance.[43, 97] By using intra-arterial epinephrine, however, the radiologist can enhance the angiographic staining of the primary tumor; although not yet proved, it is possible that this phenomenon occurs primarily with neoplasms in the intestine.[43] Angiography is indicated in the diagnosis of the primary lesion when the clinical evidence points to a carcinoid tumor but the barium studies are not diagnostic.[43] Preoperative evaluation for liver metastases is another clear indication for this study.

Leiomyosarcomas, as well as the rare fibrosarcomas and malignant schwannomas, are highly vascular neoplasms and are therefore amenable to diagnosis by arteriography.[44] These tumors are supplied by large, sometimes multiple, feeding arteries, and their prominent draining veins fill early. The tumor mass itself may contain many irregular tumor vessels, develop a dense tumor stain, and pool contrast medium in its venules. The well-defined margins of hypervascularity correspond to the size of the tumor. It is usually not possible to determine angiographically whether the neoplasm is benign or malignant, but all the larger masses, particularly if their diameter exceeds 7 cm, are best considered malignant preoperatively. Only if the entire border of the mass is irregular and it obtains parasitic blood flow from retroperitoneal or parietal vessels can the angiographer confidently predict that it is malignant. Angiography is particularly indicated in patients with leiomyosarcomas and bleeding.[44] Another indication for angiography is for the investigation of a mesenteric mass of unknown etiology. When an apparent hepatoma has been demonstrated in the liver, the angiographer should proceed directly to perform a superior mesenteric angiogram because of the identical angiographic appearances of a metastatic leiomyosarcoma from the small bowel and a hepatoma.[44]

Localization and Staging

The main purpose of radiology in the staging and localization of a known malignancy in the small bowel is to determine whether or not the neoplasm has metastasized to the lung, abdominal lymph nodes, or liver. Stereo posteroanterior and lateral chest radiographs and full tomograms are, therefore, mandatory in any patient with a malignant small bowel neoplasm.

Only when the patient has a malignant lymphoma does bipedal lymphograpy aid in detecting para-aortic nodal metastases. Careful evaluation of the small bowel series will often reveal the presence of large mesenteric and retroperitoneal node masses.

A small bowel neoplasm that extends into the retroperitoneum can displace or obstruct the ureters or the kidneys. The physician should, therefore, request an excretory urogram as a routine part of the investigation of any patient.

Hepatic angiography is an excellent method for detecting certain kinds of metastases from the small bowel (see Chapter 9).[42–44, 63] Metastases to the liver may appear more or less vascular than the surrounding parenchyma, or they may have the same vascularity.[63] Vascular metastases stand out as dense, white, coin-like areas against the generally increased whiteness of the liver substance itself. Metastases that are less

vascular than the liver appear as black holes against the general whiteness of the liver in the capillary phase of the angiogram. Before the radiologist can detect them, their measured diameter usually exceeds 2 cm.[63] Unfortunately, either normal or cirrhotic hepatic parenchyma may contain defects in the capillary or hepatogram phase that can simulate metastases. When the vascularity of the metastases is the same as that of the liver, radiologists can make the diagnosis only if they recognize displacements of normal vessels by tumor; this is difficult to do until the metastases are quite large.[63] Adenocarcinoma metastases can fit either the "less vascular" or the "equally vascular" categories.[63] If the angiographer extends the investigation of primary small bowel leiomyosarcomas and carcinoids to include the liver, the results may be most rewarding. Although hepatic metastases from carcinoid tumors are usually richly vascularized, the "tumor stain" during angiography will increase if *epinephrine* is administered through the catheter.[43]

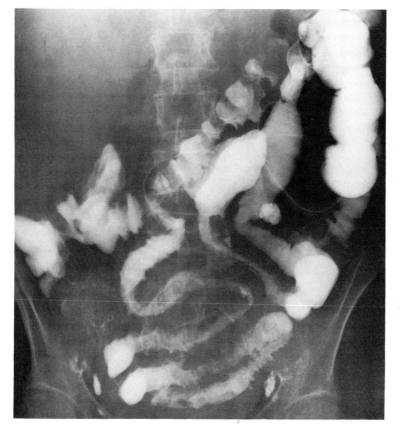

Figure 8–10 Radiation-induced enteritis. Barium outlines the distal small bowel and the proximal colon, to the level of the splenic flexure . The luminal caliber of the small bowel is markedly decreased. In some areas, the normal mucosal fold pattern is effaced; in others, submucosal thickening is present. The small bowel loops are rigid, and their walls are greatly thickened. Multiple nodules are present that *simulate* metastases; these are best seen in the lowermost loop in the pelvis.

Radiologic Follow-up

The key role of radiology in helping to ascertain the success of tumor control, as well as to assess recurrence, metastasis, or post-treatment complications, has been covered in the section on clinical follow-up. Frequently, a patient who has had a small bowel tumor resected presents 6 to 12 months later with an unusual appearance on a small bowel examination that could represent either recurrent tumor or a defect caused by the surgery itself. To obviate this dilemma, the patient's primary physician should refer every patient who has had small bowel surgery to the radiologist for a baseline small bowel series 4 weeks after surgery. It cannot be stressed too strongly that this simple precaution might prevent a considerable amount of confusion at a later date. Only by knowing what defects and deformities remain as the direct result of surgery will the radiologist feel confident that additional changes probably represent a tumor recurrence.

Radiation-induced enteritis, either acute or chronic, may develop in patients treated intensively with radiation therapy (Fig. 8–10). Ileus is the usual finding in acute radiation enteritis, and it will often resolve with conservative therapy.[92] The cardinal small bowel roentgenographic findings in chronic radiation-induced enteritis are: (1) fold thickening caused by submucosal fibrosis or edema; (2) nodular mucosal filling defects secondary to irregular submucosal thickening; (3) bowel wall thickening and rigidity; (4) stenosis; and (5) changes in the mesentery, including kinking, tacking, and pooling of barium in matted-together small bowel loops. Sometimes these findings may closely simulate metastatic disease. If any doubt exists as to the nature of the lesions, a laparotomy may be indicated; rarely, patients thought to be dying of recurrent malignancy have been shown to have radiation-induced enteritis with no evidence of neoplasm at autopsy.[92]

References

1. Third National Survey of the National Cancer Institute. CA, 25:11, 1975.
2. Darling, R. C., and Welch, C. E.: Tumors of the small intestine. N. Engl. J. Med., 260:397–408, 1959.
3. Cohen, A., McNeil, D., Terz, J. J., et al.: Neoplasms of the small intestine. Am. J. Dig. Dis., 16:815–824, 1971.
4. Kyriakos, M.: Malignant tumors of the small intestine. J.A.M.A., 229:700–702, 1974.
5. Good, C. A.: Tumors of the small intestine: Caldwell lecture, 1962. Am. J. Roentgenol. Radium Ther. Nucl. Med., 89:685–705, 1963.
6. McPeak, C. J.: Malignant tumors of the small intestine. Am. J. Surg., 114:402–411, 1967.
7. Ackerman, L. V., and del Regato, J. A.: Cancer. Diagnosis, Treatment and Prognosis. 4th ed. St. Louis, C. V. Mosby Co., 1970, pp. 465–479.
8. Mohandas, D., Chandra, R. S., Srinivasan, V., et al.: Liposarcoma of the ileum with secondaries in the liver. Am. J. Gastroenterol., 58:172–176, 1972.
9. Mir-Madjlessi, S. H., Farmer, R. G., and Hawk, W. A.: Villous tumors of the duodenum and jejunum. Report of four cases and review of the literature. Am. J. Dig. Dis., 18:467–476, 1973.
10. Jones, S. E., Fuks, Z., Bull, M., et al.: Non-Hodgkin's lymphomas. IV. Clinicopathological correlation in 405 cases. Cancer, 31:806–823, 1973.
11. Dorfman, R. F., and Kim, H.: Relationship of histology to site and to prognosis in Hodgkin's disease and non-Hodgkin's lymphomas. Front. Radiation Ther. Onc., 9:196–202, 1974.
12. Ferris, R. A., Hakkal, H. G., and Cigtay, O. S.: Radiological manifestations of North American Burkitts lymphoma. Am. J. Roentgenol. Radium Ther. Nucl. Med., 123:614–629, 1975.
13. Meyers, M. A., and McSweeney, J.: Secondary neoplasms of the bowel. Radiology, 105:1–11, 1972.
14. Silberman, H., Crichlow, R. W., and Caplan, H. S.: Neoplasms of the small bowel. Ann. Surg., 180:157–161, 1974.
15. Rubin, P.: Current concepts in cancer. Cancer of the gastrointestinal tract. E. Small intestine. Diagnosis and treatment. J.A.M.A., 299:699, 1974.
16. Higgins, P. M., Lehman, G., and Morton, H. S.: Perforation of jejunal and ileal neoplasm. A survey of the literature and case reports. Can. J. Surg., 6:338–347, 1963.
17. Starr, G. F.: Pathologic features of smooth-muscle tumors. J.A.M.A., 229:1219–1220, 1974.
18. Ureles, A. L.: Diagnosis and treatment of malignant carcinoid tumor. J.A.M.A., 229:1346–1348, 1974.
19. Van Sickle, D. G.: Carcinoid tumors. Cleve. Clin. Q., 39:79–86, 1972.
20. Oates, J. A., Pettinger, W. A., and Doctor, R. B.: Evidence for release of bradykinin in carcinoid syndrome. J. Clin. Invest., 45:173–198, 1966.
21. Mengel, C. E., and Shaffer, R. D.: Carcinoid syndrome. In Holland, J. F., and Frei, E. (eds.), Cancer Medicine. Philadelphia, Lea and Febiger, 1973, pp. 1584–1594.
22. Murray-Lyon, I. M., Rake, M. O., Marshall, A. K., et al.: Malignant carcinoid tumor with gangrene of the small intestine. Br. Med. J., 4:770–771, 1973.
23. Brown, N. K., and Smith, M. P.: Neoplastic diathesis of patients with carcinoid. Report of a case with four other neoplasms. Cancer, 32:216–222, 1973.
24. Moertel, C. G., and Dockerty, M. B.: Familial occurrence of metastasizing carcinoid tumors. Ann. Intern. Med., 78:389–390, 1973.
25. Levinson, J. D., and Kirsner, J. B.: Infiltrative diseases of the small bowel and malabsorption. Am. J. Dig. Dis., 15:741–766, 1970.

26. Rappaport, H., Ramot, B., Hulu, N., et al.: The pathology of so-called Mediterranean abdominal lymphoma with malabsorption. Cancer, 29: 1502–1511, 1972.

27. Haghighi, P., and Nasr, K.: Primary upper small intestinal lymphoma (so-called Mediterranean lymphoma). Pathol. Annu., 8:231–255, 1973.

28. Eidelman, S.: Abdominal lymphoma with malabsorption. J.A.M.A., 229:1103–1104, 1974.

29. Marshak, R. H., Hazi, C., Lindner, A. E., et al.: Small bowel in immunoglobulin deficiency syndromes. Am. J. Roentgenol. Radium Ther. Nucl. Med., 122:227–240, 1974.

30. Bonomo, L., Dammacio, F., Marano, R., et al.: Abdominal lymphoma and alpha chain disease. Am. J. Med., 52:73–86, 1972.

31. Rambaud, J. C., and Matuchansky, C.: Alpha-chain disease: Pathogenesis and relation to Mediterranean lymphoma. Lancet, 1:1430–1432, 1973.

32. Reid, J. D.: Intestinal carcinoma in the Peutz-Jeghers syndrome. J.A.M.A., 229:833–834, 1974.

33. Ross, J. E., and Mara, J. E.: Small bowel polyps and carcinoma in multiple intestinal polyposis. Arch. Surg., 108:736–738, 1974.

34. Schofield, P. F.: Intestinal malignancy and Crohn's disease. Proc. R. Soc. Med., 65:783–784, 1972.

35. Frank, J. D., and Shorey, B. A.: Adenocarcinoma of the small bowel as a complication of Crohn's disease. Gut, 14:120–124, 1973.

36. Beachley, M. C., Lebel, A., Lankau, C. A., Jr., et al.: Carcinoma of the small intestine in chronic regional enteritis. Am. J. Dig. Dis., 18:1095–1098, 1973.

37. Saeed, W., Kim, S., and Burch, B. H.: Development of carcinoma in regional enteritis. Arch. Surg., 108:376–379, 1974.

38. Asch, T., and Seaman, W. B.: Idiopathic steatorrhea and small-bowel cancer. Radiology, 100:271–275, 1971.

39. Kenwright, S.: Coeliac disease and small bowel carcinoma. Postgrad. Med. J., 48:673–677, 1972.

40. Miller, R. E., and Provines, R. L.: Tumors of the small bowel: Complete reflux small-bowel examination. Am. J. Gastroenterol., 45:40–49, 1966.

41. Miller, R. E.: Retrograde small-bowel examination. J.A.M.A., 229:1500–1501, 1974.

42. Boijsen, E., Kaude, J., and Tyl, E. N. U.: Radiologic diagnosis of ileal carcinoid tumors. Acta. Radiol. (Diagn.) (Stockh.), 15:65–82, 1974.

43. Goldstein, H. M., and Miller, M.: Angiographic evaluation of small intestinal carcinoid tumors: Value of epinephrine. Radiology, 115:23–28, 1975.

44. Itzchak, Y., Adar, R., Mozes, M., et al.: Angiographic diagnosis of leiomyomatous small bowel tumors. Angiologica, 10:310–317, 1973.

45. Polga, J. P., Sargent, J., and Dickinson, P.: Positive intestinal scan caused by carcinoid tumor. J. Nucl. Med., 15:365–366, 1974.

46. Adler, S., Parthasarathy, K. L., Bakshi, S. P., et al.: Gallium-67 citrate scanning for the localization and staging of lymphomas. J. Nucl. Med., 16:255–260, 1975.

47. Frühmorgen, P.: Endoscopy of the small bowel. Radiology, 14:404–408, 1974.

48. Kossoff, G., Garrett, W. J., and Radovanovich, G.: Gray scale echography in obstetrics and gynecology. Australas. Radiol., 18:63–111, 1974.

49. Kossoff, G.: Progress in pulse-echo techniques. In deVlieger, M., and McCready, V. R. (eds.), Ultrasonics in Medicine. Amsterdam, Exerpta Medica, 1974, pp. 37–42.

50. Wagai, T.: Advances in ultrasonotomography and its clinical evaluation. In deVlieger, M., and McCready, V. R. (eds.), Ultrasonics in Medicine. Amsterdam, Excerpta Medica, 1974, pp. 186–190.

51. Conn, H. O., and Yesner, R.: A re-evaluation of needle biopsy in the diagnosis of metastatic cancer of the liver. Ann. Intern. Med., 59:53–61, 1963.

52. Schaeffer, J., and Schiff, L.: Liver function tests in metastatic tumor of the liver: Study of 100 cases. Gastroenterology, 49:360–363, 1965.

53. Sjoerdsma, A., Weissbach, H., Terry, L. L., et al.: Further observations on patients with malignant carcinoid. Am. J. Med., 34:5–15, 1957.

54. McCready, V. R.: Scintigraphic studies of space-occupying liver disease. Semin. Nucl. Med., 2:108–127, 1972.

55. Fee, H. J., Prokop, E. K., Cameron, J. L., et al.: Liver scanning in patients with suspected abdominal tumor. J.A.M.A., 230:1675–1679, 1974.

56. Taylor, K. J. W., Carpenter, D. A., and McCready, V. R.: Gray scale echography in the diagnosis of intrahepatic disease. J. Clin. Ultrasound, 1: 284–287, 1973.

57. Taylor, K. W., Carpenter, D. A., and McCready, V. R.: Comparison of ultrasound and radioisotope examination in the diagnosis of hepatobiliary disease. J. Clin. Ultrasound, 2:264, 1974.

58. Taylor, K. J. W., Carpenter, D. A., and McCready, V. R.: Ultrasound and scintigraphy in the differential diagnosis of obstructive jaundice. J. Clin. Ultrasound, 2:105–116, 1974.

59. Sauer, R., Fahrlander, H., and Fridrich, R.: Comparison of the accuracy of liver scans and peritoneoscopy in benign and malignant primary and metastatic tumors of the liver. Scand. J. Gastroenterol., 8:389–394, 1973.

60. Berci, G., Shore, M., Panish, J., et al.: The evaluation of a new peritoneoscope as a diagnostic aid to the surgeon. Ann. Surg., 178:37–44, 1973.

61. Johri, J. P., and Peschile, C.: Combined peritoneoscopy and liver biopsy in the diagnosis of hepatic neoplasm. Gastroenterology, 63:1016–1019, 1974.

62. Ash, S. R., and Manfredi, F.: Directed biopsy using a small endoscope. Thoracoscopy and peritoneoscopy simplified. N. Engl. J. Med., 291: 1398–1399, 1974.

63. Reuter, S. R., and Redman, H. C.: Gastrointestinal Angiography. Philadelphia, W. B. Saunders, 1972, pp. 87–123.

64. Kreel, L., Jones, M. B., and Travill, A. S.: A comparative study of arteriography and scintillation scanning in space-occupying lesions of the liver. Br. J. Radiol., 41:401–411, 1968.

65. du Priest, R. W., Haines, J. E., Rösch, J., et al.: A comparison of scintiscans and arteriograms for identifying metastatic intrahepatic tumors. Surg. Gynecol. Obstet., 136:705–710, 1973.

66. Fu, Y. S., and Perzin, K. H.: Lymphosarcoma of the small intestine. A clinicopathologic study. Cancer, 29:645–659, 1972.

67. Gillett, D. J., and Smith, R. C.: Treatment of the

carinoid syndrome by hemihepatectomy and radical excision of the primary lesion. Am. J. Surg., 128:95–99, 1974.

68. Zakariai, Y. M., Quan, S.H.O., and Hajdu, S. I.: Carcinoid tumors of the gastrointestinal tract. Cancer, 35:588–591, 1975.

69. Ravry, M., Moertel, C. G., Schutt, A. J., et al.: Usefulness of serum carcinoembryonic antigen (C.E.A.) determinations during anticancer therapy for long-term follow-up of gastrointestinal carcinoma. Cancer, 34:1230–1234, 1974.

70. Turner, M. D.: Carcinoembryonic antigen. J.A.M.A., 231:756–758, 1975.

71. Holyoke, E. D.: Editor's interview: Present and probable uses of C.E.A. CA, 25:22–26, 1975.

72. Marshak, R. H., and Lindner, A. E.: Radiology of the Small Intestine. Philadelphia, W. B. Saunders, 1970.

73. Carlson, H. C., and Good, C. A.: Neoplasms of the small bowel. In Margulis, A. R., and Burhenne, H. J. (eds.), Alimentary Tract Roentgenology. 2nd ed. St. Louis, C. V. Mosby, 1973, pp. 865–902.

74. Osborn, A., and Friedland, G. W.: A radiological approach to the diagnosis of small bowel disease. Clin. Radiol., 24:281–301, 1973.

75. Goldstein, H. M., Poole, J. G., Rosenquist, C. J., et al.: Comparison of methods for acceleration of small intestinal radiographic examination. Radiology, 98:519–523, 1971.

76. Bradfield, G. P., and Chrispin, A. R.: The 90 minute follow through: a simple technique for examination of the small intestine. Br. J. Radiol., 38:691–693, 1965.

77. Dodds, W. J., Lydon, S. B., Stewart, E. T., et al.: Value of the tilt upside-down maneuver for roentgen examination of pelvic small bowel loops. Am. J. Roentgenol. Radium Ther. Nucl. Med., 123:412–414, 1975.

78. Poole, G. J.: A new roentgenographic method of measuring the retrogastric and retroduodenal spaces: Statistical evaluation of reliability and diagnostic utility. Radiology, 97:71–81, 1970.

79. Bancks, N. H., Goldstein, H. M., and Dodds, G. D.: The roentgenologic spectrum of small intestinal carcinoid tumors. Am. J. Roentgenol. Radium Ther. Nucl. Med., 123:274–280, 1975.

80. Meyers, M. A.: Metastatic seeding along the small bowel mesentery. Roentgen features. Am. J. Roentgenol. Radium Ther. Nucl. Med., 123:67–73, 1975.

81. Kaplan, H. S.: Hodgkin's Disease. Cambridge, Harvard University Press, 1972, p. 169.

82. Bennett, M. H., and Millett, Y. L.: Nodular sclerosing lymphosarcoma. A possible new clinico-pathological entity. Clin. Radiol., 20:339–343, 1969.

83. Millett, Y. L., Bennett, M. H., Jelliffe, A. M., et al.: Nodular sclerotic lymphosarcoma. A further review. Br. J. Cancer, 23:683–692, 1969.

84. Uribe, A. R., and Rappaport, H.: Malignant lymphoma, histiocytic type with sclerosis (sclerosing reticulum cell sarcoma). Cancer, 29:946–953, 1972.

85. Dorfman, R. F.: Personal communication, 1975.

86. Ostermiller, W. E., Jr., and Joergenson, E. J.: Carcinoid tumors of the small bowel. Arch. Surg., 93:616–619, 1966.

87. Norfray, J., Calenoff, L., and Zanon, B., Jr.: Aneurysmal lymphoma of the small intestine. Am. J. Roentgenol. Radium Ther. Nucl. Med., 119:335–341, 1973.

88. Hazzi, C. G., Lindner, A. E., and Marshak, R. H.: Diffuse lymphosarcoma of the intestine. Am. J. Gastroenterol., 60:74–80, 1973.

89. Selier, G.: Unusual roentgen presentation of a carcinoid tumor of the ileum. Am. J. Gastroenterol., 57:459–464, 1972.

90. Swischuk, L. E.: Mucosal patterns in diffuse diseases of the small bowel. Med. Radiogr. Photogr., 47:34–40, 1971.

91. Dunnick, R., Harell, G. S., and Parker, B.: "Bull's-eye lesions" of the stomach and small bowel. To be published.

92. Stein, L. A., and Margulis, A.: The spheroid sign. A new sign for accurate differentiation of intramural masses. Am. J. Roentgenol. Radium Ther. Nucl. Med., 123:420–426, 1975.

93. Mason, G. R., Dietrich, P., Friedland, G. W., et al.: The radiological findings in radiation-induced enteritis and colitis. A review of 30 cases. Clin. Radiol., 21:232–247, 1970.

94. Donaldson, S. S., Jundt, S., Ricour, C., et al.: Radiation enteritis in children. A retrospective review, clinicopathological correlation and dietary management. Cancer, 35:1167–1178, 1975.

95. Friedland, G. W., and Filly, R.: Intestinal tuberculosis in a child living in an affluent society. Pediatr. Radiol., 2:199–202, 1974.

96. Campbell, W. L., Green, W. M., and Seaman, W. B.: Inflammatory pseudotumor of the small intestine. Am. J. Roentgenol. Radium Ther. Nucl. Med., 121:305–311, 1974.

97. Gold, R. E., and Redman, H. C.: Mesenteric fibrosis simulating the angiographic appearance of ileal carcinoid tumor. Radiology, 103:85–86, 1972.

Chapter Nine

LIVER, GALLBLADDER, BILIARY DUCTS, PANCREAS, AND SPLEEN

CLINICAL CONSIDERATIONS

Presenting Signs and Symptoms

Primary or metastatic malignancies of the liver and spleen, as well as tumors of the gallbladder, pancreas, and some tumors of the bile ducts, often follow similar clinical courses.[1-16] Many of them are asymptomatic for a long period, or cause nonspecific symptoms such as fatigue, weakness, nausea, anorexia, fatty food intolerance, diarrhea, upper abdominal fullness or pain, and moderate weight loss. When hepatocarcinomas or gallbladder carcinomas develop in patients afflicted with cirrhosis, hemachromatosis, or chronic cholecystopathy, the tumors' first symptoms are usually hidden by those of the basic disease. Early clinical signs are often nonexistent or are of minor degree, such as slight enlargement of the liver or gallbladder, or minor jaundice. Conversely, tumors that cause early obstruction of the biliary system, such as carcinoma of the duodenal ampulla and tumors that secrete hormones, usually become manifest at an early stage. Jaundice, often of the intermittent type, and enlargement of the gallbladder and liver appear early in ampullary carcinoma. Endocrine tumors of the pancreas can manifest themselves through hyperglycemia, the ulcerative Zollinger-Ellison syndrome, or chronic diarrhea. Flushing of the skin, diarrhea, or asthma may occur with carcinoid metastases in the liver.

Progression of symptoms and signs offers qualitative and quantitative reflections of growth of the tumor, destruction of the affected organ, and involvement of the surrounding structures and organs. Upper abdominal pain, progressive weight loss, jaundice, pruritus, gallbladder distention, hepatomegaly, splenomegaly, and a palpable tumor mass are common. Fever, diarrhea, gastrointestinal bleeding, ascites, peripheral edema, migratory thrombophlebitis, and neuropsychiatric disturbances are less frequent manifestations of these malignancies.

Upper abdominal pain can be severe in carcinoma of the body or tail of the pancreas when there is infiltration of the peripancreatic neural plexi. The pain often has a postural pattern and radiates to the midback. In tumors of the liver, gallbladder, and spleen, the pain usually appears at a later stage of the disease, is located in the right or left upper quadrant, and sometimes radiates to the shoulder or subscapular area. Progressive loss of weight, common to all the malignancies under discussion, is most rapid in pancreatic carcinoma because of impaired digestion, malabsorption, and anorexia. Jaundice, often accompanied (and sometimes preceded) by pruritus, almost always occurs at some stage of biliary, pancreatic, and hepatic malignancies. In carcinoma of the head of the pancreas, jaundice often appears without pain and progresses rapidly. In bile duct or gallbladder carcinomas, it may be intermittent in type, may be less progressive, and is often associated with pain. An enlarged, palpable gallbladder with obstructive jaundice (Courvoisier's sign) is often found in association with carcinomas of the common bile duct, the duodenal ampulla, and the head of the pancreas. Hepatomegaly or splenomegaly may be impressive in both primary and metastatic tumors. On palpation, affected livers or spleens are hard, irregular, grossly nodular, and often tender. A palpable, irregular primary tumor mass is usually a late finding in carcinoma of the pancreas or gallbladder.

Gastrointestinal bleeding can occur from gastroesophageal varices secondary to extension of hepatic or pancreatic malignancies into the portal circulation and occlusion of the portal or splenic vein. Peripheral edema can result from inferior vena caval obstruction in the later stages of hepatic malignancies. Fever often accompanies primary hepatic and splenic tumors, and occasionally occurs in patients with biliary carcinomas. Migrating thrombophlebitis and neuropsychiatric disturbances are occasional prominent manifestations of carcinoma of the pancreas.

Differential Diagnosis

For years the diagnosis of malignancies of the liver, gallbladder, bile ducts, pancreas, and spleen was a dark area in the realm of oncology. Because of the late appearance of major symptoms and signs and the lack of sensitive examination methods, diagnoses were usually possible only in the late stages of disease, and often only after laparotomy. Thus, surgery was mostly palliative in nature, often confined to the relief of obstructive jaundice. Tumor resection, except in the case of carcinomas of the duodenal ampulla and endocrine tumors of the pancreas, was rarely attempted and cures were almost nonexistent.

New imaging techniques employing radionuclides or ultrasound, as well as new methods for the roentgenographic visualization of the biliary ducts, pancreatic ducts, and visceral arteries and veins, have greatly improved matters. With the proper use and experienced interpretation of these procedures, most tumors are now subject to early detection, better staging, and accurate assessment of operability (Tables 9–1 and 9–2).[17–21]

Crucial to successful early diagnosis is the prompt use of the appropriate diagnostic methods. Here the clinician has the primary responsibility, upon recognizing the possibility of tumor, to seek the indicated diagnostic measures, even when clinical findings are minor or atypical. Noninvasive screening procedures are used first; however, their diagnostic limitations have to be kept in mind in evaluating the results. In suspected hepatic or splenic malignancy, radionuclide imaging is a primary screening method (Fig. 9–1). Gray-scale ultrasonography also has high diagnostic potential in this connection (Fig. 9–2). Intravenous cholangiography is indicated in suspected gallbladder and bile duct lesions if major jaundice is absent. Radionuclide imaging, ultrasonography, and barium upper gastrointestinal studies are important screening procedures in suspected pancreatic malignancy (Fig. 9–3). Hypotonic duodenography is indicated when carcinoma of the duodenal

Table 9–1 Accuracy of Angiography in Diagnosing Hepatic, Splenic, and Pancreatic Tumors*

| Tumor Location | Number of Patients | Correct Diagnosis | | False-negative Diagnosis |
		NUMBER	PERCENTAGE	
Liver	75	73	97	2 metastatic tumors with simultaneous obstructive jaundice
Spleen	7	7	100	—
Pancreas	68	65	95	2 avascular islet cell tumors, 1 carcinoma with simultaneous pancreatitis and pancreatolithiasis

*Total of 150 consecutive proven cases at University of Oregon Health Sciences Center.

Table 9–2 Accuracy of Angiography in Excluding Hepatic and Pancreatic Tumors*

Organ	Number of Patients	Correct Diagnosis		False-positive Diagnosis
		Number	Percentage	
Liver	38	37	97	1 hepatitis with microabscesses
Pancreas	12	10	83	1 aberrant pancreas, 1 enlarged lymph node

*Total of 50 consecutive proven cases at University of Oregon Health Sciences Center.

ampulla or pancreatic head is suspected (Fig. 9–4).

If a patient has minor or atypical symptoms and screening procedures lead to positive or suspicious findings, invasive special radiologic procedures of higher accuracy are then used, as needed, for reaching a definitive diagnosis. Special procedures, however, should be applied early and as the initial investigations in patients who have clinical symptoms or signs that are highly suspicious or indicative of a malignancy. Angiography is used for diagnosis of hepatic and splenic tumors (Figs. 9–7 to 9–11, 9–22). The diagnosis of gallbladder, bile duct, and ampullary malignancies usually entails endoscopic retrograde or transhepatic cholangiography, and occasionally angiography (Figs. 9–5, 9–6, and 9–21). Angiography and endoscopic retrograde pancreatography play the leading role in the diagnosis of pancreatic cancer (Figs. 9–12 to 9–20). Employed singly or in combinations, these special procedures make possible an accurate diagnosis of most of the malignancies under discussion.

In the differential diagnosis of malignancies of the liver, gallbladder, biliary ducts, pancreas, and spleen, malignancies of other organs such as the stomach, duodenum, transverse colon, or kidney, as well as nonneoplastic diseases of an inflammatory, degenerative, or vascular origin, also have to be considered. Hepatitis, cirrhosis, benign liver tumors (angiomas, adenomas), or cysts and liver abscesses must be differentiated from hepatic malignancy. Chronic cholecystitis, primary biliary cirrhosis, gallbladder adenomatosis, biliary tract stones, strictures, and sclerosing cholangitis must be differentiated from biliary malignancy. Chronic

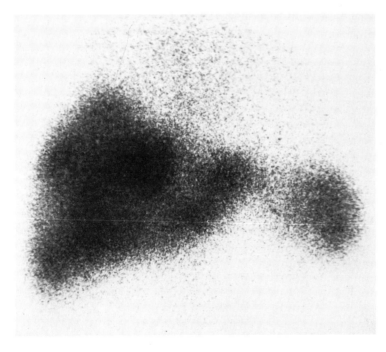

Figure 9–1 Multiple liver metastases from a colon carcinoma. Technetium-99m sulphur colloid scan reveals nonhomogeneous liver image with several defects.

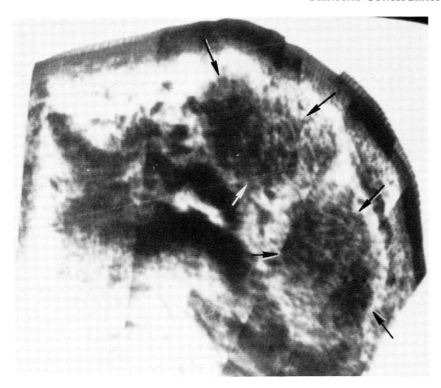

Figure 9–2 Multifocal hepatocellcarcinoma manifested clinically by fever and weight loss. B-mode ultrasonogram shows two major space-occupying lesions in the liver, with internal echoes (arrows)

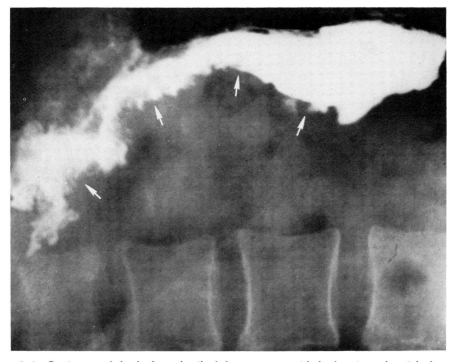

Figure 9–3 Carcinoma of the body and tail of the pancreas, with back pain and weight loss as the main clinical symptoms. Barium study of the stomach in translateral projection demonstrates enlargement of the retrogastric space (anterior stomach displacement) and tumor invasion of the posterior gastric wall (arrows).

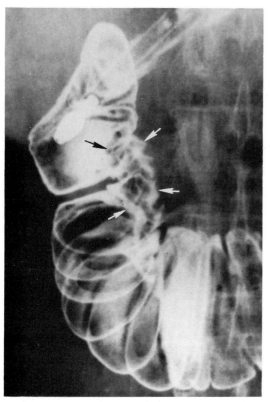

Figure 9–4 Carcinoma of the head of the pancreas presenting clinically with minor obstructive jaundice. Hypotonic duodenography shows irregularity of the medial contour of the descending duodenum with destruction of mucosa (arrows).

pancreatitis and pancreatic pseudocysts must be distinguished from carcinoma of the pancreas and, similarly, nonmalignant splenomegaly (as in portal hypertension, chronic inflammatory diseases, and lymphomyeloproliferative diseases) from splenic malignancy. Here, while the history and other clinical and laboratory findings are of great differential value, radiologic examinations are often required for a definitive answer. Selection of radiologic procedure(s) must depend on the specific clinical question(s) to be answered. Routine studies may occasionally be sufficient; however, the special procedures mentioned above often have to be used.

Therapeutic Decisions and Staging

The radical surgical resection of malignancies of the liver, gallbladder, bile ducts, pancreas, and spleen usually is a complex problem requiring detailed preoperative in-

formation about the tumor, including its type, location, size, and degree of extension, as well as the relation of the tumor to surrounding organs including major visceral arteries (celiac, hepatic, superior mesenteric arteries), portal trunks (portal, splenic, superior mesenteric veins), and the inferior vena cava (Figs. 9–8 and 9–14). Appraisal of the status of the noninvolved parts of the affected organs and their detailed vascular anatomy may also be of crucial importance in planning surgery, particularly of the liver and pancreas. The vascular anatomy in the upper abdomen, particularly anomalies of the hepatic arteries, also must be revealed prior to surgery. Angiography and cholangiopancreatography answer many of these questions. Complementary diagnostic techniques such as barium studies of the adjacent organs, inferior vena cavography, and direct portography may be necessary to obtain optimal information about tumor extension.[5, 6, 9–12, 14, 16]

Specific questions about the location of certain tumors often arise. In hepatic malignancies, the assessment of operability and decisions on the possibility of segmental or lobar hepatectomy require specific knowledge regarding the presence of segmental or lobar involvement, extension into the portal vein and inferior vena cava, and extensive involvement of the liver by diseases such as cirrhosis or hepatitis.[9] In evaluation of the operability of gallbladder carcinomas, an accurate assessment of the tumor's relation to the liver, colon, duodenum, portal vein, hepatic artery, and bile ducts is critical. Decisions about therapy and the choice of an appropriate surgical procedure for bile duct carcinoma must be based on information about its size, location and hepatic extension and the status of biliary ducts above the occlusive tumor (Figs. 9–5 and 9–6). Resectability of pancreatic carcinoma requires noninvolvement by tumor of the major celiac, hepatic, and superior mesenteric arteries, the portal, superior mesenteric, and left renal veins, and the inferior vena cava, as well as freedom from hepatic metastases and spread into the porta hepatis. In endocrine tumors of the pancreas, knowledge about multiplicity and the exact location of tumor(s), particularly with respect to distinguishing between location in the head and the tail of the pancreas and detecting the presence of liver metastases, is crucial in operative planning. In splenic malignancies, informa-

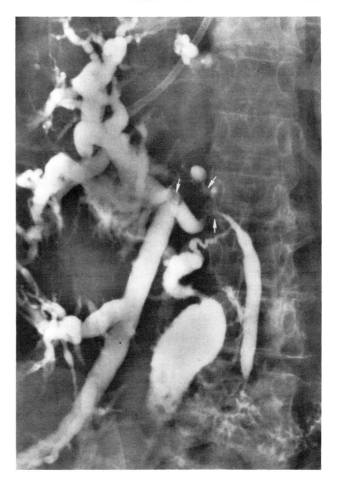

Figure 9–5 Carcinoma of the hepatic duct extending into the liver, with obstructive jaundice. Transjugular cholangiogram shows advanced, irregular obstruction of the hepatic duct (lower arrow), with deformity of the right and occlusion of the left main hepatic branches (arrows) and dilatation of the intrahepatic ducts in the right lobe.

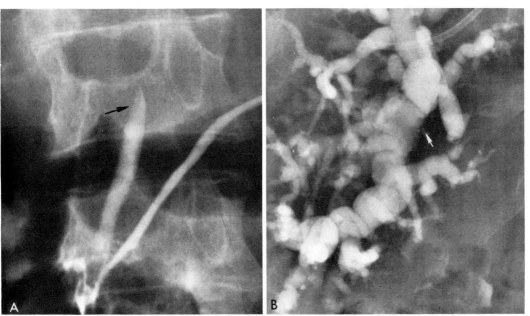

Figure 9–6 Bile duct carcinoma with occlusion of the common bile duct, presenting clinically with obstructive jaundice. A, Endoscopic retrograde cholangiogram shows distal margin of lesion occluding the common bile duct (arrow). B, Transjugular cholangiogram demonstrates proximal level of occlusion of the hepatic duct at the hepatic hilum (arrow), with extensive dilatation of the intrahepatic ducts.

tion about extension of tumor into the splenic flexure, the greater curvature of the stomach, the tail of the pancreas, and the left kidney is needed to evaluate operability and to plan surgery.

Even if a malignancy is judged inoperable because of its size, location or extension, diagnostic evaluation should be undertaken concerning its vascularity, arterial supply, and infiltrative nature, since, in some instances (including liver metastases from colonic or breast carcinomas), good clinical palliation may be achieved by selective intra-arterial infusions of chemotherapeutic agents.

Clinical Follow-up

Patients who have undergone radical or palliative operations, chemotherapy, or radiation therapy are usually examined at frequent intervals clinically. The reappearance (or increase) of symptoms and signs such as pain, weight loss, jaundice, and palpable mass is often indicative of recurrence or progression of malignancy. After extensive and radical surgery such as lobar hepatectomy or total pancreatectomy, however, some symptoms such as pain or diarrhea may persist, making the diagnosis of early tumor recurrence difficult. Similarly, it is sometimes difficult to differentiate clinically between progressive tumor growth (or recurrence) and the complications of a surgical procedure such as a subphrenic or perihepatic abscess, as well as the complications of radiation or chemical therapy. When this is a problem, radiologic follow-up, including ultrasound and radionuclide imaging, upper gastrointestinal barium study, cholangiography, and visceral angiography, may be of great value. (See also the section on radiologic follow-up later in this chapter.) These studies can help to detect early tumor recurrence, tumor progression or regression, and treatment complications. Radionuclide and ultrasound imaging and visceral angiography are indicated in the follow-up of hepatic malignancies. Upper gastrointestinal study and angiography are procedures of choice following pancreatic surgery (Fig. 9–9). Cholangiography done via a T-tube placed at surgery, or by means of endoscopic (via the duodenum) retrograde injection,

aids in the follow-up of patients who have had surgery for biliary malignancies.

RADIOLOGIC CONSIDERATIONS

Presenting Radiographic Signs

RADIONUCLIDE SCANNING

Radionuclide scanning is an important screening procedure for the diagnosis of hepatic, splenic, and pancreatic malignancies.[21–28] Technetium-99m sulfur colloid is used for the liver and spleen, and selenomethionine-75 for the pancreas. Normal organs exhibit evenly distributed radioactivity and cast homogeneous images. Tumors show up as focal defects, sometimes detectable even when they are as small as 2 to 3 cm in diameter (Fig. 9–1). However, the finding of focal defects is not specific, since these may appear in any lesion associated with parenchymal destruction, such as infarction, abscess, cyst, and cirrhosis. Anomalous organ configuration and pressure deformities from diseased adjacent organs and structures may also be difficult to distinguish from intrinsic defects. An unequivocally normal scan, however, constitutes a relatively credible finding. A suspicious or abnormal scan underscores the further need for appropriate special procedures.

ULTRASONOGRAPHY

The ultimate role of B-mode ultrasonography (echography) in the diagnosis of the malignancies under discussion remains to be established, but as a screening procedure it has the advantage of being simple, noninvasive, and nonionizing.[19–31] In this technique, a narrow beam of high frequency sound is used to scan the area in question. Reflected sound from various anatomic interfaces is reproduced as a cross-sectional image. Depending on the sensitivity and other parameters of the system, the normal liver and spleen are relatively free of internal echoes except for their hilar areas, and the normal pancreas is usually indistinguishable from contiguous retroperitoneal structures. Solid tumors can often be visualized as space-occupying lesions with scattered internal echoes (Fig. 9–2). An infiltrative tumor can exhibit irregular margins. Cystic fluid-filled spaces can usually be distinguished from neoplastic masses. Lesions less than 3 cm in diameter are usually not detectable. With further technical development, including the new gray-scale technique, the diagnostic value of ultrasonography will continue to increase. As with radionuclide scanning, however, nonspecificity is a problem with ultrasonography. The differentiation of benign solid tumors and granulomatous lesions from sonically similar malignant tumors is usually not possible and is not likely to become so.

UPPER GASTROINTESTINAL BARIUM STUDY

Conventional barium radiographic study of the stomach and duodenum has long been, and remains, the most common screening procedure for pancreatic cancer.[17, 18, 32–34] Unfortunately, its sensitivity is low. Although upper gastrointestinal examinations occasionally detect small tumors, especially those close to the duodenal wall, they usually show only carcinomas that are large enough to cause gross pancreatic enlargement and secondary infiltration or displacement of surrounding structures. Enlargement of the retrogastric space, deformity of the antrum or posterior gastric wall, and widening of the duodenal loop with medial wall irregularity are the most frequently encountered findings in pancreatic carcinoma and are seen in about 50 per cent of tumors (Fig. 9–3).[33, 34]

HYPOTONIC DUODENOGRAPHY

In this examination, an anticholinergic drug or glucagon is given to reduce the muscle tone and peristaltic activity of the duodenum.[17, 18, 35–77] With this induced immobility and with controlled distention of the duodenum with barium sulfate and air, anatomic abnormalities of the duodenum, the adjacent pancreatic head, and the duodenal papilla become more visible than in a conventional gastrointestinal study. Hypotonic duodenography is indicated particularly in the evaluation of patients with jaundice. It has a diagnostic accuracy rate of about 75 per cent in cancer of the pancreatic head and about 90 per cent in ampullary cancer.[35–37] Irregularity of the medial contour of the descending duodenum, with irregular spiculation of the wall and mucosal destruction, are often seen in carcinomas of the head of the pancreas (Fig. 9–4). Pancreatitis, however, may sometimes be difficult to distinguish from malignancy. An ampullary carcinoma can often be delineated as a mass protruding into the duodenal lumen.

INTRAVENOUS CHOLANGIOGRAPHY

Intravenous cholangiography may be indicated for patients with suspected gallbladder or bile duct malignancy.[17, 18, 38, 39] The biliary system usually can be visualized only in patients with serum bilirubin levels below 3 mg per 100 ml. Early carcinoma of the gallbladder can be seen as an irregular filling defect within this viscus. A bile duct carcinoma may appear as a localized ductal stenosis with dilatation of the proximal biliary system. Although tomography can improve the anatomic detail in intravenous cholangiography, a more direct, instrumental approach may be needed to resolve doubts (see the sections on endoscopic retrograde cholangiopancreatography and transhepatic cholangiography).

ANGIOGRAPHY

Angiography is the primary preoperative diagnostic procedure in malignancies of the liver, spleen, and pancreas, and may be of great value in gallbladder carcinoma.[18, 19, 21, 39–53] When performed by percutaneous vascular catheterization, the risk is low. Significant local complications at the site of catheter introduction (such as femoral artery thrombosis requiring surgical thrombectomy) occur in less than 0.3 per cent of patients. The high sensitivity of angiography, when properly performed, is related to the vascularity of the tumor. Highly vascular tumors (particularly metastatic carcinoids in the liver and some islet cell tumors) as small as 5 mm in diameter can be visualized; avascular tumors in the liver and pancreas are likely to be visible only when their diameter exceeds 2 cm. Angiographic accuracy in

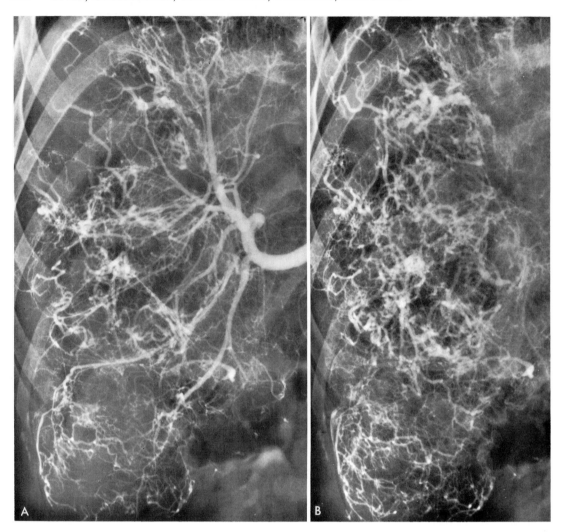

Figure 9–7 Diffuse hepatocellcarcinoma involving the whole right lobe of the liver. Abdominal fullness and hepatomegaly were the main clinical manifestations. Selective hepatic angiogram. *A,* Arterial phase reveals destruction of the normal arterial architecture and extensive tumor neovascularity. *B,* Early capillary phase accentuates tumor neovascularity, which consists of multiple bizarre, intermingled tumor vessels and vascular lakes.

hepatic and splenic tumors ranges from 80 to 95 per cent.[19–21] Optimal results require the use of "superselective" catheterization of the smaller arterial branches, including direct injections of contrast medium into the hepatic or splenic arteries. In the diagnosis of pancreatic tumors, angiographic studies that are limited to injection of the major trunks of the celiac and superior mesenteric arteries are accurate in about 60 per cent of cases and usually permit only the detection of larger tumors.[52] Direct (superselective) injections into the pancreatic branch (dorsal pancreatic; gastroduodenal; pancreaticoduodenal) arteries increase the diagnostic accuracy rate

of angiography to 95 per cent and permit the detection of much smaller tumors.[52] An evaluation of the angiographic findings by an experienced radiologist is essential for correct diagnosis in this rather difficult area. Advanced occlusive atherosclerotic disease may occasionally prevent satisfactory angiographic study.

Malignancies of the liver and spleen show up on angiograms as mass lesions causing displacement, encasement, or occlusion of adjacent "normal" vessels; they exhibit intrinsic tumor vessels to a variable degree. Hepatic carcinoma usually displays multiple, bizzare tumor vessels, vascular lakes, and arteriovenous shunts within the tumor (Figs. 9–7 and 9–8). Cholangiocarcinoma may cause minor tumor neovascularity, but more often causes invasion of adjacent vessels. Primary splenic tumors usually are moderately vascular (see Fig. 9–22). Hepatic or splenic metastases from hypernephromas, carcinoids, islet cell pan-

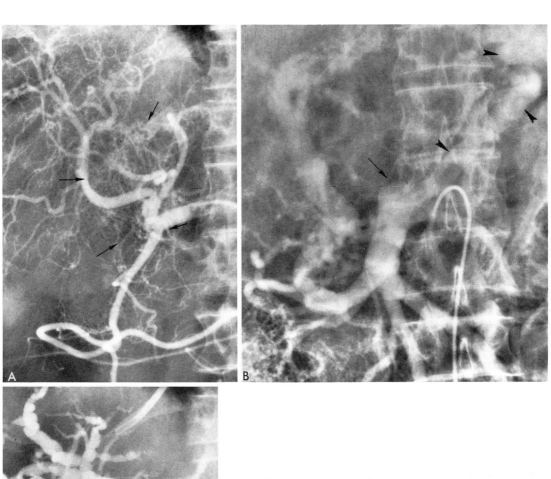

Figure 9–8 Hepatocellcarcinoma extending into the porta hepatis and presenting clinically with obstructive jaundice. *A,* Selective hepatic angiogram reveals displacement of the main hepatic branches. Tumor neovascularity extends from the liver into the porta hepatis (arrows). *B,* Venous phase of selective superior mesenteric angiogram demonstrates occlusion of the portal vein at its origin (arrow) and retrograde filling of an enlarged gastric coronary vein (lower arrowhead), with gastroesophageal varices (upper two arrowheads). *C,* Transjugular cholangiogram shows enlargement of intrahepatic ducts, compression of the main hepatic ducts (upper arrow), and advanced irregular and multifocal obstruction of the extrahepatic ductal system (lower 3 arrows).

creatic tumors, or carcinomas of the breast, colon, or thyroid are often hypervascular and thus are revealed by the presence of irregular tumor vessels during the arterial phase of the examination and by a dense tumor blush during the capillary phase (Figs. 9–9 and 9–10). The metastases of bronchogenic, esophageal, gastric, and non–islet cell pancreatic carcinomas are usually hypovascular and are revealed by vascular displacement and encasement during the arterial phase, but they mainly appear as defects within the liver or spleen during the capillary phase of the study (Fig. 9–11).

Neoplastic arterial or venous encasement and vascular occlusion are characteristic signs of pancreatic carcinoma (Figs. 9–12 to 9–14). Small intrapancreatic arteries are involved at an early stage of the disease; larger cancers also affect the peripancreatic arteries and veins. Intrinsic tumor vascularity is not prominent in ordinary pancreatic adenocarcinomas; pancreatic cystadenocarcinomas, on the other hand, display extensive neovascularity (Fig. 9–15). Islet cell tumors, both benign and malignant, are often hypervascular and exhibit a typical tumor blush in 60 to 70 per cent of cases (Figs. 9–16 and

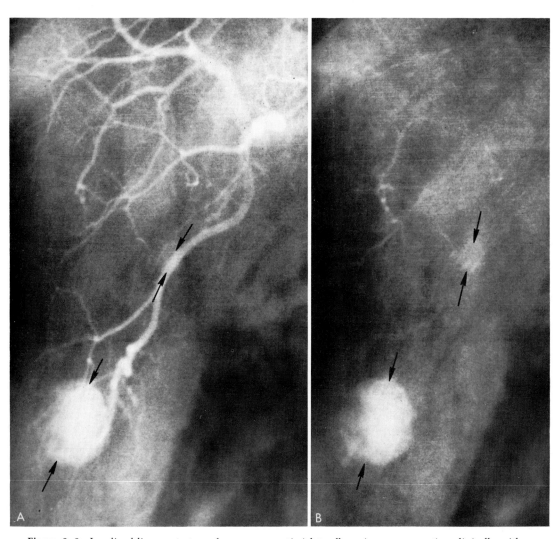

Figure 9–9 Localized liver metastases from a pancreatic islet cell carcinoma, presenting clinically with recurrence of hyperinsulinism three years after total pancreatectomy. Partial hepatectomy subsequently cured the patient (eight years follow-up). Selective hepatic angiogram. *A*, Arterial phase reveals two tumor blushes in the right lobe (arrows). *B*, Early capillary phase makes tumor blushes more obvious (arrows). Size of larger tumor is 2 cm and the smaller tumor 8 mm.

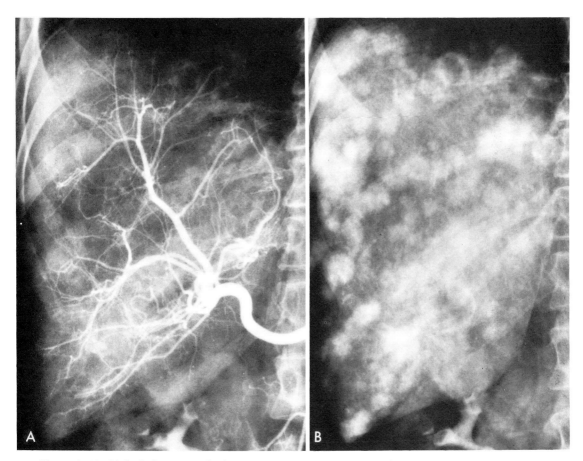

Figure 9–10 Multiple hypervascular liver metastases in a patient with breast carcinoma presenting clinically with hepatomegaly. Selective hepatic angiogram. *A,* Arterial phase reveals stretching and displacement of multiple medium-sized and small hepatic branches. *B,* Capillary phase demonstrates multiple small metastases (3 to 15 mm in size) in the form of dense tumor blushes.

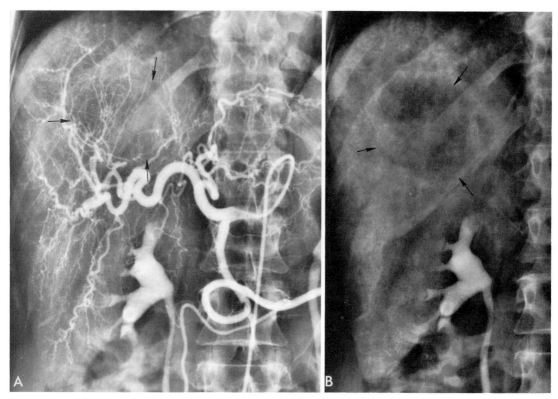

Figure 9–11   Solitary, large, hypovascular metastasis of a leiomyosarcoma in the right lobe of the liver. No clinical symptoms. Selective hepatic angiogram. *A,* Arterial phase reveals displacement and stretching of hepatic branches around a hypovascular focus in the upper part of the right lobe (arrows). *B,* Capillary phase demonstrates a rounded defect measuring 5 cm in diameter (arrows).

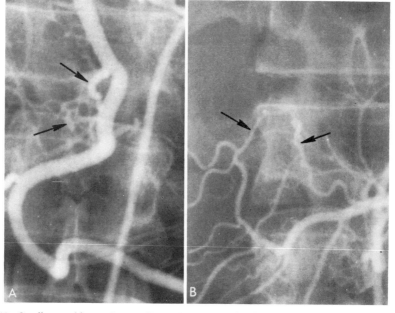

Figure 9–12   Small operable carcinoma (2 cm in size) in the head of the pancreas, clinically manifested by minor jaundice. Pancreatic angiogram. *A,* Close-up view of a selective gastroduodenal angiogram reveals localized tumor encasement of the pancreaticoduodenal arteries (arrows). *B,* Close-up view of a selective inferior pancreaticoduodenal angiogram confirms the localized encasement of small arteries (arrows) in the same area of the head of the pancreas.

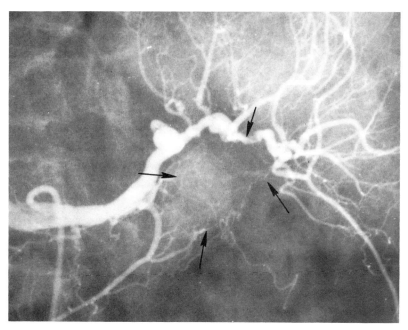

Figure 9–13 Small carcinoma in the tail of the pancreas (2 by 3 cm in size), with back pain as the only clinical symptom. Selective splenic angiogram reveals tumor invasion of the distal splenic artery (uppermost arrow), as well as occlusion of several small pancreatic arteries (arrows) by tumor.

9–17). The larger ones may contain irregular tumor vessels and, if malignant, often show irregular, blurred tumor margins. Hypovascular islet cell tumors are recognized by their mass effects on adjacent pancreatic arteries.

Gallbladder carcinoma is usually manifested by early invasive changes in the cystic artery branches, mild neovascularity, and, in particular, by an irregular blush during the capillary phase of the angiogram at the site of a localized thickening in the gallbladder wall. Larger tumors usually display moderate neovascularity, and tend to invade surrounding organs and vascular structures.

ENDOSCOPIC RETROGRADE CHOLANGIOPANCREATOGRAPHY (ERCP)

In endoscopic retrograde cholangiopancreatography (ERCP) a side-viewing fiberduodenoscope is used to cannulate the duodenal papilla (papilla of Vater) and opacify the biliary or pancreatic ducts with contrast agent.[54–56] During the peroral introduction of the endoscope, additional information is obtained about the stomach,

duodenum, and duodenal papilla. Direct or brush biopsy of visualized mucosal lesions, as well as samples of pancreatic juice or bile for laboratory tests (culture, cytology, carcinoembryonic antigen), can also be obtained during the study. With experience, the success rate in cannulating the papilla is about 90 per cent; however, sometimes only one duct system (pancreatic *or* biliary) can be visualized. ERCP has now become the primary preoperative diagnostic procedure for malignancies of the bile ducts and gallbladder and is used also in virtually all instances of unexplained obstructive jaundice. Bile duct carcinoma is demonstrated by retrograde cholangiography as a localized biliary stenosis or obstruction (Fig. 9–6). The stenosis may be smooth or irregular, and the proximal bile ducts are usually distended. With complete occlusion, only the distal portion of the common bile duct is visualized by this retrograde technique. In their early stages, gallbladder carcinomas appear as irregular, polypoid filling defects. In the later stages of the disease with local extension of the tumor, the gallbladder usually does not fill while the visualized common bile duct appears displaced and narrowed, occasionally exhibiting irregular margins.

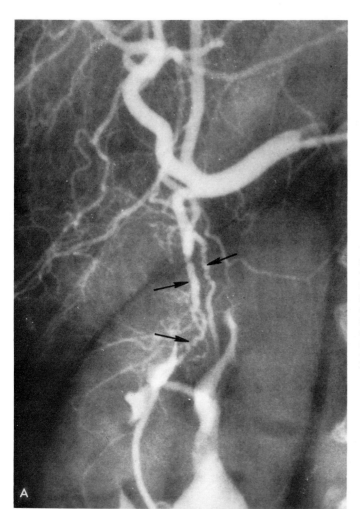

Figure 9–14   Inoperable carcinoma of the head of the pancreas, presenting clinically with weight loss, jaundice, and gastrointestinal bleeding. *A,* Selective hepatic angiogram demonstrates advanced tumor infiltration (encasement) of the gastroduodenal artery and its pancreaticoduodenal branches (arrows). *B,* Venous phase of selective celiac angiogram shows tumor invasion and segmental occlusion of the portal vein (arrows), with multiple small venous collaterals.

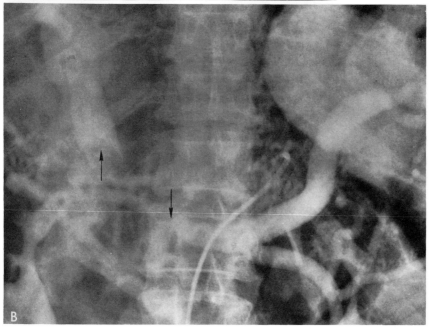

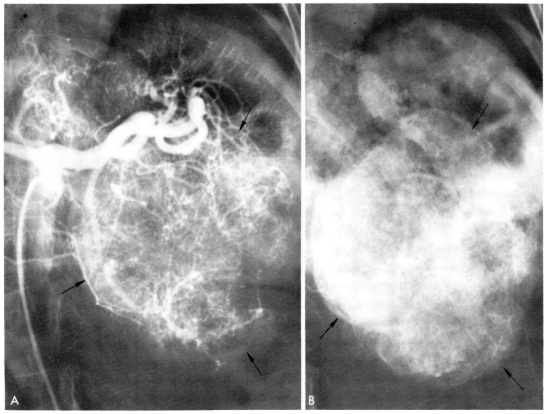

Figure 9–15 Cystadenoma of the tail of the pancreas presenting clinically with abdominal distress and a mass. Selective celiac angiogram. *A*, Arterial phase reveals hypervascular tumor, 10 by 12 cm in size (arrows). *B*, Capillary phase of the same angiogram shows nonhomogeneous tumor blush (arrows), containing several defects.

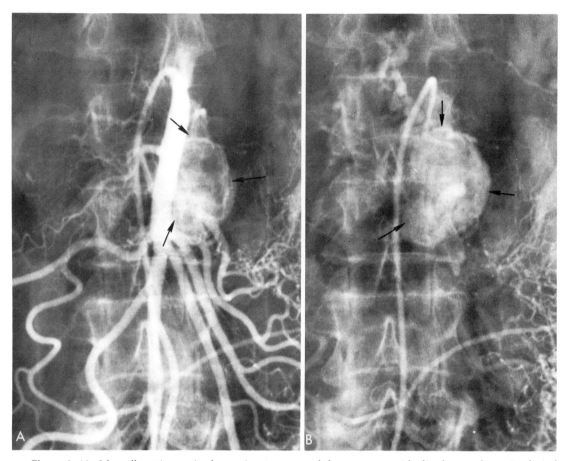

Figure 9–16   Islet cell carcinoma in the uncinate process of the pancreas, with diarrhea as the main clinical symptom. Selective superior mesenteric angiogram. *A,* Arterial phase shows hypervascular tumor blush (arrows), 4 by 3 cm in size. *B,* Early capillary phase (2 seconds later than *A);* tumor blush is more obvious (arrows).

In the diagnosis of pancreatic cancer, ERCP complements angiography. It is indicated when angiography does not give an adequate answer, either because of technical failure to visualize the pancreatic vessels directly or because diagnostically specific findings are not present. Irregular, localized narrowing of one or more major pancreatic ducts, with saccular dilatation of smaller periphral ducts, on ERCP is considered typical for pancreatic cancer (Fig. 9–18). Complete occlusion of the involved ducts is often seen, particularly with larger tumors (Fig. 9–19).

TRANSHEPATIC CHOLANGIOGRAPHY

Transhepatic cholangiography may be performed by the percutaneous (transperi-

toneal), peritoneoscopic, or transjugular (transvenous) approach.[59–63] The transjugular approach, in which a catheter-needle system is introduced percutaneously by means of the internal jugular vein through the right atrium into an hepatic vein, and a needle is then introduced through the vascular catheter into the liver to enter the biliary system, is more elaborate,* but it is safer since it eliminates the risks of hemoperitoneum and bile peritonitis. Transhepatic cholangiography is indicated in patients with obstructive jaundice, when the biliary system could not be opacified by ERCP or when complete ductal occlusion limits roentgenographic visualization to the distal hepatic or common

---

*This study (transjugular cholangiography) is not widely available in most centers, at present.

bile duct (Fig. 9–6). Visualization of the proximal, prestenotic, and distended biliary system is essential for operative planning and is the usual objective of a transhepatic study in these situations.

The site of a demonstrated bile duct occlusion is ordinarily identical to that of the tumor. Carcinoma of the bile ducts generally causes occlusion near the hepatic hilum, while carcinoma of the pancreas leads to occlusion in the middle or distal common bile duct (Figs. 9–6, 9–19A, and 9–20). Carcinoma of the duodenal papilla causes obstruction of the extreme distal segment of the common bile duct and dilatation of the whole biliary system. Neoplastic ductal occlusion may be conical or irregular in configuration, as opposed to a calculus, which gives a typical convex defect within the duct on the cholangiogram.

Differential Diagnosis

Proper application and skilled interpretation of the foregoing special examinations make accurate differential diagnosis possible

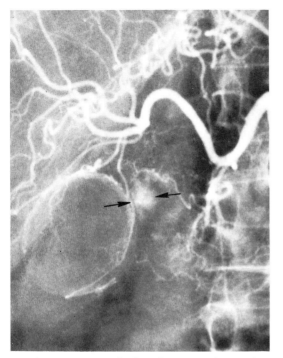

Figure 9–17   Small islet cell tumor within an aberrant pancreas in the descending duodenum, causing Zollinger-Ellison syndrome. Close-up view of selective celiac angiogram reveals tumor blush 8 mm in diameter (arrows).

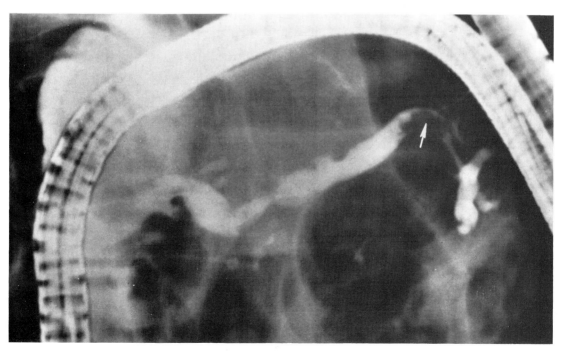

Figure 9–18   Carcinoma of the tail of the pancreas, with back pain as the main clinical symptom. Endoscopic retrograde pancreatogram shows severe, irregular stenosis of the distal pancreatic duct (arrow).

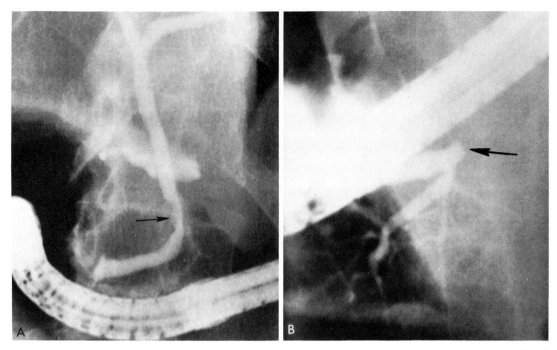

Figure 9–19 Carcinoma of the head of the pancreas, with diarrhea and weight loss as the main clinical symptoms. *A,* Endoscopic retrograde cholangiogram reveals displacement and localized, irregular narrowing of the distal common bile duct (arrow). *B,* Endoscopic retrograde pancreatogram demonstrates complete occlusion of the main pancreatic duct (arrow).

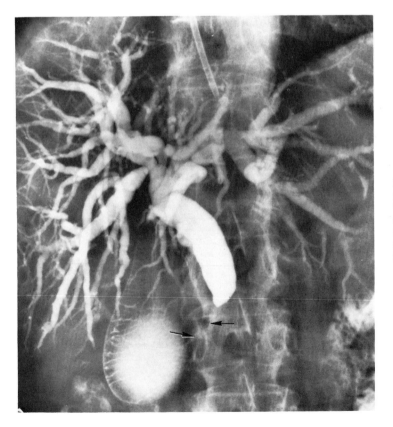

Figure 9–20 Carcinoma of the head of the pancreas, manifested clinically by obstructive jaundice. Transjugular cholangiogram shows subtotal obstruction of the distal common bile duct (arrows), with dilatation of the whole biliary system.

in most cases. For patients in whom tumors coexist with other disease(s), additional studies may be necessary.

Angiography usually allows the differentiation of primary or secondary hepatic malignancies from benign tumors (angiomas, adenomas), cysts, focal nodular hyperplasia, regenerative nodules, liver abscesses, infarcts, and diffuse liver diseases including cirrhosis and hepatitis. Difficulty may arise in differentiating a solitary tumor, with central necrosis, from an abscess. The angiographic diagnosis of hepatic metastases within a cirrhotic liver also may offer a serious problem. In this situation, small hypovascular metastases may not be demonstrable without exploratory laparotomy and biopsy.

Nontumorous biliary tract diseases such as cholecystitis, biliary calculi, gallbladder adenomatosis, and diffuse sclerosing cholangitis are not difficult to distinguish from malignancies of the gallbladder and bile ducts by means of cholangiography. However, benign biliary strictures and *localized* sclerosing cholangitis, affecting the common or hepatic bile ducts, may closely resemble bile duct carcinomas. Here, complementary selective angiography is of great value when it demonstrates neoplastic invasion of the hepatic artery or one of its branches (Fig. 9–21). Unfortunately, vascular invasion is usually a relatively late finding, and the above problems in differential diagnosis may require laparotomy and open biopsy.

Pancreatic carcinoma is readily distinguished from a pseudocyst on angiography; its differentiation from chronic pancreatitis is more difficult but is usually possible. The localized changes of irregular encasement and occlusion of pancreatic vessels seen in carcinoma differ from the diffuse, more regular vascular changes associated with chronic pancreatitis. When carcinoma develops in a pancreas that is already affected by chronic atrophic pancreatitis, a pre-existing reduction in the vasculature may make the differentiation difficult or impossible. Angiography ordinarily permits a differentiation to be made between pancreatic islet cell tumors and other processes with a similar appearance, such as inflammatory lymph nodes or foci of aberrant splenic tissue.

In the differential diagnosis of splenic malignancies, angiography again plays a significant role, helping to distinguish them by virtue of their tumor neovascularity from splenomegaly due to passive congestion, blood dyscrasias, or inflammation (Fig. 9–22). In the spleen as in the liver, the differentiation between a necrotic tumor and an abscess may be difficult, however.

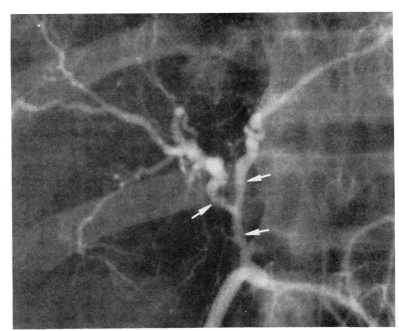

Figure 9–21 Bile duct carcinoma clinically manifested by minor, recurrent obstructive jaundice. Close-up view of a selective hepatic angiogram reveals tumor encasement of the hepatic artery and its branches (arrows).

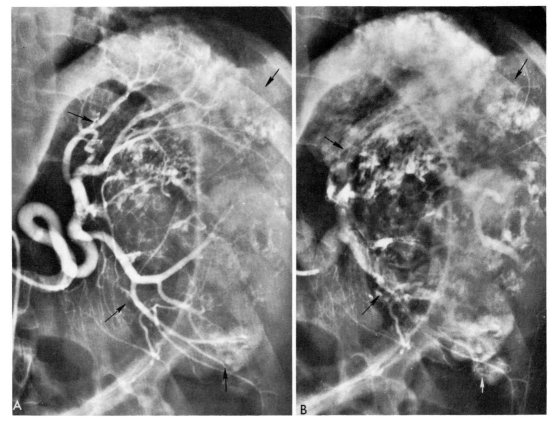

Figure 9–22   Reticulum cell sarcoma of the spleen, presenting clinically with fever, left upper quadrant pain, and mass. Selective splenic angiogram (arrows indicate tumor size). *A,* Arterial phase reveals stretching and displacement of intrasplenic branches and multiple, irregular tumor vessels. *B,* Capillary phase: tumor neovascularity is more obvious.

Localization and Staging

Various special roentgen examination methods, particularly angiography, are useful in locating and establishing the nature of malignancies and also in providing prognostic information about their size, spread, plurality, and extension to surrounding organs and structures.[17–19, 39–53] Angiographically, determination of the location and extent of a tumor is based on the ability to visualize its blood supply (Fig. 9–17). Thus, while a localized tumor gets its entire supply from the organ primarily involved, as a tumor invades surrounding tissues it tends to parasitize the adjacent blood supply and this may be recognizable angiographically.

Direct tumor invasion may also be reflected angiographically through changes caused by the neoplastic infiltration of adjacent vascular structures and organs. Malig-

nancies of the liver, particularly primary hepatomas, frequently invade the portal vessels and the inferior vena cava (Fig. 9–8). Tumors in the right hepatic lobe extend into the right colonic flexure or the right kidney, those in the left lobe into the spleen and stomach. Gallbladder carcinomas can erode into the liver, portal vein, right colonic flexure, or duodenum. Pancreatic carcinomas often involve the celiac artery and its branches, the splenic and portal veins, the mesentery and its vessels, the duodenum, the stomach, and occasionally the spleen, the left kidney, and the inferior vena cava (Fig. 9–14). Splenic malignancies tend to extend into the stomach, the tail of the pancreas, and the left colonic flexure.

Tumor invasion may cause characteristic angiographic changes consisting of irregular vascular encasement or occlusion. These invasive changes are distinguishable from simple pressure displacements of adjacent vessels caused by an expansive tumor growth. Direct tumor extension into the surrounding organs and vital vessels such as the celiac, hepatic, and superior mesenteric arteries, and the portal and superior mesenteric veins, usually precludes radical surgery (Figs. 9–8 and 9–14)

In evaluating tumor extension, other types of examination may be needed to add to the information provided by the studies already discussed. Barium examination can be useful in connection with the possible spread of tumors into the stomach, duodenum, and colon. An assessment of the relationship of a tumor to the major trunks of the portal circulation can usually be based upon the venous phase of visceral angiography. Should this be inadequate, *direct* portography can be performed by means of splenoportography (direct percutaneous splenic puncture and injection of contrast medium into the spleen), by transhepatic portal vein catheterization (following transperitoneal or transjugular puncture of the liver), or by umbilical vein catheterization (after surgical reopening of the umbilical vein). At times, inferior vena cavography may be a useful adjunct to evaluate the relationship of a tumor to the cava, including direct extension of hepatic malignancies via the hepatic veins.

In the preoperative evaluation of the vascular anatomy of the upper abdomen, it is important that attention be directed to the possible presence of major vascular anomalies in order to provide a guide for the surgeon. The liver is supplied relatively often, at least in part, by aberrant hepatic arteries arising from the superior mesenteric or the left gastric arteries, and less commonly from other visceral arteries or the aorta. Specific knowledge of such anatomic variations can be crucial to the safe performance of surgery. It is also important in planning selective arterial infusions of chemotherapeutic agents.

Radiologic Follow-up

Evaluation of results and complications of surgery, irradiation, or chemotherapy and the detection of tumor recurrence are the principal indications for radiologic follow-up studies. In the patient with primary or secondary liver malignancies, radionuclide imaging offers a starting point. Scanning performed after chemotherapy can show progression or decrease in metastases and in overall liver size. After partial hepatectomy, scanning easily permits an assessment of compensatory hypertrophy of the remaining liver parenchyma. In youthful patients, total restoration of the original liver mass may take place within a year. Posthepatectomy recurrence of hepatic tumors can also be diagnosed by scanning; however, a nonhomogeneous liver image, occasionally associated with compensatory hypertrophy, may make the *early* diagnosis of tumor recurrence difficult and uncertain. Angiography is preferable to scanning when a detailed evaluation of the liver is required. With successful chemotherapy of liver metastases, angiography reveals the diminished size and vascularity of individual tumors, with associated necrosis and fibrosis, as well as decreased overall liver size. When compensatory liver hypertrophy occurs following partial hepatectomy, the arteries in the residual parenchyma enlarge in diameter and in length, and they spread apart in association with the hypertrophy.[64] Tumor recurrence is also readily recognizable by angiography, especially with hypervascular malignancies; resurgent neovascularity similar to that in the previously resected tumor is the typical finding.

In patients who have undergone radical pancreatic surgery, upper gastrointestinal study allows an evaluation of the reconstituted upper gastrointestinal tract. In the diagnosis of tumor recurrence, however, barium studies have a low order of sensitivity, because the differentiation of changes caused by surgery from those caused by tumor recurrence is difficult. Angiography affords a much higher level of diagnostic accuracy. Like the original malignancy, a recurrent pancreatic tumor may cause angiographic evidence of vascular invasion and tumor neovascularity. Familiarity with what has been done at surgery is essential to making a distinction between postsurgical changes and tumor recurrence. The angiographic follow-up of patients after pancreatic surgery should always include, specifically, a careful search for liver metastases. This is particularly important in patients with islet cell tumors, in which recurrent clinical symptoms can be caused by localized liver metastases that can then be excised (Fig. 9–9). In postoperative patients who develop primary or recurrent obstructive jaundice, transhepatic cholangiography may be indicated in order to show the site of obstruction and the anatomy of the proximal biliary system.

Following biliary surgery, patients are often studied by cholangiography through a T-tube that has been left in place. When this is not applicable and an indication for cholangiography exists, the endoscopic retrograde technique can be employed. While progressive ductal stenosis can be caused by persistent or recurrent tumor, it may be difficult to differentiate tumor from benign postsurgical scarring. When complete occlusion of the reconstructed bile duct develops postoperatively, transhepatic cholangiography will be required to evaluate the biliary system above the obstruction.

References

1. Berk, J. E., and Priest, R. J.: Tumors of the liver. *In* Bockus, H. L. (ed.), Gastroenterology. 3rd ed., vol. 3. Philadelphia, W. B. Saunders, 1965.
2. Berk, J. E., and Haubrich, W. L.: Tumors of the pancreas. *In* Bockus, H. L. (ed.), Gastroenterology. 3rd. ed., vol. 3. 1965.
3. Carey, L. C.: Islet cell tumors of the pancreas. *In* Carey, L. C. (ed.), The Pancreas. St. Louis, C. V. Mosby, 1973.
4. Cohn, E. M.: Tumors of the gallbladder and bile ducts. *In* Bockus, H. L. (ed.), Gastroenterology. 3rd ed., vol. 3. Philadelphia, W. B. Saunders, 1965.
5. DeBakey, M. E., and Jordan, G. L.: Surgery of the liver. *In* Schiff, L. (ed.), Diseases of the Liver. 3rd ed. Philadelphia, J. B. Lippincott, 1969.
6. Dowdy, G. S.: The Biliary Tract. Philadelphia, Lea and Febiger, 1969.
7. Dreiling, D. A., and Greenstein, A.: Diagnosis of pancreatic disease. *In* Carey, L. C. (ed.) The Pancreas. St. Louis, C. V. Mosby, 1973.
8. Gall, E. A.: Tumors of the liver. *In* Schiff, L. (ed.), Diseases of the Liver. Philadelphia, J. B. Lippincott, 1969.
9. Jordan, G. L.: Benign and malignant tumors of the pancreas and the periampullary region. *In* Howard, J. M. (ed.), Surgical Diseases of the Pancreas. Philadelphia, J. B. Lippincott, 1960.
10. Puestow, C. B.: Surgery of the Biliary Tract, Pancreas, and Spleen. Chicago, Year Book Medical Pub., 1964.
11. Schwartz, S. I.: Surgical Diseases of the Liver. New York, McGraw-Hill, 1964.
12. Smith, R.: The Surgery of Pancreatic Neoplasms. Edinburgh and London, E. S. Livingston, Ltd., 1953.
13. Solan, M. J., and Jackson, B. T.: Carcinoma of the gallbladder: A clinical appraisal and review of 57 cases. Br. J. Surg., 58:593–597, 1971.
14. Warren, K. W., and Jefferson, M. F.: Carcinoma of the exocrine pancreas. *In* Carey, L. C. (ed.), The Pancreas. St. Louis, C. V. Mosby, 1973.
15. Williams, R. D., and Fisch, Y. C.: Diseases of the gallbladder and extrahepatic bile ducts. *In* Schiff, L. (ed.), Diseases of the Liver. Philadelphia, J. B. Lippincott, 1969.
16. Wilson, S. D.: Ulcerogenic tumors of the pancreas: The Zollinger-Ellison syndrome. *In* Carey, L. C. (ed.), The Pancreas. St. Louis, C. V. Mosby, 1973.
17. Eaton, S. B., Jr., and Ferrucci, J. T., Jr. (eds.): Radiology of the Pancreas and Duodenum. Philadelphia, W. B. Saunders, 1973.
18. Rösch, J.: Roentgenology of the Spleen and Pancreas. Springfield, Ill., Charles C Thomas, 1968.
19. Rösch, J.: Arteriography in the diagnosis of tumors of the liver, spleen, and pancreas. *In* Tumor Diagnosis. Chicago, Year Book Medical Pub., 1975.
20. Short, W. F., Bron, K. M., Eaton, S. B., et al.: Pancreatic evaluation by roentgenography, ultrasound, and radioisotopes. *In* Carey, L. C. (ed.), The Pancreas. St. Louis, C. V. Mosby, 1973.
21. DuPriest, R. W., Haines, J. E., Rösch, J., et al.: A comparison of scintiscans and arteriograms for identifying metastatic intrahepatic tumors. Surg. Gynecol. Obstet. 136:705–710, 1973.
22. Haynie, T. P., Ajmani, S. K., and Johns, M. F.: Liver, spleen, and pancreas scanning. *In* Tumor Diagnosis. Chicago, Year Book Medical Pub., 1975.
23. Landman, S., Polcyn, R. E., and Gottschalk, A.: Pancreas imaging—is it worth it? Radiology, 100:631–636, 1971.
24. Potsaid, M. S.: Radionuclide pancreatography. *In* Eaton, S. B., Jr., and Ferrucci, J. T., Jr. (eds.), Radiology of the Pancreas and Duodenum. Philadelphia, W. B. Saunders, 1973.
25. Lunia, S., Parthasarathy, K. L., Bakshi, S., et al.: An evaluation of 99m Tc-sulfur colloid liver scintiscans and their usefulness in metastatic workup: A review of 1,424 studies. J. Nucl. Med., 16:62–65, 1975.
26. De Nardo, G. L., Stadalnik, R. C., DeNardo, S. J., et al.: Hepatic scintiangiographic patterns. Radiology, 111:135–141, 1974.
27. Drum, D. E., and Christacopoulos, J. S.: Hepatic scintigraphy in clinical decision making. J. Nucl. Med., 13:908–914, 1972.
28. Rossi, P., and Gould, H.: Angiography and scanning in liver disease. Radiology, 96:553–561, 1970.
29. Leopold, G. R.: Ultrasonic B-scanning in the evaluation of abdominal malignancy. *In* Tumor Diagnosis. Chicago, Year Book Medical Pub., 1975.
30. Filley, R. A., and Freimanis, A. K.: Echographic diagnosis of pancreatic lesions. Radiology, 96:575–582, 1970.
31. Walls, W. J., Gonzalez, G., Martin, N. L., et al.: B-scan ultrasound evaluation of the pancreas. Radiology, 114:127–134, 1975.
32. Eyler, W. R., Clark, M. D., and Rian, R. L.: An evaluation of roentgen signs of pancreatic enlargement. J.A.M.A., 181:967–971, 1962.

33. Larsen, R. A., and Pedersen, A.: Roentgenologic findings in the stomach and duodenum in cancer of the pancreas. Acta Radiol. (Stockh.), 45:459–469, 1956.

34. Moseley, R. D.: Roentgen diagnosis of pancreatic disease. Arch. Intern. Med., 107:31–36, 1961.

35. Jacquemet, P., Liotta, D., and Mallett-Guy, P.: The Early Radiological Diagnosis of Diseases of the Pancreas and Ampulla of Vater: Elective Exploration of the Ampulla of Vater and the Head of the Pancreas by Hypotonic Duodenography. Springfield, Ill., Charles C Thomas, 1965.

36. Bilbao, M. K., Rösch, J., Frische, L. H., et al.: Hypotonic duodenography in the diagnosis of pancreatic disease. Semin. Roentgenol., 3:280–287, 1968.

37. Eaton, S. B., Benedict, K. T., Ferrucci, J. T., et al.: Hypotonic duodenography. Radiol. Clin. North Am., 8:125–137, 1970.

38. Bragg, D. G., and Evans, J. A.: Roentgen aspects of liver and biliary tract diseases. In Schiff, L. (ed.), Diseases of the Liver. Philadelphia, J. B. Lippincott, 1969.

39. Shehadi, W. H.: Clinical Radiology of the Biliary Tract. New York, McGraw-Hill, 1963.

40. Abrams, R. M., Meng, C. H., Firooznia, H., et al.: Angiographic demonstration of carcinoma of the gallbladder. Radiology, 94:277–282, 1970.

41. Baum, S., and Athanasoulis, C. A.: Angiography. In Eaton, S. B., Jr., and Ferrucci, J. T., Jr. (eds.), Radiology of the Pancreas and Duodenum. Philadelphia, W. B. Saunders, 1973.

42. Boijsen, E.: Selective hepatic angiography in primary and secondary tumors of the liver. Rev. Int. Hepatol., 15:385–398, 1965.

43. Boijsen, E., and Samuelsson, L.: Angiographic diagnosis of tumors arising from the pancreatic islets. Acta Radiol., 10:161–176, 1970.

44. Bookstein, J. J., Reuter, S. R., and Martel, W.: Angiographic evaluation of pancreatic carcinoma. Radiology, 93:757–764, 1969.

45. Gray, R. K., Rösch, J., and Grollman, J. H.: Arteriography in the diagnosis of islet-cell tumors. Radiology, 97:39–44, 1970.

46. Lunderquist, A.: Angiography in carcinoma of the pancreas. Acta Radiol. (Diagn.) (Suppl.), 235: 1965.

47. Nebesar, R. A., Pollard, J. J., and Stone, I. D.: Angiographic diagnosis of malignant disease of the liver. Radiology, 86:284–292, 1966.

48. Pollard, J. J., Fleischli, D. J., and Nebesar, R. A.: Angiography of hepatic neoplasms. Radiol. Clin. North Am., 8:31–41, 1970.

49. Reuter, S. R., and Redman, H. C.: Gastrointestinal Angiography. Philadelphia, W. B. Saunders, 1972.

50. Reuter, S. R., Redman, H. C., and Bookstein, J. J.: Differential problems in the angiographic diagnosis of carcinoma of the pancreas. Radiology, 96:93–99, 1970.

51. Rösch, J., and Steckel, R. J.: Selective angiography of the abdominal viscera. In Hanafee, W. N., et al. (eds.), Golden's Diagnostic Radiology, Section 18, Selective Angiography. Baltimore, Williams & Wilkins, 1972.

52. Rösch, J., and Holman, C.: Superselective arteriography of the pancreas. In Anacker, H. (ed.), Efficiency and Limits of Radiologic Examination of the Pancreas. Stuttgart, Thieme Verlag, 1975.

53. Tylén, U.: Accuracy of angiography in the diagnosis of carcinoma of the pancreas. Acta Radiol., 14:449–466, 1973.

54. Weiss, H. D., Anacker, H., Wiesner, W., et al.: Duodenoscopic pancreatography. Radiology, 106:333–339, 1973.

55. Short, W. F.: Pancreatography. In Eaton, S. B., Jr., and Ferrucci, J. T., Jr. (eds.), Radiology of the Pancreas and Duodenum. Philadelphia, W. B. Saunders, 1973.

56. Katon, R. M., Lee, T. G., Parent, J. A., et al.: Endoscopic retrograde cholangiopancreatography. Am. J. Diag. Dis., 19:295–306, 1974.

57. Vennes, J. A.: Endoscopic visualization of pancreatic and bile ducts in malignant disease. In Tumor Diagnosis. Chicago, Year Book Medical Pub., 1975.

58. Legge, D. A., and Carlson, H. C.: Cholangiographic appearance of primary carcinoma of the bile ducts. Radiology, 102:259–266, 1972.

59. Seldinger, S. I.: Percutaneous transhepatic cholangiography. Acta Radiol. (Diagn.) (Suppl.), 253: 1966.

60. Mujahed, L., and Evans, J. A.: Percutaneous transhepatic cholangiography. Radiol. Clin. North Am., 4:535–545, 1966.

61. Hanafee, W., and Weiner, M.: Transjugular percutaneous cholangiography. Radiology, 88:35–39, 1967.

62. Weiner, M., and Hanafee, W. N.: A Review of transjugular cholangiography. Radiol. Clin. North Am., 8:53–68, 1970.

63. Rösch, J., Lakin, P. C., Antonovic, R., et al.: Transjugular approach to liver biopsy and transhepatic cholangiography. N. Engl. J. Med., 289:227–231, 1973.

64. Bengmark, S., Engevik, L., Rosengren, K.: Angiography of the regenerating human liver after extensive resection. Surgery, 65:590–596, 1969.

Chapter Ten

COLON AND RECTUM

JAMES E. YOUKER, M.D., AND WYLIE J. DODDS, M.D.

The large bowel is the most common site for the development of a life-threatening malignancy in man. Approximately 15 per cent of all malignant tumors and 75 per cent of intestinal cancers originate in the colon, rectum, or anus.[1] Primary colorectal malignancies include carcinomas, sarcomas (including lymphomas), and carcinoid tumors (Table 10–1). Carcinoma, by far the most common colon malignancy, afflicts almost 100,000 individuals in the United States each year and causes 48,000 deaths.[2] Colorectal cancer causes more deaths than any other form of malignancy. Statistically, one person in every hundred will develop a colon carcinoma during his adult life.

Although colorectal malignancy poses a serious threat, physicians should not be pessimistic. The overall five-year survival rate for patients with cancer of the colon is only about 30 to 40 per cent, but a survival rate of 65 per cent is achieved in individuals who do not have regional lymph node metastases at the time of surgery.[3–5] Unfortunately, the cure rate for colon carcinoma has not changed significantly during the past 30 years. Despite this disturbing fact, three of every four afflicted individuals *might* be cured if their lesions were detected early enough.[5] For this reason, an improved rate of colon cancer detection should be the concern of all physicians evaluating patients with intestinal complaints.[6, 7]

COLON CARCINOMAS

Incidence

Eighty to 90 per cent of colon carcinomas develop in patients who are between 50 and 70 years of age, with a mean age of about 60 years.[3, 8, 9] The incidence is equal in both sexes. Marked differences exist in the incidence of colon carcinoma in different parts

Table 10–1. Classification of Large Bowel Tumors

Malignant Neoplasms

Primary
1. Carcinoma
   a. Adenocarcinoma
      1. Medullary
      2. Papillary
      3. Villous
      4. Mucinous
      5. Scirrhous
      6. Adenocanthoma
   b. Epithelioma
      1. Squamous cell
      2. Basal cell
   c. Cloacogenic

2. Sarcoma
   a. Lymphoma
      1. Reticulum cell (histiocytic)
      2. Lymphocytic
      3. Hodgkin's disease
      4. Follicular (nodular)
   b. Leiomyosarcoma
   c. Fibrosarcoma
   d. Myxosarcoma
   e. Angiosarcoma
   f. Rhabdomyosarcoma
   g. Hemangiopericytoma
   h. Plasmacytoma

3. Carcinoid
4. Malignant melanoma

Secondary
1. Direct extension (from stomach, pancreas, or kidney)
2. Hematogenous

Benign Neoplasms

Epithelial
1. Adenoma
2. Papilloma
3. Villous adenoma

Intramural
1. Lipoma
2. Leiomyoma
3. Hemangioma, lymphangioma
4. Neurofibroma, fibroma
5. Ganglioneuroma
6. Mesothelioma
7. Granular cell myoblastoma
8. Teratoma

Non-neoplastic Tumors

Juvenile polyp
Endometriosis
Enterocystoma
Duplication
Cyst

200

of the world. The incidence is greatest in Scotland, relatively high in the United States, and low in Africa and Japan. These geographic differences seem to be best explained by environmental rather than racial differences. For example, Japanese and Africans living in the United States have the same incidence rate for colon carcinoma as other Americans. On the basis of these observations, Burkitt recently suggested that the genesis of colon carcinoma was primarily related to diet.[41] Intraluminal colonic carcinogens do not appear to accumulate in people eating high-residue, low-carbohydrate diets that cause relatively frequent, bulky stools.

Identification of high-risk groups of patients is important.[10–13] Virtually all patients with familial multiple polyposis and Gardner's syndrome will develop colon carcinoma if not treated by prophylactic colectomy. The malignant potential of the small bowel polyps associated with the Peutz-Jegher's syndrome is low, but these patients have a greater risk of developing colon carcinoma than do individuals in the general population. There is also an increased incidence of colon cancer in patients who have a history of previous colon carcinoma, chronic ulcerative colitis, or an immunologic disorder featuring agammaglobulinemia.[10] Individuals from certain families that have a high incidence of cancer are more likely to develop colon cancer.

Presenting Signs and Symptoms

The cardinal clinical symptoms of colon carcinoma are rectal bleeding, change in bowel habits, and abdominal discomfort or pain. The patient may also complain of a palpable abdominal mass or weight loss. Clinical rectal bleeding generally varies from blood-streaked stools to melena; massive hemorrhage is unusual in colon carcinoma. Subclinical bleeding resulting in guaiac-positive stool occurs commonly. Consequently, testing stools for occult blood offers promise as a screening technique. Changes in bowel habits may include diarrhea, constipation, thin pencil-like stools, or constipation alternating with diarrhea. Abdominal pain as a presenting sign may be related to defecation, but it generally tends to be dull and persistent.

In a given patient, the symptoms and signs of large bowel cancer depend on several factors such as the lesion's anatomic location, size, and stage, as well as the presence of complications. Left-sided carcinomas usually surround and constrict the relatively narrow lumen of the left colon, thereby causing obstructive symptoms. Abdominal distress accompanied by constipation or narrowed stool caliber is common. Rectal bleeding, generally bright red, is noted with the stool. Insidious anemia seldom occurs. Lesions in the rectum are often associated with red blood coating the stool, a sensation of incomplete evacuation, tenesmus, and mucous diarrhea. Pain is generally a late symptom.

In contrast to left-sided lesions, symptoms associated with right-sided colon cancers are vague, variable, and of late occurrence. Insidious weakness from chronic occult blood loss is common, and the patient may incidentally note an abdominal mass. Bowel habits are altered in only one third of patients, the most common complaint being diarrhea.[14] Because the right colon is larger in width than the left, and its contents are more liquid, obstructive symptoms are uncommon unless the tumor involves the iliocecal valve or causes intussusception. Many patients have unexplained weight loss.

Similar to cancers of the right colon, cancers of the transverse colon often produce insidious, late, and nonspecific symptoms.[15] The frequency of obstructive symptoms, however, is somewhat greater.

Complications

Complications associated with colon cancer are predictable from a knowledge of colon cancer growth patterns and modes of spread. Such complications are directly related to the bulk of the primary tumor, local tumor extension through the colon wall, and distant metastases.

As with carcinoma elsewhere in the alimentary tract, colon carcinoma may assume stenotic, ulcerative, polypoid, or diffuse forms. Occasional local complications include gross hemorrhage and obstruction. Fecal impaction or pseudomembranous colitis may develop proximal to a colon cancer, causing either partial or complete obstruction. Protein-losing enteropathy or hypokalemic diarrhea suggests the presence of a villous lesion (adenoma or carcinoma). Right-sided lesions may obstruct the appendix and cause symptoms similar to those of acute appendicitis or cecal volvulus.

Whereas right-sided carcinomas tend to be polypoid, growing intraluminally with only slight wall infiltration, left colon lesions often are infiltrating, stenosing growths that extend through the bowel wall and invade the surrounding peritoneal tissues. The latter process may cause frank perforation,[16] but walled-off perforation[17] and fistula formation are more common. The patient may present clinically with an unexplained flank, perinephric, retroperitoneal, intra-abdominal, or abdominal wall abscess.[18] A fistula between the colon and the stomach may result. Subcutaneous emphysema or a cutaneous sinus that drains fecal material may also occur. The tumor may extend outside the colon and cause small bowel obstruction, bladder dysfunction, or splenic vein occlusion. As the tumor breaks through the serosa, metastatic peritoneal implantation may occur. Gravitational seeding leads to pelvic masses (Blumer's shelf) and to ovarian involvement.

More commonly, metastases spread by direct lymphatic or venous invasion. Lymphatic metastatic deposits occur first in regional nodes and then spread to remote glands. Because the colon veins drain into the portal system, the liver contains tumor in most fatal cases.[19] Colon cancer may also cause systemic effects such as dermatomyositis, eosinophilic pulmonary infiltrates, or the hormonally induced hyperglycemia of Cushing's syndrome (i.e., an "ectopic" endocrine effect).[20–23]

Evidence of hepatomegaly should be carefully sought, and a palpable abdominal mass may be present, especially with carcinoma of the right or transverse colon. Abdominal examination may also disclose tumor involvement of the abdominal wall, an umbilical metastasis, ascites, or, rarely, cutaneous venous collaterals secondary to portal obstruction. Additionally, metastases may cause enlargement of the inguinal or supraclavicular lymph nodes ("sentinel" nodes). In the case of hepatic metastases, jaundice may occur. Subcutaneous metastatic lesions occur in 1 to 3 per cent of patients.[24] Rare immune-type skin reactions may be present, and other skin manifestations of colon cancer include acanthosis nigricans, erythema multiforme bullosum, pemphigoid, urticaria, and reticulohistiocytosis.[25] Additionally, there may be evidence of the cutaneous lesions associated with familial polyposis syndromes such as Gardner's syndrome.

Differential Diagnosis

Because the symptoms of colon cancer are numerous and varied, colon cancer may mimic a wide variety of intra-abdominal disorders. Depending on the existing clinical features, colon cancer may simulate functional intestinal disorders, diverticulosis, diverticulitis, inflammatory bowel disease, ischemic disease of bowel, noncarcinomatous large bowel malignancies (see Table 10–1), or benign small bowel tumors.

The diagnosis of large bowel carcinoma can be made by digital examination of the rectum in 15 per cent of all cases.[26] In the remaining patients, the preoperative diagnosis of colon cancer is established primarily by endoscopic and roentgenographic methods. Both types of examination should be obtained in all patients being evaluated for possible colon malignancy.

The differential diagnosis of a colonic mass may be difficult and varies with the morphology of the lesion under consideration. The various morphologic forms of colon cancer and the differential diagnosis of each form are discussed in the following sections. Correlation of the *clinical* picture with the roentgenographic appearance of the lesion is often helpful, but biopsy is usually required to obtain a definitive diagnosis. Many lesions may be reached by sigmoidoscopy and most are accessible by colonoscopy. Currently, laparotomy is seldom necessary for diagnosis alone.

Presenting Radiographic Signs

Diagnosis with roentgenographic examination of the colon depends on multiple factors, including appropriate patient selection, adequate colon cleansing, suitable contrast medium, thorough fluoroscopic observation, proper filming technique, quality equipment, careful film scrutiny, and expert interpretation. Although the radiologist is directly involved in all aspects of the examination, the referring physician must also share the responsibility for ensuring appropriate patient selection. The clinician should always provide the pertinent clinical information so that the radiologist can determine whether to perform a barium enema or pneumocolon air contrast examination. The clinician and radiologist must work together to provide their patients with an effective colon cleansing regimen, since a poorly prepared colon represents the most common cause of an inadequate colon examination.

On barium enema examination, colon cancer may appear as one of several different morphologic types: (1) a constricting lesion, (2) a large endophytic mass, (3) an exophytic, extraluminal mass, (4) a long, narrowed segment, or (5) a discrete intraluminal polyp(s). The statistical probability of carcinoma and the differential diagnosis are determined by the type of morphologic abnormality present and the clinical findings.

Constricting colonic cancers are usually annular and resemble an "apple core" or "napkin ring," with luminal narrowing, contour irregularity, ulceration, and overhanging margins at the junctions with nor-

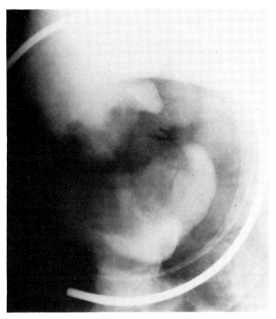

Figure 10–1 Annular carcinoma of the right colon.

mal bowel (Figs. 10–1 and 10–2). Lesions with this morphology are almost always carcinomas, and they occur generally in the left colon. A persistent, localized area of muscle contraction may occasionally simulate an annular tumor, but the luminal contours are smooth and the narrowing seldom persists on a second examination. Occasionally,

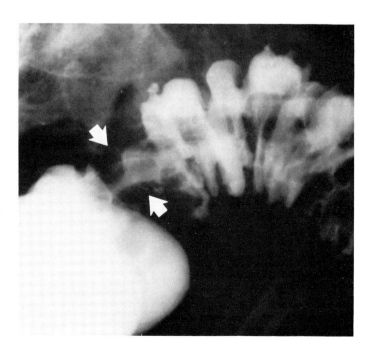

Figure 10–2 Annular carcinoma (arrows) at the rectosigmoid junction. The overhanging margins distinguish this lesion from a segmental narrowing caused by diverticulitis. In addition, the contour of the lesion did not change after Pro-Banthine was given intravenously.

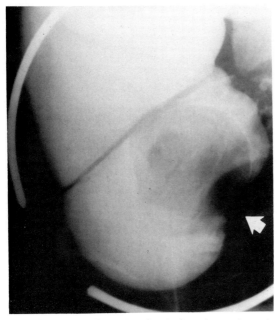

Figure 10–3 Large intraluminal carcinoma (arrow) arising in the cecum.

annular primary carcinomas can also be simulated by diverticulitis, adhesions, tuberculosis, ameboma, carcinoid,[27] tumor extension from a neighboring structure, hematogenous metastases, serosal implants in the bowel, or an unrecognized earlier surgical anastomosis.

Large exophytic colon carcinomas (Fig. 10–3) tend to occur in the right colon and the rectum. Such tumors have an irregular, nodular, or lobulated luminal contour, often producing a fungating appearance. Discrete mucosal ulcers may also be seen in the tumor. A frond-like contour suggests a villous adenoma, many of which are malignant. Villous tumors often develop in the rectosigmoid colon (Fig. 10–4), and may cause diarrhea, electrolyte depletion, or protein-losing enteropathy because large volumes of interstitial fluid are lost from the papillary surface of the lesion. Other rarer varieties of primary bowel malignancies with a seeming predilection for the anorectal region include epidermoid carcinomas, cloacogenic tumors, melanomas, and carcinoids. Stippled calcification (Fig. 10–5) observed roentgenographically within a colonic mass suggests a mucinous adenocarcinoma, a vicious malignancy that occurs in somewhat younger individuals and has a poorer prognosis because it is commonly associated with abdominal carcinomatosis.[28, 29] Other entities to be considered in the differential diagnosis of intraluminal colonic masses are sarcomas and metastatic lesions, as well as

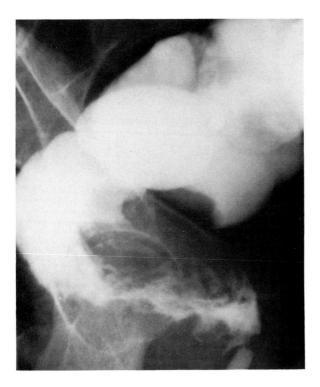

Figure 10–4 Rectal villous adenocarcinoma. The correct diagnosis is suggested by the irregular, frond-like contours of the lesion.

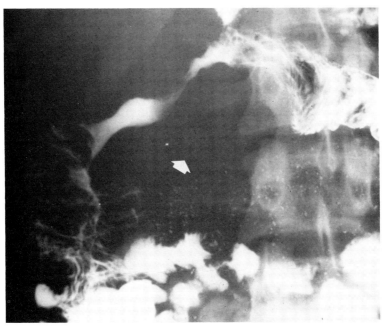

Figure 10–5 Mucinous adenocarcinoma involving the entire hepatic flexure in a 25-year-old housewife. The initial diagnosis was an inflammatory lesion, but the presence of stippled tumoral calcifications (arrow) suggests the correct diagnosis.

large benign lesions. A colonic mass with an exquisitely smooth luminal contour suggests a benign intramural lesion, such as a lipoma or leiomyoma.

Exophytic lesions growing outside the bowel lumen often may become very large before the patient experiences any clinical symptoms. Although more characteristic of bowel sarcomas, this growth pattern may occasionally occur with a primary carcinoma. The amount of associated intraluminal tumor observed within the bowel may vary. Carcinoma that is associated with a walled-off bowel perforation may also cause an extraluminal mass. The differential diagnosis of extraluminal colonic masses includes diverticulitis, intra-abdominal abscess, foreign body perforation, hematoma, endometriosis, cyst, invading tumor from a neighboring structure, hematogenous metastases, and peritoneal tumor implants.

Colon cancer may rarely present as a long, narrowed segment of bowel, appearing more like an inflammatory lesion than a carcinoma (Figs. 10–5 and 10–6). This uncommon and confusing entity, known as linitis plastica or scirrhous carcinoma of the colon, has a particularly poor prognosis.[30] The sigmoid colon and rectum are the sites most frequently reported. Even the symptoms of

this form of cancer suggest inflammatory disease, with mild lower abdominal pain, weight loss, and diarrhea.[31] The diagnostic difficulties are heightened by the fact that 20 per cent of reported cases of scirrhous carcinoma have occurred in patients with known ulcerative colitis.[30] Great care must be taken to exclude the much more common entity of "linitis plastica" caused by metastases to the colon from a primary stomach or gallbladder tumor. The barium enema in linitis plastica of the colon reveals a long, narrow colonic segment with tapered ends, rather than the usual overhanging margins of a carcinoma. The involved segment is rigid and lacks the irritability (and changeable caliber) usually seen in inflammatory lesions. The mucosa usually remains intact, although complete effacement of the colonic folds may occur in the central portion of the lesion. Other areas of the lesion may show a distorted mucosal pattern, with scalloping and "thumbprinting," or a very coarse, cobblestone-like appearance secondary to the thickened folds. The differential diagnosis includes vascular disease of the bowel, metastases, segmental ulcerative colitis, granulomatous colitis, diverticulitis, radiation-induced change, or endometriosis.

Colon tumors presenting as polypoid

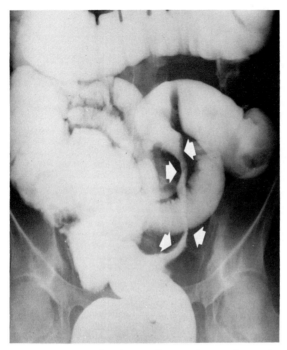

Figure 10–6 Scirrhous adenocarcinoma (arrows) in a 22-year-old female, causing narrowing over a long segment of the sigmoid. The initial diagnosis was segmental granulomatous colitis.

lesions protruding into the bowel lumen are encountered frequently in barium enema examinations, particularly during the investigation of rectal bleeding. The polyp may have a stalk of variable length. In the vast majority of patients these lesions are benign and represent either hyperplastic polyps or adenomatous polyps. Polypoid tumors with prominent villous or frond-like elements have a much higher incidence of malignancy. Some colon cancers, however, may present a smooth or gently lobulated polypoid appearance (Figs. 10–7 and 10–8). Debate exists over whether such carcinomas represent malignant transformation in a pre-existing benign polyp, or whether a small polypoid carcinoma has developed de novo. Therefore, a small polypoid lesion discovered on the barium enema presents a diagnostic dilemma: a carcinoma cannot be excluded with absolute certainty, but the possibility of malignancy may be so small as to rule against operative intervention. Fiberoptic colonoscopy greatly expands our ability to diagnose these lesions definitively, but this option is not yet available in every area of the country. Consequently, the radiologist is still called upon to assess the possibility of malignancy in polypoid colon lesions. The incidence of malignancy for polypoid lesions 1.2 cm or less in size is only 1 or 2 per cent. Polypoid lesions greater than 2 cm in diameter, however, have a 20 per cent chance of being malignant.[32] Other features associated with a high incidence of malignancy are a rough surface of the polyp, irregularity of the polyp base, and rapid growth.[32, 33] Small

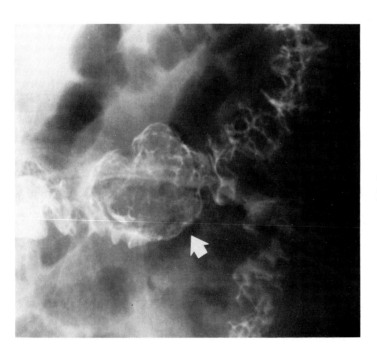

Figure 10–7 Post-evacuation roentgenogram demonstrating a polypoid carcinoma (arrow) in the distal transverse colon.

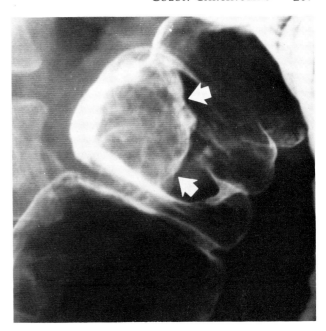

Figure 10–8 Sessile carcinoma (arrows) of the transverse colon shown on pneumocolon (barium–air contrast) examination.

polypoid *carcinomas* also tend to be flat or sessile with a broad attachment to the bowel wall (Fig. 10–9). Their rapid growth and early invasion of the bowel wall probably are responsible for their sessile form. Conversely, the presence of a long stalk strongly suggests a benign lesion.

Endoscopic Examination

Because of their tendency to develop in the distal colon, many colon cancers may be diagnosed by proctosigmoidoscopy. Different series report that 50 to 75 per cent of all colorectal carcinomas are located 25 cm or less from the anus, which is within reach of the sigmoidoscope. In practice, the sigmoidoscope is not always inserted to its full 25 cm; nevertheless, a high percentage of colon carcinomas, probably more than 50 per cent, may be visualized by sigmoidoscopy.[3, 6, 9, 26] Despite the efficacy of proctoscopy and widespread publicity by the American Cancer Society, proctosigmoidoscopy remains woefully underutilized. Regretfully, many physicians rely on the roentgenographic examination alone to evaluate the large bowel. We believe that both types of examination should be obtained in all patients with suspected colonic disease.

During the past few years, new instrumentation and techniques have been developed for examining the entire colon by colonoscopy.[34] Using long flexible fiberoptic scopes, experienced colonoscopists can now examine the colon all the way to the cecum in about 90 per cent of patients. This instrument also allows biopsy for tissue diagnosis and electrosurgical removal of most polypoid lesions less than 2 cm in size. Despite the fact that colonoscopy represents an important advance in the diagnostic evaluation and treatment of colonic neoplasms, this new modality cannot replace conventional sigmoidoscopy and the barium enema. Currently, colonoscopy is not a suitable method for screening large numbers of patients because of its high cost, the relatively long procedure time, and a significant rate of incomplete examinations (about 10 per cent). For selected *high-risk* patients, however, with known or suspected colonic lesions, colonoscopy greatly aguments conventional diagnostic modalities. Laparotomy no longer remains the sole option for definitive diagnosis of lesions beyond the reach of the sigmoidoscope. Colonoscopy, however, is not without hazard.[35] The most common complication is perforation of the colon, which occurs in 0.4 to 1.9 per cent of colonoscopic examinations. The radiographic identification of extraluminal gas may be crucial

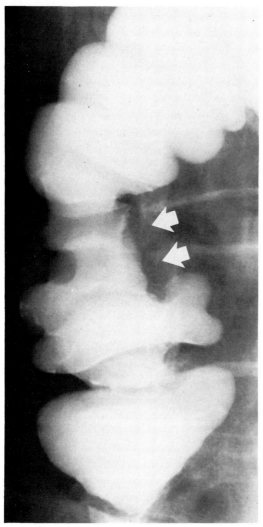

Figure 10–9 Flat sessile adenocarcinoma (arrows) of the ascending colon.

in the diagnosis of perforation. Other complications include bleeding, mesosigmoid hematoma, splenic avulsion, and impaction of the instrument.

Laboratory Methods

Testing the stools for occult blood is an accepted method of detecting colon cancer. The method developed by Greegor, which utilizes commercially available guaiac-impregnated slides, is simple and inexpensive.[36] It requires that the patient be restricted to a meat-free, high-residue diet during the period of stool collection. The initial experience in 900 patients reveals that 5 per cent of those studied had one or more of the slides positive for occult blood. One in five of the patients with a positive slide proved to have carcinoma of the colon.

Exfoliative cytology in the colon has had far less impact on the diagnosis of colon cancer than it has had on diagnosis in other areas of the body (such as the uterine cervix). Adequate specimens, free from debris, are difficult to obtain. Laboratory personnel have been understandably unenthusiastic about handling large numbers of fecal specimens.

A variety of techniques for obtaining cytologic specimens have been developed including direct smears, flotation followed by millipore filtration, differential centrifugation, smears of silicone casts of the colon, and saline washes.[37] Positive results have been obtained using specially designed instruments employing saline lavage with simultaneous suction.[38] This technique is done in conjunction with sigmoidoscopy. An accuracy of 75 per cent has been demonstrated for sigmoid and left colon lesions.

The utilization of immunodiagnostic techniques for the detection of circulating carcinoembryonic antigens (CEA) in patients with colon cancer has created enormous enthusiasm.[37, 39-43] Early reports suggested great specificity,[39] but recent evidence indicates that the technique is not specific for colon cancer. Elevated levels of carcinoembryonic antigen may be seen in malignancies of the gastrointestinal tract, pancreas, lungs, breast, prostate, ovary, and urinary bladder. Elevation of CEA also may be seen in benign conditions such as cirrhosis, ulcerative colitis, and granulomatous bowel disease, and even in heavy smokers. However, the extent of malignant involvement is related to the degree of elevation of CEA; positive results are observed in almost all patients with colon cancer and widespread metastases. Carcinoembryonic antigen assays do have some value in evaluating treatment for colon cancer in the individual patient, since values tend to fall following successful therapy and to rise with recurrence of tumor.

Radiologic Localization and Staging

The appearance of a carcinoma on barium enema examination may give only a rough indication of the true extent of tumor. For example, submucosal tumor may extend beyond the apparent tumor margins. In addition, patients with proven primary carcinoma of the colon have a definitely increased incidence of second colon cancers (Fig. 10–10).[44–47] It is therefore imperative that the entire colon be carefully examined roentgenographically (by means of a barium enema) to exclude the possibility of a coexisting cancer. It should also be remembered that there is a higher incidence of a second colon cancer developing in these patients in the future.[45–47] Interestingly, the presence of polyps coexisting with a cancer is associated with a higher incidence of a second colon malignancy.[46, 47]

The crucial problem of identifying preoperatively colon cancer that has extended beyond the bowel wall and into regional lymph nodes represents a frustrating challenge to radiologists. Lymphography has been utilized in the diagnosis of retroperitoneal lymph node metastases but has not received wide acceptance.[48, 49] Preoperative identification of tumor spread to mesenteric as well as retroperitoneal nodes is important, because preoperative irradiation of adenocarcinomas with involved regional nodes results in a significant improvement in the five-year survival figures. Occasionally, even non-resectable tumors can be rendered

resectable by a preoperative tumor dose of 5000 rads.[50] The proper examination of a patient who is to have surgery for colon cancer should include not only a barium enema but also a chest film, intravenous pyelogram, and upper gastrointestinal series. On rare occasions, hepatic and retroperitoneal metastases can be identified by the presence of stippled calcifications on a plain abdominal radiograph. High-quality plain film studies of the abdomen are imperative if this unusual finding is to be recognized. The appearance of this typical form of tumoral calcification is almost pathognomonic of a mucus-secreting adenocarcinoma of the colon.[28, 66] "Routine" bone surveys are probably *not* warranted, unless there are local symptoms suggestive of bone metastases. Bone metastases from carcinoma of the colon are very uncommon, but when present they are frequently osteoblastic and may closely resemble primary bone tumors.[51]

Radionuclide scans using various technetium-99m labeled preparations are now the method of choice in screening for bone metastases. However, appropriate radiographs should also be used to exclude the possibility of a benign cause of any scan abnormality. Technetium-99m sulfur colloid liver scans may aid in detecting hepatic metastasis. When normal, however, liver scans are not reliable for ruling out meta-

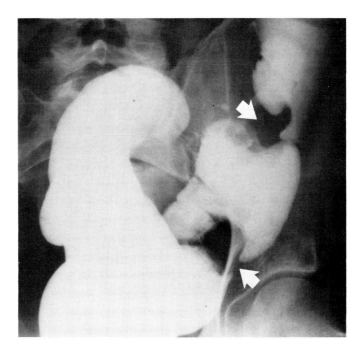

Figure 10–10 Two coexisting carcinomas (arrows) in the left colon.

static disease. Even when positive, liver scans are not specific for the diagnosis of hepatic metastases; a false-negative rate close to 30 per cent and a false-positive detection rate of between 5 and 10 per cent have been reported.[52] Gallium-67 citrate scans can sometimes demonstrate the actual primary tumor or its metastatic deposits.[53]

Abdominal ultrasound is another interesting diagnostic modality with considerable promise,[54] but its use in defining the primary colon lesion or regional lymph nodes seems limited at present. Angiography, like ultrasound, can be useful in the evaluation of hepatic metastases, but it may cause discomfort in some patients and rare fatal complications are reported.

Perhaps the most promising new modality on the horizon is whole-body scanning with computerized axial tomography. This new technique permits the visualization of soft tissues and organs without contrast material. Its clinical value in studying the brain has already been proven (see Chapter 15), and several companies are actively developing whole-body scanners that will soon become available for clinical use.

Radiologic Follow-up

The proper follow-up of the colon cancer patient after surgery is a critical aspect of good cancer management. Early detection of recurrent tumor is important; one half of patients dying from colon cancer may succumb to complications of *local* disease, such as intestinal or ureteral obstruction. The development of distant metastatic disease may be excluded by the same diagnostic tools as are used preoperatively. The radiographic barium enema examination, with either single or double (air) contrast technique, is used to evaluate the anastomotic site and to detect a possible second primary colon cancer. However, numerous authors have emphasized the difficulty of distinguishing between a surgical deformity of the bowel and recurrent cancer.[55, 56] *Therefore, it is helpful to obtain a baseline barium enema examination about three months after surgery, for use in later comparisons when the patient may develop symptoms of recurrent tumor.* Studies performed less than three months after surgery often have a confusing

appearance because of edema and other early postoperative changes. As a rule, benign surgical deformities in the bowel tend to be circumferential, whereas recurring cancer at the resection line may involve the bowel asymmetrically. Although bowel wall granulomas may create similar defects, all changes on contrast examination, regardless of how small, should be treated with suspicion. Attention should also be directed to the detection of a new primary cancer in the remaining colon. Agnew and Cooley, in a postoperative barium study of anastomotic sites in 111 patients taken from a group of 574 colon cancer patients, found 12 recurrent lesions and 6 new colon cancers.[57]

COLON SARCOMAS

Although sarcomas constitute only a small percentage of colon malignancies, these lesions are important because they have a better prognosis than carcinomas. A variety of colon sarcomas occur (Table 10–1), but the two most common are *lymphoma* and *leiomyosarcoma*. On roentgenographic examination, a colon sarcoma is frequently misdiagnosed as a carcinoma.

Primary Lymphoma

In the largest series yet reported, *primary colonic lymphoma* is stated to be more than twice as common as large bowel lymphoma occurring in association with malignant lymphoma elsewhere in the body.[58] Non-Hodgkin's colonic lymphomas are the most frequent type; Hodgkin's disease is rare as a primary entity in the large bowel. These tumors arise primarily in young and middle-aged adults, and there is a male to female ratio of 2 to 1. The clinical symptoms are usually gradual in onset. The most common presenting symptom is abdominal pain, often cramping in type and usually most intense over the site of the tumor. Other common symptoms include weight loss, abdominal mass, and constitutional symptoms such as weakness or easy fatigability. Bowel obstruction occurs in less than one quarter of the patients, and gastrointestinal bleeding is relatively uncommon.

The cecum, which is affected in more than half the cases, represents the most common site of primary colonic lymphoma. The cecal tumor often extends into the adjacent terminal ileum or ascending colon. The next most common location is the rectosigmoid colon. As with colon carcinoma, a second primary lymphoma may sometimes be present. Colon lymphomas also present in a variety of forms: polypoid, ulcerating, annular, and diffuse infiltrating (Fig. 10–11). These lesions are often large when they first become apparent, accounting for the frequent clinical finding of a palpable abdominal mass. In contrast to colon carcinomas, sarcomas (including lymphomas) incite negligible fibrosis and often grow away from the bowel lumen. Consequently, bowel obstruction is relatively uncommon.

Morphologically, colon lymphomas may suggest carcinoma, inflammatory lesions, or even polyposis.[59] As a rule, however, the radiographic findings closely simulate carcinoma. Two forms of presentation are of special interest. Because these tumors often attain large size, large central ulcerations and excavations in continuity with the bowel lumen are common. The neoplastic process may therefore seem to enlarge the intestinal lumen, causing the appearance of "aneurysmal dilatation" of the bowel. In other patients with colonic lymphoma, diffuse submucosal nodularity throughout the colon may simulate hereditary polyposis syndromes.

The pretreatment examination of a patient with primary lymphoma is similar to that for colon carcinoma, but lymphography and gallium-67 abdominal scanning, in particular, should be considered. Extension of primary lymphoma beyond the bowel wall or involvement of local nodes adversely affects the prognosis. Following surgical treatment, augmented with radiation in some instances, the prognosis for primary colon lymphoma is somewhat better than for colon carcinoma. A five-year survival rate of 55 per cent was reported for one large series.[58]

Primary Leiomyosarcoma

Primary leiomyosarcomas of the colon demonstrate no sex or age predilection. The clinical symptoms are similar to those of colon lymphoma, except that bleeding is somewhat more common. In contrast to lymphoma, which tends to involve the right

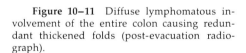
Figure 10–11 Diffuse lymphomatous involvement of the entire colon causing redundant thickened folds (post-evacuation radiograph).

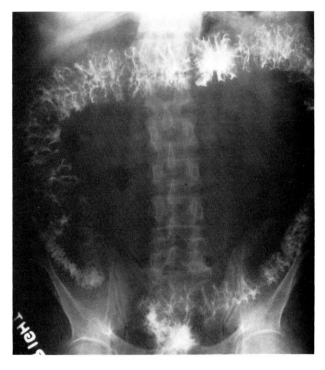

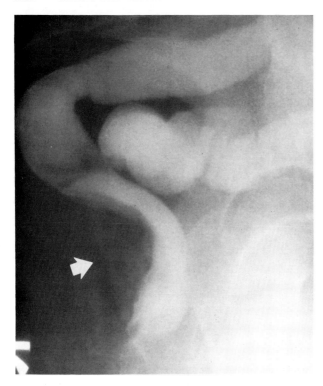

Figure 10–12 Bulky leiomyosarcoma (arrow) arising in the wall of the rectum.

colon, two thirds of large bowel leiomyosarcomas are in the rectum (Fig. 10–12). Characteristically, leiomyosarcomas are bulky, exophytic lesions.[60] These tumors often outgrow their blood supply, causing central necrosis and subsequent ulceration of the overlying mucosa. Excavation of the necrotic tumor center into the bowel lumen creates an irregular extraluminal cavity that communicates with the bowel lumen. Lymphoma, diverticulitis, or pericolonic abscess may present similar findings on radiographic examination. Roentgenographically, leiomyosarcomas cannot be distinguished absolutely from benign leiomyomas, unless metastatic lesions are evident. Even the pathologist may have difficulty differentiating between these two tumors on the basis of histologic criteria alone. Leiomyosarcomas rarely involve regional nodes; rather, they metastasize to the liver or outside the abdomen. Following surgical treatment, the five-year survival rate is about 50 per cent.

References

1. DePeyster, F. A., and Gilchrist, R. K.: Pathology and manifestations of cancer of the colon and rectum. In Turell, R. (ed.), Diseases of the Colon and Anorectum. Philadelphia, W. B. Saunders, 1969, pp. 428–452.
2. Cancer Statistics 1975. CA, 25:8–21, 1975.
3. Galante, M., Dunphy, J. E., and Fletcher, W. S.: Cancer of the colon. Ann. Surg., 165:732–744, 1967.
4. Liechty, R. D., Ziffren, S. E., Miller, F. E., et al.: Adenocarcinoma of the colon and rectum: Review of 2,261 cases over a 20-year period. Dis. Colon Rectum, 11:201–208, 1968.
5. Coller, F. A., and Regan, W. J.: Cancer of the Colon and Rectum. New York, American Cancer Society, 1963.
6. Hight, D., Kjartannsson, S., and Barillas, A. E.: Importance of early diagnosis in the treatment of carcinoma of the colon and rectum. Am. J. Surg., 125:304–307, 1973.
7. Cole, J. W.: Carcinogens and carcinogenesis in the colon. Hosp. Pract. 8:123–130, 1973.
8. Glenn, F., and McSherry, C. K.: Carcinoma of the distal large bowel: 32-year review of 1026 cases. Ann. Surg., 163:838–849, 1966.
9. Corman, M. L., Swinton, N. W., and O'Keefe, D. D., et al.: Colorectal carcinoma at the Lahey Clinic, 1962–66. Am. J. Surg., 125:424–428, 1973.
10. McKusick, V. A.: Genetics and large-bowel cancer. Am. J. Dig. Dis., 19:954–958, 1974.
11. Dodds, W. J., and Lydon, S. B.: Intestinal polyposis syndromes. CRC Crit. Rev. Clin. Radiol. Nucl-Med. 5:295–336, 1974.
12. Burdick, D., Prior, J., and Scanlon, G. T.: Peutz-Jeghers syndrome: Clinical-pathologic study of a large family with a 10-year follow-up. Cancer, 16:854, 1963.

13. Youker, J. E., Dodds, W. J., and Welin, S.: Colonic polyps. In Margulis, A. R., and Burhenne, H. J. (eds.), Alimentary Tract Roentgenology. 2nd ed., vol. 2. St. Louis, C. V. Mosby, 1973, pp. 1037–1067.

14. Scudamore, H. H.: Cancer of the colon and rectum—general aspects, diagnosis, treatment, and prognosis: A review. Dis. Colon Rectum, 12:105–114, 1969.

15. Messinger, N. H., Beneventano, T. C., Siegelman, S. S.: Interflexural carcinoma of the colon: Clinical-radiologic-pathologic correlations. Dis. Colon Rectum, 14:255–258, 1971.

16. Whelan, C. S., Furcinitti, J. F., Lavarreda, C.: Surgical management of perforated lesions of the colon with diffusing peritonitis. Am. J. Surg., 121:374–378, 1971.

17. Mathe, G., Gold, P., Gerfo, P. L., et al.: Immunology and colonic cancer. Dis. Colon Rectum, 16:339–340, 1973.

18. White, A. F., Haskin, B. J., Jenkins, C. K., et al.: Abscess of the abdominal wall as the presenting sign in carcinoma of the colon. Cancer, 32:142–146, 1973.

19. Willis, R. A.: Pathology of Tumours. 4th ed. London, Appleton-Century-Crofts, 1967.

20. Allan, R. N., Dykes, P. W., Harris, O. C., et al.: Dermatomyositis associated with hepatic secondaries from carcinoma of the colon. Gastroenterology, 62:1227–1231, 1972.

21. Boone, A. W.: Pulmonary infiltrations with eosinophilia as a manifestation of carcinoma. Dis. Chest, 55:341–344, 1969.

22. Montgomery, J. A., and Berne, C. J.: Gastrointestinal tract neoplasms with dependent hypoglycemia. Case report. Am. J. Surg., 127:737–739, 1974.

23. Miura, K., Demura, H., Sato, E., et al.: A case of ACTH-secreting cancer of the colon. J. Clin. Endocrinol. Metab., 31:591–595, 1970.

24. Hardin, W. J.: Unusual manifestations of malignant disease of the large intestine. Surg. Clin. North Am., 52:287–298, 1972.

25. Rosato, F. E., Shelley, W. B., Fitts, W. T., Jr., et al.: Nonmetastatic cutaneous manifestations of cancer of the colon. Am. J. Surg., 117:277–281, 1969.

26. O'Donnell, W. E., Day, E., and Venet, L.: Early Detection and Diagnosis of Cancer. St. Louis, C. V. Mosby, 1962.

27. Crittenden, J. J., Byllesby, J., and Dodds W. J.: Carcinoid tumor presenting as annular lesion in the ascending colon. Radiology, 97:85–86, 1970.

28. Rose, P. G.: Calcifications in metastases from adenocarcinoma of the colon. Acta Radiol. (Diagn.), 14:713–720, 1973.

29. Hermann, G., and Rozin, R.: Calcification in gastrointestinal carcinomata. Clin. Radiol., 15:139, 1964.

30. Wolf, B. S., and Marshak, R. H.: Linitis plastica or diffusely infiltrating type of carcinoma of the colon. Radiology, 81:502–507, 1963.

31. Raskin, M. M., and Viamonte, M., Jr.: Primary linitis plastica carcinoma of the colon. Radiology, 113:17–22, 1974.

32. Welin, S., Youker, J., and Spratt, J. S., Jr.: The rates and patterns of growth of 375 tumors of the large intestine and rectum observed serially by double contrast enema studies (Malmö technique). Am. J. Roentgenol., 90:673, 1963.

33. Youker, J. E., Welin, S., Main, G.: Computer analysis in the differentiation of benign and malignant polypoid lesions of the colon. Radiology, 90:794–797, 1967.

34. Williams, C. B., Hunt, R. H., Loose, H., et al.: Colonoscopy in the management of colon polyps. Br. J. Surg., 61:673–682, 1974.

35. Meyers, M. A., and Ghahremani, G. G.: Complications of fiberoptic endoscopy. Radiology, 115:301–307, 1975.

36. Greegor, D. H.: Occult blood testing for detection of asymptomatic colon cancer. Cancer, 28:131–134, 1971.

37. Sherlock, P., and Winawer, S. J.: Modern approaches to early identification of large bowel cancer. Prospects for newer methodologies. Am. J. Dig. Dis., 19:959–964, 1974.

38. Katz, S., Sherlock, P., and Winawer, S. J.: Rectocolonic exfoliative cytology. A new approach. Am. J. Dig. Dis., 17:1109–1116, 1972.

39. Gold, P., and Greedman, S. O.: Specific carcinoembryonic antigens of the human digestive system. J. Exp. Med., 122:467–481, 1965.

40. McCartney, W. H., and Hoffer, P. B.: The value of carcinoembryonic antigen (CEA) as an adjunct to the radiological colon examination in the diagnosis of malignancy. Radiology, 110:325–328, 1974.

41. Burdette, W. J.: Newer approaches to the problem of colorectal cancer. Dis. Colon Rectum, 17:462–468, 1974.

42. Dhar, P., Moore, T., Zamcheck, N., et al.: Carcinoembryonic antigen (CEA) in colonic cancer. Use in preoperative and postoperative diagnosis and prognosis. J.A.M.A., 221:31–35, 1972.

43. Zamcheck, N., Moore, T. L., Dhar, P., et al.: Immunologic diagnosis and prognosis of human digestive tract cancer: Carcinoembryonic antigins. N. Engl. J. Med., 286:83–86, 1972.

44. Devitt, J. E., Roth-Moyo, L. A., and Brown, F. N.: Significance of multiple adenocarcinomas of the colon and rectum. Ann. Surg., 169:364–367, 1969.

45. Diamante, M., and Bacon, H. E.: Primary multiple malignancy of the colon and rectum: Report of 230 cases. Dis. Colon Rectum, 9:441–446, 1966.

46. Copeland, E. M., Jones, R. S., and Miller, L. D.: Multiple colon neoplasms. Arch. Surg., 98:141–143, 1969.

47. Ekelund, G., and Pihl, B.: Multiple carcinomas of the colon and rectum. Cancer, 33:1630–1634, 1974.

48. Chiappa, S., Bonadonna, G., Uslenghi, C., et al.: Lymphangiography in the diagnosis of retroperitoneal node metastases in rectal cancer. Br. J. Radiol., 40:584–593, 1967.

49. Meeting on Early Diagnosis, Prevention, and Human Genetics. Am. J. Dig. Dis., 19:968, 1974.

50. Rose, P. A.: Planning surgery for colon carcinoma. Surg. Clin. North Am., 50:81–92, 1970.

51. Seife, B.: Osseous metastases from carcinoma of the large bowel. Am. J. Roentgenol., 119:414–418, 1973.

52. Jhingran, S. G., Jordan, L., Johns, M. F., et al.: Liver scintigrams compared with alkaline phosphatase and BSP determination in the detection of metastatic carcinoma. J. Nucl. Med., 12:227, 1971.

53. Nash, A. G., Dance, D. R., McCready, V. R., et al.:

Uptake of gallium-67 in colonic and rectal tumours. Br. Med. J., 3:508–510, 1972.

54. Antoine, J. E.: Diagnostic oncologic imaging. Curr. Probl. Radiol., 5:18–21, 1974.

55. Fleischner, F. G., and Berenberg, A. L.: Recurrent carcinoma of the colon at the site of anastomosis. Gastroenterology, 62:1227–1231, 1972.

56. Golden, R., and Sharpe, M.: End-to-end anastomosis of the colon following resection: A roentgen study of 42 cases. Am. J. Roentgenol., 64:769–777, 1950.

57. Agnew, C. H., and Cooley, R. N.: Barium enema study of postoperative recurrences of carcinoma of the colon. J.A.M.A., 179:119–124, 1967.

58. Wychulis, A. R., Beahrs, O. H., and Woolner, L. B.: Malignant lymphoma of the colon: A study of 69 cases. Arch. Surg., 93:215–225, 1966.

59. Messinger, N. H., Bobroff, L. M., and Beneventano, T. C.: Lymphosarcoma of the colon. Am. J. Roentgenol., 117:281–286, 1973.

60. Marshak, R. H., and Lindner, A. E.: The radiology corner. Leiomyosarcoma of the colon. Am. J. Gastroenterol., 54:155–157, 1970.

Chapter Eleven

UROLOGIC TRACT

J. Duncan Craven, M.D.

CLINICAL CONSIDERATIONS

Presenting Signs and Symptoms

The most common presenting sign of cancer of the kidney, renal pelvis, ureter,[1] bladder,[2] or prostate[3] is hematuria. However, hematuria from prostatic cancer is a late finding, since most tumors begin in the posterior lobe. Coexistent benign prostatic hypertrophy, leading to bladder outlet obstruction and infection, often calls attention to the urinary tract and results in the earlier diagnosis of cancer. Coexistent calculi are common with carcinoma of the renal pelvis, and they are rare in this country with transitional cell carcinoma of the bladder (stones do occur with epidermoid carcinoma of the bladder, however). Renal carcinoma or hydronephrosis from cancer of the ureter, bladder, or prostate (rare) can also present as a lumbar mass. Cancer of the urethra is often associated in the male with increasing severity of symptoms from a long-standing urethral stricture.[4, 5]

Rectal or leg pain (caused by cancer of the bladder, prostate, or urethra) and leg edema (in tumors of the kidney, bladder, prostate, or urethra) suggest metastatic disease involving the inguinal, pelvic, or aortic nodes. Some genitourinary cancers may present initially with metastatic disease to the supraclavicular lymph glands[8] (cancer of the prostate or testicle), to the chest[9-15] (cancer of the kidney or testicle), and rarely to the bone, brain, or liver (cancer of the kidney).[1] Nearly one half of patients with

bladder carcinoma have been treated by a physician for more than a year for a benign condition.[7]

Adenocarcinoma of the kidney can masquerade as many other diseases that in turn may prompt further expensive but futile radiographic studies, as shown in Table 11–1.

Tumors of the adrenal cortex can produce Cushing's syndrome.[16-18] Cushing's syndrome that has developed over a period of a few weeks, if not factitious, must be attributed to an adrenocortical carcinoma. Hyperaldosteronism with hypertension, edema, and weakness can be seen in patients with an intrarenal tumor (juxtaglomerular cell adenoma),[19] as well as in those with adrenal neoplasm. Precocious puberty and feminization in males and amenorrhea and virilism in females also occur with adrenal tumors, especially carcinoma. Tumors of the ovary, testis (interstitial cell),[20, 21] and pituitary should usually be considered before focusing on the adrenal, however. A benign adrenal adenoma can be simply removed by means of a posterior retroperitoneal approach; however, a carcinoma should be radically removed by way of an abdominothoracic approach. Therefore, a preoperative presumptive diagnosis is highly desirable. Recurrences from adrenal carcinoma have been reported to occur more than three years after primary treatment.

Pheochromocytomas are usually single and benign and may present with labile hypertension, headaches, and sweating.[22, 23] Associated diseases have been reported, including neurofibromatosis and medullary

Table 11–1 Conditions Initially Suspected in Adenocarcinoma of the Kidney

Common Presenting Symptoms	Suspected Diagnosis	Radiologic Studies Performed
Fever of unknown origin; dysuria; hematuria weight loss	Renal tuberculosis; lymphoma	Intravenous urography, sometimes arteriography
Fatigue, night sweats,	Hepatitis; tuberculosis	Chest radiograph
Abdominal pain; bloating, colic; anorexia.	Gastrointestinal disorder	Cholecystogram, liver scan, gastroduodenal series
Weakness	Iron-deficiency anemia	Upper and lower gastro-intestinal series
Hypercalcemia (with secondary personality change)	Psychiatric disorder	Skull radiographs; brain scans
Back pain	Lumbosacral disc disease	Spine radiographs; myelography

carcinoma, and in these instances multiple tumors occasionally are encountered.[24] Familial inheritance also has occurred.[25] These tumors can occur in any location between the cervical retroesophageal region and the base of the bladder.[23] One of ten lesions are multiple or malignant, or both.

Testicular germinal malignancies present clinically as masses.[25-27] These testicular masses are often tender and simulate a mild orchitis or epididymitis, because the testicle containing the tumor may be too heavy to be protected normally from trauma by the cremasteric muscle. An associated hernia or hydrocele may delay diagnosis. Intrascrotal sarcomas can occur also at all ages.[27] Back pain (caused by metastatic lumbar lymph nodes), "acute abdomen" (owing to cryptorchid testicular carcinoma with hemorrhage or strangulation), nonspecific gastrointestinal complaints (caused by bulky celiac lymph nodes), and dyspnea (from pulmonary metastases) are rarer forms of clinical presentation.

Differential Diagnosis

The most common symptom of a genitourinary carcinoma is hematuria. Benign causes of *red* or *brown* urine are hemolytic crises (sickle cell; spherocytosis; sensitivity to penicillin, methyldopa, salicylic acid, 8-aminoquinolines, sulfonamides, or nitro-furans), anticoagulants (however, remember in these circumstances that renal cell tumors also bleed spontaneously), hemoglobinurias, stones, tuberculosis, emboli, renal aneurysms, hydatid disease, ureteroceles, hemangiomas, benign prostatic hypertrophy, cystitis, urethritis, and renal carbuncles. Diseases in neighboring organs can cause hematuria by invasion of urinary structures; examples of such diseases are carcinoma of the uterus, vagina, or colon, and certain inflammatory diseases (diverticulitis, Crohn's disease, appendicitis, salpingitis).

In considering a differential diagnosis, it is worth remembering that genitourinary tumors with the exception of testicular and Wilms' tumors, occur mainly in patients over the age of 40. (Wilms' tumor is extremely rare in adults.[28]) Papillomas of the bladder are rare in patients under the age of 25 and bladder carcinoma is rare in those under 45.

Oliguria and edema of the lower extremities caused by tumors can mimic chronic renal or cardioperipheral vascular disease. An enlarged kidney can be confused with an enlarged liver or spleen, or with a distended gallbladder. Furthermore, hydronephrosis occurring in patients over the age of 40 must always be precisely explained in order to avoid missing a carcinomatous obstruction. Carcinomas can occur in horseshoe and cystic kidneys.[29, 30] Renal or perirenal calcification does *not* rule out carcinoma. Lymphoma involving kidney substance is usually part of generalized disease, and kidney masses may also be caused by metastases from primary lesions in the breast, stomach, and lung, as well as by leukemic infiltrates. Distortion of the kidney by an adrenal or retroperitoneal cancer occurs. Kidney and stomach lesions have also metastasized to the ureter, and the pelvic ureter can be involved in continuity by cancer from rectum, cervix, bladder, and prostate.

Therapeutic Decisions and Staging

Adenocarcinoma of the kidney is often bulky and has a tendency to involve the renal vascular pedicle and to invade the colon, diaphragm, and adrenal glands, necessitating an abdominothoracic approach for exposure as well as for renal vein ligation and for successful extirpation of tumor thrombus in the renal vein or inferior vena cava. High-grade (undifferentiated) or granular cells, venous tumor thrombus, and regional lymph node metastasis are all poor prognostic factors that singly or in combination reduce the patient's chances for survival. If penetration of the renal capsule with invasion can be demonstrated *preoperatively*, preoperative irradiation should be considered. However, in all series the most important prognostic factor is whether or not all the tumor is confined within Gerota's fascia.[31-34] The rare adenocarcinoma of the kidney in children does not appear to have a different natural history or survival rate.[35, 36]

Carcinomas of the renal pelvis and ureter are consistently treacherous.[37-40] These thin viscera allow early "through-and-through" penetration by tumor. Only patients with well-differentiated tumors survive after nephroureterectomy and removal of the intravesical part of the ureter (bladder cuff). Their treatment and follow-up are complicated by the fact that one third have secondary tumors elsewhere in the urothelium at the time of diagnosis, and the urothelium remaining after surgery will often develop new tumors.

A palpable kidney (hydronephrosis) or a nonfunctioning kidney is a poor prognostic sign in primary cancer of the ureter.[39] These tumors are so rare that the clinician and radiologist must rule out secondary ureteral involvement by other tumors (of the cervix, colon, or testis), before arriving at a tentative diagnosis. High-grade (undifferentiated) histology and invasion of the ureteral musculature are poor prognostic signs. The appearance of new tumors following treatment (in one out of three patients) in the remaining urothelium (bladder, contralateral renal pelvis and ureter) has influenced some urologists to employ conservative operative procedures rather than the generally accepted total nephroureterectomy.[40, 41]

As long as cancer of the bladder has not metastasized to the regional lymph nodes, cure is possible; however, a few patients with one node positive (obturator) have been reported "cured." Lymphoma or cancer of the prostate, colon, uterus, or ovaries can simulate a primary bladder cancer clinically as well as roentgenographically, as can bladder calculi. A large suprapubic mass may indicate a urachal adenocarcinoma, which has a poor prognosis because of frequent extravesical extension.[42, 43] On the other hand, some well-differentiated carcinomas can be very bulky but still be confined to the bladder.

If searched for, *in situ* carcinoma of the bladder urothelium may be found away from the tumor in as many as one of five patients. Transurethral resection for well-differentiated superficial TIS or T1 tumors (see Table 11–2) up to 3 cm in size can result in good five-year control.

If the tumor is confined to the dome, is 4 cm or less in diameter, and is in stage T1

Table 11–2 Clinical (Cystoscopic and Pathologic*) Staging System for Carcinoma of the Bladder

TIS	Pre-invasive carcinoma, so-called carcinoma *in situ*, either papillary or sessile
T1	Tumor with infiltration of subepithelial connective tissue
T2	Tumor with infiltration of superficial muscle
T3	Tumor with infiltration of deep muscle
T4	Tumor fixed or invading adjoining organs

*Lymph node metastases (N) can only be determined reliably by an abdominal surgical procedure. Visceral metastases can be suspected by imaging techniques (M).

or T2, good control can be obtained even with partial cystectomy. It must be emphasized, however, that the proportion of patients truly suitable for partial cystectomy is 5 per cent. The great importance of histologic grade independent of stage in transitional cell carcinoma of the bladder is that it may allow one to make some treatment decisions on the basis of only transurethral tissue fragments.

The error of clinical staging as opposed to surgical staging is 20 to 30 per cent. This means that about one of five tumors clinically classified as stage T1 are pathologically stage T2, and about two of seven tumors pathologically determined to be stage T2 involve deep muscle or perivesical fat (stage T3). Roentgenographic studies to make a better distinction between superficial and deep bladder muscle invasion or extravesical extension have not been extensively used, but would be extremely helpful prior to establishing definitive therapy. Moderately undifferentiated cancers of the bladder usually have metastasized outside the bladder (to the regional nodes, lung, liver, or bones). Death caused by renal insufficiency and by urosepsis occurs frequently in the untreated patient.

Carcinoma of the male urethra is rare. Patients die of local invasion with resulting sepsis from fistula or abscess. If metastases can be ruled out initially, a total urethrectomy, a prostatovesiculectomy, and (if indicated) a cystectomy should be considered for these rare but locally invasive lesions that usually metastasize only after inadequate treatment. Patients with pelvic or inguinal node involvement have a much poorer rate of survival.[44, 45]

Adenocarcinoma of the prostate penetrates through the posterior capsule, invading the bladder, seminal vesicles, and, late in its course, the rectum. It commonly has metastasized to bone, however, at the time of diagnosis. Lymph node metastases are found in one out of five patients with stage T2 tumors and in two out of three patients with stage T3 tumors (see Table 11–3). As in bladder cancer, only rarely is cancer of the prostate that has metastasized to the nodes curable, since the eventual likelihood of visceral spread is so high.[46-50]

Clinical staging in cancer of the prostate has proved inaccurate in about one third of cases. The association of tumor size with

Table 11–3   Clinical (Palpation*) Staging System for Carcinoma of the Prostate

T1	Tumor occupying less than one half of the prostate and surrounded by palpably normal gland
T2	Tumor occupying one half or more of the prostate but not producing enlargement or deformity of the gland
T3	Tumor confined to the prostate but producing enlargement or deformity of the gland
T4	Tumor extending beyond the prostate

*Lymph node metastases (N) can only be determined reliably by an abdominal surgical procedure. Visceral metastases (M) can be suspected by imaging techniques.

metastasis is tenuous because of associated benign prostatic hypertrophy; however, of tumors weighing 35 to 150 gm, nearly 50 per cent will have positive regional nodes, and of those weighing more than 150 gm nearly 100 per cent will have positive nodes.[52] Radiation therapy rather than estrogen is now being used for stage T3 prostatic carcinoma.[53] Despite the propensity of this tumor to metastasize to nodes and bone, fully 20 per cent of patients who die of cancer of the prostate have no distant metastatic disease. Death due to causes other than cancer (often cardiovascular or respiratory disease) occurs in at least 30 per cent of patients.

Testicular tumors frequently metastasize to lymph nodes in the hilus of the ipsilateral kidney. If the spermatic cord is invaded, obturator and iliac nodes can be involved. Inguinal node metastases can also occur with tumor penetration of the tunica albuginea or invasion of the scrotum. It is well to remember, however, that previous surgical procedures in the inguinal canal or pelvis can alter lymphatic drainage patterns. Involved para-aortic nodes greater than 3 cm can rarely be completely removed in non-seminomatous tumors.[54] Preservation of sexual function is sometimes the reason for avoiding a bilateral retroperitoneal node dissection.[55] The ipsilateral para-aortic nodes are involved earlier; later, contralateral lymphatic spread can occur in one of five patients. The survival rate is best in patients with solitary and ipsilateral nodal metastases, which can be completely resected. Primary retroperitoneal seminomas and embryonal carcinomas have been reported, but some authors have subsequently found a microscopic primary in the testicle.[56, 57] Hyperthyroidism has been reported with metastatic embryonal carcinoma.[58]

Clinical Follow-up

Following retroperitoneal spread, tumors of the testicle metastasize to the thorax (lymph nodes or lung), liver, brain, and bones. Most embryonal and mixed carcinomas metastasize within the first year. Spontaneous "maturation" of pulmonary metastases and a resectable solitary pulmonary metastasis have occasionally been seen with mixed tumors.[59-62] Long-term control (cure) has been obtained even in metastatic seminomas occurring five to six years after the initial diagnosis.[63]

After radical cystectomy for bladder carcinoma, one in six patients with an ileal or sigmoid bladder will need another operation for intestinal obstruction, fistulas, or stones. New tumors can develop in the penile urethra (see above), the remaining kidney, the ureters, or even in the colon following uterosigmoidostomy.[63] The possibility of a new urothelial tumor after successful treatment of the first urothelial cancer needs emphasis inasmuch as it appears to occur in 20 per cent of patients.

The recurrence of fever, anemia, or hypercalcemia after a nephrectomy for renal carcinoma signifies that metastasis has occurred until proven otherwise. Functioning adrenal tumors should also be followed chemically after surgery; hormone elevations persisting weeks after treatment mean metastasis has occurred.

Hemorrhage, late hydronephrosis, cystitis, proctitis, contracted bladder and bladder neck, and fistulas are treatment complications that simulate recurrent tumor. Necrosis and stricture occurring after treatment of cancers of the urethra may also simulate new tumors or recurrence. Dilated urinary tracts, rectal ulceration, and strictures of the prostatic urethra can also occur after treatment for carcinoma of the prostate and should be investigated and treated vigorously when appropriate. Potential late complications from vigorous irradiation include nephritis, duodenal or gastric ulcer, enteritis (steatorrhea), neuropathy or myelopathy, and pneumonitis.

RADIOLOGIC CONSIDERATIONS

Renal Cell Carcinoma

PRESENTING RADIOGRAPHIC SIGNS

The role of radiology in confirming or refuting the diagnosis of renal cell carcinoma is paramount. The first radiologic examination should be an intravenous urogram. The scout film of the abdomen can show the shape, size, and position of the kidneys, the presence of skeletal metastases, and the size of the liver. Renal outlines are visible in 70 to 80 per cent of plain films, depending on the amount of overlying gas and feces, and this emphasizes the need for adequate bowel preparation.[65, 66] A peripheral space-occupying lesion may be seen as a localized bulge on the renal surface, whereas a mass deeper in the kidney may present as an enlarged renal pole, or even as a generalized renal enlargement replacing the normal outline. These features only indicate the presence of a space-occupying lesion in the kidney; the differential diagnosis must include neoplasm, cyst, abscess, hematoma, and miscellaneous rare conditions. The most common problem is the differentiation of cyst from tumor. The differentiation of renal from extrarenal masses is also a frequent matter of practical concern.

The plain film also will show whether calcification is present in relation to the mass. If so, this favors the diagnosis of neoplasm.[67-69] Calcification has been found in up to 3 per cent of simple cysts and tends to be curvilinear and marginal, whereas calcification may occur in 10 to 35 per cent of renal cell carcinomas, in which it may be curvilinear or amorphous. In any single case, therefore, it is wise to presume that the presence of calcification in relation to a mass implies that it is a neoplasm, unless proved to the contrary by the subsequent examinations. Confusing appearances may result from calcification, for example, in a tuberculous lesion, adenoma, aneurysm of the renal artery, or an adrenal lesion.

Once the plain films have been evaluated, contrast medium is given intravenously and the urogram completed. A detailed description of the refined technique achieved in the last few years is inappropriate in this text, but it can be summarized as the use of larger amounts of contrast medium, nephrotomography, and the use of external compression of the lower abdomen to produce adequate distension of the ureters, pelves, and calyces. A careful and complete intravenous urogram should ensure complete demonstration of the upper renal tracts, including both kidneys and the entire ureters.

The urographic appearances of the calyces and pelvis in the presence of a space-occupying lesion will vary depending on the site of the mass. A small peripheral mass may cause a bulge on the kidney surface but not reach deeply enough into the parenchyma to affect the calyces. A mass lying more centrally in the parenchyma will displace and distort the adjacent calyces, and even the pelvis, by extrinsic pressure on these structures. Some calyces may be elongated, some may be totally obstructed, and the infundibula may appear "cut off." In other situations a major calyx may be partially obstructed with dilatation of its associated minor calyces. A tumor may be so large at the time of initial discovery that it has replaced most of the kidney, causing a loss of the normal kidney shape. Under these circumstances the intravenous urogram may show only a few grossly distorted calyces or none at all ("nonfunctioning" kidney), and this implies that the pelvis or the renal vein is obstructed by the mass. When venous obstruction is present, commonly caused by direct venous extension of the renal cell carcinoma, collateral veins dilate and occasionally may be seen indenting the outer margins of the ureter.

Nephrotomography, tomography of the kidneys performed after the injection of a large bolus of intravenous contrast medium, is now considered an essential part of the intravenous urogram.[70-74] Its value is twofold. First, it will demonstrate the renal outlines with precision. Second, it will show the density of the mass following the contrast injection and help to distinguish a cyst from a tumor. Cysts will show as radiolucent defects, being totally avascular; depending on their location they may have a hairline-thin wall and a clearly defined beak-like margin of displaced renal tissue adjacent to the cyst, where it projects from the kidney surface. Most renal cell carcinomas, on the other hand, will show the same or slightly increased density compared with the surrounding parenchyma.[75] Some, however, undergo extensive central necrosis or hemorrhage, which will on occasion mimic the appearance of a cyst, but the wall in this case will appear thick.[76] If strict radiographic criteria are used, the accuracy of diagnosis of a cyst by contrast nephrotomography may be as high as 95 per cent.[77]

The choice of subsequent procedures will depend on the accepted mode of practice at each individual hospital. The following is an approach that will yield a high rate of accurate diagnosis with a minimum of investigation.

Following the intravenous urogram with nephrotomography, cysts may be distinguished from solid lesions by the use of diagnostic ultrasound. Ultrasonic echoes are produced by tissue interfaces, and by this means an ultrasonic image of the kidneys may be built up by repeated scans. No echoes, however, are produced by homogenous fluid, and so in the case of a cyst an echo-free region will become obvious. Even with high amplification levels a cyst will not "fill in," and its margins, especially anteriorly, will become much more clearly defined. However, a solid mass of whatever nature will behave quite differently: echoes will occur from within the mass even when it contains areas of cystic degeneration. At the present time the accuracy rate of sonography alone in differentiating cysts from solid tumors is 90 to 95 per cent.[78, 79]

If the intravenous urogram and the ultrasound examination suggest a renal cyst that is not immediately adjacent to the renal pelvis (see later), the next diagnostic investigation should be percutaneous cyst puncture and aspiration of cyst fluid.[80] A method of ultrasonically guided cyst puncture has also been described.[81] The cyst fluid is sent for cytologic examination, and contrast medium (with or without air for double contrast) is introduced into the cyst. Radiographs are then exposed in multiple projections to show that the cyst wall is smooth. The combination of negative cytologic examination of the cyst fluid and the demonstration of a smooth internal wall of the cyst, plus confirmation by direct superimposition of the visualized cyst and the films from the urogram showing that the whole space-occupying lesion has been demonstrated, will establish the lesion as a benign cyst and avoid the need for arteriography. It is also essential that the cytologist be satisfied with the quality of the specimen received before a negative result is accepted as final.

A parapelvic renal cyst is central in location and has a direct relationship to the large vessels at the renal hilum, and so should be approached with caution. In this situation many prefer to undertake renal angiography as the next diagnostic step.

Much has been written about the coexistence of cyst and tumor in the same kidney. This is a rare coincidence (probably no more than about 1 per cent), and the entity of tumor tissue within a simple renal cyst is extremely rare.[82-85] If the radiologist strictly adheres to the criteria outlined above, cystic degeneration of a hypernephroma will not be diagnosed as simple cyst.

If the ultrasound examination shows a solid lesion, or is in any way atypical for a cyst, the next diagnostic step should be renal angiography.[86] There is one situation, however, in which the presence of a solid space-occupying lesion does not make an angiogram mandatory. This is when the mass is produced by a large septum of Bertin (cortical rest, or "pseudotumor") (Fig. 11–1).[87, 88] Septa of Bertin exist in the normal kidney as projections of normal cortex between adjacent renal pyramids. The septum is normally slightly thinner than or equal in thickness to the peripheral cortex, but occasionally may be wider and displace adjacent calyces in a manner mimicking a space-occupying lesion. These enlarged septa of Bertin frequently occur at the junction of the upper one-third and lower two-thirds of the kidney, do not produce a bulge of the renal surface (but may be associated with an overlying indentation of the renal margin), and may appear as a well-defined density on a nephrotomogram in the nephrogram phase.[87, 88] They are particularly common in this situation in the duplex (double collection system) kidney.[89] Usually, their characteristic location, their association with duplex kidney, and their appearance on nephrotomography is sufficient to make the diagnosis. Occasionally there is

enough doubt to merit an arteriogram, which is pathognomonic: the renal vessels and their branches are entirely normal, and skirt around the enlarged septum without evidence of the abnormal vessels and capillary "blush" seen in neoplasms. Acquired pseudotumors also exist and may be produced by hematoma, infarct, or focal hypertrophy adjacent to a region of chronic pyelonephritis.[90]

Renal angiography is the technique by which a catheter is passed under local anesthesia percutaneously via the femoral artery (or rarely the axillary artery, if the iliac vessels are stenosed) into the aorta for *aortography* and later into the orifice of a renal artery for *selective renal angiography*. The value of selective arteriography is that the vascular supply to a single kidney can be demonstrated in the finest detail in isolation. The angiographic appearance of most renal cell carcinomas (94 per cent) is pathognomonic (Fig. 11–2).[91] (See differential diagnosis section, however, for caution about the appearance of angiomyolipoma.) Most renal cell carcinomas are supplied with many small arteries that branch irregularly and do not taper normally, but show variations of their luminal caliber, rarely with aneurysmal dilatations, and empty into large capillary spaces through which the blood flow is slow. This process gives a characteristic appearance of "puddling" of the contrast material. In addition, because arteriovenous connections develop in the tumor, early venous filling is commonly seen. In the capillary phase, the tumor opacification is not necessarily uniform. Larger nonopacified areas represent cystic necrosis or hemorrhage. Occasionally, nonopacified areas are caused by the fact that the blood supply of part of the tumor is derived from an adjacent, nonrenal artery (for example, the inferior phrenic, lumbar, or adrenal artery). These extrarenal supplies can be demonstrated by selective injection of the appropriate branch from the aorta, but their presence does not necessarily imply perinephric extension of the tumor through the fascial planes.[92, 93] Of more practical value to the surgeon is an assessment of the extent to which the tumor has spread proximally in the renal vein (Fig. 11–3). Venous extension has already occurred in 30 to 50 per cent of patients at the time of radical nephrectomy, and on occasion tumor

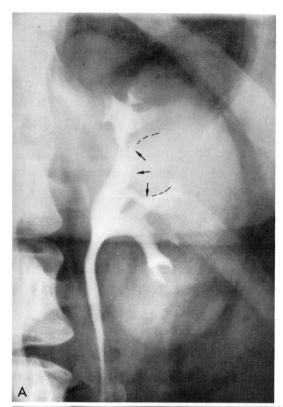

Figure 11–1 Renal cortical rest (pseudo-tumor, enlarged septum of Bertin) in a 24-year-old female with hematuria. *A,* The intravenous urogram shows a space-occupying lesion (arrows) in the middle segment of the left kidney. Angiography shows the typical changes of a cortical rest or enlarged septum of Bertin. There are no abnormal vessels (*B*), and in the capillary phase (*C*) the enlarged septum of Bertin shows a uniform increase of density equal to that of the overlying cortex. Note also that other septa are visible, and these are of the usual width.

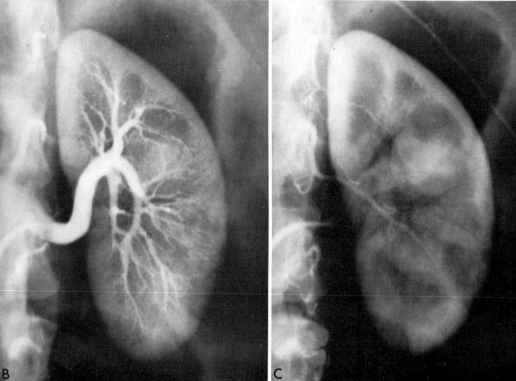

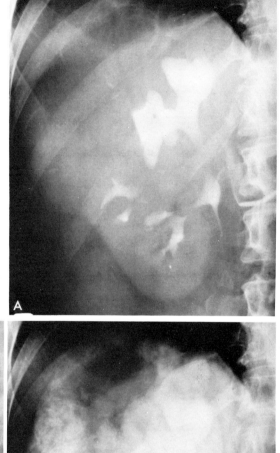

Figure 11–2 Renal cell carcinoma. *A*, The lower calyces are displaced, the renal pelvis is compressed, and the upper calyces are partly obstructed by a large space-occupying lesion involving the upper two thirds of the right kidney. In the angiogram a typical pathologic circulation is demonstrated in the arterial phase (*B*) and in the capillary phase (*C*). The apparent defect in the upper pole of the tumor (*C*) was subsequently shown to be supplied by a nonrenal artery. The same appearances could occur if this defect were caused by necrosis or hemorrhage. The inferior vena cavagram was negative.

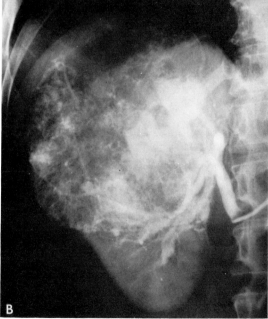

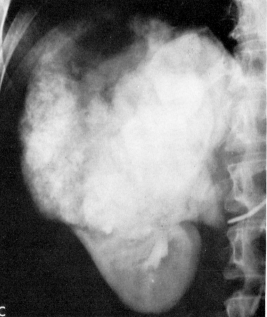

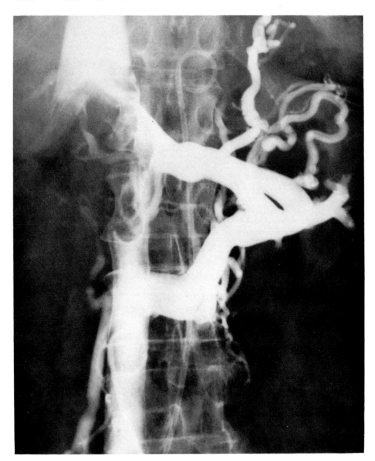

Figure 11–3 Extension of renal cell carcinoma into the inferior vena cava. The inferior vena cavagram shows a large mass severely obstructing the caval lumen. This is an extension from a large right renal cell carcinoma. The left kidney has two renal veins which provide a partial bypass of the obstructed segment. (Courtesy of J. Po, M.D. and P. Cahill, M.D.)

may extend into the inferior vena cava and even to the right atrium.[94, 95] Demonstration of filling defects within a renal vein or inferior vena cava in the late films following an arterial injection is difficult and often inaccurate, and the only sure method is to perform an inferior vena cavogram.

If the cava is clear, some examiners then advance the venous catheter into the renal vein and inject contrast material. This carries the potential danger of dislodgment of tumor emboli. If the cava is clear (as is true in 90 per cent of cases), the surgeon need not open it during radical nephrectomy but will ligate the renal vein at its entry into the cava. A decision regarding tumor spread within the renal vein can then be made by the pathologist. If tumor is present within the cava, several special surgical techniques are available to facilitate attempted resection.[96]

Most of the time renal angiography is pathognomonic in the diagnosis of renal cell carcinomas.[97-99] Six per cent of such tumors, however, are so hypovascular that they may be easily misdiagnosed (Fig. 11–4).[100] In this case further help may be obtained by the use of epinephrine, the subtraction technique, and renal venography.

Epinephrine has a marked vasoconstrictive effect on normal renal arteries.[101, 102] Tumor vessels do not respond to the same degree, and initially this was thought to be of specific diagnostic value. Unfortunately, experience has shown that this response is not specific for neoplastic vessels, but may also be seen in newly formed vessels in chronic inflammatory conditions.[103] The present practice therefore is to inject 6 to 8 μg epinephrine into the renal artery through a selective catheter followed by the injection of contrast material, in the hope that the intense vasoconstriction of normal vessels will divert more opacified blood into the less constricted vessels of hypovascular tumors, and thus they will be more easily visualized arteriographically.[104]

The subsequently obtained films may then be subjected to the subtraction technique, which is a photographic process in which all the features (bones, bowel gas, etc.) present on the preliminary film before contrast injections were made are removed (subtracted) from the angiographic film, enabling the viewer to examine more closely all opacified vessels in the absence of the "background."[105, 106]

A new opacification technique, not yet in general use, is renal venography performed by selective venous catheter injection following a renal *arterial* injection of epinephrine. The effect of the arterial epinephrine is to reduce the blood flow through the kidney and permit a more extensive retrograde filling of small renal venous tributaries. When an intrarenal tumor is present, the veins in the region will be displaced, invaded, or occluded.[107, 108]

If, despite all the above procedures, doubt still exists about the diagnosis, percutaneous needle puncture of the mass has been advocated in order to obtain a biopsy and also to inject contrast into the mass.[109] The extravasation pattern of the contrast within the mass will readily distinguish an avascular tumor from a cyst, but it must be stressed that this is not yet accepted in common practice, and many still object on the grounds that if a malignant neoplasm is present this needling technique may cause sufficient breach of the wall to permit seeding of the tumor along the needle track. However, one series of 77 punctures of renal cell carcinomas has been reported in which no local recurrence along the needle track and no worsening of prognosis occurred during a five-year follow-up period.[110]

The aim of the procedures already described is to make a correct, firm diagnosis of renal cell carcinoma, and, because the presently accepted treatment is radical nephrectomy,[111] to provide the surgeon with information about the size of the mass, the origin of its blood supply, and the presence or absence of tumor extension into the renal vein or vena cava. The opposite (normal) kidney must not be forgotten in view of the fact that renal cell carcinomas may be bilateral in about 1 per cent of cases.[112] These tumors may in fact represent two separate primaries, or a primary in one kidney with

a metastasis in the opposite kidney; in these situations, even pathologists may have difficulty making the distinction. Normally the intravenous urogram will not reveal the presence of a space-occupying lesion less than about 2 cm in diameter, but a tumor of this size or less may be demonstrable on angiography if it has the usual hypervascularity. It is clinically important that small tumors in the contralateral "normal" kidney be recognized, since new techniques of "workbench" surgery are now being elaborated in which a kidney can be surgically removed, a small lesion segmentally excised under controlled conditions outside the body, and the kidney then autotransplanted into the iliac fossa.[113, 114]

DIFFERENTIAL DIAGNOSIS

It would be inappropriate here to review the radiological features that help in differentiating renal cell carcinoma and cyst from other space-occupying lesions of the kidney such as metastases, adenoma, xanthogranulomatous pyelonephritis, abscess (acute or chronic), or hematoma.[115-122] However, renal angiomyolipoma (AML) can mimic renal cell carcinoma so completely that it deserves special mention. This lesion usually occurs in one of two groups of patients: (1) a younger group of patients (of both sexes) with tuberous sclerosis, in whom the angiomyolipoma is frequently small and bilateral and occurs in 80 per cent of the patients in this group, and (2) a group of females in the third to fifth decade of life, who have an isolated renal lesion and no other evidence of tuberous sclerosis. Of the two groups, tumors in the latter tend to be larger and more symptomatic than the former.

Radiologically, angiomyolipoma may be diagnosed in the first group when the following features are seen: a renal space-occupying lesion with a marked pathologic circulation on arteriography; obvious radiolucent regions due to the fat within the renal mass, occasionally visible on the plain abdominal film; radiologic signs of tuberous sclerosis elsewhere, such as intracranial calcifications in the basal ganglia and paraventricular regions, a honeycomb pattern on the chest radiograph, or patchy areas of sclerosis in the skeleton.[123] When the angio-

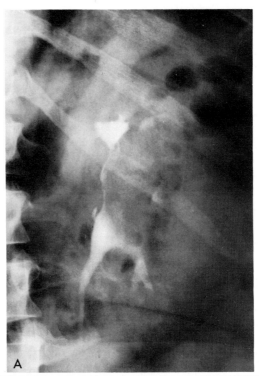

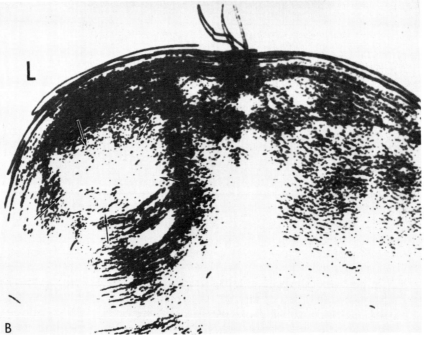

Figure 11-4   Renal cell carcinoma (hypovascular). A 46-year-old male has a large space-occupying lesion occupying the middle segment of the left kidney, as shown on the intravenous urogram (A). Ultrasound examination (B) in the prone position shows that the lesion (arrows) is atypical for a cyst because ultrasonic echoes are present within the mass.

Legend continues on the opposite page.

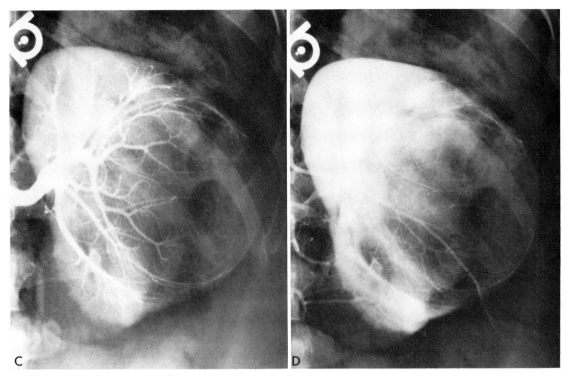

Figure 11–4 *Continued*   (C) Angiography shows displaced renal vessels but no definite neovascularity in the arterial phase. In the capillary phase (D) there is questionable puddling of contrast within the mass. Pathologic examination of the surgical specimen showed renal cell carcinoma. Preoperative diagnosis depended upon ultrasound examination. (Courtesy of J. Po, M.D., P. Cahill, M.D., and F. Sample, M.D.)

myolipoma is bilateral in the appropriate clinical context, the diagnosis becomes much easier.

In patients of the second group, however, in whom the angiomyolipoma presents as a solitary lesion without tuberous sclerosis, the radiologic signs may be identical with those already described for renal cell carcinoma; unless the fat component is seen on plain films, differential diagnosis may prove to be impossible.[124-126] However, these tumors are benign in the sense that, although local extension may occur, death from metastasis has not been reported.[127] Unfortunately, at the present time there is no preoperative solution to this diagnostic dilemma.

LOCALIZATION AND STAGING

Comparison of the value of different forms of treatment for renal cell carcinoma demands an acceptable scheme of staging. At the present time no entirely satisfactory system exists. Schemes based on surgical and pathologic findings have been proposed and a staging scheme depending on preoperative arteriographic and venographic criteria has also been suggested.[128-131] A useful clinico-roentgenologic staging system is shown in Table 11–4.

Whatever detailed staging system finally emerges, it should be noted that careful radiologic evaluation is capable of demonstrating the site of the tumor, its spread through the renal capsule, any spread into the renal vein, and the presence of distant metastases (for example, on chest and bone radiographs). Preoperative radiologic demonstration of lymphatic spread is more difficult. The regional nodes are involved in 5 to 30 per cent of cases, and occasionally in the angiogram pathologic vessels and a subsequent tumor stain may be seen within enlarged nodes. Standard lymphangiography

Table 11–4   Clinico-roentgenologic Staging System for Renal Cell Carcinoma

Tumor (T)

T1   No enlargement of kidney; urography shows minimal calyceal abnormality

T2   Kidney enlarged; perirenal fat involved, but tumor confined within Gerota's fascia

T3   Mobility of the kidney impaired on clinical and radiologic examination; renal vein involvement and/or varicocele

T4   Complete fixation of an enlarged kidney

Nodes (N)

N1   Regional nodes enlarged; may be suspected from lymphogram or angiogram

Metastases (M)

M1   Distant metastases present (liver, adrenal, lung, contralateral kidney)

M1a Single metastasis only

M1b Multiple metastases

has not been found to be helpful, inasmuch as the regional nodes of the kidney are usually not visualized at all, and some of the para-aortic nodes may be bypassed. At the present time, it would therefore seem that accurate staging should be based on a *combination* of the results of preoperative radiology, the operative observations, and careful examination of the surgical specimen.

TREATMENT CONSIDERATIONS

Radical nephrectomy is the presently accepted form of treatment for renal cell carcinoma. Preoperative radiation therapy has not yet been assigned a definite place, but this is under national cooperative study.[132-134] The results from isolated cases suggest that preoperative radiation therapy may cause shrinkage of the tumor, make the operation easier, and improve the five-year survival rate. It is interesting to note that this type of management depends on the absolute accuracy of the radiologic diagnosis, a situation that has only been achieved in the last few years.

Infarction of the tumor by selective catheterization of the feeding vessels fol-

lowed by injection of artificial emboli ("interventional radiology") is a tempting possibility, both for those patients who are too ill to undergo an operation and for those in whom the vascularity or extent of the tumor may make the operation unduly hazardous. This procedure has been done, and there are reports of success in the literature.[135-138] One danger lies in the arteriovenous connections within the tumor that might allow small embolic particles to reach the systemic circulation. The advantages of a relatively "bloodless' field, and a potential reduction of the likelihood of tumor emboli from the renal vein occurring during operation, are obvious. It seems certain that many advances in interventional radiology will emerge in the next few years and that this approach will gain wider acceptance.

RADIOLOGIC FOLLOW-UP

Routine chest radiographs, bone scans, and bone radiographs if bone pain or an abnormal scan occurs, are indicated for the follow-up of a treated patient together with repeat intravenous urograms at appropriate intervals. The intravenous urogram will show the development of any mass in the remaining kidney (not necessarily a second primary) and may show signs of a recurring mass in the nephrectomy site. In the latter situation angiography may be required to demonstrate the mass adequately, if further treatment is contemplated.

As a rare event spontaneous regression of a primary renal cell carcinoma may occur, or metastases may regress following surgical removal of the primary renal cell carcinoma.[139-143] The reason for these occurrences is not clear, but hormones or immune mechanisms that may exert biological control of the cancer are being investigated. It is important to note that radiographic disappearance of metastases does not necessarily indicate that the microscopic tumor has been eradicated, but at least implies that the tumor growth process has been controlled.[144]

Renal Lymphoma

The occurrence of lymphoma as a primary renal lesion is so rare that it will not be discussed further. However, infiltration of the kidneys during the course of lymphoma already diagnosed in other sites, occurs quite commonly. In a large series of autopsies the kidneys were involved in 13 per cent of cases of Hodgkin's disease, in 38.5 per cent of lymphosarcoma without bone marrow involvement, in 63 per cent of lymphosarcoma with bone marrow involvement, and in 46 per cent of reticulum cell sarcoma.[145] Bilateral renal involvement is much more common than is unilateral involvement.

The accuracy of radiologic diagnosis depends entirely upon the extent of renal involvement.[146] When the renal infiltration is minimal, whether generalized or localized, the intravenous urogram may be normal. If the infiltration is extensive and generalized the intravenous urogram will show an enlarged kidney with a smooth outline, and either a normal pelvicalyceal pattern or calyces that appear stretched and attenuated. The same morphologic change can occur *without* renal parenchymal involvement when para-aortic glands that are enlarged from deposits of lymphoma press on and occlude, or partially occlude, the renal veins. Renal venous obstruction with its resulting generalized edema of the kidney will mimic generalized infiltration. If the infiltration is localized and large enough, the intravenous urogram will show the presence of one or more space-occupying lesions. The investigation of these masses follows the steps outlined in the previous section, but the diagnosis is frequently obvious when the presence of lymphoma elsewhere is already known. Arteriography of these lesions does not show a pathognomonic appearance, as the lesions tend to be hypovascular.[147]

Lymphoma may also involve other levels of the urinary tract. The ureter may be displaced laterally in the middle and lower lumbar region by a mass of enlarged lymphomatous nodes, and as a rare event large lymphomatous masses in the true pelvis may cause extrinsic pressure on the bladder.

Uroepithelial Tumors

Uroepithelial tumors of the kidney are less common than parenchymal malignan-cies, comprising 7 to 8 per cent of all renal tumors compared with 83 per cent in the case of renal cell carcinomas. The majority occur in patients in the age range of 40 to 70 years; histologically, transitional cell carcinoma comprises 85 per cent of this group, with the incidence of squamous carcinoma being 15 per cent. Males are affected two to three times more frequently than females. Tumors of these cell types occur at all levels, from the renal calyx to the bladder, and they may also occur in the prostatic urethra. They may be multiple when first diagnosed, or new tumors may develop subsequently; this favors the theory that the tumors may arise multifocally because of a basic instability of the entire transitional cell epithelium.

Clinically, there is no specific presenting symptom complex, but hematuria is common and is present in up to 90 per cent of cases. Radiologically, these neoplasms present as mass lesions in the wall of the collecting system of the upper urinary tract or the bladder, with a variable amount of infiltration into the surrounding tissue. Radiologic investigation can assist both in the diagnosis of the tumor by showing the presence of a plaque in the wall or nodule projecting into the lumen, and in the process of staging by showing to some degree the extent of deep invasion.

RENAL PELVICALYCEAL CARCINOMA

A uroepithelial neoplasm within the kidney is indicated on the intravenous urogram by the presence of a filling defect with an irregular margin projecting directly into the lumen of a calyx or the renal pelvis (Fig. 11–5). This alone is not pathognomonic; occasionally, similar appearances may be produced by a non-opaque calculus, proteinaceous cast, aberrant renal papilla, vascular impression or arteriovenous malformation, sloughed papilla, or a blood clot in the renal pelvis. It is imperative that the diagnosis be confirmed with certainty because the proper surgical treatment involves nephroureterectomy together with excision of a cuff of bladder around the corresponding ureteric orifice. For this reason, and because the uroepithelium of the opposite collecting system and bladder may be involved with tumors too small to be detected

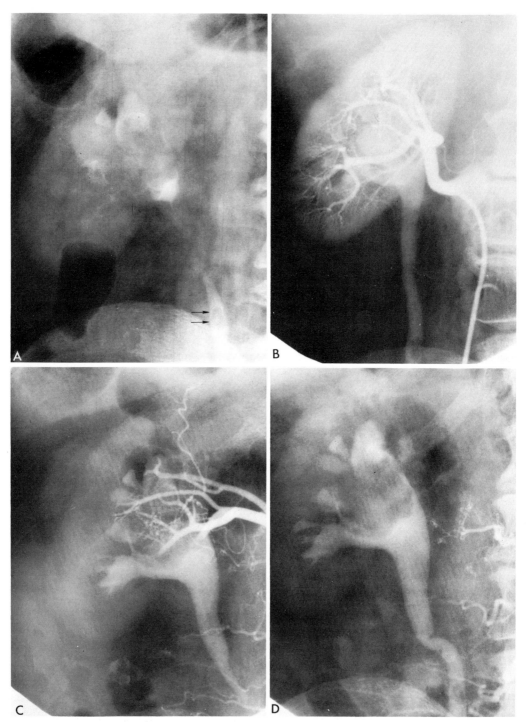

Figure 11–5   Carcinoma of the renal pelvis. *A,* The intravenous urogram shows a large filling defect within the pelvis and upper calyx. There is also an oval filling defect in the lumen of the ureter above the iliac crest (arrows). *B,* Angiography shows possible neovascularity in the region of the mass, with otherwise normal renal arterial supply. *C,* Following arterial epinephrine, the neovascularity is preferentially demonstrated. *D,* A later phase of the angiogram illustrates the filling defect. The vessels are numerous but extremely fine and beaded, and they are only seen with certainty after the epinephrine injection. After nephroureterectomy the mass was proved to be transitional cell carcinoma, and the filling defect in the ureter was a second tumor of similar histology.

by the intravenous urogram, preoperative cystoscopy followed by bilateral ureteric catheterization for the purpose of retrograde pyelography and urine collections for cytology are essential.[148]

A recent development that has improved the accuracy of cytologic diagnosis is the use of a brush biopsy technique.[149] A small version of a bottle brush may be passed up the lumen of the ureteric catheter and under fluoroscopic control rubbed over the surface of the tumor. Cells that cling to the brush can be examined by conventional cytologic techniques.

A special situation exists when hematuria is severe. The presence of excessive amounts of blood clot in the collecting system may make the intravenous urogram impossible to interpret and the cytologic examination difficult. Therefore cystoscopy may be required first to lateralize the site of bleeding. Later, if the hematuria subsides, a definitive intravenous urogram, retrograde pyelogram, and urine collection for cytology can be carried out.

Epithelial carcinomas of the calyces or renal pelvis usually present as a filling defect within the lumen. The growth may be of sufficient size to obstruct a calyx or even the renal pelvis at the ureteropelvic junction. In the first instance the appearance will mimic an "amputated calyx" caused by tuberculosis. In the second instance the appearance will be that of a "nonfunctioning" kidney caused by any chronic and high-grade pelviureteric obstruction. In this situation, or when the tumor has infiltrated the renal parenchyma so widely that it has produced a nonfunctioning kidney by massive renal tissue replacement, renal angiography may be helpful (see the following discussion).

Uroepithelial tumors are poorly vascularized and therefore present a problem for angiographic diagnosis unless meticulous selective renal angiographic technique is used.[150] In about 80 per cent of cases, the presence of a poorly vascularized mass can be established, however, and the main angiographic features are: (1) enlargement of the pelviureteric artery branch(es) of the renal artery, (2) a fine tumor neovascularity with a localized homogeneous blush in the capillary phase, (3) vessel encasement, and (4) the absence of arteriovenous shunting in the tumor. Rarely, the epithelial neoplasm will have infiltrated the kidney widely, in which case the presence of arterial encasement is an important sign in differentiating it from a hypovascular renal cell carcinoma. On the other hand, if the neoplasm has caused complete obstruction at the pelviureteric junction, the angiogram will show (in addition to the tumor) attenuated intrarenal vessels arching over and around the dilated calyces with generalized diminution of renal parenchymal thickness, an appearance pathognomonic of severe hydronephrosis. The renal vein is not commonly involved in transitional or squamous cell carcinomas of the kidney, and if the patient presents with a nonfunctioning kidney it is more likely to be caused by renal parenchymal replacement or urinary obstruction than by renal vein obstruction.[151] The opposite is true for renal cell carcinoma.

CARCINOMA OF THE URETER

Primary carcinoma of the ureter may occur in association with carcinoma of the uroepithelium elsewhere (renal pelvis or bladder), but it is rare as a solitary lesion.[152, 153]

Presenting Radiographic Signs. Radiologically, carcinoma of the ureter presents in one of two ways, either as an intraluminal mass (60 per cent) or as an irregular stricture caused by infiltration of the wall of the ureter over a short segment (40 per cent) (Fig. 11–6). In the first case, and when the mass is small, both the intravenous urogram and the retrograde ureterogram may be required to delineate the small, irregular filling defect that partly fills the lumen of the ureter. If the mass is large, the ureteric lumen will be obstructed, and delayed films (up to 24 hours following the injection) from the intravenous urogram may be required to demonstrate the upper irregular margin of the tumor. The lower margin of the tumor in these cases can only be demonstrated by a retrograde ureterogram, and it has been noted that in this type of lesion the ureter immediately below the malignant lesion is often dilated and provides space for the ureteric catheter to coil.[154] Contrasted with this is the situation in which a stone is impacted, below which the ureter is contracted. When the neoplasm presents as an irregular ureteral stricture, a variable degree of obstruction will result.

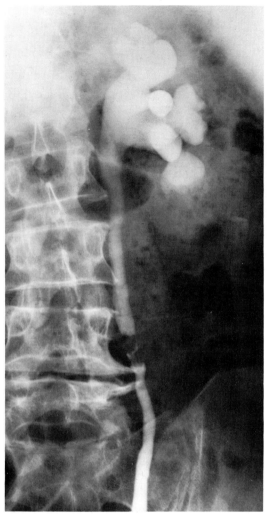

Figure 11–6   Carcinoma of the ureter in a 54-year-old male with a long history of recurrent bladder tumor. This retrograde examination shows a mass with an irregular surface severely obstructing the lumen of the ureter in its middle segment with resultant hydronephrosis. Pathologic examination revealed transitional cell carcinoma.

When obstruction occurs as a result of a ureteral lesion, and when an intravenous urogram is unsuccessful and a retrograde pyelogram is not possible, direct antegrade pyelography should be considered.[155-157] With the patient prone, a needle is introduced percutaneously in the region of the costovertebral angle and directly through the paravertebral muscles into the dilated renal pelvis. Ultrasound guidance of the needle may be helpful. Urine can then be withdrawn for cytology, and contrast medium can be instilled to demonstrate the collecting system up to the point of obstruc-

tion. In this way the upper margin of an obstructing lesion can be visualized, and the presence of any other intraluminal lesions can also be demonstrated. Another situation in which the technique of direct antegrade pyelography can be of great value is in those cases of ureteric obstruction in which there has been previous rerouting of the urine either by a Bricker procedure (ileal loop) or by ureterosigmoidostomy, for example following cystectomy for carcinoma of the bladder. In these cases if the intravenous urogram shows no excretory function, antegrade pyelography is the *only* procedure available by which the urinary collection system above the obstruction may be visualized.

Differential Diagnosis.   When carcinoma of the ureter presents as an infiltrating, intramural plaque, the radiologic appearance is likely to be that of an irregular "stricture." Strictures of the ureter may also result from inflammatory changes secondary to impaction of a calculus, tuberculosis, fibrosis following surgery, or by involvement with an adjacent retroperitoneal process (sarcoma or retroperitoneal fibrosis), as well as by ureteric carcinoma. It is impossible to distinguish these conditions by considering the morphology of the stricture alone, and it is therefore wise to consider a stricture of the ureter in a patient whose age puts him at a high risk for cancer as a suspect malignancy in the first instance. Subsequent investigation with urine cytology, microbiology, and occasionally angiography may help.[158] Because these tumors are hypovascular it may be difficult to demonstrate the fine neovasculature at the site of the tumor fed by the periureteric vascular plexus. Here again, careful utilization of the subtraction technique to emphasize fine tumor vessels is of the utmost value. Finally, it is essential that, apart from demonstrating the lesion itself and its effects on the upper tracts, radiologic investigation in carcinoma of the ureter must also provide a full anatomic evaluation of the rest of the uroepithelium.

CARCINOMA OF THE BLADDER

Presenting Radiographic Signs.   In considering the role of radiology in the diagnosis and staging of carcinoma of the bladder, it must be emphasized at the outset that while the intravenous urogram may on occasion demonstrate an unsuspected bladder lesion or may demonstrate a lesion that is already suspected clinically, there are many false-negative results. Cystoscopy, not the urogram (or cystogram), is the definitive diagnostic procedure.[159] It is only by cystoscopy and biopsy that the diagnosis of carcinoma of the bladder can be made with confidence, and the main value of the urogram is to assess the uroepithelium of the upper tracts and to show whether the adjacent ureter is obstructed. Thus if the possibility of bladder carcinoma is raised as the result of urography, cystoscopy must be the next step together with adequate biopsy and bi-manual examination for staging purposes.

The radiologic features of bladder carcinoma fall into two groups. The transitional cell carcinoma is usually a papillary tumor presenting as a filling defect of variable size within the bladder lumen (Fig. 11–7). The squamous cell carcinoma, on the other hand, is a plaque-like lesion in the bladder wall that has a greater tendency than transitional cell carcinoma to invade deeply and

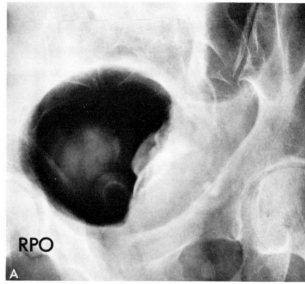

Figure 11–7 Carcinoma of the bladder in a 62-year-old female presenting with hematuria. *A,* A double-contrast cystogram shows the irregular mass on the reader's right projecting into the air-filled bladder lumen. *B* and *C,* Angiography confirms the presence of neovascularity within the mass and extending out into the perivesical tissue. The ureter is not obstructed. Pathologic examination showed infiltrating, poorly differentiated transitional cell carcinoma.

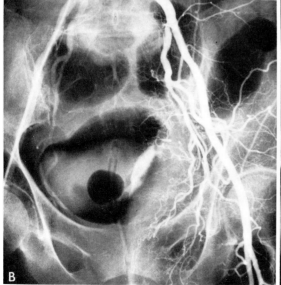

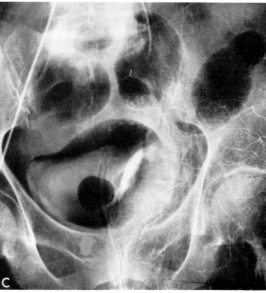

extend into the perivesical tissues.[160] This type of tumor presents radiologically as a flattening of a segment of bladder wall, which may also be displaced if extravesical extension has occurred into the adjacent tissues. The loss of wall flexibility from local tumor infiltration can be demonstrated radiologically by considering the change in outline of the opacified bladder during various stages of filling. However, this cystographic technique together with other opacification methods using double contrast (air or carbon dioxide along with positive contrast) are only of historical interest in view of the pre-eminence of cystoscopy in the establishment of the diagnosis.

Localization and Staging. In most centers the staging of bladder carcinoma depends on cystoscopy, biopsy, and bi-manual examination under general anesthesia. Radiology contributes little to this procedure in routine practice. Occasionally the perivesical fat line is visible (in 30 to 40 per cent of intravenous urograms), permitting an estimate to be made of actual bladder wall thickness; it may be increased locally at the site of a carcinoma.[161]

Pelvic arteriography has been advocated as a useful adjunct to other available methods of staging bladder carcinoma as far as local extension within the pelvis is concerned.[162] The presence of tumor tissue outside the confines of the bladder may be shown by a localized collection of abnormal "corkscrew" vessels, arteriovenous lakes, and early venous filling. The position of the neovascularity relative to the bladder, which is previously filled with a small amount of contrast and distended with gas, gives a good visual representation of the extent of extravesical tumor spread. In routine practice, however, arteriography is little used as an adjunct to staging, and reliance is placed on the biopsy and bi-manual techniques together with the subsequent surgical findings.

A technique of perivesical gas insufflation has also been advocated in which carbon dioxide is introduced into the soft tissue planes around the bladder, and at the same time the bladder lumen is outlined radiologically with double contrast.[163] By this means, localized thickenings of the bladder wall, or the presence of extension of bladder carcinoma into the adjacent soft tissues, can be demonstrated. This com-bined technique is difficult to perform, and perivesical inflammatory disease can easily mimic carcinoma. Hence its value is limited, and (as with arteriography) perivesical gas insufflation is not used routinely for the staging of bladder carcinoma.

Lower limb lymphangiography is not commonly used in staging bladder carcinoma, since the important obturator and internal iliac glands are not visualized by this means.

Differential Diagnosis. The differential diagnosis of a filling defect within the lumen of the bladder includes the possibility of a radiolucent calculus or blood clot, several rare benign tumors, and rhabdomyosarcoma (see Chapter 17). Rhabdomyosarcoma is an extremely rare bladder neoplasm in adults. It presents on cystography as a basal filling defect in the trigone region of the bladder and has no features that distinguish it from carcinoma of the bladder, or even of the prostate. Definitive diagnosis must be made by cystoscopy and biopsy.[164, 165]

Radiologic Follow-up. Radiology can assist in the period following initial treatment of a patient with bladder carcinoma by demonstrating that the rest of the uroepithelium remains normal on sequential intravenous urograms. When cystectomy with urinary diversion has been performed, follow-up studies are utilized to check the patency of the new drainage routes. The occurrence of para-aortic lymph node masses with lateral displacement of the ureters can be assessed, and concurrent chest radiographs will show whether pulmonary metastases have developed.

Carcinoma of the Prostate

Carcinoma of the prostate often arises peripherally in the gland in its posterior portion. It forms a relatively small mass, but as it enlarges it will eventually distort the prostatic urethra, base of the bladder, and seminal vesicles. Metastases to bone may occur at a time when the primary tumor is quite small, and they may even be present at the time of the initial diagnosis.

For these reasons the intravenous urogram alone is of little value in making an *early* diagnosis. Many attempts have been made to assess the size of the prostate radiologically, even when there is considerable enlargement in benign prostatic hypertrophy, but none of these methods has proved sufficiently reliable for clinical use.

Occasionally, a prostatic carcinoma may enlarge enough to cause a filling defect in the base of the bladder, even to the extent of deforming one ureteric orifice with or without obstruction of the ureter. In these cases, the intravenous urogram is of definite diagnostic and staging value.

Because the diagnostic yield from a routine intravenous urogram is small, other techniques have been explored with the hope of assisting in the early diagnosis of prostatic cancer. Bilateral vasography has been advocated.[166] In this technique cannulae are inserted into both vasa defferentia in the inguinal region, and radiologic contrast medium is injected to outline the vasa defferentia, seminal vesicles, vasa efferentia, and prostatic urethra. Local extracapsular extension of prostatic carcinoma involves the vas deferens and the seminal vesicle. Their respective lumens may thereby become narrowed, irregular, and distorted. In benign prostatic hypertrophy, on the other hand, the ducts may be displaced but are usually dilated also. The vasography technique is not in widespread use, since some of the same information regarding local extension may be obtainable by careful rectal examination and needle biopsy.

Voiding cystourethrography is the accepted radiologic technique for examination of the prostatic urethra and will demonstrate deformation caused by adjacent prostatic enlargement. However, the resulting appearances are nonspecific for differentiating the cause of prostatic enlargement, and therefore voiding cystourethrography is not reliable in the diagnosis of prostatic carcinoma.

Although radiologic examinations are of little direct value in diagnosing the primary lesion in carcinoma of the prostate, they are extremely valuable in assessing the presence of metastases in bone and lungs. Up to 90 per cent of the metastases in bone are osteoblastic, the most common sites being the pelvis, upper femora, and lumbar spine. Osteoblastic bone metastases frequently present as focal lesions, but occasionally they involve an entire bone such as a vertebral body. The other 10 per cent may be entirely osteolytic, or mixed osteo-

blastic and lytic. In an older male presenting with purely osteoblastic metastases, the most likely primary site is the prostate; however, the same picture may occur occasionally with metastases from carcinomas of the bronchus or the gastrointestinal tract. The main differential diagnosis is Paget's disease. However, in this condition the overall size of the affected bone is generally increased, and the cortex is usually widened and split by linear lucencies. These features will enable a distinction to be made from prostatic metastases in most cases, but if doubt still exists a percutaneous needle biopsy of the bone under fluoroscopic control will settle the issue. Occasionally, in renal failure, in myeloid metaplasia (accompanied by a large spleen), and in widespread prostatic metastases, the skeleton will react to produce a *generalized* increase in density. The accompanying clinical, hematologic, and biochemical features will help in the differentiation; in renal failure other radiologic features of renal osteodystrophy may also be visible, such as those of osteomalacia and secondary hyperparathyroidism.

Pulmonary metastases are less common in prostatic cancer, occurring in only 5 to 10 per cent of cases and presenting in a nonspecific way as multiple rounded nodules.

After prostatectomy, follow-up intravenous urograms are indicated to assess the bladder, the prostatic cavity, and the condition of the distal ureters. Voiding cystourethrograms and urethral pressure/flow studies may be required in the small group of patients in whom persistent incontinence follows operation. The occurrence and progression of bone and pulmonary metastases can be determined by sequential bone scans and radiographs.

Whereas conventional radiology has little to offer in the diagnosis of primary prostatic carcinoma before it has involved the bladder or ureter, ultrasound examination is now being widely explored and the early results are very promising.[167] They suggest that this mode of examination eventually will prove an extremely useful adjunct for the diagnosis of prostatic disease in general.

Carcinoma of Male Urethra

These are rare tumors, with 50 to 60 per cent being located in the bulbomembranous portion and approximately one third in the distal penile urethra. The majority (65 to 75 per cent) are squamous cell carcinomas.[168] The next most common type is transitional cell carcinoma, and the least common is adenocarcinoma arising in the periurethral glands (found most commonly adjacent to the bulb).

Radiologically these carcinomas present as nonspecific strictures, and only when the stricture is grossly irregular or is associated with adjacent filling defects (tumor nodules) in the urethral lumen can the true diagnosis be suggested with any assurance. The urethra can be demonstrated radiologically by voiding cystourethrography (which presupposes catheterization of the bladder either through the urethra or by suprapubic percutaneous puncture of the bladder) or by retrograde urethrography utilizing some form of penile clamp. The latter procedure is good for demonstrating the normal distensibility of the urethra up to the external sphincter. However, because of contraction of the sphincter during the retrograde procedure the prostatic urethra is inadequately distended by the contrast medium and cannot be examined.

The diagnosis of carcinoma of the urethra, therefore, depends first on suspecting it, and second on a careful clinical evaluation that includes taking note of bleeding associated with obstructive symptoms, palpation of a mass, careful urethroscopic examination, and cytologic evaluation of a penile discharge. Radiology confirms that a stricture exists and may occasionally indicate features of the stricture that are not typical for a purely benign condition.

There is no adequate technique for examining the urethra radiologically in the female.

Carcinoma of the Seminal Vesicles

These are extremely rare, and the same comments about the limited role of radiology in the primary diagnosis apply as were made regarding carcinoma of the prostate. The intravenous urogram will rarely show any abnormality but is required for screening and as a baseline for follow-up studies. On occasion a mass may be visible in the base of the bladder and may even involve one ureteric orifice, but in this situation the differential diagnosis from primary bladder carcinoma, carcinoma of the prostate, or carcinoma of adjacent organs extending into the bladder is not possible. Metastasis to bone is uncommon; when it occurs, it is usually lytic in nature.

Tumors of the Testes

At the present time radiologic methods are not used in the diagnosis of the primary tumor, but are regularly used in detecting metastases to the iliac and para-aortic nodes.[169] Pedal lymphangiography is definitive in demonstrating the presence of metastases in these nodes, but the primary drainage node from tumors of the left testicle (located near the left renal vein) is not usually opacified. The intravenous urogram may demonstrate lateral displacement of the ureter(s) by involved nodes if they are large enough (Fig. 11–8), and it may even show enlargement of the kidney with reduced function if the nodes press on the renal vein (with or without accompanying thrombosis). Occasionally, the investigation of both these situations may be supplemented further by inferior vena cavography and bilateral selective renal venography.[170]

Tumors of the Adrenal

Until recently adrenal enlargement (caused by hyperplasia or localized space-occupying lesions—hematomas, cysts, tumors, and others) could only rarely be demonstrated by using plain abdominal films to show a soft tissue mass in the adrenal area, the intravenous urogram to show an "adrenogram" effect during the nephrogram phase or to show inferior displacement of a kidney resulting from the adjacent suprarenal mass, or the retroperitoneal insufflation of gas to show the kidney and adrenal surrounded by negative contrast (gas). Nephrotomography including the adrenal areas was introduced subsequently with an increased diagnostic yield.[171]

Extensive experience with these techniques, however, has shown them to be deficient in demonstrating the smaller le-

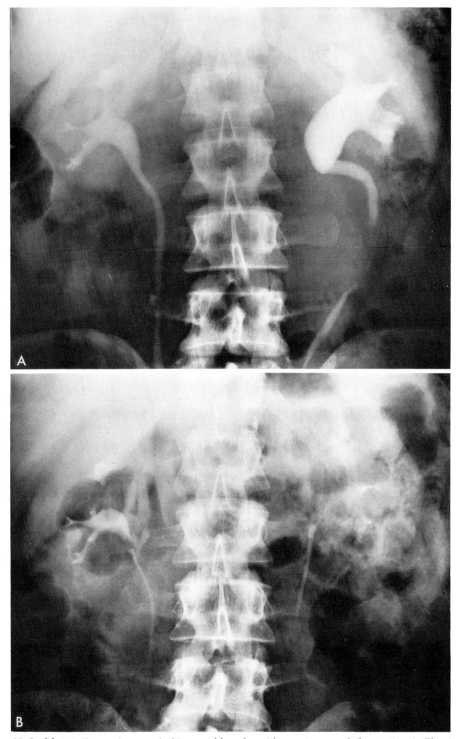

Figure 11–8 Metastatic seminoma. A 36-year-old male with seminoma of the testis. *A*, The intravenous urogram shows a large retroperitoneal mass displacing the left ureter with partial obstruction and hydronephrosis. *B*, Following a course of radiation therapy, the intravenous urogram returned to normal with disappearance of the mass.

sions in the adrenals, and this disappointment has given impetus to the development of selective adrenal arteriography,[172, 173] selective adrenal venography,[174, 175] and adrenal venous sampling for hormonal assay purposes. Used in a systematic manner in expert hands (this aspect cannot be overemphasized), these new techniques can now provide the clinician with a much more definitive diagnosis of adrenal pathology than was previously possible.[176]

The choice and the order of performance of these delicate and often very difficult and time-consuming examinations will depend to a large extent on the presenting clinical picture. When pheochromocytoma is suspected clinically and confirmed by an elevated level of urinary catecholamines, the first radiologic examination should be aortography: 90 per cent of these tumors are hypervascular with characteristic enlarged feeding arteries, a reticular network of small, irregular, and tortuous vessels, and a tumor "blush."[177, 178] In 10 per cent of cases bilateral tumors are present. A word of caution is appropriate here. Acute hypertensive crisis with death has been reported following aortography,[179] and therefore this examination should not be done for diagnosis but rather for localization of the tumor once its presence is known from other investigations. In such cases the patient should be prepared for four to five days with appropriate adrenergic blocking agents before the aortogram.[180] In 10 per cent of cases the pheochromocytoma lies in the sympathetic chain *outside* the adrenals, requiring pelvic and thoracic arteriography following a negative abdominal aortogram.

Only in the case of a hypovascular pheochromocytoma (10 per cent of cases) will selective adrenal venography be necessary and with the same precautions as outlined above. At the same time, blood sampling from the adrenal veins and from the vena cava above and below the renal veins can be carried out for catecholamine assay. When a pheochromotytoma is present the adrenal veins in the gland will be displaced and will show varying degrees of obliteration and alteration of the normal venous architecture. This abnormal venous pattern is in no way pathognomonic of pheochromocytoma, but will occur to a varying degree with any intra-adrenal mass. However, if a carcinoma of the adrenal is present, invasion of the veins may also be visible, presenting as intraluminal filling defects. The plain films will show calcification within the mass in one third of adrenal carcinomas. If an aldosteronoma is present the tumor will usually be less than 2 cm in diameter, and therefore great care is needed in interpreting small changes in the adrenal venogram.[181-183]

With the exception of the normally hypervascular pheochromocytomas and some adrenal carcinomas, all other localized adrenal masses tend to be normo- or hypovascular, with or without an associated hormonal syndrome. Following the intravenous urogram and nephrotomography, the choice of angiographic procedure will depend on clinical assessment. Selective adrenal venography has the added advantage of permitting venous sampling for hormonal assay. When adrenal carcinoma is the suspected diagnosis there is some advantage in doing arteriography first because it can be followed by hepatic angiography, using the same catheter, to investigate the possibility of hepatic metastases. Ultrasound shows particular promise in identifying suprarenal cystic lesions.

In summary, the radiologist can help in the investigation of the adrenal by identifying a space-occupying lesion, occasionally by using an intravenous urogram but relying mainly on arteriography or venography. Through the venous catheter, he can also provide selective samples of adrenal venous blood for hormonal assay. The sequence of specialized procedures will be chosen as outlined above, but whenever there is doubt it is good practice to start with arteriography.

FUTURE CONSIDERATIONS

Investigation of lesions of the renal tracts with new cross-sectional body imaging techniques such as gray-scale ultrasound and computerized axial tomography will undoubtedly increase the precision of roentgenographic diagnosis in the areas of the bladder, prostate, seminal vesicles, and intrapelvic female genital tract. These added capabilities are greatly needed in view of limitations in imaging with routine radiographic techniques in these regions. However, it will always be of importance to visualize the entire urologic tract in order to select areas which need further detailed study by tomographic imaging methods. It follows, therefore, that the radiologic procedures outlined in the foregoing sections will continue to be of major importance in making clinical and radiologic decisions.

References

1. Lucke, B., and Schlumberger, H. G.: Tumors of the kidney, renal pelvis and ureter. *In* Atlas of Tumor Pathology. Washington, D.C., Armed Forces Institute of Pathology, 1957.
2. Friedell, G. H., and Mcauley, R. L.: Untreated bladder cancer: 31 autopsy cases. J. Urol., *100*:293–296, 1968.
3. Cook, G. B., and Watson, F. R.: Events in the natural history of prostate cancer: Using salvage curves, mean age distributions and contingency coefficients. J. Urol., *99*:87–96, 1968.
4. Guinn, G. A., and Ayala, A. G.: Male urethral cancer: Report of 15 cases including a primary melanoma. J. Urol., *103*:176–179, 1970.
5. Kaplan, W., Bulkley, G. J., and Grayhack, J. T.: Carcinoma of the male urethra. J. Urol., *98*: 365–371, 1967.
6. Kiely, J. M.: Hypernephroma—The internist's tumor. Med. Clin. North Am., *50*:1067–1083, 1966.
7. Leadbetter, W. F.: Cystectomy. *In* Cooper, P. (ed.), The Craft of Surgery. 2nd ed. Boston, Little, Brown, pp. 1521–1538.
8. Butler, J. J., Howe, C. D., and Johnson, D. R.: Enlargement of the supraclavicular lymph nodes as the initial sign of prostatic carcinoma. Cancer, *27*:1055–1063, 1971.
9. Hewitt, C. B.: Renal carcinoma: A clinical challenge. *In* King, J. S., Jr. (ed.), Renal Neoplasia. Boston, Little, Brown, 1967, pp. 3–12.
10. Thackray, A. C.: The pathology and spread of renal adenocarcinoma. *In* Riches, E. (ed.), Tumors of the Kidney and Ureter. Baltimore, Williams and Wilkins, 1964, pp. 72–86.
11. Mostofi, F. K.: Pathology and spread of renal cell carcinoma. *In* King, J. S., Jr. (ed.), Renal Neoplasia. Boston, Little, Brown, 1967, pp. 41–85.
12. Van der Werf-Messing, B.: Spread of testicular tumours. Clin. Radiol., *22*:125–132, 1971.
13. Pierce, G. B., and Abell, M. R.: Embryonal carcinoma of the testis. *In* Sommers, S. C. (ed.), Pathology Annual 1970. New York, Appleton-Century-Crofts, 1970.
14. Varkarakis, M. Merris, C., Gaeta, J., et al.: Non-seminomatous testicular tumor: Comparison of treatment. Urology, *3*:684–688, 1974.
15. Gilbert, H. A., Shapiro, R., Kagan, A. R., et al.: Recurrence patterns in the non-seminomatous germinal testicular tumors: Implications for treatment. Submitted for publication.
16. Orth, D. N., and Liddle, G. W.: Results of treatment in 108 patients with Cushing's syndrome. N. Engl. J. Med., *285*:243, 1971.
17. Hayes, M. A., and Goldenberg, I. S.: Operative treatment of adrenal cortical hyperfunctioning diseases. Ann. Surg., *154*:33, 1961.
18. Scott, H. W., Jr., Foster, J. H., Rhamy, R. K., et al.: Surgical management of adrenocortical tumors with Cushing's syndrome. Ann. Surg., *173*: 892, 1971.
19. Conn, J. W., Cohen, E. L., Lucas, C. P., et al.: Primary reninism: Hypertension, hyperreninemia, and secondary aldosteronism due to renin-producing juxtaglomerular cell tumors. Arch. Intern. Med., *130*:682–296, 1972.
20. Tamoney, H. J., Jr., and Noriega, A.: Malignant interstitial cell tumor of the testis. Cancer, *24*:547–551.
21. Johnstone, G.: Prepubertal gynaecomastia in association with an interstitial-cell tumour of the testis. Br. J. Urol., *39*:211–220, 1967.
22. Egdahl, R. H., and Chobanian, A. V.: Acute pheochromocytoma. Surg. Clin. North Am., *66*:645–652, 1966.
23. Fries, J. G., and Charberlin, J. A.: Extra-adrenal pheochromocytoma: Literature review and report of a cervical pheochromocytoma. Surgery, *60*:268–279, 1968.
24. Sipple, J. H.: The association of pheochromocytoma with carcinoma of the thyroid gland. Am. J. Med., *31*:163–166, 1961.
25. Hume, D. M.: Pheochromocytoma in the adult and in the child, Am. J. Surg., *99*:458–496, 1960.
26. Notter, G., and Ranuud, N. E.: Treatment of malignant testicular tumours. Acta Radiol. (Ther.), *2*:273–301, 1964.
27. Skinner, D. G., and Leadbetter, W. F.: The surgical management of testis tumors. J. Urol., *106*:84–93, 1971.
28. Olsen, B. S., and Bischoff, A. J.: Wilms' tumor in an adult. Cancer, *25*:21–25, 1970.
29. Malek, R. S., Litz, D. C., Culp, O. S., et al.: Malignant tumors of solitary kidneys. Mayo Clin. Proc., *47*:180–188, 1972.
30. McQuiggan, M. C., and Cerny, J. C.: Wilms' tumor in a horseshoe kidney. J. Urol., *93*:445, 1965.
31. Priestley, J. T.: Survival following removal of malignant renal neoplasm. J.A.M.A., *113*:902, 1939.
32. Del Regato, J. A., and Kagan, A. R.: Basic considerations in radiotherapy of renal carcinomas. *In* King, J. S., Jr. (ed.), Renal Neoplasia. Boston, Little, Brown, 1967, pp. 547–557.
33. Glenn, J. F.: Discussion: Renal cell carcinoma in the human being. *In* King, J. S., Jr. (ed.), Renal Neoplasia. Boston, Little, Brown, 1967, pp. 149–158.
34. Varkarakis, M. J., Bhanalaph, R., Moore, R. H., et al.: Prognostic criteria of renal cell carcinoma. J. Surg. Oncol., *6*:97–106, 1974.
35. Yates-Bell, A. J., and Cardell, B. S.: Adenocarcinoma of the kidney in children. Br. J. Urol., *43*:399–402, 1971.
36. Dehner, L. P., Leestma, J. E., and Price, E. B.: Renal cell carcinoma in children: A clinico-pathologic study of 15 cases and review of the literature. J. Pediatr., *76*:358–368, 1970.
37. Wagle, D. G., Moore, R. H., and Murphy, G. P.: Primary carcinoma of the renal pelvis. Cancer, *33*:1642–1648, 1974.
38. Bloom, N. A., Vidone, R. A., and Lytton, B.: Primary carcinoma of the ureter: A report of 102 new cases. J. Urol., *103*:590–598, 1970.
39. Beck, A. D., Heslin, J. E., Milner, W. A., et al.: Primary tumors of the ureter: Diagnosis and management. J. Urol., *683*:102, 1969.

40. Williams, C. B., and Mitchell, J. P.: Carcinoma of the ureter—A review of 54 cases. Br. J. Urol., 45:377–387, 1973.

41. McDonald, J. R., and Priestley, J. T.: Carcinoma of renal pelvis: Histopathologic study of seventy-five cases with special reference to prognosis. J. Urol., 51:245–258, 1944.

42. Back, A. D., Gaudin, H. J., Bonham, D. G.: Carcinoma of the urachus. Br. J. Urol., 42:555–562, 1970.

43. Whitehead, E. D., and Tessler, A. N.: Carcinoma of the urachus. Br. J. Urol., 43:468–476, 1971.

44. Duncan, W., and Jackson, S. M.: The treatment of early cancer of the penis with megavoltage X-rays. Clin. Radiol., 23:246–248, 1972.

45. Mewaishy, G. A., and Deeley, T. J.: Radiotherapy in the treatment of carcinoma of the penis. Br. J. Radiol., 41:519–552, 1968.

46. Arduino, L. J., Bailar, J. C., Becker, L. E., et al.: Carcinoma of the prostate: Treatment comparisons. J. Urol., 98:1967.

47. Flocks, R. H.: Present status of interstitial irradiation in managing prostatic cancer. J.A.M.A., 210:328–330, 1969.

48. Belt, E., and Shroeder, F. H.: Total perineal prostatectomy for carcinoma of the prostate. J. Urol., 107:91–96, 1972.

49. Schoonees, R., Palma, L. D., Gaeta, J. F., et al.: Prostatic carcinoma treated at categorical center: Clinical and pathologic observation. N.Y. State J. Med., 72:1021–1027, 1972.

50. Arnheim, F. K.: Carcinoma of the prostate: A study of the postmortem findings in 176 cases. J. Urol., 61:599–603, 1948.

51. Hilaris, B. S., Whitmore, W. F., Batata, M. A., et al.: Radiation therapy and pelvic node dissection in the management of cancer of the prostate. Am. J. Roentgenol. Radium Ther. Nucl. Med., 121:832–838, 1974.

52. Flocks, R. H., and Cheng, S. F.: Combination therapy for prostatic carcinoma. J. Iowa Med. Soc., 58:125–129, 1968.

53. Del Regato, J. A.: Radiotherapy of tumors of the urinary tract. Am. J. Roentgenol. Radium Ther. Nucl. Med., 121:467–472, 1974.

54. Biswamay, R., Hajdu, S., and Whitmore, W. F., Jr.: Distribution of retroperitoneal lymph node metastases in testicular germinal tumors. Cancer, 33:340–348, 1974.

55. Smithers, D. W., Wallace, D. M., and Austin, D. E.: Fertility after unilateral orchidectomy and radiotherapy for patients with malignant tumors of the testis. Br. Med. J., 4:77–79, 1973.

56. Abell, M. R., Fayos, J. V., and Lampe, I.: Retroperitoneal Germinomas (seminomas) without evidence of testicular involvement. Cancer, 18:273–290, 1972.

57. Meares, E. M., Jr., and Briggs, E. M.: Occult seminoma of the testis masquerading as primary extragonadal germinal neoplasms. Cancer, 30:300–306, 1972.

58. Steigbigel, N. H. Oppenheim, J. J., Fishman, L. M., et al.: Metastatic embryonal carcinoma of the testis associated with elevated plasma TSH-like activity and hyperthyroidism. N. Engl. J. Med., 271:345–350, 1964.

59. Snyder, R. N.: Completely mature pulmonary metastasis from testicular teratocarcinoma: Case report and review of literature. Cancer, 24:810–819, 1969.

60. Skinner, D. G., Leadbetter, W. F., and Wilkins, E. W.: The surgical management of testis tumors metastatic to the lung: A report of 10 cases with subsequent resection of from one to seven pulmonary metastases. Trans. Am. Assoc. Genitourin. Surg., 62:183–190, 1970.

61. Smithers, D., Wallace, E. N., and Wallace, D. M.: Radiotherapy for patients with tumours of the testicle. Br. J. Urol., 43:83–92, 1971.

62. Smithers, D. W.: Chemotherapy for metastatic teratomas of the testis. Br. J. Urol., 44:217–228, 1972.

63. Friedman, M., and Purkayastha, M. C.: Recurrent seminoma: The management of late metastasis, recurrence, or a second primary tumor. Am. J. Roentgenol. Radium Ther. Nucl. Med., 83:25–42, 1960.

64. Preissig, R. S., Barry, W. F., and Lester, R. G.: The increased incidence of carcinoma of the colon following ureterosigmoidostomy. Am. Roentgenol. Radium Ther. Nucl. Med., 121: 806–810, 1974.

65. Ettinger, A., and Elkin, M.: Value of plain film in renal mass lesions (tumors and cysts). Radiology, 62:372–382, 1954.

66. Hodson, C. J.: Chapter 4. In Black, D. A. K., Renal Disease. Philadelphia, F. A. Davis, 1967, p. 136.

67. Cannon, A. H., Zanon, B., Jr., and Karras, B. G.: Cystic calcification in the kidney: Its occurrence in malignant renal tumors. Am. J. Roentgenol. Radium Ther. Nucl. Med., 84: 837–848, 1960.

68. Phillips, T. L., Chin, F. G., and Palubinskas, A. J.: Calcification in renal masses: An eleven-year survey. Radiology, 80:694–794, 1963.

69. Daniel, W. W., Jr., Hartman, G. W., Witten, D. M., et al.: Calcified renal masses: A review of ten years experience at the Mayo Clinic. Radiology, 103:503–508, 1972.

70. Evans, J. A., Dubilier, W., Jr., and Monteith, J. C.: Nephrotomography—A preliminary report. Am. J. Roentgenol. Radium Ther. Nucl. Med., 71:213–223, 1954.

71. Witten, D. M., Greene, L. F., and Emmet, J. L.: An evaluation of nephrotomography in urologic diagnosis. Am. J. Roentgenol. Radium Ther. Nucl. Med., 90:115–123, 1963.

72. Greene, L. F., Segura, J. W., Hattery, R. R., et al.: Routine use of tomography in excretory urography. J. Urol., 110:714–720, 1973.

73. Bosniak, M. A.: Nephrotomography: A relatively unappreciated but extremely valuable diagnostic tool. Radiology, 113:313–321, 1974.

74. Evans, J. A.: Nephrotomography: 20 years later. Radiology, 113:483–484, 1974.

75. Chynn, K. Y., and Evans, J. A.: Nephrotomography in the differentiation of renal cyst from neoplasm: A review of 500 cases. J. Urol., 83:21–24, 1960.

76. Bosniak, M. A., and Faegenburg, D.: The thick-wall sign: An important finding in nephrotomography. Radiology, 84:692–698, 1968.

77. Evans, J.: The accuracy of diagnostic radiology. J.A.M.A., 204:223–226, 1968.

78. Leopold, G. R., Talner, L. B., Asher, W. M., et al.: Renal ultrasonography: An updated approach to the diagnosis of renal cyst. Radiology, *109*: 671–678, 1973.

79. Hately, W., and Whitaker, R. H.: How accurate is diagnostic ultrasound in renal disease? Br. J. Urol., *45*:468–473, 1973.

80. Lindblom, K.: Percutaneous puncture of renal cysts and tumors. Acta Radiol., *27*:66–72, 1946.

81. Goldberg, B. B., and Pollack, H. M.: Ultrasonically guided renal cyst aspiration. J. Urol., *109*: 5–7, 1973.

82. Emmet, J. L., Levine, S. R., and Woolner, L. B.: Co-existence of renal cyst and tumour: Incidence in 1,007 cases. Br. J. Urol., *35*:403–410, 1963.

83. Pearlman, C. K.: Coexisting renal carcinoma and cyst. *J. Int. Coll. Surg.*, *41*:620–631, 1964.

84. Lang, E. K.: Coexistence of cyst and tumor in the same kidney. Radiology, *101*:7–16, 1971.

85. Brannan, W., Miller, W., and Crisler, M.: Coexistence of renal neoplasms and renal cysts. South. Med. J., *55*:749–752, 1962.

86. Lang, E. K.: Roentgenographic Diagnosis of Renal Mass Lesions. St. Louis, Warren H. Green, 1971.

87. Azimi, F., and Bryan, P. J.: Familial occurrence of renal pseudotumour due to enlarged column of Bertin in two brothers and their first cousin. Clin. Radiol., *25*:467–474, 1974.

88. Green, W. M., Pressman, B. D., McClennan, B. L., et al.: "Column of Bertin": Diagnosis by nephrotomography. Am. J. Roentgenol. Radium Ther. Nucl. Med., *116*:714–723, 1972.

89. Hartman, G. W., and Hodson, C. J.: The duplex kidney and related abnormalities. Clin. Radiol., *20*:387–400, 1969.

90. King, M. C., Friedenberg, R. M., and Tena, L. B.: Normal renal parenchyma simulating tumor. Radiology, *91*:217–222, 1968.

91. Watson, R. C., Fleming, R. J., and Evans, J. A.: Arteriography in the diagnosis of renal carcinoma: Review of 100 cases. Radiology, *91*: 888–897, 1968.

92. Sprayregan, S.: Parasitic blood supply of neoplasms. Radiology, *106*:529–535, 1973.

93. Buist, T. A. S.: Parasitic arterial supply to intracapsular renal cell carcinoma. Am. J. Roentgenol. Radium Ther. Nucl. Med., *120*:653–659, 1974.

94. McDonald, J. R., and Priestley, J. T.: Malignant tumors of the kidney: Surgical and prognostic significance of tumor thrombosis of the renal vein. Surg. Gynecol. Obstet., *77*: 295–306, 1943.

95. Skinner, D. G., Pfister, R. F., and Colvin, R.: Extension of renal cell carcinoma into the vena cava: The rationale for aggressive surgical management. J. Urol., *107*:711–716, 1972.

96. McCullough, D. L., and Talner, L. B.: Inferior vena caval extension of renal carcinoma: A lost cause? Am. J. Roentgenol. Radium Ther. Nucl. Med., *121*:819–826, 1974.

97. Freed, S. Z., Caplan, L. H., and Bosniak, M. A.: The role of renal arteriography in the management of renal carcinoma. Surg. Gynecol. Obstet., *123*:1303–1308, 1966.

98. Kahn, P. C., Wise, H. M., and Robbins, A. H.: Complete angiographic evaluation of renal cancer. J.A.M.A., *204*:753–757, 1968.

99. Schreiber, M. H., and Rea, V. E.: The resectability of carcinoma of the kidney: Analysis of roentgen signs in 63 histologically verified cases. Am. J. Roentgenol. Radium Ther. Nucl. Med., *104*:343–349. 1968.

100. Becker, J. A., Fleming, R., Kanter, I., et al.: Misleading appearances in renal angiography. Radiology, *88*:691–700, 1967.

101. Abrams, H. L., Boijsen, E., and Borgstrom, K. E.: Effect of epinephrine on the renal circulation. Angiographic observations. Radiology, *79*: 911–922, 1962.

102. Abrams, H. L.: The response of neoplastic renal vessels to epinephrine in man. Radiology, *82*: 217–224, 1964.

103. Kahn, P. C., and Wise, H. M., Jr.: Simulation of renal tumor response to epinephrine by inflammatory disease. Radiology, *89*:1062–1064, 1967.

104. Kahn, P. C., and Wise, H. M., Jr.: The use of epinephrine in selective angiography of renal masses. J. Urol., *99*:133–138, 1968.

105. Zeides des Plantes, B. G.: Subtraktion: Eine roentgenographische methode zur separaten abbildung bestimmter teile des objects. Fortschr. Geb. Roentgenstr. Nuklearmed., *52*: 69–79, 1935.

106. Hanafee, W., and Stout, P.: Subtraction technic. Radiology, *79*:658–661, 1962.

107. Kahn, P. C.: Selective venography in renal parenchymal disease. Radiology, *92*:345–349, 1969.

108. Rösch, J.: Personal communication, 1975.

109. Stevens, G. M., and Jackman, R. J.: Renal tumor diagnosis by contrast spread patterns following antegrade injection. Personal communication, 1975.

110. von Schreeb, T., Arner, O., Skovsted, G., et al.: Renal adenocarcinoma. Is there a risk of spreading tumour cells in diagnostic puncture? Scand. J. Urol. Nephrol., *1*:270–276, 1967.

111. Grabstald, H.: The extent of nephrectomy for renal cell cancer. J.A.M.A., *204*:9–15, 1968.

112. Bastable, J. R. G.: Bilateral carcinoma of the kidneys. Br. J. Urol., *32*:60–68, 1960.

113. Calne, R. Y.: Treatment of bilateral hypernephromas by nephrectomy, excision of tumor, and autotransplantation. Lancet, *2*:1164–1167, 1973.

114. Sachs, S. A., Petritsch, P. H., Linde, R., et al.: Renal autotransplant: Future use of a new perfusate. Am. J. Surg., *128*:402–407, 1974.

115. Bosniak, M. A., Stern, W., Lopez, F., et al.: Metastatic neoplasm to the kidney. Radiology, *92*: 989–993, 1969.

116. Ben-Menachem, Y., Marcos, J., Wallace, S., et al.: Angiography of renal metastases. Br. J. Radiol., *47*:869–974, 1974.

117. Rabinowitz, J. G., Wolf, B. S., and Goldman, R. H.: Roentgen features of renal adenomas. Radiology, *84*:263–269, 1965.

118. McKenzie, K. R.: Xanthogranulomatous pyelonephritis: Confusion with renal carcinoma. J. Urol., *92*:261–262, 1964.

119. Beachley, M. C., Ranniger, K., and Roth, F. J.: Xanthogranulomatous pyelonephritis. Am. J. Roentgenol. Radium Ther. Nucl. Med., *121*: 500–517, 1974.

120. Koehler, P. R.: The roentgen diagnosis of renal inflammatory masses—Special emphasis on angiographic changes. Radiology, *112*:257–266, 1974.

121. Craven, J. D., Hardy, B., Stanley, P., et al.: Acute renal carbuncle: The importance of preoperative angiography. J. Urol., 3:727–731, 1974.

122. Sukthomya, C., and Levin, B.: Pseudotumors of kidney secondary to anticoagulant therapy. Radiology, *88*:701–703, 1967.

123. Green, G. J.: The radiology of tuberose sclerosis. Clin. Radiol., *19*:135–147, 1968.

124. Viamonte, M., Jr., Ravel, R., Politano, V., et al.: Angiographic findings in a patient with tuberous sclerosis. Am. J. Roentgenol., *98*:723–733, 1966.

125. Clark, R. E., and Palubinskas, A. J.: The angiographic spectrum of renal hamartoma. Am. J. Roentgenol., *114*:715–721, 1972.

126. Becker, J. A., Kinkhabwala, M., Pollack, H., et al.: Angiomyolipoma (hamartoma) of the kidney. An angiographic review. Acta Radiol. (Diagn.), *14*:561–568, 1973.

127. Price, E. B., Jr., and Mostofi, F. K.: Symptomatic angiomyolipoma of the kidney. Cancer, *18*: 761–774, 1965.

128. Flocks, R. H., and Kadesky, M. C.: Malignant neoplasms of the kidney: An analysis of 353 patients followed five years or more. J. Urol., *79*:196–201, 1958.

129. Petkovic, S. D.: An anatomical classification of renal tumors in the adult as a basis for prognosis. J. Urol., *81*:618–623, 1969.

130. Robson, C. J., Churchill, B. M., and Anderson, W.: The results of radical nephrectomy for renal cell carcinoma. J. Urol., *101*:297–301, 1969.

131. Lang, E. K.: Arteriographic Assessment and staging of renal-cell carcinoma. Radiology, *101*: 17–27, 1971.

132. Rubin, P.: Comment: National cooperative studies. Adjuvant radiotherapy. J.A.M.A., *204*:232–233, 1968.

133. Riches, E.: The place of irradiation. J.A.M.A., *204*: 230–231, 1968.

134. Riches, E. W.: Factors in the prognosis of carcinoma of the kidney. J. Urol., *79*:190–195, 1958.

135. Lang, E. K.: Superselective arterial catheterization of tumors of the urogenital tract: A modality used for perfusion with chemotherapeutic agents and infarction with radioactive pellets. J. Urol., *104*:16–25, 1970.

136. Almgard, L. E., Fernström, Haverling, M., et al.: Treatment of renal adenocarcinoma by embolic occlusion of the renal circulation. Br. J. Urol., *45*:474–479, 1973.

137. Goldin, A. R., Naude, J. H., and Thatcher, G. N.: Therapeutic percutaneous renal infarction. Br. J. Urol., *46*:133–135, 1974.

138. Turner, R. D., Rand, R. W., Bentson, J. R., et al.: Ferro magnetic silicone necrosis of hypernephromas by selective vascular occlusion to the tumor: A new technique. Submitted for publication.

139. Bartley, O. and Hultquist, G. T.: Spontaneous regression of hypernephromas. Acta Pathol. Microbiol. Scand., *27*:448–460, 1950.

140. Eveson, T. C., and Cole, W. H.: Spontaneous regression of adenocarcinoma of the kidney (hypernephroma). *In* Boyd, W. (ed.), Spontaneous Regression of Cancer. Springfield, Ill., Charles C Thomas, 1966, pp. 11–87.

141. Goodwin, W. E.: Regression of hypernephromas. J.A.M.A., *204*:609, 1968.

142. Rubin, P.: Comment: Are metastases curable? J.A.M.A., *204*:612–613, 1968.

143. Bloom, H. J. G.: Hormone-induced and spontaneous regression of metastatic renal cancer. Cancer, *32*:1066–1071, 1973.

144. Jenkins, G. D.: Final report: Regression of pulmonary metastasis following nephrectomy for hypernephroma: Thirteen-year followup. J. Urol., *94*:99–100, 1965.

145. Richmond, J., Sherman, R. S., Diamond, H. D., et al.: Renal lesions associated with malignant lymphomas. Am. J. Med., *32*:184–207, 1962.

146. Lalli, A. F.: Lymphoma and the urinary tract. Radiology, *93*:1051–1054, 1969.

147. Seltzer, R. A., and Wenlund, D. E.: Renal lymphoma. Arteriographic studies. Am. J. Roentgenol. Radium Ther. Nucl. Med., *101*:692–695, 1967.

148. Grace, D. A., Taylor, W. N., Taylor, J. N., et al.: Carcinoma of the renal pelvis: A 15-year review. J. Urol., *98*:566–569, 1968.

149. Gill, W. B., Lu, C. T., and Thomsen, S.: Retrograde brushing—A new technique for obtaining histological and cytological material from ureteral, renal pelvic, and renal calyceal lesions. J. Urol., *109*:573–576, 1973.

150. Rabinowitz, J. G., Kinkhabwala, M., Himmelfarb, E., et al.: Renal pelvic carcinoma. Radiology, *102*:551–554, 1972.

151. Becker, J. A.: Transitional cell carcinoma of the renal pelvis: Causes of non-visualization on excretory urography. J. Urol., *101*:280–282, 1969.

152. Williams, C. B., and Mitchell, J. P.: Carcinoma of the ureter—A review of 54 cases. Br. J. Urol., *45*:377–387, 1973.

153. Riches, E. W., Griffiths, I. H., and Thackray, A. C.: New growths of the kidney and ureter. Br. J. Urol., *23*:297–338, 1951.

154. Bergman, H., Friedenberg, R. M., Sayegh, V.: New roentgenologic signs of carcinoma of the ureter. Am. J. Roentgenol. Radium Ther. Nucl. Med., *86*:707–717, 1961.

155. Casey, W. C., and Goodwin, W. E.: Percutaneous antegrade pyelography and hydronephrosis. J. Urol., *74*:164–173, 1955.

156. Ogg, C. S., Saxton, H. M., Cameron, J. S.: Percutaneous needle nephrostomy. Br. Med. J., 4: 657–660, 1969.

157. Sherwood, T., Doyle, P. T., and Williams, D. I.: Antegrade pyelography in adults and children. Proc. R. Soc. Med., *67*:1210–1215, 1974.

158. Boijsen, E.: Angiographic diagnosis of ureteric carcinoma. Acta Radiol. (Diagn.), *57*:172–176, 1962.

159. Emmett, J. L., and Witten, D. M.: Clinical Urography. Philadelphia, W. B. Saunders, 1971, p. 1257.

160. McDonald, J. R., and Thompson, G. J.: Carcinoma of the urinary bladder: A pathologic study with special reference to invasiveness and vascular invasion. J. Urol., *61*:435–445, 1948.

161. Franksson, C., and Lindblom, K.: Roentegnographic signs of tumor infiltration of the wall of the urinary bladder. Acta Radiol. (Diagn.), *37*:1–7, 1952.

162. Lang, E. K.: Roentgenographic Diagnosis of Bladder Tumors. Springfield, Ill., Charles C Thomas, 1968.

163. Bartley, O., and Eckerbom, H.: Perivesical insufflation of gas for determination of bladder wall thickness in tumors of the bladder. Acta Radiol. (Diagn.), *54*:241–250, 1960.

164. Evans, A. T., and Bell, T. E.: Rhabdomyosarcoma of the bladder in adult patients: Report of three cases. J. Urol., *94*:573–575, 1965.

165. Joshi, D. P., Wessely, Z., Seery, W. H., et al.: Rhabdomyosarcoma of the bladder in an adult: Case report and review of the literature. J. Urol., *96*:214–217, 1966.

166. Vestby, G. W.: Vasoseminal vesiculography in hypertrophy and carcinoma of the prostate. Acta Radiol. (Diagn.), *50*:273–284, 1958.

167. King, W. W., Wilkiemeyer, R. M., Boyce, W. H., et al.: Current status of prostatic echography. J.A.M.A., *226*:444–447, 1973.

168. Kaplan, G. W., Bulkley, G. J., and Grayhack, J. T.: Carcinoma of the male urethra. J. Urol., *98*: 365–371, 1967.

169. Cook, F. E., Jr., Lawrence, D. D., Smith, J. R., et al.: Testicular carcinoma and lymphangiography. Radiology, *84*:420–426, 1965.

170. Baum, S., Bron, K. M., Wexler, L., et al.: Lymphangiography, cavography, and urography. Radiology, *81*:207–218, 1963.

171. Hartman, G. W., Witten, D. M., and Weeks, R. E.: The role of nephrotomography in the diagnosis of adrenal tumors. Radiology, *86*:1030–1034, 1966.

172. Kahn, P. C., and Nickrosz, L. V.: Selective angiography of the adrenal glands. Am. J. Roentgenol. Radium Ther. Nucl. Med., *101*:739–749, 1967.

173. Alfidi, R. J., Gill, W. M., and Klein, H. J.: Arteriography of adrenal neoplasms. Am. J. Roentgenol. Radium Ther. Nucl. Med., *101*:739–749, 1967.

174. Starer, F.: Percutaneous suprarenal venography. Br. J. Radiol., *38*:675–681, 1965.

175. Reuter, S. R., Blair, A. J., Schteingart, D. E., et al.: Adrenal venography. Radiology, *89*:805–814, 1967.

176. Lecky, J. W.: Section 18, Selective Angiography. In Robbins, L. L. (ed.), Diagnostic Radiology. Baltimore, Williams & Wilkins, 1960, pp. 170–203.

177. Meaney, T. F., and Buonocore, E.: Selective arteriography as a localizing and provocative test in the diagnosis of pheochromocytoma. Radiology, *87*:309–314, 1966.

178. Zelch, J. V., Meaney, T. F., and Belhobek, G. H.: Radiologic approach to the patient with suspected pheochromocytoma. Radiology, *111*: 279–284, 1974.

179. Saltz, N. J., Luttwak, E. M., Schwartz, A., et al.: Danger of aortography in the localization of pheochromocytoma. Ann. Surg., *144*:118–123, 1956.

180. Rossi, P., Young, I. S., and Panke, W. F.: Techniques, usefulness, and hazards of arteriography of pheochromocytoma. Review of 99 cases. J.A.M.A., *205*:547–553, 1968.

181. Conn, J. W.: Part II. Primary aldosteronism, a new clinical syndrome. Part I. Painting background. J. Lab. Clin. Med., *45*:6–17, 1955.

182. Melby, J. C., Spark, R. F., Dale, S. L., et al.: Diagnosis and localization of aldosterone-producing adenomas by adrenal-vein catheterization. N. Engl. J. Med., *277*:1050–1056, 1967.

183. Kahn, P. C., Kelleher, M. D., Egdahl, R. H., et al.: Adrenal arteriography and venography in primary aldosteronism. Radiology, *101*:71–78, 1971.

Chapter Twelve

FEMALE GENITAL TRACT

Harvey Gilbert, M.D.

Modern gynecologic oncology is concerned with better identification of the sites of treatment failure, exact delineation of disease extent (staging) before treatment, and more aggressive curative as well as palliative treatment for tumors of the female reproductive tract. Diagnostic radiology may facilitate solutions in all three major areas of concern.

These aims of modern oncology have led to the introduction of a number of controversial radiologic and nonradiologic techniques. The standard chest radiograph, intravenous pyelogram, gastrointestinal contrast studies, liver scanning techniques, radiographic bone surveys, and radionuclide bone scans, as well as cystoscopy, cystography, laparoscopy, and culdoscopy, are widely used and are accepted procedures in selected cases. On the other hand, lymphography (lymphangiography), pelvic venography, pelvic arteriography, diagnostic surgical staging, hysterography, diagnostic ultrasound, and "tumor-specific" radionuclide scanning all have produced controversy regarding the appropriateness of their application. The following sections discuss radiologic techniques that are clinically important and especially identify contrast techniques that might be effective in gaining useful information for actual treatment decisions.

CLINICAL CONSIDERATIONS

Presenting Signs and Symptoms

Patients with vulvar carcinoma may present with a bleeding papillary ulcerative growth and may have a long history of pruritus vulvae, secondary infection, atrophic or hypertrophic leukoplakia, Bowen's disease, or atypical vulvar skin.[1-7] Vaginal bleeding and palpable pelvic masses may be the presenting symptoms of vaginal, cervical, uterine, or ovarian tumors. Urethral carcinoma may first manifest itself as dysuria and urethrorrhagia.

It is well to remember that vaginal masses may represent primary vaginal carcinoma, extensions of cervical and uterine tumors, or metastases from *any* gynecologic site as well as from kidney, breast, or colon primary tumor.[1, 8, 9] Similarly, urethromeatal masses may be either primary tumors or extensions of bladder, cervical, or uterine malignancies.[2] Adolescent females with lateral vaginal adenosis and a mass,[10] and young girls with botryoid vaginal masses, are highly suspect for adenocarcinoma and sarcoma, respectively.[1, 5] It is important to recognize that vaginal masses are frequently missed with the bivalved speculum (causing late diagnosis).[8, 10, 12]

Adnexal masses are found clinically in primary tubo-ovarian malignancies and in the granulosa-theca ovarian tumors that are sometimes associated with uterine malignancy.[13, 14] Ascites or abdominal distension secondary to intestinal obstruction is commonly associated with ovarian malignancy (with and without diffuse peritoneal seeding), as well as with advanced uterine corpus malignancy.[6, 7, 13-16]

An acute abdomen may be the presenting clinical picture in a patient with a twisted ovarian tumor, with a ruptured viscus in a malignancy (choriocarcinoma or pseudo-myxoma peritoneii following rupture of a mucinous ovarian tumor), or with acute intestinal obstruction secondary to ovarian and uterine malignancies that seed the peritoneum.[6, 13, 15, 17, 18] Weight loss and anemia may be the result of many gyne-cologic diseases including malignancies, but dyspareunia and postcoital spotting may be the first indications of a vaginal or cervical tumor.[4, 9] Virilization *or* increas-ing feminization can be caused by an ovarian stromal malignancy.[13, 19, 20] Pelvic pain, uremia, leg edema, and obstipation are most commonly associated with an advanced cervical, uterine, or ovarian lesion that al-ready involves structures outside the pri-mary site (lymph nodes, ureters, nerve plexi).[2, 13, 21-25]

Hydronephrosis is common in ad-vanced cervical and vaginal lesions, occur-ring occasionally in uterine corpus malig-nancies.[26] Retroperitoneal node metastases may cause ureteral displacement without obstruction.[27] Bladder and rectal invasion are late findings in cervical and vaginal malignancies.[7, 28]

Dyspnea and hemoptysis occurring in the presence of a pelvic mass are likely to be associated with metastatic choriocarci-noma, late carcinoma of the uterus, or a dis-seminated pelvic sarcoma.[29-31] Pleural ef-fusion can be caused by ascites from meta-static ovarian carcinoma or, occasionally, from another gynecologic primary tumor.[32, 33] Metastatic involvement of the brain, liver, and bone in gynecologic malignancies is less common, with the highest incidence in patients with lymphomas, sarcomas, mela-nomas, or choriocarcinomas of the reproduc-tive system and with endometrial carcinoma.[1] However, bone metastasis is not rare in advanced carcinoma of the cervix.

Molar pregnancy and persistently high gonadotropin titers precede choriocarcinoma in most cases; less commonly, normal or abortive non-molar pregnancies may also lead to this malignancy.[29] Invasive mole (chorioadenoma destruens) and chorio-carcinoma, jointly considered as gestational trophoblastic disease, are usually detected by a history of molar pregnancy, failure of gonadotropin titer to return to normal fol-lowing mole removal, and less frequently by the local or distant symptoms previously enumerated.[29, 31]

Differential Diagnosis

The differential diagnosis of any adeno-carcinoma involving the reproductive system should include metastatic disease from a primary lesion of the kidney, breast, intestinal tract, or another gynecologic site.[5, 15] Poorly differentiated anaplastic tu-mors of the reproductive tract might also represent a primary sarcoma or a lym-phoma.[6, 34]

Vaginal bleeding, of course, can also result from nonmalignant hemopathy (thrombocytopenia or a coagulation dis-order), leukemic infiltrate of the reproductive mucosa, or uterine fibroids or hormonal disorders (including functioning ovarian tumors).[13, 19, 35] Vaginal masses could repre-sent benign müllerian cystic disease or granulomatous disease, as well as leukemic infiltration or metastatic disease.[4, 9] Meta-static disease to the vagina is in fact more common than the rare primary vaginal malignancy and is the principal diagnosis to exclude when lesions are detected simul-taneously in the ovary, cervix, or vulva.[1, 6] However, in children the rare botryoid embryonal vaginal tumor should be dif-ferentiated carefully from other small cell tumors metastatic to the vagina.[3]

The differential considerations with adnexal masses should include inflammatory tubo-ovarian disease, pedunculated fibroids, metastatic tumors in the ovaries (especially if noncystic and bilateral), and lymphoma (always disseminated), as well as the wide spectrum of benign ovarian masses and primary ovarian malignancies (epithelial, stromal, and germinal tumors).[5, 13, 14] The differential considerations in palpable pelvic masses may also include (in addition to metastatic disease) pelvic kidney, re-dundant colon, diffuse tubo-ovarian in-flammation, fibroids, distended bladder, hematometria, and primary bladder and bowel malignancies.[4, 6, 7, 36, 37] The differ-ential diagnosis of unexplained virilization or feminization must include pituitary and adrenal tumors,[9, 32] as well as gonadal neo-plasms.

It must be remembered that ascites in middle-aged or elderly women can also re-sult from tuberculosis, cirrhosis, pancreatic insufficiency, and other benign diseases such as an ovarian fibroma (Meigs' syn-drome), as well as other (nongynecologic) primary and secondary abdominal malignant tumors.[33, 38, 39] Other sites of primary cancers that metastasize to the reproductive tract include the stomach, pancreas, intestine, breast, lung, or esophagus (all rare, except breast).[1, 13]

Nonmalignant causes of an acute abdomen in a patient with a pelvic mass include ovarian torsion with an ovarian cyst or benign tumor, acute pelvic inflammatory disease, pyometrium, and colonic diverticular disease.[4]

Differential diagnoses to consider (besides tumor in the lung parenchyma) when dyspnea develops in a patient who has a pelvic malignancy include fluid retention secondary to a hormonally functioning ovarian tumor,[32] concurrent congestive heart failure or chronic lung disease, severe ascites elevating the diaphragm, a large pleural effusion, or tracheal compression secondary to metastatic mediastinal nodes.[6] Occasionally, a pleural effusion (sometimes chylous) in a patient who has a gynecologic malignancy may be associated with abdominal carcinomatosis alone (that is, without malignant pleural involvement).[13] In addition to metastasis, a solitary lung lesion or a solitary mass in any other visceral organ may of course be caused by a second primary cancer arising there, or the lesion may be inflammatory and should be evaluated further before it is labeled as metastatic.[40]

A histologic distinction between invasive molar disease (chorioadenoma destruens) and choriocarcinoma is not essential with present treatment policies, and vigorous treatment of a persistently elevated gonadotropin titer in both forms of gestational trophoblastic disease is now accepted.[29, 31] Neither a hysterectomy nor a repeat dilatation and curettage is required.[31] A lung mass in a patient with a greatly elevated gonadotropin titer is almost pathognomonic of choriocarcinoma (it only rarely indicates an invasive mole), especially with the history of a recent molar pregnancy. However, other rare causes of persistent moderately elevated gonadotropin titers are known.[41]

Therapeutic Decisions and Staging

Clinical staging should not have to be altered after appropriate treatment is begun, and, especially for patients with cervical carcinoma, all of the appropriate staging studies should *precede* treatment. Furthermore, the determination of the presence or absence of regional metastatic lymph node involvement is critical to the successful treatment of the patient with a gynecologic malignancy.[2]

The incidence of bilateral inguinal lymph node metastases in vulvar carcinoma is related to the primary lesion's size (common, when the primary is greater than 3 cm), depth of invasion (common, when the primary is deeper than 5 mm), and histologic grade. However, false-positive inguinal node involvement may result from superinfection.[42] Involvement of deep pelvic nodes without inguinal metastases in vulvar carcinoma is extremely rare, but may occur with urethral or clitoral invasion.[5, 6, 7, 11, 43, 44]

Inguinal nodes may also become involved clinically when primary *or* secondary vaginal malignancies involve the lower third of the vagina.[9] However, vaginal and cervical primaries commonly tend to involve the iliac nodes first (in 15 per cent of cases in which the primary tumor is confined to the cervix, and in 40 to 50 per cent of cases in which there is extensive parametrial involvement), followed by secondary metastatic spread to the periaortic nodes (in 20 per cent of cases in which the primary lesion is advanced). Uterine carcinomas in a fundal location spread initially to the periaortic nodes, whereas lesions in the lower uterine segment (especially the endocervix) lead first to metastatic involvement of the iliac nodes. Ovarian epithelial malignancies actually tend to metastasize initially to the periaortic nodes, but the first clinically apparent spread is usually to the peritoneum and the omentum (tumor implants) or to contiguous pelvic organs (except with dysgerminoma).[14, 32] Sarcomas of all gynecologic sites (including botryoid tumors and stromal sarcomas) and ovarian germinal malignancies tend to metastasize hematogenously to the lungs and viscera, with lymphogenous spread playing only a secondary role.[2]

It appears that conscientious treatment of groin nodes in patients with vulvar malignancies (radical vulvectomy and groin dissection), and of iliac nodes in those with cervical and vaginal primaries, has improved survival rates.[3, 6, 7, 28, 45] Attempts to cure known periaortic node disease in any female pelvic malignancy (with the exception of dysgerminoma, discussed below) are of questionable value and must be regarded as investigational at present.[2, 27] Treatment or surgical staging of involved lymph nodes with endometrial and ovarian cancers has not conclusively improved survival rates except for patients with the radiosensitive ovarian dysgerminoma.[2, 36] In addition to establishing or ruling out nodal involvement, prognosis and therapeutic decisions are based on several factors. In patients with vaginal lesions, involvement of the adjacent paravaginal tissue reduced survival by one third. In those with cervical primaries, the prognosis is greatly improved with confinement of the lesion to the cervix (survival rate of more than 80 per cent). Extension of cervical cancer (Table 12–1) into the parametrium reduces the five-year survival rate to 40 to 60 per cent, and extension to the lower third of the vagina, the pelvic sidewalls, the bladder, or the rectum reduces it to 10 per cent. Increase in the extent of the primary disease also parallels an increase in regional node involvement (see preceding discussion).[2, 3, 6, 13, 28, 45, 47, 48]

The prognosis for patients with endometrial carcinoma is related to the degree of histologic differentiation, the presence of myometrial invasion, and the occurrence of tumor extension into the endocervix (see Table 12–2).[2, 5, 6, 49, 50] Ovarian cancer rarely may coexist with an endometrial malignancy.[13]

Patients with sarcomas of the female genital tract have a universally poor prognosis except when the disease is confined to a previously benign uterine leiomyoma, or when discovered while still limited to an endometrial polyp. The sarcomas, along with primary genital melanomas, lymphomas, and anaplastic carcinomas, are vicious in their behavior, with rapid local, lymphatic, intra-abdominal, and distant hematogenous spread.[1, 4, 6, 13]

A good prognostic sign in a patient with an epithelial ovarian tumor is lack of stromal invasion, low histologic grade, and known confinement to one or both ovaries.[13, 15, 38] In a teratoma the presence of mature histologic elements and the absence of solid (noncystic) areas is favorable.[13, 32, 39, 51, 52] If a stromal malignancy is a pure thecoma the prognosis is better. (See Table 12–3.) Gross extraovarian spread of ovarian malignancies to nongynecologic structures carries a poor prognosis, but, paradoxically, the presence of moderate ascites alone seems to have little deleterious effect on the prognosis of a patient who has otherwise early ovarian disease.[38]

Involvement of the paracervical segment of the ureter, with resulting hydronephrosis, is especially serious (decreasing the survival rate by more than 50 per cent) in otherwise early cervical or vaginal carcinoma.[26, 53] In general, parametrial extension is significant (especially if it is nodular) when associated with primary cervical and vaginal lesions, but paracervical induration may occasionally be inflammatory and cause the tumor to be categorized in a higher stage (the induration may also increase during irradiation).[4, 54-56]

The occurrence of radicular leg pain or

Table 12–1   Clinical Staging System and Treatment of Carcinoma of Cervix

Stage	Extent of Disease	Subclassification	Treatment
0	In situ		Surgery
I	Confined to cervix	a. Microinvasion b. All other	Surgery or radiation therapy
II	Extending beyond cervix (central pelvic disease)	a. Vaginal fornix involved b. Parametrium, but not extending to pelvic sidewall	Radiation therapy
III	Extending beyond cervix (advanced pelvic disease)	a. Lower vagina involved b. Nodular pelvic sidewall involvement	Radiation therapy (surgery possible for IIIa)
IV	Invading adjacent viscera and/or extrapelvic extension	a. Clinical bladder or rectum involvement b. Outside pelvis	Radiotherapy for local involvement (surgery possible for IVa if parametrium minimally involved)

Table 12–2   Clinical-Surgical Staging and Treatment of Carcinoma of Uterus

Stage	Extent of Disease	Subclassification	Treatment	Adjunctive Measures
I	Confined to corpus of uterus	a. Uterus sounds up to 8 cm b. Uterus sounds above 8 cm	Surgery	Radiation for poor prognostic types
II	Extends to endocervix or cervix		Radiation and surgery	
III	Extends outside uterus, but confined to true pelvis	a. Adnexal mass b. Parametrial spread	a. Surgery b. Radiation therapy	Progestational agents
IV	Extends outside pelvis		Pelvic radiation and progesterone	

leg edema, or the recent appearance of cutaneous venous collaterals, is usually indicative of pelvic nerve plexus or lymphovascular involvement in patients with late cervical, vaginal, vulvar, or uterine malignancies, and in these cases radiation or surgery is of little help.[5, 58-60]

Rarely, ascites may not indicate extraovarian spread, and the establishment of peritoneal tumor seeding or positive ascitic fluid cytology by laparotomy or endoscopy (especially in otherwise early disease) is essential for accurate staging. Similarly, as mentioned earlier, pleural effusion associated with ascites occasionally may not be caused by direct pleural tumor involvement. Careful evaluation of the lungs and liver for metastatic involvement is particularly important in patients with aggressive pelvic sarcomas, lymphomas, germinal ovarian carcinomas, melanomas, and gestational trophoblastic disease.[40]

The prognosis in gestational trophoblastic disease is considerably worse if gonadotropin titers (luteinizing hormone) are greater than 100,000 international units or if liver, lung or brain is involved.[3, 61] If titers do not return to normal with treatment, this may be evidence for resistant tumor foci in the uterus (most likely), or in the liver or brain (the latter is best detected with a lumbar tap and titers specific for cerebrospinal fluid[29, 62]).

Clinical Follow-up

Most treatment failures in carcinoma of the vulva (11 per cent of all operable cases) become manifest within three years;[3, 7] 60 per cent of these are recurrences within the vulva[44] and a number are still treatable. However, 25 per cent of treatment failures

Table 12–3   Surgical-Pathological Staging and Treatment of Carcinoma of Ovary

Stage	Extent of Disease	Subclassification	Treatment	Adjunctive Treatment
I	Growth limited to one ovary (a), or to both ovaries (b)*	1. Tumor has smooth surface 2. Malignant papillations on surface	Surgery	Radiation and chemotherapy
II	Extra-ovarian growth, but confined within pelvis	a. Confined to gynecologic organs b. Extragynecologic extension*	Surgery and radiation	Chemotherapy
III	Intra-abdominal spread		Chemotherapy and possible "debulking" surgery	Radiation as needed
IV	Distant metastases		Chemotherapy	Surgery for complications; radiation as needed

*The additional presence of malignant ascites is subclassification "c."

occur after five years.[44] Many apparent recurrences may actually represent post-treatment complications, infection, phlebitis, and urinary complications without active cancer.[2] Leg edema from a tumor recurrence in the lymphatics may be difficult to distinguish from benign post-lymphadenectomy changes. Only rarely is treatment failure in vulvar carcinoma manifested initially as distant (non-regional) disease. Urethral carcinoma recurrences are also usually local, with 15 per cent of recurrences presenting in distant sites only.[11] In a reported series of 135 patients with genital melanomas, only 21 have survived, and early disseminated disease predominates.[5]

Vaginal squamous cell carcinoma recurrences are often local,[1] with metastatic tumor appearing in inguinal nodes only when the vulva has been invaded by the primary lesion.[63] A total of 80 per cent of all treatment failures in this disease occur within four years, and 25 per cent of these involve distant metastases.[63] Two thirds of late (post-treatment) vaginal fistulas are due to recurring or persistent vaginal cancer.[9] Effective treatment in the latter cases is difficult.[2, 9, 63] In one series, only 5 out of 108 patients with vaginal adenocarcinoma had local recurrences; 11 developed distant metastases.[10] A number of the former were still successfully treated. Most of the patients who died had involvement of pelvic lymph nodes at the time of the original diagnosis of the disease.[10]

Most endometrial carcinoma recurrences first become manifest within the abdomen or the pelvis (60 per cent); most of these are metastatic nodes or peritoneal implants.[1] Vaginal recurrences, more common in the poor prognostic group, still occur in 1 to 3 per cent of cases in spite of routine postoperative irradiation.[2, 5, 28] Suburethral recurrences indicate concurrent disseminated disease, but vaginal apex recurrences with endometrial carcinomas can still be treated in one third of the cases.[2] Distant disease (usually in the lung) occurs only in 15 to 30 per cent of all the initial treatment failures, and because of the occasional hormonal sensitivity of these metastases they should be carefully searched for.[2] Otherwise, periodic pelvic examination is adequate, with an intravenous pyelogram every two years. Recurrence of endometrial carcinoma with bone pain, ascites, or leg edema occasionally responds to hormones or to local irradiation.[5, 16, 20] Common metastatic sites in ultimate treatment failures are lung (30 per cent), liver (30 per cent), and peritoneum (30 per cent).[1]

Most cervical carcinoma recurrences present within four years.[64] Regional, surgically treatable recurrences occur in only 2 to 3 per cent of early-stage cervical cancers; an abnormal intravenous pyelogram signals the recurrence in 96 per cent of these patients.[5, 26] Symptoms of pelvic pain, bleeding, discharge, and an enlarging mass may also indicate recurrence.[65] (Note that a residual mass of scar tissue may also persist in a cured patient.[25]) Symptoms such as sciatic leg pain or unilateral leg edema, and clinical or radiologic findings such as pelvic sidewall nodularity, weight loss, pelvic and periaortic nodal disease, or especially pulmonary metastasis, are contraindications to late pelvic exenteration.[66-68] Only 2 to 15 per cent of patients with recurrences of cervical carcinoma present only with metastases in distant sites, whereas 30 per cent of these patients have local *plus* distant disease. Among the sites of cervical carcinoma recurrence are the lung (15 to 20 per cent), bone (10 to 20 per cent), and liver (15 to 20 per cent).[1] Differentiating the bleeding, painful mass of a recurrence from pelvic radiation injury (with diarrhea, tenesmus, cystitis, and malodorous discharge) is at times extremely difficult, and identifying late radiation small bowel injury presenting as obstruction, malabsorption, fistula, or pain may be equally difficult, utilizing all available methods.[5, 59, 65, 70-76] Almost any radiologic finding or suspicious pelvic symptoms in the postirradiation period can be caused by a tumor recurrence as well as by a late radiation effect.[5, 77, 78]

Ovarian tumors that recur following chemotherapy, radiation, or surgery will usually do so initially within the abdomen or pelvis. Certain patients whose disease completely responded to chemotherapy can justifiably be subjected to a "second-look" operation, for resection of residual disease or for consideration of a decision to stop the drug treatment.[6, 36] The recurrences that can be treated surgically are found mainly in patients who were treated initially only with unilateral oophorectomy or even a segmental ovarian "cyst" removal, and in whom the recurrence is located in the uterus or the remaining ovary.[6, 14, 36] Of the ovarian tumors, only sarcomas, teratomas, and dysgerminomas recur in significant percentages *outside* the abdomen (usually within one year).[4, 32, 51, 79] Epithelial ovarian malignancies do not recur at distant sites without a coexisting regional recurrence, and the liver is the site of metastasis in less than 10 per cent of recurrences.[4] Granulosa cell tumors may recur late, but the first recurrence is always intra-abdominal.[5, 19, 35] Pelvic outlet obstruction, with bouts of intestinal obstruction, cachexia, or ascites, may herald the recurrence. Pleural effusion may occur eventually in any recurrent ovarian malignancy of epithelial origin.

RADIOLOGIC CONSIDERATIONS

Presenting Radiographic Signs

With gynecologic tumors, a simple anteroposterior radiograph ("flat plate") of the abdomen *may* reveal: (1) soft tissue mass densities in the pelvis or lower abdomen; (2) calcifications in a uterine fibroid or a serous ovarian tumor, or teeth in a cystic teratoma (Fig. 12–1); (3) the ground-glass appearance of ascites with effacement of properitoneal fat lines and bulging of the flanks; (4) dilated loops of bowel secondary to intestinal obstruction from a large pelvic mass or from omental or serosal tumor seeding (nonobstructive ileus may also be observed with an acute abdomen, associated with a ruptured or twisted viscus in a trophoblastic or ovarian malignancy); or (5) the absence of a fetal skeleton with a large molar pregnancy.[1, 5, 7, 8, 78]

On the other hand, chest radiographs may first reveal the nodular parenchymal metastases of metastatic choriocarcinoma, teratoma, endometrial carcinoma, pelvic sarcoma, and melanoma, or the pleural effusion secondary to ovarian ascites or to metastatic disease from any gynecologic site.[1, 2, 5, 8, 78] The patterns of parenchymal lung involvement are variable: interstitial

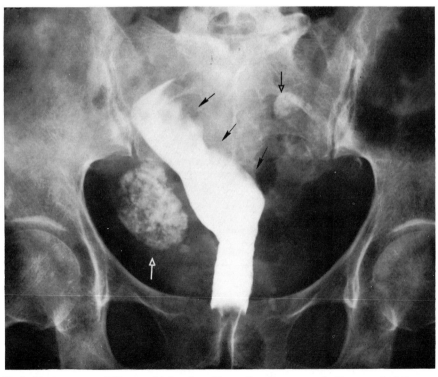

Figure 12–1 Hysterogram of 80-year-old female with cardiac disease precluding surgical therapy. Histologic diagnosis was "mixed Mullerian sarcoma," and a large pelvic mass was palpable. The large uterine tumor mass occluded the lumen (arrows), and incidental calcified subserosal fibroids also were present (open arrows).

or nodular deposits occur with metastatic gynecologic carcinomas, and patients with sarcomas have occasional large "golf-ball" nodules. Solitary lung metastases are most common in patients with endometrial and cervical primaries.[40]

For the patient who is difficult to examine and is suspected to have a pelvic cyst or neoplasm, pelvic pneumography or laparoscopy might demonstrate a mass that deserves surgical evaluation.[78] (This usually is not helpful in distinguishing benign from malignant disease, however.) A "routine" intravenous pyelogram performed for another purpose occasionally might reveal obstructed or deviated ureters secondary to direct parametrial tumor extension from a cervical or vaginal primary, or to regional periaortic node metastases from a pelvic primary.[78] Only rarely will a pelvic primary malignancy other than a sarcoma come to attention *initially* as hepatic, osseous, or central nervous system disease.[1]

Differential Diagnosis

The primary diagnosis of pelvic malignancies is rarely made by radiologic means. Furthermore, most radiologic diagnostic studies in this body region make a limited contribution toward further distinguishing a benign from a malignant lesion.[78] Pelvic pneumography, laparoscopy, and hysterography are therefore rarely indicated for the primary purpose of diagnosing pelvic cancer, but they may be helpful in examining the patient who is obese or otherwise difficult to palpate when one desires confirmation of a suspicious but indefinite pelvic mass or requires preoperative assistance in distinguishing a uterine from an adnexal mass. (Fig. 12–1).[5, 32] However, these studies carry at least a theoretical risk of seeding tumor or rupturing a cystic mass.[6, 14, 72] The author has not used these techniques and prefers diagnostic laparotomy as a more direct and effective measure to use when dealing with a known mass and a suspected pelvic malignancy.

The role of radiology in the differential diagnosis of gynecologic masses is primarily in separating primary pelvic malignancies from those that originated at other sites, and, conversely, in detecting concurrent extra-pelvic lesions and determining whether they too are neoplastic (i.e., metastatic) or are instead unrelated to the pelvic mass. However, in connection with the second role, no patient should be denied possible curative treatment exclusively on the basis of a solitary radiologic or scan finding.

In distinguishing primary gynecologic malignancies and their metastases preoperatively from malignant and benign diseases arising at other sites, the most critical examinations are the chest radiograph, clinical breast examination (sometimes supplemented with mammography), the intravenous pyelogram, and upper and lower gastrointestinal series.[6, 78] The preoperative evaluation of the ascitic abdomen or a known or ill-defined pelvic mass should also include liver function tests, radionuclide liver scan, bone scan, and proctosigmoidoscopy. Ultrasound B scans may be helpful in distinguishing solid from cystic pelvic masses and in evaluating suspected hepatic metastases.

After abdominal extension and extra-abdominal disease have been ruled out radiologically and clinically, the patient with a pelvic mass of suspected adnexal origin should not be subjected to paracentesis since she must undergo laparotomy in any event for a definitive diagnosis and resection of bulk disease, surgical clipping of any residual disease, and cytologic study of peritoneal fluid.[5, 32]

Preoperative chest radiographs in a patient presenting with a pelvic mass may reveal massive mediastinal/hilar adenopathy associated with a lymphoma, pleural fluid associated with osteoblastic metastases that in turn may point toward a disseminated breast carcinoma, or evidence of unsuspected noncancerous conditions.[4] They may also reveal lung metastases from an endometrial, tubal, or (rarely) uterine cervical primary (Fig. 12–2), as well as metastases from a breast, gastrointestinal, melanoma, or lymphoma primary with a concurrent pelvic mass.[1, 5, 6] The solitary lung nodule or mediastinal/hilar mass may be evaluated further with lung or mediastinal tomography, and if found to be the only site of extrapelvic disease should be biopsied using any of the following appropriate methods: (1) percutaneous needle biopsy (under radiologic control) if the lesion is accessible; (2) mediastinoscopy, if the radiologically

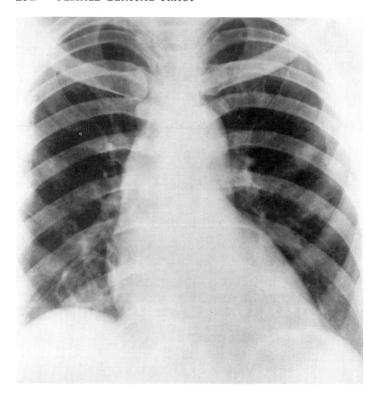

Figure 12–2 Chest roentgenogram. Cavitating metastasis in right lower lobe of lung from squamous carcinoma of uterine cervix.

visible adenopathy is right paratracheal or anterior mediastinal; (3) bronchoscopy or bronchographic brush biopsy if the tumor deposit appears to be related to major bronchi;[31] or (4) thoracotomy if the aforementioned methods prove nonproductive.[40] In a patient with a diagnosis of genital carcinoma, an associated primary carcinoma of the lung may also be the cause of a solitary lung lesion.

A pleural effusion without lung parenchymal or mediastinal lesions on the chest radiograph should be examined cytologically and biochemically for evidence of carcinoma.[5, 6, 14] Both pleural biopsy and pleural fluid cytology may be necessary to rule out metastatic disease from breast or ovarian carcinoma, and radiologic guidance with the image amplifier is often indicated. However, an effusion that is negative for malignant cells after three diagnostic thoracenteses probably indicates that there is no metastatic disease to the pleura. Persistently elevated chorionic gonadotropin titers in women of childbearing age, together with an appropriate history, have replaced most other differential diagnostic procedures in distinguishing metastatic

pulmonary trophoblastic disease from other causes of lung nodules on the chest radiograph.[29, 41, 78]

The intravenous pyelogram serves two purposes in contributing to a differential diagnosis of a pelvic mass: (1) the detection of an unsuspected primary urologic malignancy, and (2) detection of para-aortic or parametrial spread secondary to a suspected gynecologic malignancy (see Figure 12–3).

While assisting the clinician in making a differential diagnosis between a primary gynecologic lesion and metastatic spread to the pelvis from another primary site, upper gastrointestinal and small bowel contrast studies may reveal the intrinsic defects of a primary or metastatic lymphoma, multiple metastatic gastrointestinal lesions from a melanoma, a primary stomach carcinoma, or a gastrointestinal carcinoid.[2, 5, 7, 13, 78] Similarly, a gastrointestinal series may also reveal the extrinsic gastrointestinal effects of a large retroperitoneal lymphoma, sarcoma, or pancreatic carcinoma, as well as partial intestinal obstruction or bowel defects caused by abdominal carcinomatosis.[24, 72, 73, 75, 76] (See the sections on staging and follow-up.)

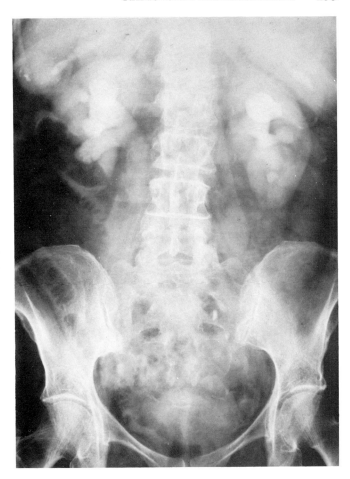

Figure 12–3 Clinically, this patient had stage Ib carcinoma of the cervix. However, IVP demonstrates bilateral hydronephrosis and hydroureters, indicating more extensive disease than suspected and a more adverse prognosis.

In assisting the differential diagnosis, a barium enema may reveal the intrinsic defects of a primary intestinal carcinoma, carcinoid, lymphoma, or sarcoma.[81] It may also demonstrate a rectosigmoid stricture related to previous pelvic irradiation, rectosigmoid displacement or actual mural invasion from a pelvic mass, or bowel obstruction secondary to intrinsic or extrinsic tumor involvement.[53, 70, 78]

Similarly, cystoscopy and proctoscopy may be valuable in distinguishing primary bladder or rectal carcinoma from extrinsic invasion by a primary gynecologic tumor, as well as in making the distinction between a primary urethral tumor and local extension from a bladder or vulvovaginal primary.[2, 81] Hepatic and skeletal imaging by radiodiagnostic and radionuclide methods are discussed in the section on localization and staging; they serve little purpose initially in arriving at a differential diagnosis.

Attempted amniocentesis followed by amniography may help to confirm the suspicion of a molar pregnancy (Fig. 12–4).[78] Often, no fluid can be aspirated in these instances.

Localization and Staging

The importance of defining the extent or stage of disease preoperatively for a patient with a gynecologic malignancy (beyond the use of physical examination and simple laboratory tests) must be linked directly to the impact that any newly derived knowledge will have on the treatment and the survival of an individual patient. This aspect unfortunately is often ignored.

The contribution of the chest radiograph has already been covered. It is worthwhile emphasizing the use of lung tomography in patients with known (or suspected)

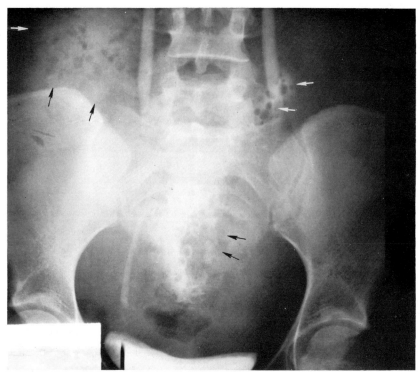

Figure 12–4 Amniogram of 28-year-old female with enlarging abdominal mass, nausea, and vomiting. Gonadotropin titer was elevated. Scout film of abdomen had revealed no fetal skeleton. Multiple circumscribed filling defects were outlined by contrast material, indicative of hydatidiform mole (arrows).

solitary pulmonary nodules, to confirm or rule out suspected lesions, to detect multiple small lesions, and to look for any signs indicating that the nodules are benign (principally small calcifications within solitary lung nodules). Intravenous pyelography is also important for proper tumor staging, for the following reasons: (1) the presence of ureteral obstruction on the intravenous pyelogram cuts expected survival rates in half, in otherwise *clinical* stage 1 or stage 2 cervical carcinomas; (2) the presence of an ectopic (horseshoe or pelvic) kidney and its function may be important in planning appropriate radiotherapy; (3) laterally deviated ureters may indicate retroperitoneal (para-aortic) nodal disease. Radionuclide renography or scintigraphy is sensitive in picking up early upper urinary obstruction, but is much less specific in delineating some of the above findings; however, renography may be helpful for repeated observation of urinary patency during and following therapy, once a baseline has been established.[82, 83]

The purpose of lymphography in tumor staging is to define the extent of metastatic pelvic and periaortic nodal involvement. However, its specificity for distinguishing node metastases from malignancies other than dysgerminomas, melanomas, and lymphomas is limited. *Non*malignant causes of apparent nodal filling defects on the lymphadenogram include fatty infiltration of one or more nodes, immunologic disorders, infection, fibrosis, and superimposition of adjacent normal nodes, among others.[84] Moderate lymphatic vessel displacement in the iliac and para-aortic chains, taken alone, may not be *pathognomonic* of tumor because of normal variations in lymphatic flow patterns; neither may a localized absence of nodes nor an apparent increased number of nodes be diagnostic.[84, 85] Moderate nodal enlargements can also be caused by benign diseases such as chronic infection, Whipple's disease, sarcoid, reactive hyperplasia, and others.[86] The preceding interpretative problems have led experienced clinical investigators to demand a constellation of two or more positive findings before diagnosing a metastatic malignancy on a lymphogram. The positive findings may include: (1) marginal filling defects involving more than one third of the lymph node;[87, 88] (2) localized lymphatic stasis at 24 hours; (3) collateralization of lymphatic drainage *around* suspicious or unfilled nodes;[89] (4) nodal enlargement;[77, 84, 85, 89, 90] and (5) failure of the lymph channels to traverse the marginal filling defects (may require tomography).[91] (See Figure 12–5.) Combining the above criteria may increase diagnostic accuracy in "positive" cases to 90 per cent (for experienced lymphographers) for histologically involved iliac or para-aortic nodes,[77] but more carefully circumscribing the criteria for a "positive" lymphogram also increases the incidence of false-negatives. It should be emphasized that the busy occasional lymphographer, who has limited experience and time for this study, will find it difficult to bring the accuracy rate of lymphography above 50 to 70 per cent in pelvic epithelial malignancies,[42, 77, 87, 91, 92, 94, 95] with the re-

sult that this study must still be relegated to an investigational status in most settings. Therefore, the only gynecologic patients for whom we presently recommend the use of the lymphogram as a decision-making (staging) examination routinely are those with pelvic lymphomas and dysgerminomas.

In vulvar lesions, the primary nodal drainage is to the inguinal nodes, and rarely to the deep pelvic nodes. Vaginal primaries drain to the iliac and superior gluteal nodes, with occasional posterior midline drainage to the sacral nodes. When there is lower vaginal-vulvar tumor extension, drainage is to the inguinal nodes. With carcinomas of the uterus or ovary, drainage is to both para-aortic and iliac nodes. Cervical lesions drain to the iliac and superior gluteal nodes.

Femoral venography can occasionally be of help in confirming suspected iliac adenopathy, especially in the patient with leg edema; however, the information gained is often nonspecific.[94, 97] Demonstration of *complete* femoral or iliac vein obstruction may be diagnostic of local malignant in-

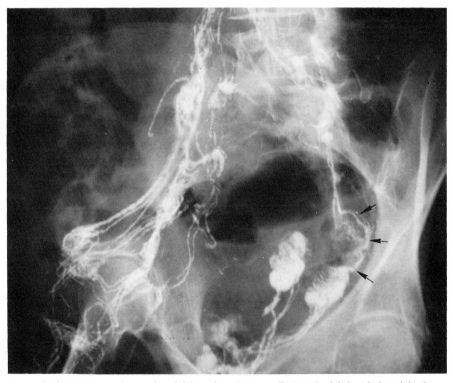

Figure 12–5 Early injection phase of pedal lymphangiogram. Patient had left-sided pedal edema, as well as left-sided hydronephrosis and a past history of stage I, well-differentiated carcinoma of the uterus. Delayed (24-hour) films showed a suspicious area of non-filled nodes in the left iliac chain. However, only this early oblique view revealed the other critical finding: circumvention of lymphatic channels around the replaced, metastatic left iliac lymph nodes (arrows).

volvement in an appropriate clinical context, but the clinical diagnosis itself may also be obvious by this time. Selective retrograde ovarian venography has been of no particular assistance as a staging procedure to evaluate parametrial extension from a cervical primary.[93]

Inferior vena cavography for evaluation of nodes in the right paravertebral and celiac axis areas is plagued with artifacts in interpretation, including possible confusion with benign masses or venous anomalies. The method is of relatively low sensitivity as well as specificity.[78, 97] Ordinarily, none of these venous opacification techniques is clinically useful for making treatment decisions, in our opinion.

Pelvic arteriography has also been found by most authors to be unreliable in tumor *staging* and in distinguishing benign from malignant disease.[70, 77, 96] The reasons are: (1) normal variations in arterial anatomy, (2) the normal high degree of vascularity of the pelvis, and (3) the frequent "characteristic" alterations (corkscrew vessels and "tumor vessels") produced by many benign (particularly inflammatory) conditions.[77, 78, 96] Pelvic arteriography for staging, therefore, remains investigational except for identifying persistent foci of trophoblastic disease in the uterus or in the liver (Fig. 12–6).[78]

Hysterography (per vaginal injection of radiologic contrast material into the uterus) is useful only occasionally in defining a pelvic mass for the radiotherapist in a patient who cannot undergo an operation for medical reasons (Fig. 12–1).[78] Cystography may help to define tumor extent in pelvic embryonal sarcoma of childhood (Fig. 12–7), but cystoscopy alone is sufficient in most cases for the important task of ruling out mucosal or submucosal bladder involvement by cervical or vaginal tumors in adults.[78]

Upper and lower gastrointestinal examinations with barium can be helpful in staging a pelvic malignancy, especially for investigating possible rectosigmoid invasion, as well as for evaluating all patients with gastrointestinal symptoms (obstipation, bleeding, or a suspected fistula). A small bowel series can also be helpful following hysterectomy and prior to intensive pelvic irradiation, to ascertain the presence of dependent and fixed small bowel in the pelvic radiation field.

Exploratory laparotomy has been found to provide much more accurate staging of

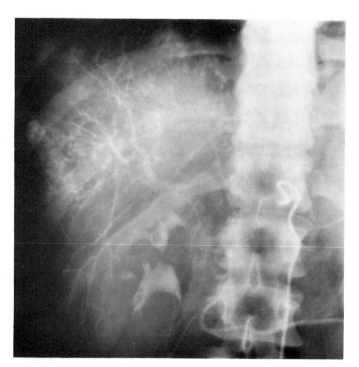

Figure 12–6 Hypervascular metastatic choriocarcinoma in right lobe of the liver, defined by hepatic arteriography (late arterial phase of arteriogram). The patient was a 31-year-old female with a persistently elevated chorionic gonadotropin titer following adequate chemotherapeutic trial.

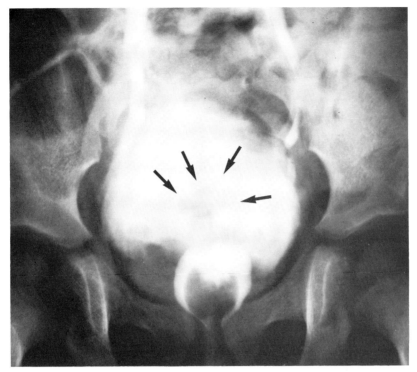

Figure 12–7 Cystogram in child showing multiple, faint filling defects within body of bladder (arrows), from embryonal botryoid sarcoma. (The large filling defect in trigone region is a Foley catheter.)

the disease in patients with cervical and vaginal carcinomas, although positive proof of patient benefit, in the form of an actual increase in survival rates, is not yet available. With *clinical* examination alone, an under-staging inaccuracy for para-aortic nodal involvement and an over-staging inaccuracy for local pelvic extension (because of inflammatory adnexal disease) have been noted in various series.[54, 56, 92, 99]

Radiologic screening studies for determining skeletal involvement are not routinely recommended for staging gynecologic malignancies, but bone scanning, correlated with special radiographic views of "positive" areas, can certainly be helpful in the symptomatic patient. A solitary bone lesion should not be accepted unequivocally as being metastatic disease without a biopsy, which can sometimes be accomplished by the use of a percutaneous cutting needle under fluoroscopic control. When a gynecologic malignancy does metastasize to bone, osseous symptoms and involvement of multiple bones are the rule. However, it is not rare for locally extensive cervi-

cal carcinoma to metastasize hematogenously to a single bone, often to a vertebral body.

Routine screening of the clinically normal liver (nuclide scans; possibly ultrasound) for tumor involvement is probably valuable in pelvic sarcomas, ovarian teratocarcinomas, lymphomas, and dysgerminomas, and endometrial cancers, but liver scanning and hepatic angiography may be indicated only with advanced disease in other gynecologic tumors. A "positive" liver scan is usually nonspecific and will indicate the need for a biopsy for histologic confirmation in most instances. An isolated elevation in serum alkaline phosphatase may be of assistance in diagnosing liver involvement, if distinctly abnormal and unassociated with any bone disease.

Alleged "tumor-specific" radionuclide scans (gallium; bleomycin) are not yet of demonstrated clinical utility in evaluating metastatic liver involvement except in an investigational setting. Ultrasonic techniques are also not yet of demonstrated efficacy as decision-making modalities in the staging of pelvic tumors.[5, 100]

Radiologic Follow-up

Following treatment, the radiologic contribution to the detection of tumor recurrence or extension rests heavily upon the follow-up chest radiograph, which may reveal the common, early pulmonary metastases of a gynecologic sarcoma, the later-appearing lung deposits from a carcinoma of the endometrium, the pleural effusion associated with an ovarian carcinoma, or the unusual and late lung parenchymal or hilar metastasis from a carcinoma of the cervix. It is important to keep in mind that a pleural effusion with an ovarian primary may not *necessarily* contain malignant cells.[5] Furthermore, solitary pulmonary nodules may represent a second malignancy or even a benign lesion.[40] Comparison with earlier chest films is mandatory. Tomography to detect calcification or cavitation in lung nodules should precede attempted removal or biopsy of these lesions. Whereas lung cavitary lesions are often inflammatory in nature, it is important to remember that metastatic lymphomas, choriocarcinomas, and squamous cell tumors in the lungs (including metastatic carcinoma of the cervix; see Figure 12–2) not uncommonly will cavitate.

Intravenous pyelography should be performed yearly following definitive treatment of cervical and upper vaginal carcinomas for the first three years (more frequently if abnormal) and as often as clinically indicated thereafter.[26, 82] It should be employed following the treatment of other pelvic malignancies only as specifically indicated. An abnormal intravenous pyelogram (caused by ureteral obstruction or deviation) developing *after* definitive radiation treatment should be regarded as evidence of a recurrence; only 2 per cent of these abnormalities are caused by radiation damage alone.[26] Cystography may of course be helpful in following the bladder mass of an embryonal botryoid sarcoma after radiation and chemotherapy (Fig. 12–7).[78]

Post-treatment liver function tests, along with oral cholecystography or intravenous cholangiography, are indicated when right upper quadrant pain, hepatomegaly, hypoalbuminemia, or jaundice appears. With severe jaundice and an extrahepatic biliary obstructive pattern, transhepatic cholangiography, retrograde cholangiography through the duodenal fiberscope, peritoneoscopy, or some combination of these studies may be required. Liver scans are unequivocally helpful in these cases only if the patient does not drink alcohol, does not have diabetes, and does not have pre-existing nonmalignant liver disease.[72] Both serologic tests and radionuclide liver scans are helpful in *screening* the patient being considered for pelvic exenteration who presents with a pelvic recurrence after receiving primary treatment. Hepatic angiography may add further information in patients in whom the screening tests prove to be equivocal or "positive." Anemia following treatment, without known blood loss, deserves an open bone marrow biopsy for ruling out myelophthisis from metastatic tumor.[6] Unexplained weight loss is indicative of recurrent disease until proved otherwise, and an assiduous clinical and radiologic search, utilizing any of the means already mentioned, should be undertaken to make the diagnosis.[5]

When specifically indicated by symptoms or clinical findings, post-treatment barium enemas are helpful in distinguishing intrinsic from extrinsic colorectal pathology, including a pelvic tumor recurrence. In addition, proctosigmoidoscopy is especially useful in detecting postirradiation enteritis or proctitis (the incidence of this complication is related to dose, dose-rate, and the method of irradiation). Chronic radiation enteritis may appear radiologically as a short-segment rectal or sigmoid constriction, as a fistula, or as an ulcer 10 cm or more from the anus.[70] With treated ovarian carcinomas, a small bowel series may also be helpful in distinguishing late radiation enteritis producing malabsorption, abdominal distress, obstipation, anorexia, or vomiting, from bowel adhesions or from an obstruction caused by omentoperitoneal tumor seeding.[5, 24, 73–75] However, because of an understandable tendency to intervene surgically rather early for constrictive small bowel injury or obstruction, this diagnostic problem is often resolved in practice by laparotomy. A post-treatment upper gastrointestinal series may also detect gastric ulcers secondary to para-aortic nodal irradiation (or even to pelvic irradiation) when there is a long, dependent J-shaped stomach.

Lymphograms, venograms, or arteriograms may be especially difficult to interpret following irradiation or extensive abdomino-pelvic surgery. Nodal fibrosis, lymphatic vessel obstruction, or deviation of lymph chains with associated pools of extravasation ("lymphoceles") may be found simply as sequelae to treatment.[5, 59, 77, 78] However, Wallace feels that an observed deviation of lymph channels is caused only by tumor.[91]

Lymphography is practically impossible to interpret in a patient who has undergone radical vulvectomy and may be very difficult technically to perform in a patient who has an edematous lower extremity. However, post-treatment lymphograms may be particularly helpful in following a patient with an ovarian dysgerminoma.[89, 90] It is also important to remember to take abdominal films on follow-up visits for treated patients who have already undergone a pretreatment lymphogram for staging: the nodes often remain opacified for months or even years following the initial study, and minimal changes in size or position of iliac or para-aortic nodes on follow-up visits may be indicative of a tumor recurrence. Pelvic pain (usually denoting a recurrence) in the cervical cancer patient should be evaluated initially with pelvic plain films and an intravenous pyelogram, and, if still negative, a pelvic bone scan.

Ascites in a patient who has been treated for uterine or ovarian carcinoma is indicative of tumor recurrence, with little need for radiologic evaluation after paracentesis and cytology have been performed.[4] However, surgery may occasionally still be performed by some clinicians if the palpable recurrent tumor is localized,[6] and a laparotomy might be indicated also if ascites is accompanied by intestinal obstruction. Radiologic studies required in these cases are the same as those utilized in primary diagnosis and staging of the disease.

The rate of treatment success for patients with vaginal apex recurrences from primary uterine carcinomas is high, and an effort to screen out metastatic disease in the liver and lung by all available means is indicated.[2, 30] Suburethral recurrences, however, usually have associated distant disease.[1, 2, 30]

Choriocarcinoma may be followed during and after treatment with gonadotropin titers and chest films only.[29, 41, 102] Specialized radiologic studies of the liver, skeleton, brain, and uterus (see Figure 12–3) are performed when titers do not return to normal or localized symptoms occur.[29, 61, 78]

CONCLUSION

Radiologic diagnostic studies have an important place in the detection, differential diagnosis, pretreatment staging and post-treatment follow-up of patients with gynecologic malignancies. Nevertheless, it is important to avoid the trap of using these studies to defer needed decisions or to satisfy clinical curiosity. Radiologic examinations, when applied, must have demonstrated usefulness in the context of specific clinical problems; they should be employed judiciously and only to arrive at judgments that have practical therapeutic significance for the individual patient.

References

1. Hertig, A. T., Gore, H.: Tumors of the female sex organs, part II: Tumors of the vulva, vagina, and uterus. *In* Atlas of Tumor Pathology. Washington, D.C., Armed Forces Institute of Pathology, 1960.
2. Plentl, A. A., and Friedman, E. A.: Lymphatic System of the Female Genitalia. Philadelphia, W. B. Saunders, 1971.
3. Rutledge, F.: The vagina. *In* Holland, J. F., and Frei, E.: Cancer Medicine. Philadelphia, Lea & Febiger, 1973, pp. 1743–1746.
4. Ackerman, L., and del Regato, J.: Cancer: Diagnosis, Treatment, and Prognosis. 4th ed. St. Louis, C. V. Mosby, 1970.
5. DiSaia, P. J., Morrow, C. P., and Townsend, D. E.: Synopsis of Gynecologic Oncology. Los Angeles County/University of Southern California Medical Center. To be published.
6. Barber, H., and Graber, E. (eds.): Gynecological Oncology. Baltimore, Williams & Wilkins, 1970.
7. DiSaia, P. J., Morrow, C. P., and Townsend, D. E.: Cancer of the vulva. Calif. Med., *118*:13–18, 1973.
8. Hummer, W. K., Mussey, E., Decker, D. G., et al.: Carcinoma in situ of the vagina. Am. J. Obstet. Gynecol., *108*:1109–1116, 1970.
9. Murphy, W. T.: Primary carcinoma of the vagina. *In* Deeley, T. J. (ed.), Modern Radiotherapy: Gynaecological Cancer. Reading, Mass., Butterworths, 1971, p. 214.
10. Herbst, A. L., Robboy, S. J., Scully, R. E., et al.: Clear-cell adenocarcinoma of the vagina and cervix in girls: Analysis of 170 registry cases. Am. J. Obstet. Gynecol., *119*:713–724, 1974.

11. Grabstald, H., Hilaris, B., Henschke, U., et al.: Cancer of the female urethra. J.A.M.A., *197*: 835–842, 1966.

12. Laufe, L. E., and Bernstein, E. D.: Primary malignant melanoma of the vagina. Obstet. Gynecol., *37*:148–154, 1971.

13. Novak, E. R., and Woodruff, J. D. (eds.): Novak's Gynecologic and Obstetric Pathology. 7th ed. Philadelphia, W. B. Saunders, 1974.

14. Griffiths, C. T.: Ovary and fallopian tube. *In* Holland, J. F., and Frei, E., Cancer Medicine. Philadelphia, Lea & Febiger, 1973, pp. 1710–1720.

15. Aure, J. C., Hoeg, K., and Kolstad, P.: Clinical and histologic studies of ovarian carcinoma: Long-term follow-up of 990 cases. Obstet. Gynecol., *37*:1–9, 1971.

16. Strickland, P.: The treatment of carcinoma of the body of the uterus. *In* Deeley, T. J. (ed.), Modern Radiotherapy: Gynaecological Cancer. Reading, Mass., Butterworths, 1971, p. 167.

17. Bellingham, F. R.: Choriocarcinoma: Clinician beware. Med. J. Aust., *1*:587–593, 1967.

18. Easley, J. D., and Fletcher, G. H.: Analysis of the treatment of stage I and II carcinomas of the uterine cervix. Am. J. Roentgenol. Radium Ther. Nucl. Med., *111*:243–248, 1971.

19. Novak, E.: Feminizing gonadal stromal tumors: Analysis of the granulosa-theca cell tumors of the ovarian tumor registry. Obstet Gynecol., *38*:701–713, 1971.

20. Schellhas, H. F.: Malignant potential of the dysgenetic gonad, part I and part II. Obstet. Gynecol., *44*:298–309, 1974.

21. Currie, D. W.: Operative treatment of carcinoma of the cervix. J. Obstet. Gynaecol. Br. Commonw., *78*:385–405, 1971.

22. Pilleron, J. P., Chavanne, G., Durand, J. C., et al.: L'apport de la lymphographie dans la colpohystérectomie élargie pour cancer du dol. Etude de 100 cas. Mem. Acad. Chir. (Paris), *92*:641–647, 1966.

23. Boyes, D. A., Worth, A. J., and Fidler, H. K.: Results of treatment of 4,389 cases of preclinical cervical squamous carcinoma. *J. Obstet. Gynaecol. Br. Commonw.*, *77*:769–780, 1970.

24. Eleventh Annual M. D. Anderson Symposium on Cancer, Chicago, Year Book Medical Publishers, 1969.

25. Ulfelder, H.: Ultra-radical surgery in pelvic cancer. Seventh National Cancer Conference Proceedings. Philadelphia, J. B. Lippincott, 1973, pp. 239–241.

26. Waggoner, C. M., and Spratt, J. S.: Prognostic significance of radiographic ureteropathy before and after irradiation therapy for carcinoma of the cervix uteri. Am. J. Obstet. Gynecol., *105*:1197–1200, 1969.

27. Nelson, J. H., Macasaet, M. A., Lu, T., et al.: The incidence and significance of para-aortic lymph node metastases in late invasive carcinoma of the cervix. Am. J. Obstet. Gynecol., *118*:749–755, 1974.

28. Gusberg, S.: Corpus uteri. *In* Holland, J. F., and Frei, E., Cancer Medicine. Philadelphia, Lea & Febiger, 1973.

29. Bagshawe, K. D.: The treatment of trophoblastic tumors. *In* Deeley, T. J. (ed.), Modern Radio-therapy: Gynaecologic Cancer. Reading, Mass., Butterworths, 1971, p. 228.

30. Boronow, R. C.: Editorial comment: A fresh look at corpus cancer management. Obstet. Gynecol., *42*:448–451, 1973.

31. Li, M. C.: Trophoblastic disease: Natural history, diagnosis and treatment. Ann. Intern. Med., *74*:102–112, 1971.

32. Scully, R. E.: Recent progress in ovarian cancer. Human Pathol., *1*:73–98, 1970.

33. Sall, S.: The treatment of ovarian cancer. *In* Ariel, I. (ed.), Progress in Clinical Cancer. Vol. 5. New York, Grune & Stratton, 1973, pp. 249–262.

34. Chorlton, I., Norris, H. J., and King, F. M.: Malignant reticuloendothelial disease involving the ovary as a primary manifestation. Cancer, *34*:397–407, 1974.

35. Engle, R. B.: Roentgen treatment of granulosa cell carcinoma of the ovary. Am. J. Roentgenol. Radium Ther. Nucl. Med., *80*:5, 1958.

36. Kottmeier, H. L.: Ovarian cancer with special regard to radiotherapy. *In* Deeley, T. J. (ed.), Modern Radiotherapy: Gynaecologic Cancer. Reading, Mass., Butterworths, 1971.

37. Schiller, H. M., and Silverberg, S. G.: Staging and prognosis in primary carcinoma of the fallopian tube. Cancer, *28*:389–395, 1971.

38. Pomerance, W.: Factors influencing survival in ovarian carcinoma. Am. J. Obstet. Gynecol., *96*:418–424, 1966.

39. Woodruff, J. Metastatic ovarian tumors. Am. J. Obstet. and Gynecol., *107*:202–209, 1970.

40. Saegesser, F., Besson, A., and Kajai, F.: Pulmonary coin lesions and metastases. *In* Saigesser, F., and Pettavel, J. (eds), Surgical Oncology. Baltimore, Williams & Wilkins, 1971.

41. Weintraub, B. D., Rosen, S. W.: Ectopic production of human chorionic somatomammotropin by nontrophoblastic cancers. J. Clin. Endocrinol. Metab., *32*:94–101, 1971.

42. Way, S.: Carcinoma of the vulva. *In* Deeley, T. J. (ed.), Modern Radiotherapy: *Gynaecologic Cancer.* Butterworths, 1971, pp. 203–213.

43. Franklin, E. W., III: Prognostic factors in epidermoid carcinoma of the vulva. Obstet. Gynecol., *37*:892–901, 1971.

44. Goperud, D. R.: Carcinoma of the vulva. Am. J. Obstet. Gynecol., *100*:550–553, 1968.

45. Hsu, C. T., Cheng, Y. S., and Su, S. C.: Prognosis of uterine cervical cancer with extensive lymph node metastases. Am. J. Obstet. Gynecol., *114*:954–962, 1972.

46. Kagan, A. R.: Adenocarcinoma of the uterine cervix. Am. J. Obstet. Gynecol., *117*:464–468, 1973.

47. Gusberg, S. B., Yannopoulos, K., and Cohen, C. J.: Virulence indices and lymph nodes in cancer of the cervix. Am. J. Roentgenol. Radium Ther. Nucl. Med., *111*:273–277, 1971.

48. Pilleron, J. P., Durand, J. C., and Lenoble, J. C.: Carcinoma of the uterine cervix, stage I and II, treated by radiation therapy and extensive surgery (1000 cases). Cancer, *29*:593–596, 1972.

49. Nelson, J. H.: Uterine cervix. *In* Holland, J. F., and Frei, E. (eds.), Philadelphia, Lea & Febiger, 1973, pp. 1733–1742.

50. Keller, D., Kempson, R. L., Levine, G., et al.:

Management of the patient with early endometrial carcinoma. Cancer, 33:1108–1116, 1974.

51. Caruso, P. A., Marsh, M. R., Minkowitz, S., et al.:
An intense clinicopathologic study of 305
teratomas of the ovary. Cancer, 27:343–348,
1971.

52. Rogers, L. W., Julian, C. G., and Woodruff, J. D.:
Mesonephroid carcinoma of the ovary: A study
of 95 cases from the Emil Novak Ovarian
Tumor Registry. Gynecol. Oncol. 1:76–89, 1972.

53. Frick, H. C.: The place for hysterectomy. J.A.M.A.,
193:119, 1965.

54. Uckmakli, A., and Bonney, W.: Exploratory laparotomy as routine pretreatment investigation in cancer of the cervix. Radiology, 104:371–377,
1972.

55. Piver, M. S., Wallace, S., and Castro, J. R.: The accuracy of lymphangiography in carcinoma of
the uterine cervix. Am. J. Roentgenol. Radium
Ther. Nucl. Med., 111:278–283, 1971.

56. Van Nagell, J., Roddick, J. W., and Lowin, D. M.:
The staging of cervical cancer: Inevitable dis-
crepancies between clinical staging and
pathologic findings. Am. J. Obstet. Gynecol.,
110:973–978, 1971.

57. Easson, E.: Cancer of the Uterine Cervix. Philadelphia, W. B. Saunders, 1973.

58. Parker, R. T.: Radical hysterectomy and pelvic
lymphadenectomy, with and without preoperative radiotherapy for cervical cancer.
Am. J. Obstet. Gynecol., 99:933–943, 1967.

59. Krieger, J. S., and Embree, H. K.: Pelvic exenteration. Cleve. Clin. Q., 36:1–8, 1969.

60. Ketcham, A. S., Deckers, P. J., Sugarbaker, E. V.,
et al.: Pelvic exenteration for carcinoma of the
uterine cervix: A fifteen year experience.
Cancer, 26:513–521, 1970.

61. Hammond, C. B., Borchert, L. G., Tyrey, L., et al.:
Treatment of metastatic trophoblastic disease:
Good and poor prognosis groups. Am. J.
Obstet. Gynecol., 115:451–457, 1973.

62. Brace, K.: The role of irradiation in the treatment
of metastatic trophoblastic disease. Radiology,
91:540–544, 1968.

63. Perez, C. A., Arneson, A. N., Galakatos, A., et al.:
Malignant tumors of the vagina. Cancer, 31:
36–44, 1973.

64. Campos, J. L.: Mortality trends in carcinoma of
the cervix uteri. J. Chronic Dis., 24:701–709,
1971.

65. Kurohara, S. I.: Post-irradiational recurrent epidermoid carcinoma of the uterine cervix.
Am. J. Roentgenol. Radium. Ther. Nucl. Med.,
3:249–259, 1971.

66. Creasman, W. T., Rutledge, F.: Preoperative evaluation of patients with recurrent carcinoma of
the cervix. Gynecol. Oncol., 1:111–118, 1972.

67. Ketcham, A. S., Hoye, R. C., Taylor, P. T., et al.:
Radical hysterectomy and pelvic lymphaden-
ectomy for carcinoma of the uterine cervix.
Cancer, 28:1272–1277, 1971.

68. Rubin, P.: Cancer of the cervix, stage IV and recurrent carcinoma. J.A.M.A., 194:273, 1965.

69. Paunier, J. P., Delclos, L., and Fletcher, G. H.:
Causes, time of death and sites of failure in
squamous cell carcinoma of the uterine cervix.
Radiology, 88:555–562, 1967.

70. Gray, M. J., and Kottmeier, H. L.: Rectal and bladder injuries following radium therapy for

carcinoma of the cervix at the radiumhemmet.
Am. J. Obstet. Gynecol., 74:1294, 1957.

71. Reddi, P. R., Nussbaum, H., Wollin, M., et al.:
Treatment of carcinomas of the uteri with
special reference to radium system. Obstet.
Gynecol., 43:238–247, 1974.

72. Covington, E.: Pitfalls in liver photoscans. Am. J.
Roentgenol. Radium Ther. Nucl. Med., 109:
745–748, 1970.

73. Jones, T. E.: Benign Stricture of the intestine due
to irradiation. Surg. Clin. North Am., 19:
1185–1194, 1939.

74. Mason, G. R., Guernsey, J. M., and Hanke, G. E.:
Surgical therapy for radiation enteritis. Oncology, 22:241–257, 1968.

75. Warren, S., and Friedman, N. B.: Pathology and
pathologic diagnosis of radiation lesions in
the gastrointestinal tract. Am. J. Pathol., 18:
499–513, 1942.

76. Wiley, H. M., and Sugarbaker, E. P.: Roentgenographic changes in the small intestine, surgical aspects. Cancer, 3:629–640, 1950.

77. Averette, H., LeMaire, W., and LePage, J.: Lymphography, arteriography and venography in
gynecologic cancer. Clin. Obstet. Gynecol.,
12:372–397, 1969.

78. Stevens, M.: The female reproductive system. In
Atlas of Tumor Radiology. Chicago, Year Book
Medical Publishers, 1971.

79. Azoury, R. S.: Primary ovarian sarcoma: Report
of 43 cases from the Emil Novak Ovarian Tumor Registry. Obstet. Gynecol., 37:920–941,
1971.

80. Herman, P. G., et al.: A physiologic approach to
lymph flow in lymphography. Am. J. Roentgenol. Radium Ther. Nucl. Med., 91:1207–1215,
1964.

81. Meschan, I.: Roentgen Signs in Clinical Practice.
Philadelphia, W. B. Saunders, 1966.

82. Patricio, M. B., Baptista, A. M.: Renographic
analysis in radiation therapy of cancer of the
uterus. Acta Radiol. (Ther.), 7:97–107, 1968.

83. Jenkins, D. J.: The radioisotope renogram in carcinoma of the cervix. 44:441–444, 1971.

84. Viamonte, M., Altman, O., Parks, R., et al.: Radi-
ographic-pathologic correlation in the interpretation of lymphangioadenograms. Radiology, 80:903–916, 1963.

85. Baum, S., Bron, K. M., Wexler, L., et al.: Lymphangiography, cavography and urography. Radiology, 81:207–218, 1963.

86. Johnsrude, I. S.: Refresher course in lymphography.
Chicago, Radiologic Society of North America
Meeting, Nov. 29, 1971.

87. Fischer, H. W.: Interpretation of normal and abnormal lymphograms. Cancer Chemother.
Rep., 52:119–123, 1968.

88. Wallace, S., and Jackson, L.: Diagnostic criteria
for lymphangiographic interpretation of
malignant neoplasia. Cancer Chemother.
Rep., 52:125–145, 1968.

89. Abrams, H. L., Takahashi, M., and Adams, D.:
Usefulness and accuracy of lymphangiography
in lymphoma. Cancer Chemother. Rep., 52:
157–170, 1968.

90. Viamonte, Manuel: Interpretation of lymphangiograms. Cancer Chemother. Rep., 52:147–155.

91. Piver, M. S., Wallace, S., and Castro, J. R.: The
accuracy of lymphangiography in carcinoma

of the uterine cervix. Am. J. Roentgenol. Radium Ther. Nucl. Med., *111*:273–283, 1971.

92. Averette, H. E.: Exploratory celiotomy for surgical staging of cervical cancer. Am. J. Obstet. Gynecol., *113*:1090–1096, 1972.

93. Helander, C. G., and Lindbom, A.: Retrograde pelvic venography. Acta Radiol., *51*:401–414, 1959.

94. Lang, E. K., and Greer, J.: The value of pelvic arteriography for the staging of carcinoma of the cervix. Radiology, *92*:1027–1034, 1969.

95. Hagen, S., and Bjorn-Hansch, R.: Lymphography in the treatment of carcinoma of the vulva. Acta Radiol., *2*:609–618, 1971.

96. Lee, K. F., Greening, R., Kramer, S., et al.: The value of pelvic venography and lymphography in the clinical staging of carcinoma of the uterine cervix: Analysis of 105 proven cases. Am. J. Roentgenol. Radium Ther. Nucl. Med., *111*:284–296, 1971.

97. Doppman, J. L., and Chretien, P.: Visceral pelvic venography in carcinoma of the cervix. Radiology, *98*:405–418, 1971.

98. Petty, W. M., Teaford, A. K., Park, R. C., et al.: Angiographic evaluation of early carcinoma of the cervix. Gynecol. Oncol., *1*:211–219, 1973.

99. Piver, M. S., and Barlow, J. J.: Para-aortic lymphadenectomy, aortic node biopsy and aortic lymphangiography in staging patients with advanced cervical cancer. Cancer, *32*:367–370, 1973.

100. Thompson, H. E.: Ultrasonic diagnostic procedures in obstetrics and gynecology. J. Clin. Ultrasound, *1*:160–171, 1973.

101. Schaffer, B., Koehler, P. R., Daniel, C. R., et al.: A critical evaluation of lymphangiography. Radiology, *80*:917–930, 1963.

102. Tow, S. H.: The pulmonary lesion in chorion carcinoma. (Symposium of Chorion Carcinoma.) Proc. R. S. Med., *60*:239–240, 1967.

Chapter Thirteen

BREAST

RICHARD H. GOLD, M.D.

It is a cruel paradox that while the breast is the female organ most accessible to palpation, half of breast carcinomas go undetected and hence untreated until they have already undergone regional or disseminated metastasis. Cancer of the breast may be curable when the lower axillary nodes contain microscopic metastasis; yet it remains the leading cause of cancer deaths in American women. The average diameter of a mammary carcinoma that has been accidentally discovered by the patient is 3.5 cm; a tumor of this size is accompanied by axillary lymph node metastases in 65 per cent of cases and is associated with a five-year survival rate of only 50 per cent. Smaller carcinomas are less frequently accompanied by axillary lymph node metastases, and in the absence of node metastases a five-year survival rate greater than 80 per cent may be attained.

Physicians are able to palpate a centrally located (deep) breast mass as small as 1 cm in diameter, but mammography (radiography of the breast), utilizing film or xeroradiographic images, can disclose the presence of an even smaller carcinoma—a lesion not yet symptomatic or palpable, still localized, and hence potentially curable.

Mammography performed in combination with physical examination promises to become a major factor in decreasing the number of deaths caused by cancer of the breast. In a group of 20,000 women screened by both methods for the Health Insurance Plan of Greater New York, there were one-third less deaths from breast cancer over a

five-year follow-up period than there were in another group of women screened by physical examination alone.[1] One third (44 of 132) of the cancers detected in the combined screening program were discovered by mammography after the physical examination had revealed no tumor. Only one of these 44 women with nonpalpable, asymptomatic tumors died of breast cancer during the five-year follow-up period. Preliminary data from the Breast Cancer Screening Demonstration Program sponsored jointly by the American Cancer Society and the National Cancer Institute imply that a combination of mammography and physical examination will yield at least 10 patients with mammary carcinomas per 1,000 asymptomatic women screened, and that 75 per cent of these patients will have axillary lymph nodes that are free of tumor.[2]

Some drawbacks of past mammographic screening surveys have been: (1) their relatively great expense, especially in relationship to the low yield of cancers detected; (2) the reluctance of surgeons to perform a biopsy of a radiographically suspicious lesion in the absence of a mass; and (3) the difficulty of detecting cancer in breasts that contain little fat. When screening programs are undertaken through a team approach encompassing the radiologist, surgeon, and pathologist, and when mammography is combined directly with physical examination, the cancer detection rate rises.[3] Survey mammography for the detection of nonpalpable, asymptomatic cancer produces the greatest yield in identified high-risk

263

groups: women who have, or have had, cancer in the contralateral breast, women with a history of breast cancer on the maternal side of the family, and women who have papillomatosis or atypical intraductal hyperplasia (diagnosed by a previous biopsy).

MAMMOGRAPHY

Indications for Mammography

Of the many indications for mammography, two are outstanding. It should be part of the preoperative evaluation of any woman over 35 years of age who is slated to undergo breast surgery for a mass of unknown etiology. In that particular situation, mammography is indicated not so much for examination of the clinically obvious lesion that is soon to receive a definitive evaluation by the pathologist, but rather to evaluate fully both breasts for signs of cancer. If ominous findings are detected through mammography in an area other than the area scheduled to undergo biopsy, a specimen of the radiographically suspicious area could be taken along with one of the clinically obvious lesion. This indication for mammography is valid whether the clinically obvious lesion is thought to be benign or malignant. The case for a mammogram becomes even stronger if the known lesion is suspected to be malignant, since carcinoma occurs bilaterally and simultaneously in at least 10 per cent of cases. The second outstanding indication for mammography is in the serial evaluation of a woman with a past history of breast cancer.[4] The chance of a carcinoma arising eventually in her contralateral breast is many times greater than that of breast carcinoma occurring in the general population of women. Annual (or biannual) mammographic examinations of women in high-risk groups permit serial comparisons, which favor the detection of subtle changes signifying early cancer.

The Mammographic Examination

The mammographic examination ideally is combined with: (1) an interview of the patient in which a detailed history relating to breast disease is obtained, and (2) a thorough physical examination of the breasts and axillae in the manner described by Haagensen.[5] Clinical examination alone or mammography alone will permit detection of only about half the cancers that can be discovered through the use of both modalities in combination. Just as mammography cannot replace a thorough physical examination, the physical examination cannot replace mammography. Moreover, a negative mammogram *or* a negative physical examination should never deter the performance of a biopsy on a suspicious lesion that has been detected by either method. Unfortunately, mammography cannot be relied upon always to differentiate benign from malignant disease. Thus, we urge biopsy (or cyst aspiration) of all *solitary* masses regardless of their mammographic appearance. If an apparent cyst cannot be aspirated, biopsy of the mass should be performed. Biopsy is especially important in women over 60 years of age, because in that age group twice as many solitary breast lesions are malignant as are benign.[6]

The mammographic examination includes mediolateral, cephalocaudal, and sometimes axillary views of both breasts. The mediolateral and cephalocaudal views, being at right angles to each other, permit the mammographer to make a three-dimensional assessment that allows suspicious lesions to be localized not only by breast quadrant, but also by their "clock-face" location and relative depth. The axillary view is not obtained routinely because it results in more radiation exposure to the skin than the other views and seldom provides information about the lymph nodes that is not readily obtainable through clinical palpation. Lymph node metastases arising from mammary carcinoma rarely exhibit the tell tale radiographic evidence of "malignant" calcifications (see the section on calcifications). Furthermore, the apparent size of axillary lymph nodes displayed radiographically is a poor measure of metastatic involvement; small nodes may harbor metastases while large ones may be free of tumor. The presence of indurated or fixed axillary lymph nodes, as felt by the hand of the examiner, is far more conclusive evidence of metastasis than the radiographic image of nodes in the axillary view.

MAMMOGRAPHIC ANATOMY

The breast is composed of 8 to 12 lobes of glandular tissue located between superficial and deep layers of the superficial fascia. Each lobe drains through a separate duct, the orifice of which is in the nipple. The lobules and lobes of glandular tissue are separated from each other by thin sheaths of fibrous connective tissue. Once the glandular tissue has atrophied or has undergone transformation into fat with advancing age or childbearing, the connective tissue sheaths can be seen end-on in mammograms (Fig. 13–1). However, in contradistinction to the relatively radiolucent (fatty) breasts of older women, those of adolescents have an almost homogeneous, exaggerated radiopacity, because they contain only a small amount of fat in relation to the glandular tissue.

Breast tissue is normally distributed in a pattern that is bilaterally symmetric on mammograms (Fig. 13–2). Asymmetry of the breast patterns may result from dysplasia (fibrocystic disease), prior surgical excision, or, most important, deposition of fibrous connective tissue in response to a carcinoma (Figs. 13–3 and 13–4). Cooper's ligaments are peripheral, toothlike projections of breast tissue within fibrous processes that extend from the skin to the superficial layer of superficial fascia (Fig. 13–1). Cooper's ligaments, also called the breast suspensory ligaments, are important because carcinoma may evoke fibrosis in their vicinity, causing them to shorten. This condition is the usual basis for skin retraction associated with an underlying carcinoma. Similarly, elaboration of fibrous tissue by the breast in response to an underlying carcinoma may thicken the walls of the ducts, increasing their prominence on mammograms (Fig. 13–5) and eventually causing them to shorten, with resultant nipple retraction.

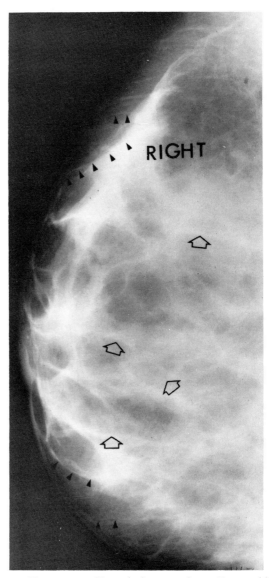

Figure 13–1 Normal breast of a 43-year-old woman, para 2, showing Cooper's ligaments (arrowheads) and interlobar connective tissue sheaths (open arrows). Much of the radiopaque glandular tissue has atrophied, having been replaced by fat. The capability of mammography to record the shadow of a carcinoma or any other breast lesion is largely dependent upon the presence of sufficient fat to serve as a contrasting radiolucent background.

CALCIFICATIONS

A circumscribed cluster of numerous tiny, finely stippled, angular, lacy, or branching calcifications on a mammogram is characteristic, but not absolutely diagnostic, of a malignancy (Figs. 13–5 and 13–6). Unfortunately, cancer of the breast exhibits mammographic evidence of such calcifications in no more than one half of cases. Moreover, a commonly occurring benign disorder—sclerosing adenosis—may also manifest finely stippled calcifications (Fig. 13–7), although the tiny "benign" calcifications are usually rounder in shape, and tend to be fewer in number and more scat-

Text continued on page 269.

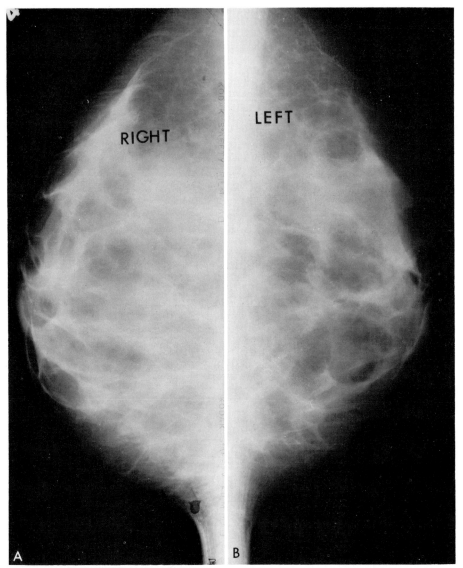

Figure 13–2 Normal right (*A*) and left (*B*) breasts, (same case as illustrated in Figure 13–1). Mammograms reveal a normal, bilaterally symmetric tissue pattern.

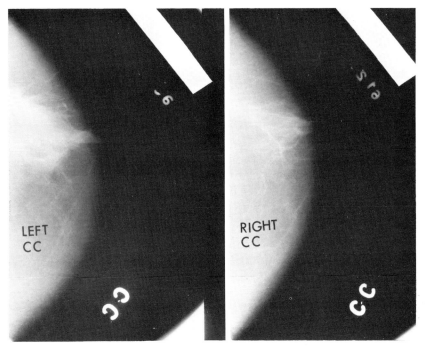

Figure 13–3 Carcinoma, left. Direct comparison between the right and the left breasts of a woman, aged 63, reveals *asymmetry* of the tissue pattern. Increased prominence of the stroma of the left breast reflects fibrous tissue proliferation incited by an underlying carcinoma. Asymmetrical prominence of ducts or stroma should provoke a careful search for an underlying malignancy.

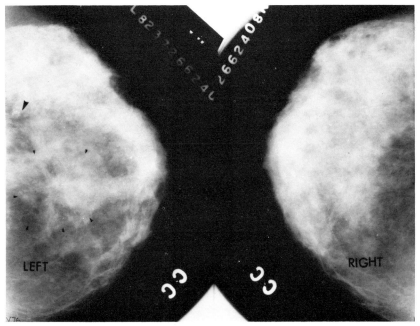

Figure 13–4 Nonpalpable carcinoma, left, in an asymptomatic woman. Views of both breasts reveal diffuse nodularity, signifying mammary dysplasia. An area of duct prominence and fibrillary, fibrous tissue proliferation on the left (encircled by small arrowheads) results from a carcinoma. A 5 mm cluster of tiny calcifications (large arrowhead), although suspicious for carcinoma, was actually in an area of sclerosing adenosis.

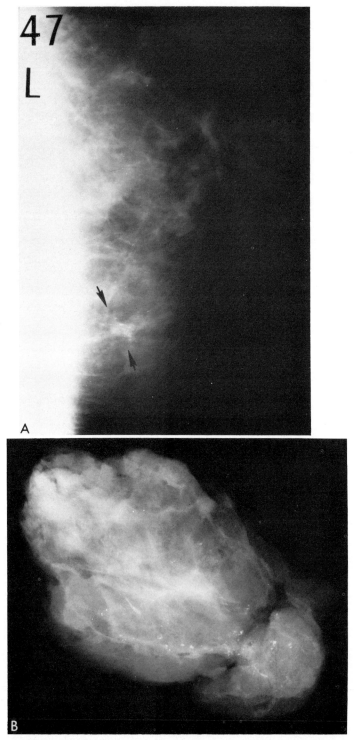

Figure 13–5 Carcinoma *in situ*, in a woman aged 47. *A*, This asymptomatic, nonpalpable lesion was found in preoperative mammograms prior to the planned excision of a benign lesion of the contralateral breast. The stippled calcifications (arrows) and the prominent duct that bisects the calcifications are both highly suspicious signs of malignancy. *B*, A radiograph of the surgical specimen confirmed that the suspicious lesion had indeed been biopsied. Some of the calcifications in the specimen assume a characteristic branching pattern as they follow the course of small ducts.

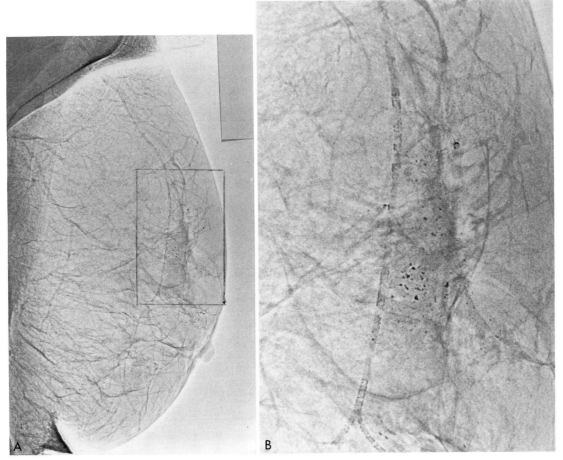

Figure 13–6 Carcinoma, signified by tiny, angular calcifications and mild distortion of breast architecture. *Xeroradiograph* (*A*) and close-up view of enclosed area (*B*) reveal the calcifications in greater detail, as well as an adjacent artery (vertical) containing two broken parallel lines of calcium in its wall. (Courtesy of John Wolfe, M. D.)

tered in distribution than the calcifications of carcinoma. Intraductal papillomas may contain a rosette pattern of several small, coarse calcifications that may at times mimic those of malignancy. Scattered, ring-shaped, or coarse linear calcifications reflect secretory disease, a very common benign disorder, also termed duct ectasia because the observed calcifications are located in dilated segments of ducts (Fig. 13–8). Fibroadenoma, the most common solid benign tumor of the breast, may hyalinize and calcify with advancing maturity; the calcifications are usually large and amorphous, and may replace the tumor completely (Fig. 13–9). Calcified arteries in the breast appear as broken parallel lines of calcium (Fig. 13–6 *B*).

All suspicious clusters of punctate calcifications on mammography deserve an excision biopsy, with the expectation that in many cases they will be found to result not from a malignancy but from benign disease—usually sclerosing adenosis. Similarly, localized duct prominence and other alterations of breast architecture on the mammogram that could possibly signify a desmoplastic reaction require biopsy. Until recently, resection of a quadrant of the breast was frequently necessary. To reduce the size of the specimen of tissue that must be removed for the biopsy and to improve the accuracy of localization of suspicious findings, percutaneous localization with a long 25-gauge needle may be

Text continued on page 272.

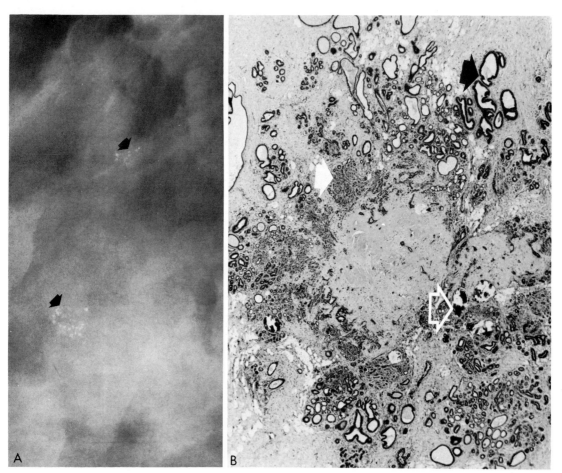

Figure 13–7 Sclerosing adenosis. *A,* Close-up view of a mammogram reveals two clusters of punctate calcifications (arrows) that resemble those of malignancy. Biopsy with specimen radiography is frequently required to exclude carcinoma (see text). *B,* Histologic section revealed lobules (closed white arrow) that are distorted by dense fibrous connective tissue surrounding a large, central, hyalinized scar. Intraductal calcification (appearing black) is localized by open arrow. Dilated ducts lined by hyperplastic epithelium are signified by the black arrow (hematoxylin and eosin stain, × 4). (From Gold, R. H., Montgomery, C. K., and Rambo, O. N.: Significance of margination of benign and malignant infiltrative mammary lesions: Roentgenographic-pathologic correlation. Am. J. Roentgenol. Radium Ther. Nucl. Med., *118:* 881–894, 1973.)

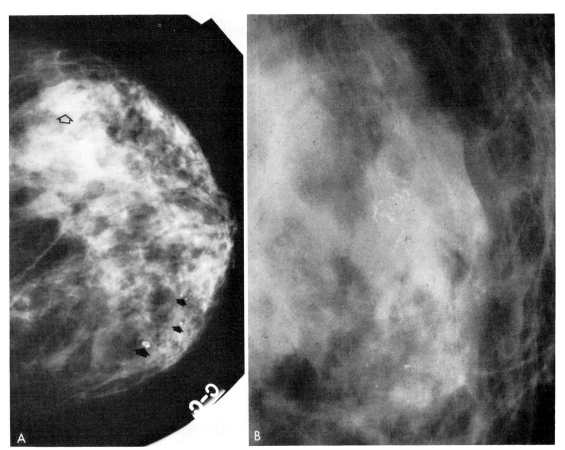

Figure 13–8 Benign ring-shaped calcifications (lower solid arrows) reflecting benign secretory disease (duct ectasia) and delicate, lacy, branching calcifications (upper open arrow) consistent with carcinoma. *A*, Mammogram. *B*, Close-up view of the upper cluster of malignant calcifications.

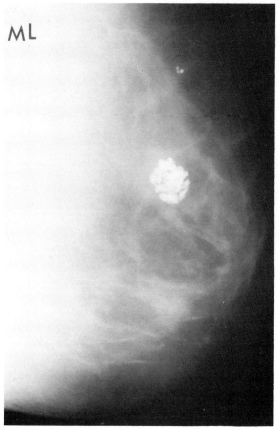

Figure 13–9 Calcified fibroadenoma. The entire tumor has become hyalinized, and the resultant calcification is characteristically coarse and amorphous.

performed just prior to surgery.[7] This is done by estimating the position of the suspicious area from its appearance in cephalocaudal and mediolateral views and then directing the needle tip toward it. The needle is inserted all the way to its hub. Repeat mammograms are then obtained with the needle in place. If the needle is in or near the suspicious area, it is taped securely in place to serve as a landmark for the surgeon. Alternatively, a drop of methylene blue may be injected near the lesion, and the needle then withdrawn, the dye acting as a surgical landmark.

SPECIMEN RADIOGRAPHY

Breast biopsy is followed by specimen radiography. Should the mammograms be the sole preoperative evidence for a malignancy, it is necessary for a radiograph to be made of the surgical specimen to confirm that the suspicious area has indeed been excised (Fig. 13–10). If radiographs of the specimen fail to reproduce the suspicious mammographic findings (i.e., calcifications), excision of additional tissue followed by radiography is required until the findings finally are corroborated. The patient therefore remains on the operating table until the specimen has been radiographed and the radiograph processed and reviewed. The surgeon is notified by the mammographer as to the presence or absence of the previously identified findings within the specimen. Only permanent histologic sections should be relied upon for diagnosis of tumors less than 0.5 cm in diameter. The histopathologic differentiation of *in situ* lobular or ductal *microinvasive* carcinoma from atypical epithelial hyperplasia demands proper fixation and cellular detail. These minimal carcinomas could conceivably limit the extent of surgery required. It is obvious that the surgeon, the mammographer, and the pathologist must cooperate in this team effort.[8, 9]

The final diagnosis is always based upon permanent histologic sections obtained primarily from the site or sites of suspicious calcifications, localized within the specimen by the mammographer in the following manner. Following the analysis of a frozen section of a small lesion that has the gross consistency of malignancy, the remaining excised tissue is cut into slices by the pathologist, the slices are numbered, and once again a radiograph is made (Fig. 13–10 C and D). The mammographer identifies for the pathologist the radiographically suspicious region within each slice that is likely to provide the most fruitful area for permanent histologic sections. The permanent sections are processed and examined within 24 to 36 hours. If additional surgery is necessary, it may then be undertaken after further consultation with the patient and with added confidence in the diagnosis.

OBSTACLES TO MAMMOGRAPHIC DETECTION OF CANCER

The capability of mammography to outline the actual shadow of a carcinoma, prominent ducts, alterations in architec-

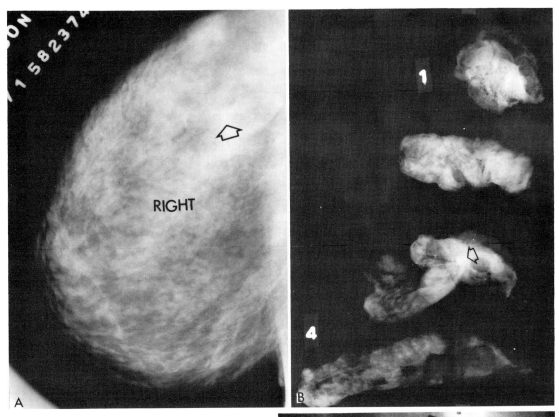

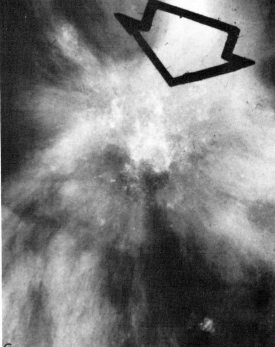

Figure 13–10 Carcinoma. *A,* In the mammogram, faint area of fibrillary desmoplastic reaction (arrow) and associated calcifications (too faint to reproduce) signify a carcinoma. The lesion was occult clinically, possibly because of diffuse nodularity throughout the breast reflecting mammary dysplasia. The resulting nodular radiopacity may also easily mask a malignancy in mammograms. Subsequent radiography of the operative specimen revealed that the suspicious area had been excised. The specimen was then cut into slices by the pathologist and re-radiographed. *B,* "Bread-loaf" slices: The mammographer can now alert the pathologist to the area (arrow) in each slice that is likely to provide the most rewarding tissue for permanent histologic sections. *C,* Close-up view of calcifications and fibrillary reaction in specimen from *B.* The calcifications are tiny and are so numerous that they appear confluent centrally.

ture, or in fact any lesion is largely dependent upon the presence of sufficient fat in the breast to serve as a contrasting radiolucent background. Mammography may detect an obvious carcinoma only a few millimeters in diameter in an atrophied breast in which all glandular tissue has been replaced by fat. On the other hand, breasts that are packed with dense glandular tissue, such as those of young, nulliparous, pregnant, or lactating women, and breasts manifesting severe mammary dysplasia may contain a large carcinoma that is completely masked by the dense tissue that surrounds it (Fig. 13–11).

Mammary dysplasia (fibrocystic disease) probably results from an exaggeration and distortion of changes that normally occur during the menstrual cycle. For some reason, in the dysplastic breast monthly involution of these changes cannot keep pace with cyclic breast tissue proliferation. At least four histologic patterns occur with so much overlap that it is usually impossible to detect one pattern in the absence of the others: (1) adenosis (lobular hyperplasia), (2) cysts (resulting from duct dilation), (3) fibrosis of stroma, and (4) intraductal epithelial hyperplasia.

Pregnancy and lactation result in excessive proliferation of glandular tissue and a corresponding increase in radiographic density. Since the increased density may mask underlying pathology, mammography during pregnancy or lactation should be considered as being of limited value. While

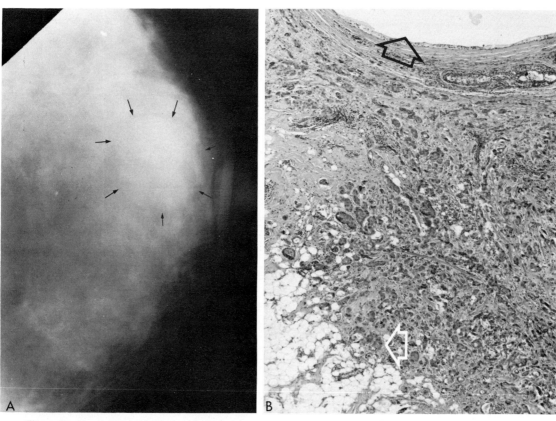

Figure 13–11 *A,* Breast packed with dense mammary dysplastic tissue containing a 2 cm benign cyst (arrows) and a carcinoma that is completely masked in the mammogram by dysplastic tissue. The lack of fat in such breasts leads to extreme difficulty in detecting carcinomas. *B,* Histologic section. Macrocyst formation (open black arrow) and duct ectasia coexist with cords and nests of carcinoma cells (open white arrow) infiltrating the mammary fat (hematoxylin and eosin stain, × 40). (From Gold, R. H., Montgomery, C. K., and Rambo, O. N.: Significance of margination of benign and malignant infiltrative mammary lesions: Roentgenographic-pathological correlation. Am. J. Roentgenol. Radium Ther. Nucl. Med., *118:*881–894, 1973.)

this limitation must be appreciated, *any* rapidly enlarging mass during pregnancy or lactation is an indication for mammography. The low-energy mammography x-ray beam is largely absorbed by the breast and film holder and, when well-coned, does not affect the abdomen.

MAMMOGRAPHIC FEATURES OF CANCER

Mammographic signs of possible *early* cancer (asymptomatic, localized in the breast, nonpalpable, and without clinical signs) include a circumscribed cluster of stippled calcifications, a segmental prominence of one or more ducts, and a localized distortion of breast architecture (Figs. 13–4, 13–5, and 13–6).[10] Any or all of these signs may become manifest in the absence of any mammographic evidence of a mass, which usually signifies that the local disease is more advanced. As stated, the peculiar

calcifications characterizing malignancy tend to be clustered, numerous, finely stippled, and angular, lacy, or branching (Figs. 13–5 and 13–6), and the localized prominence of ducts and distortion of breast architecture result primarily from the deposition of reactive fibrous tissue within the duct walls and surrounding stroma (Figs. 13–3, 13–4, and 13–5).

Carcinoma, while tending initially to grow slowly and occasionally to remain intraductal (noninvasive or *in situ*) for years (Fig. 13–5), eventually invades the ductal basement membrane. After the breast stroma is invaded, the velocity of tumor growth tends to increase. The vast majority of these tumors are designated simply as *infiltrating duct carcinomas* and are also known as *scirrhous carcinomas* because of the prominent desmoplastic reaction that they incite. The resulting fibrosis creates a characteristic rock-hard induration clinically.

The key mammographic feature dis-

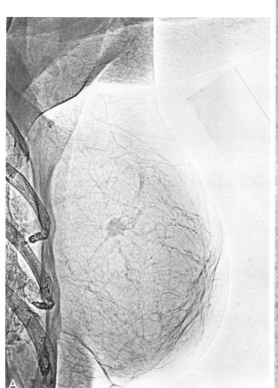 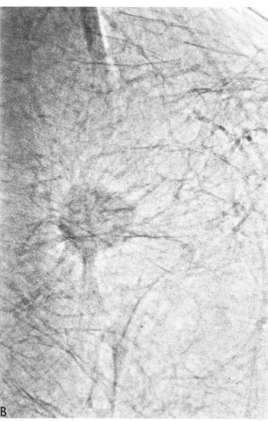

Figure 13–12   Typical irregular margin of infiltrating (scirrhous) duct carcinoma. *A,* Xeroradiograph. *B,* Close-up view discloses peripheral tendrils of fibrous tissue radiating into the surrounding fat. (Courtesy of John Wolfe, M. D.)

tinguishing a carcinoma that is large enough to form a mass from most benign breast masses is the irregular margin of the carcinoma (Figs. 13–12 and 13–13).[11] This irregularity reflects aggressive local infiltration of the carcinoma into the surrounding tissue. The majority of mass-forming carcinomas are highly infiltrative pathologically and appear so mammographically (Fig. 13–13). Even cancers that infiltrate the breast only slightly, typically appear irregular or indistinct in outline on a mammogram (Fig. 13–14). A high degree of correlation exists between the mammographic and pathologic appearances of the carcinoma margins.[12–14] Axillary lymph node metastasis occurs more frequently with carcinomas that appear highly infiltrative on mammograms.[15] Highly infiltrative carcinomas (Fig. 13–13) incite a striking desmoplastic reaction and also correspond to the

"irregular" carcinomas described by Lane and associates,[16] to the "scirrhous" type described by Ingleby and Gershon-Cohen,[13] and to the "stellate growth pattern" reported by Gallager and Martin.[14] Gross examination of cross-sections of these tumors reveals a firm, white, gritty mass of irregular contour, with tendrils radiating into the surrounding tissue. Microscopic examination discloses nests and cords of tumor cells encased within, and infiltrating together with, the fibrous stroma into the adjacent breast tissue. Minimally infiltrative carcinomas (Fig. 13–14) correspond to the "well-delimited" tumor type described by Lane and associates,[16] the "circumscribed" type described by Ingleby and Gershon-Cohen,[13] and to the "knobby growth pattern" reported by Gallager and Martin.[14] Minimally infiltrative carcinomas macroscopically tend to appear more circumscribed, microscopically are

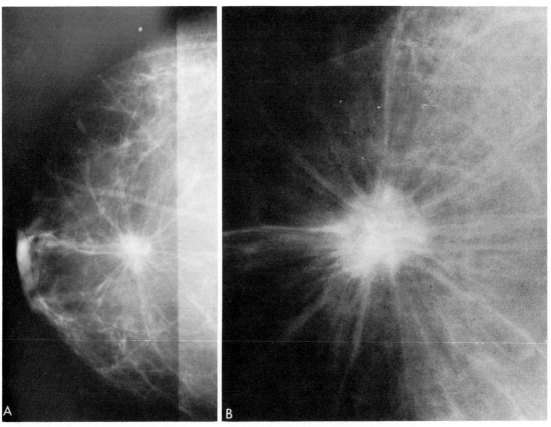

Figure 13–13 *A,* Highly infiltrative carcinoma characterized mammographically by spiculation over its entire periphery and prominent ducts between tumor and nipple. *B,* Close-up view.

more cellular, and are less desmoplastic than highly infiltrative carcinomas. While highly infiltrative carcinomas tend upon palpation to feel larger than their observed dimensions in the mammographic image, minimally infiltrative carcinomas, because they incite less desmoplastic reaction, tend to feel the same size by palpation as they appear in mammograms.

Lobular carcinoma, a less common type of breast cancer, may be noninvasive or invasive and is difficult to detect mammographically. *Comedocarcinoma* forms solid plugs of tumor cells (in ducts), which frequently calcify. Comedocarcinoma may be invasive, or it may extend throughout much of the duct system and still remain entirely intraductal (noninvasive).

In contrast to the infiltrative character of most carcinomas, the great majority of discrete benign masses — cysts and fibroadenomas — appear pathologically, and hence mammographically, to be sharply circumscribed (Fig. 13–15). On occasion, however, a carcinoma may be so well circumscribed that it resembles a benign lesion, both clinically and mammographically. It is therefore prudent to perform excision biopsy (or to attempt cyst aspiration) of all solitary masses in women who are at risk for cancer, regardless of the mammographic features. Examples of these uncommon well-circumscribed carcinomas include *medullary carcinoma* (a cellular tumor that grows slowly, manifests a lymphocytic response, infiltrates minimally, and is frequently associated with a favorable prognosis, even when large) and *colloid (mucinous) carcinoma* (also slowly growing, with a relatively favorable prognosis).

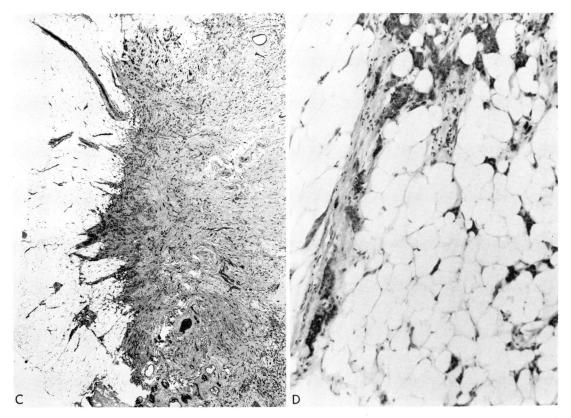

C   D

Figure 13–13 *Continued   C,* Histologic section shows strikingly irregular boundary between the carcinoma and the surrounding fat (hematoxylin and eosin stain, × 10). *D,* Higher magnification reveals infiltration of the mammary fat by small nests of tumor cells accompanying the fibrous tendrils (hematoxylin and eosin stain, × 40). (From Gold, R. H., Montgomery, C. K., and Rambo, O. N.: Significance of margination of benign and malignant infiltrative mammary lesions: Roentgenographic-pathological correlation. Am. J. Roentgenol. Radium Ther. Nucl. Med., *118*:881–894, 1973.)

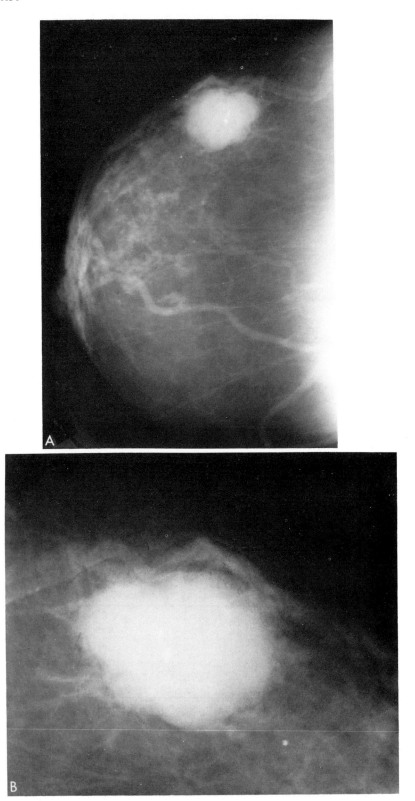

Figure 13–14 Slightly infiltrative carcinoma characterized by an irregular margin without spiculation. *A,* Mammogram. The flecks of calcium within the tumor are *atypical* of malignancy because of their paucity and their coarse nature (relatively large size). Unilateral venous prominence, as seen here, may be associated with carcinoma but is frequently a normal variation. *B,* Close-up view.

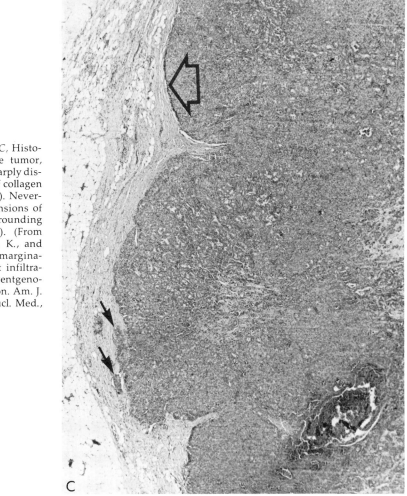

Figure 13–14 *Continued C,* Histologic section reveals that the tumor, along much of its margin, is sharply dissociated from the thin layer of collagen that surrounds it (open arrow). Nevertheless, small finger-like extensions of tumor extend into the surrounding fibrous tissue (small arrows). (From Gold, R. H., Montgomery, C. K., and Rambo, O. N.: Significance of margination of benign and malignant infiltrative mammary lesions: Roentgenographic-pathological correlation. Am. J. Roentgenol. Radium Ther. Nucl. Med., *118*:881–894, 1973.)

MAMMOGRAPHIC DIFFERENTIAL DIAGNOSIS

Cysts are more common than solid benign lesions and result from localized duct dilatation. Inasmuch as the fluid within the cyst is under tension, the distended cyst wall has a smooth, sharp border (Fig. 13–15). Cysts are usually round or oval, while fibroadenomas may appear lobulated.

Fibroadenoma is the most common solid benign tumor of the breast. A fibroadenoma consists of a hypocellular, fibroblastic stroma containing numerous glandular epithelial clefts. The peak incidence rate for fibroadenoma is in patients less than 25 years of age. A fibroadenoma of the breast may grow rapidly during adolescence, pregnancy,

or the menopause. With advancing age, it may degenerate, undergo hyalinization, and develop coarse calcifications within it (Fig. 13–9).

Cystosarcoma is a rare tumor that bears pathologic similarities to fibroadenoma, except that it has a more cellular stroma. Cystosarcoma grows rapidly and frequently attains large size before the patient seeks the aid of a physician. Although the tumor may invade adjacent normal breast tissue, the invasion tends to be limited in extent, and the tumor rarely undergoes metastasis. Whereas a fibroadenoma may be locally excised, cystosarcoma merits excision of a wide margin of normal breast tissue, sometimes including the nipple. A bulky cystosarcoma may cause pressure necrosis of the

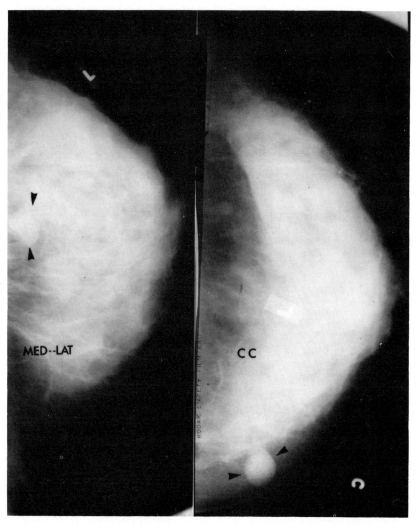

Figure 13–15 Benign mass (cyst) characterized by a smooth, sharp border in mediolateral and cephalocaudal views. The cyst is outlined by the subcutaneous fat into which it projects, as shown on the second view; were it located in the center of this breast, where fat tissue is scant, it would probably go undetected by mammography.

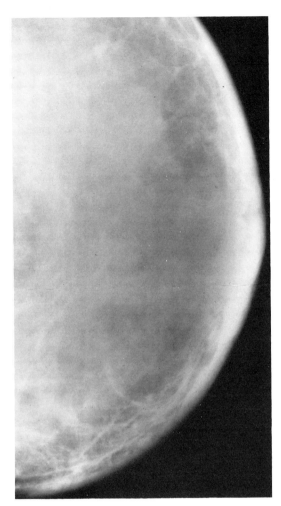

Figure 13–16 Diffuse skin thickening resulting from breast abscess. Although carcinoma with lymphatic permeation must always be considered first among the causes of diffuse skin thickening, the most common benign cause is breast abscess. Edema within the breast masks the underlying pathology, prohibiting a distinction between the two major differential diagnostic possibilities. (From Gold, R. H., Montgomery, C. K., Minagi, H., and Annes, G. P.: The significance of mammary skin thickening in disorders other than mammary carcinoma: A roentgenologic-pathologic correlation. Am. J. Roentgenol. Radium Ther. Nucl. Med., 112:613–621, 1971.)

skin, but the skin usually is not actually invaded by the tumor.

Sclerosing adenosis competes with abscess (see next paragraph) as the most commonly occurring benign disorder of the breast that is apt to be *mis*diagnosed mammographically as malignant.[17] Sclerosing adenosis usually appears in mammograms as an ill-defined, widespread, mottled, and nodular process or, after coalescence of the nodules, as an extensive, homogeneous soft tissue density with indistinct margins.[12, 18] Tiny flecks of calcium (which are usually fewer in number but similar in size to those found in association with an infiltrating carcinoma) may permeate the lesion, resulting in the need for a biopsy to exclude malignancy (Fig. 13–7).

Breast abscess causes diffuse thickening of the skin of the breast, a sign that often signifies lymphatic permeation from an underlying primary carcinoma. Although carcinoma must always be entertained first among the causes of diffuse skin thickening, breast abscess must also be considered and frequently can be excluded only by biopsy. The abscess may be surrounded by intense edema, leading to a mammographic appearance that simulates a carcinoma (Fig. 13–16).

Fat necrosis is a nonsuppurative inflammatory process that occurs most often in the fatty, pendulous breasts of middle-aged women. The disorder may simulate carcinoma clinically and mammographically.[19, 20] Fat necrosis may follow trauma, or it may result from stagnation of the contents of a duct with subsequent erosion of the ductal epithelium and, finally, extrusion of the intraductal debris into the surrounding fat. A similar auto-irritative phenomenon is thought to be the cause of plasma cell mastitis (see next paragraph). The mammographic appearance of fat necrosis is sometimes characterized by a "mass" with irregular margins simulating an infiltrating carcinoma. Thickening and retraction of the overlying skin may even occur, just as it does in association with some carcinomas.[21]

Plasma cell mastitis is yet another benign disorder that may simulate carcinoma clinically and mammographically.[22] Clues to the diagnosis of plasma cell mastitis include a tendency to subareolar location and to bilaterality.[23] Plasma cell mastitis probably results from inflammation of a duct secondary to obstruction by inspissated necrotic material. Extrusion of the material into the periductal stroma leads to a sterile, chronic inflammatory process. The desmoplastic reaction of plasma cell mastitis and the reaction that accompanies infiltrating carcinoma may be remarkably similar. In both disorders this reaction often results in fixation and retraction of the overlying skin and nipple.

OTHER TECHNIQUES FOR DETECTION

Radiographic Techniques

Although conventional mammographic techniques using industrial x-ray film continue to be widely employed in the United States, two recently introduced variations have already gained strong support: *xeroradiography*, which does not require x-ray film and usually employs a tungsten target as the x-ray source, and *low-dose mammography*, which employs x-ray film and one or two high-definition intensifying screens contained within a vacuum cassette to reduce patient exposure, and, ideally, an x-ray tube with a molybdenum target. With both techniques, *compression* of the breast during the radiographic exposure is essential if optimal results are to be achieved. Compression diminishes the thickness of the breast, thus decreasing the amount of scattered radiation with a resulting improvement in image detail. Both xeroradiography and low-dose film mammography result in significantly less exposure to the breast than conventional mammography with industrial film.

Xeroradiography does not make use of film to record an image, but instead employs an electrically charged aluminum plate coated with vitreous selenium, a semiconductor.[24] Upon exposure to x-rays, charges leak from the plate in proportion to the amount of x-rays passing through the breast and striking each portion of the plate. An electrostatic image of the breast is thus recorded upon the charged plate. The image is made visible ("developed") by application to the plate of oppositely charged, blue powder granules. The blue image is then transferred to paper and coated with plastic. Xeroradiography is an advance over conventional film mammography because it provides an image of superior detail. The improvement in image detail is a result of increased concentration of blue powder granules along the edges or boundaries of anatomic (and pathologic) structures—a feature called edge enhancement. This feature of xeroradiography permits an exceptional display of tiny malignant calcifications, mammary ducts, peripheral extensions of a breast cancer, and minor architectural alterations in the breast that could signify cancer. A disadvantage of xeroradiography, in comparison to film mammography, is a relative deficiency in image contrast between large soft tissue areas that have different radiographic densities. (See Figures 13–6 and 13–12.)

Low dose film mammography utilizes one or two high-definition intensifying screens enclosed together with a film in a cassette; the film is sensitive to light emitted by the intensifying screen(s) during the x-ray exposure.[25] The film and screen are held in intimate contact by a vacuum, which diminishes diffusion of the light emitted by the screen. A resulting image of high contrast and excellent detail highlights the differing radiographic densities of fat, fibroglandular tissue, and minute calcifications in the breast. An average exposure requires only a fraction of a second, and is approximately one-eighth the patient exposure dose required for conventional film mammography. The combination of a very short exposure and high film contrast results in a detailed image that reveals the skin as well as internal breast structures with equal clarity. For best results, the low-dose film-screen combination should be employed with a molybdenum tube target as the source of x-rays, and the breast should be compressed during the radiographic exposure.

Ductal cytology with contrast injection mammography has received only preliminary evaluation as an adjunct to ordinary mammography and physical examination for the earlier detection of cancer.[26] When carried to completion these two complementary techniques (breast duct aspiration for cytology, followed by injection of contrast material into individual ducts) require great technical skill and are time consuming. However, in women at high risk for breast cancer, especially those with nodular and radiographically dense breasts that are difficult to evaluate clinically as well as mammographically, duct cytology with contrast injection mammography is a promising diagnostic modality. Initial aspiration of the nipple with a suction device is followed by cytologic examination of the pooled duct secretions. Secretions can be obtained in this way from over 75 per cent of women who have no clinical evidence of breast disease. In the event of *abnormal* cytology in the pooled secretions, selective catheterization of each tiny duct is followed by aspiration to localize the pathologic breast lobe or, should a duct not produce secretions, by duct perfusion with isotonic saline and collection of the individual duct washings for cytologic examination. Radiopaque contrast material is then injected into individual ducts and radiography is performed to outline the actual site of duct pathology within the breast.

Non-Radiographic Techniques

Thermography is a quick, simple, reproducible, noninvasive, and innocuous test that *does not require exposure to ionizing radiation* and that augments the value of mammography and physical examination in the detection of breast cancer.[27] Thermography involves the visual display of infrared emission from the breast; therefore, it depicts minimal temperature variations at the skin surface. The resulting picture or pattern primarily represents the heat of blood in superficial veins. The heat is conveyed to these veins from the deep mammary veins by way of the intermediary subareolar venous plexus. The temperature

of blood in the deep veins of the breast is directly influenced by increased temperature of the tissues in close proximity, including certain benign and malignant lesions.

Because the deeper veins in the breast are thickly insulated by overlying fat and fibroglandular tissue, heat within them can be detected only when it is carried by blood flow to the subareolar venous plexus and the superficial veins. Thus, while a malignant pathologic process located just beneath the skin may, by virtue of direct heat emission, yield an overlying "hot spot" on the thermogram, *no* direct spatial relationship may exist between the site of a deep pathologic process and the resultant increase in subareolar and superficial venous heat in the thermographic image.

Slight asymmetry of the thermographic heat patterns between the right and left breast is the rule rather than the exception. This asymmetry results from the varying distribution and depth of the superficial venous systems of the two breasts. As the depth of the veins increases, so does their insulation from the external infrared detector. Thus, one or more veins located just beneath the skin of one breast will appear warmer than corresponding veins located

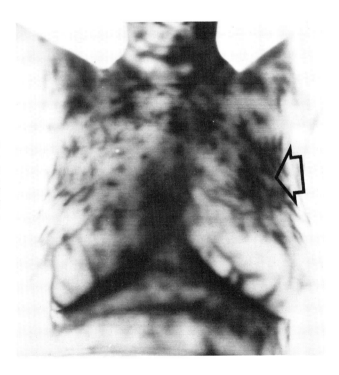

Figure 13–17 Abnormal left thermogram resulting from carcinoma. Dark areas are relatively "hot" and white areas "cold" on this study. The thermogram discloses localized temperature elevation in the upper hemisphere of the left breast. This finding takes the form of "hot" streaks, which follow the course of superficial veins draining the cancerous breast.

slightly deeper in the contralateral breast. The disparity in the depth of the superficial veins undoubtedly accounts for some false-positive thermograms. This pitfall may be avoided by direct observation of the skin of the breasts during physical examination, to determine in which breast the veins appear bluer and, therefore, less deeply situated.

Any (or all) of the following criteria are indicative of a "positive" breast thermogram: (1) a localized homogeneous area of intense heat, called a "hot spot," (2) an abnormally prominent venous heat pattern in one breast, as compared to the other breast, or (3) a *diffuse* increase in heat in one breast as compared to the other.

The major shortcomings of thermography are its acknowledged deficiencies in diagnostic specificity and sensitivity. A "positive" thermogram may reflect benign *or* malignant disease. Up to 50 per cent of thermograms that appear abnormal occur in the absence of a carcinoma. On the other hand, false-negative thermograms (thermograms that are negative in the presence of carcinoma) occur in up to 40 per cent of cases of non-palpable breast cancers. At the present time the consensus is that, if thermography is to be used at all, it should definitely be utilized only *in combination with* mammography and physical examination. The three procedures are complementary to each other and are not competitive. It is our opinion that a woman with a positive thermogram, in combination with negative physical and mammographic examinations, should be re-examined by thermography and physical examination after six months. In the event that the thermogram remains positive, mammography should be repeated in an attempt to detect a carcinoma that previously may have been occult, both clinically and mammographically.

Diagnostic ultrasound is useful in evaluating palpable masses, especially in breasts that are nodular and thus difficult to evaluate clinically and mammographically.[28] The outlines of the ultrasonic image of a scirrhous carcinoma are characteristically irregular with tiny internal echoes; images of fibroadenomas and medullary carcinomas both have slightly irregular borders and few internal echoes; cysts have smooth borders and no internal echoes, and are associated with strong echoes posterior to their posterior margins. Ultrasound thus may permit differentiation of solid from cystic masses, but in its present state of development *cannot* detect small masses including, especially, early cancers. Recent advances in gray-scale ultrasonography could conceivably lead to increased efficiency in detecting smaller lesions.

Scintigraphic scans of the breast with technetium-99m pertechnetate[29] or bleomycin labeled with indium-111 have undergone preliminary trials as an aid to the diagnosis of palpable masses, but the number of patients studied thus far is too small to evaluate the usefulness of these techniques.

Proton radiography and ultrasonic holography of the breast are two additional techniques that show potential promise, but for now they must be regarded as experimental and impractical for clinical use.[30, 31]

STAGING AND FOLLOW-UP

A modification of the TNM classification of the extent of cancer of the breast is shown in Table 13–1. The stage of the disease is assessed by clinical and radiographic methods. Minimal cancer of the breast (preinvasive, and carcinomas less than 0.5 cm in diameter) can only be diagnosed after histopathologic exam. TIS is used to designate carcinoma *in situ* or Paget's disease of the nipple with no demonstrable tumor. Although T1 (see Table 13–1) refers to lesions 2 cm or less in diameter, it should be recognized that minimal cancer of the breast, nonpalpable, asymptomatic, 0.5-cm lesions, and *in situ* carcinomas ought to be placed in another category since the prognosis is excellent (five-year survival rate of 90 per cent). The mammographic size of the lesion is more accurate than the clinical measurement; therefore, physicians routinely using mammography may have more patients with tumors classified as T1 or T2 than physicians who do not use mammography routinely.

There is no argument that many mammary carcinomas have distant metastases at the time the patient undergoes surgery. However, our ability to detect them in an

Table 13–1   Staging System for Carcinoma of the Breast

Tumor

TIS   Preinvasive carcinoma (*in situ*), noninfiltrating intraductal carcinoma, or Paget's disease of the nipple with no demonstrable tumor
T1a   Tumor 2 cm or less in greatest dimension with no fixation
T1b   Same as T1a but with fixation to underlying pectoral muscle or fascia
T2   Tumor from 2–5 cm (a and b as above)
T3   Tumor greater than 5 cm (a and b as above)
T4   Tumor of any size with *extension* to chest wall or *skin* (skin retraction does not alter classification)

Nodes

N0   No palpable homolateral axillary nodes
N1   Movable axillary nodes
N2   Fixed axillary nodes
N3   Supraclavicular or infraclavicular nodes or edema of arm

Metastasis

M0   No distant metastases
M1   Distant metastases including skin involvement beyond the involved breast area

Stages

Stage I   T1, N0, M0
Stage II   T1 or T2, N1, M0
Stage III T3 or T4, or N2 or N3, M0
Stage IV   M1

---

asymptomatic patient whose disease is classified as stage I or stage II by pathological examination is very poor. Skeletal surveys and bone scans of patients whose disease is stage I or stage II clinically are ordered out of habit, but their low yield suggests that they could be omitted. The patient with clinical stage III or stage IV disease should have an extensive diagnostic examination including liver and bone scans.

At the time of the *first recurrence,* an extensive examination is indicated, especially if the interval from mastectomy is less than two years. Unfortunately, extensive imaging examinations in asymptomatic high-risk patients (stage III, stage IV, and recurrence) are not rewarding. This is disappointing, since metastases will arise in the majority of these patients within five years of mastectomy.

Lymphography plays a limited role in the staging of breast cancer, because microscopic (nonpalpable) metastases to the axillary lymph nodes are not revealed in the lymphogram. Moreover, none of the internal mammary nodes and only some of the axillary nodes are opacified in upper limb lymphography. Direct injection of radiologic contrast material into a breast lymphatic channel to outline the lymph node drainage is rarely performed, since it requires an extreme degree of perseverance and technical skill.

PULMONARY AND PLEURAL METASTASES

Blood-borne metastases from breast cancer occur predominantly in the pleura, bone, lungs, and liver.[32] Metastases carried by the blood to the lungs tend to appear nodular in chest radiographs, while those that spread through lymph channels (lymphangitic) tend to produce a ray-like pattern spreading from the hila into the lung fields and branching peripherally into a fine web-like pattern (Fig. 13–18). Horizontal septal lines near the peripheral pleural surface of the lungs, also called "Kerley B" lines, frequently occur on chest radiographs when there has been lymphangitic tumor spread. The diagnosis of lymphangitic metastasis is a medical emergency and can only be successfully treated by multi-agent chemotherapy. Most blood-borne pleural metastases from breast carcinoma, usually presenting as pleural effusion, represent secondary spread from metastases in the liver. Seeding of the pleural surfaces may also occur directly from the subpleural lymphatics and lead to pleural effusion; a solitary pulmonary metastasis from cancer of the breast is rare. If it has been more than four years since the mastectomy was performed, a new primary neoplasm or benign lesion should be considered in the evaluation of a solitary pulmonary nodule.

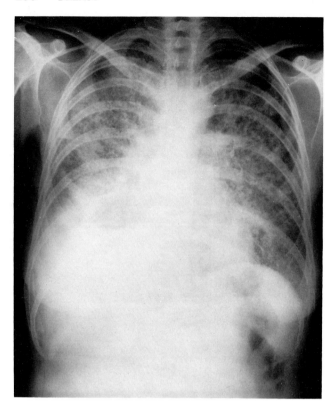

Figure 13–18 Perihilar interstitial lung "infiltrates" representing lymphangitic spread of breast cancer, from the mediastinum peripherally into both lung fields. A malignant right pleural effusion is also present.

BONE METASTASES

In a woman of age 40 or older, a destructive focus in bone should be considered metastatic until proved otherwise. Carcinoma of the breast must be excluded first, even when the physical examination does not reveal a mass. Bone metastases usually go undetected by routine radiography until they are far advanced locally. Radionuclide *bone scans* and scintigrams, however, may arouse suspicion of bone metastases long before they become visible radiographically. Since a localized increase in radionuclide uptake alone, demonstrated on bone scan, is a nonspecific finding, bone needle biopsy of the abnormal area should be undertaken to provide histologic confirmation of suspected metastatic involvement. Breast metastases may arise in any bone, including the short tubular bones of the hands and feet, but they predominate in the vertebrae, ribs, pelvis, skull, and the proximal segments of the proximal long bones — in summary, in the bones that retain red marrow in adulthood. The majority of metastases are initially osteolytic; however, some may combine osteolytic and osteoblastic features, and a few are *purely* osteoblastic (sclerotic), even in the absence of treatment. Osseous repair brought about by hormonal therapy, endocrine ablation, or multi-agent chemotherapy may cause an osteolytic (motheaten or permeated) metastatic pattern to convert to an osteoblastic one. Pathologic fractures are uncommon sequelae of pure osteoblastic metastases, but they frequently accompany the larger osteolytic lesions. A positive bone marrow aspirate is a poor prognostic sign, because it implies diffuse skeletal metastasis.

References

1. Strax, P., Venet, L., and Shapiro, S.: Value of mammography in reduction of mortality from breast cancer in mass screening. Am. J. Roentgenol. Radium Ther. Nucl. Med., *117*:686–689, 1973.
2. Rauscher, F. J., Jr.: Report to the Profession from the Breast Cancer Task Force. Bethesda, Maryland, National Cancer Institute, Sept. 30, 1974.
3. Dowdy, A. H., Barker, W. F., Lagasse, L. D., et al.: Mammography as a screening method for the examination of large populations. Cancer, *28*:1558–1562, 1971.

4. Missakian, M. M., Witten, D. M., and Harrison, E. G. Jr.: Mammography after mastectomy: Usefulness in the search for recurrent carcinoma of the breast. J.A.M.A., *191*:1045–1048, 1965.

5. Haagensen, C. D.: Diseases of the Breast. 2nd ed. Philadelphia, W. B. Saunders, 1971.

6. Clark, R. L., Copeland, M. M., Egan, R. L., et al.: Reproducibility of the technic of mammography (Egan) for cancer of the breast. Am. J. Surg., *109*:127–133, 1965.

7. Threatt, B., Appelman, H., Dow, R., et al.: Percutaneous needle localization of clustered mammary microcalcifications prior to biopsy. Am. J. Roentgenol. Radium Ther. Nucl. Med., *121*:839–842, 1974.

8. Dowdy, A. H., Lagasse, L. D., Sperling, L., et al.: A combined screening program for the detection of carcinoma of the cervix and carcinoma of the breast. Surg. Gynecol. Obstet., *131*:93–98, 1970.

9. Egan, R. L., Ellis, J. T., and Powell, R. W.: Team approach to the study of diseases of the breast. Cancer, 23:847–854, 1969.

10. Wolfe, J. N.: Analysis of 462 breast carcinomas. Am. J. Roentgenol. Radium Ther. Nucl. Med., *121*:846–853, 1974.

11. Witten, D. M.: The Breast: An Atlas of Tumor Radiology. Chicago, Year Book Medical Publishers, 1969.

12. Gold, R. H., Montgomery, C. K., and Rambo, O. N.: Significance of margination of benign and malignant infiltrative mammary lesions: Roentgenographic pathological correlation. Am. J. Roentgenol. Radium Ther. Nucl. Med., *118*:881–894, 1973.

13. Ingleby, H., and Gershon-Cohen, J.: Comparative Anatomy, Pathology, and Roentgenology of the Breast. Philadelphia, University of Pennsylvania Press, 1960, pp. 309–376.

14. Gallager, H. S., and Martin, J. E.: The study of mammary carcinoma by mammography and whole organ sectioning: Early observations. Cancer, 23:855–873, 1969.

15. Gold, R. H., Main, G., Zippin, C., et al.: Infiltration of mammary carcinoma as an indicator of axillary node metastasis: A preliminary report. Cancer, 29:35–40, 1972.

16. Lane, N., Goksel, H., Salerno, R. A., et al.: Clinicopathologic analysis of the surgical curability of breast cancers: A minimum 10-year study of a personal series. Ann. Surg., 153:483–498, 1961.

17. Egan, R. L.: Mammography and breast diseases. *In* Robbins, L. L. (ed), Golden's Diagnostic Radiology. Baltimore, Williams & Wilkins, 1970, p. 233.

18. Urban, J. A., and Adair, F. E.: Sclerosing adenosis. Cancer, 2:625–634, 1949.

19. Adair, F. E., and Munzer, J. T.: Fat necrosis of the female breast: Report of 110 cases. Am. J. Surg., 74:117–128, 1947.

20. Minagi, H., and Youker, J. E.: Roentgen appearance of fat necrosis in the breast. Radiology, 90:62–65, 1968.

21. Gold, R. H., Montgomery, C. K., Minagi, H., et al.: The significance of mammary skin thickening in disorders other than primary carcinoma: A roentgenologic-pathologic correlation. Am. J. Roentgenol. Radium Ther. Nucl. Med., *112*:613–621, 1971.

22. Haagensen, C. D.: Mammary-duct ectasia: Disease that may simulate carcinoma. Cancer, 4:749–761, 1951.

23. Gershon-Cohen, J., and Ingleby, H.: Secretory disease and plasma-cell mastitis in female breast: Roentgenologic and pathologic studies. Surg. Gynecol. Obstet., 95:497–504, 1952.

24. Wolfe, J. N.: Xerography of the breast. Radiology, 91:231–240, 1968.

25. Ostrum, B. J., Becker, W., and Isard, H. J.: Low-dose mammography. Radiology, *109*:323–326, 1973.

26. Silverstein, M. J., Sartorius, O. W., and Zarem, H.: Pertinent pathology. *In* Goldwyn, W. (ed.), Plastic and Reconstructive Surgery of the Breast. Boston, Little, Brown, 1975.

27. Isard, H. J., Becker, W., Shilo, R., et al.: Breast thermography after four years and 10,000 studies. Am. J. Roentgenol. Radium Ther. Nucl. Med., *115*:811–821, 1972.

28. Jellins, J., Kossoff, G., Buddee, F. W., et al.: Ultrasonic visualization of the breast. Med. J. Aust., *1*:305–307, 1971.

29. Villareal, R. L., Parkey, R. W., and Bonte, F. J.: Experimental pertechnetate mammography. Radiology, *111*:657–661, 1974.

30. Steward, V. W., and Koehler, A. M.: Proton radiography in the diagnosis of breast carcinoma. Radiology, *110*:217–221, 1974.

31. Anderson, R. E., and Curtin, H. R.: Ultrasonic holography. A promising medical imaging tool. Radiology, *109*:417–421, 1973.

32. Fraser, R. G., and Paré, J. A. P.: Diagnosis of Diseases of the Chest: An Integrated Study Based on the Abnormal Roentgenogram. Philadelphia, W. B. Saunders, 1970, pp. 792–803, 1150–1152.

Chapter Fourteen

BONE AND SOFT TISSUE

RICHARD H. GOLD, M.D.

CLINICAL CONSIDERATIONS

Presenting Signs and Symptoms

Pain and swelling at the site of a malignant tumor in a limb may be indistinguishable from the symptoms and signs of a benign tumor or inflammatory process. Clinical factors that imply an unfavorable prognosis include fever in a patient with Ewing's sarcoma, hemoglobin below 6 gm/100 ml in one with myeloma, underlying Paget's disease in a patient with osteosarcoma, and a short clinical history of rapid growth or regional lymphadenopathy in a patient who has any sarcoma. Osteosarcoma has a better prognosis if it is superficial (parosteal) in location or if it occurs in the mandible (see Chapter 4). Pathologic fractures complicate primary malignant bone tumors infrequently, occurring more commonly with aggressive metastatic lesions (from the breast, lung, kidney, or thyroid). Internal fixation of a grossly destructive peripheral bone lesion should be undertaken electively *before* fracture occurs.

Patients with primary bone tumors sometimes have a history of recent trauma that may seem insignificant relative to the pain, discomfort, and swelling that ensued. Resolving hematoma, arthritis, neuritis, or bursitis is frequently the initial clinical diagnosis, and the early roentgenograms may be negative even in retrospect. In the presence of symptoms, failure to demonstrate roentgenographic abnormalities does not eliminate the possibility of a malignant tumor. This is especially true of vertebral bodies, which contain much cancellous bone that may in turn conceal roentgenographic evidence of tumor destruction.

Chondrosarcomas may arise in a patient who has a benign cartilage tumor, Ollier's disease (multiple enchondromatosis), or multiple hereditary exostoses (see section on radiographic features). Furthermore, fibrous dysplasia may rarely give rise to a fibrosarcoma, and Paget's disease occasionally evolves into fibrosarcoma or osteosarcoma. Bone or soft-tissue sarcomas have also developed after many years in areas that had been heavily irradiated during the treatment of angiofibromas, giant cell tumors, retinoblastomas, and other tumors.

Differential Diagnosis

Careful examination of roentgenograms can direct the surgeon to the extraosseous portion of a bone tumor that may be most productive in reaching the histologic diagnosis. Pitfalls for the pathologist include "sampling errors," which may yield tissue that appears benign histologically from a roentgenographically obvious bone sarcoma (motheaten or permeated radiologic pattern; large soft-tissue mass; and so forth). Some neoplasms such as giant cell tumors may be misdiagnosed by *both* the radiologist and the pathologist, because the ordinary predictive patterns for benignancy or malig-

288

nancy are frequently in error. Stress fracture, traumatic myositis ossificans or subperiosteal ossification, aneurysmal bone cyst, and other lesions of benign origin may at times be mistaken (clinically, pathologically, or radiographically) for a malignant bone tumor. Biopsy should consist of a generous specimen from the growing edge of the lesion, and the pathologist should always be provided with the roentgenograms and pertinent clinical information.

Therapeutic Decisions and Staging

The critical issue in deciding upon appropriate therapy (and determining the prognosis) for patients with bone or soft-tissue sarcomas is the presence or absence of lung metastases. Although posteroanterior and lateral chest films with tomograms provide the only reliable preoperative means of detecting lung metastases (see Chapter 3), "microscopic" metastases from an osteogenic sarcoma primary can occasionally be inferred from positive lung scans made following the injection of a bone-seeking radionuclide. Metastases of primary bone tumors to another bone (particularly Ewing's tumor, but less frequently osteogenic sarcoma) can also be detected or confirmed by this means, together with appropriate radiographic studies. In those unfortunate individuals with advanced metastases, the presence of respiratory symptoms or multiple foci of pain and swelling may make dissemination obvious. However, if *any* doubt remains that dispersed lesions actually do represent metastatic disease from a known primary sarcoma, percutaneous or open biopsy must be undertaken. A solitary lung nodule in a patient with a malignant bone or soft-tissue tumor may be a noncalcified granuloma, hamartoma, or even a primary pulmonary carcinoma.

As stated later in this chapter (see the section on lymphography) regional lymph node metastases with peripheral sarcomas may be more common than is generally appreciated. At a minimum, careful palpation of the regional nodes (neck, axillary, or inguinal) is therefore mandatory before planning treatment.

Clinical Follow-up

The same considerations that guide the preoperative examination (staging) of a patient with a primary bone or soft-tissue sarcoma must also govern the posttreatment follow-up evaluation. Specifically, the presence or absence of metastases, particularly in the lungs, is of paramount importance in determining prognosis, treatment, and the need for institution (or reinstitution) of intensive therapy. For slowly growing metastases (long tumor size "doubling-times"), segmental lung resections have occasionally been performed, usually followed by adjunctive chemotherapy, immunotherapy, or both.

Following intensive irradiation of a malignant bone lesion, whether primary or metastatic, diminution in pain is the earliest sign of a therapeutic response; roentgenographic healing, on the other hand, may take weeks or months to become manifest. In certain benign conditions, including multiple cartilaginous tumors, giant cell tumor, and Paget's disease of bone, a rapid increase in local pain or swelling makes additional studies mandatory to rule out malignant degeneration. Careful posttreatment surveillance of an irradiated bone lesion, with attention to the development or persistence of local pain and swelling, will permit detection of tumor radioresistance or radionecrosis. Surgical excision or amputation may then be indicated, or, in the case of destructive metastatic lesions in weight-bearing bones, prophylactic internal fixation may be used to forestall a pathologic fracture. Pain in an amputation stump also warrants careful investigation; the clinical differential considerations here include local tumor recurrence, causalgic pain, local infection, or a poorly-fitting prosthesis.

RADIOLOGY OF MALIGNANT BONE TUMORS

Primary malignant bone tumors are uncommon, with a yearly incidence in the United States of only 2 cases per 100,000 population. Distinguishing a benign primary tumor of bone from a malignant one is sometimes difficult. Microscopy plays a discriminating role, but histologic features of malignancy are sometimes manifested by tumors that neither metastasize nor invade locally. Moreover, a single biopsy specimen may be unrepresentative of the most malignant part of a tumor. The radiographic examination is a complementary diagnostic tool that, while frequently not yielding a specific diagnosis, nevertheless serves to permit assessment of the relative aggressiveness or indolence of a tumor. Indeed, most experienced bone pathologists refrain from basing a diagnosis of a bone tumor solely upon histology, preferring instead to correlate histologic with radiographic features before coming to a conclusion.[1]

Presenting Radiographic Signs

Roentgenologic evaluation of a bone tumor requires an analytic approach. Key emphasis is placed upon the significance of the site and pattern of bone destruction, reactive bone proliferation, and tumor matrix formation—features of paramount importance because they mirror the cellular origin and the relative quiescence or aggressiveness of the tumor. Although reactive new bone proliferation may predominate, destruction is usually antecedent and at times is the only radiographic change. Destruction is not a direct effect of the tumor, but results from osteolytic and osteoclastic stimulation by the tumor.

Obstacles to Early Diagnosis. The significance of destructive and proliferative changes in bone and the obstacles to their radiographic detection can be better appreciated after a review of the basic structure of bone. Every bone is composed of two structural components: cortical (compact) bone and cancellous (spongy) bone. Cortical bone is a continuous peripheral sheath in which no spaces can be observed radiographically, save for nutrient foramina. The sheath of cortical bone surrounds the medullary cancellous bone, which consists of a latticework of trabeculae with spaces between the trabeculae. Owing to its compactness, cortical bone is more resistant to destruction than cancellous bone. Moreover, because of the greater radiographic density of cortical bone, a minor alteration in its structure, such as a nutrient

foramen or a hairline fracture, is more easily seen in radiographs. In contradistinction, cancellous bone is masked radiographically by the denser surrounding cortex. Thus, a relatively large volume of cancellous bone must be destroyed before any change becomes apparent in standard radiographs. Tomography (body-section radiography) may help the examiner to discern the nature and extent of cancellous bone destruction. In aged patients, generalized loss of bone—particularly cancellous bone—is a natural process that further hinders radiographic detection of primary and metastatic tumor. It is therefore understandable that a malignant tumor of bone may go undetected in standard radiographs until it has attained a size large enough to erode the *cortex* (Fig. 14–1). Prior to the appearance of an abnormality in standard radiographs or tomograms, bone scans and scintigrams may reveal an abnormally increased uptake of radionuclide resulting from primary or metastatic tumor. Unfortunately, a positive bone scan is not specific for malignant neoplasm, and pathologic confirmation is usually required.

Indeed, the classic radiographic features of a primary malignant bone tumor become manifest only when the tumor is far advanced locally. These features include: (1) cortical destruction with extracortical tumor extension; (2) subperiosteal new bone that is interrupted, lamellated, or finely spiculated; (3) deposition of an isolated triangular focus or cuff of subperiosteal new bone (Codman triangle) at the boundary of the neoplasm and the cortex; and, (4) in osteosarcoma, the cloud-like mineralization of tumor osteoid. In contradistinction to malignant tumor a benign bone tumor, because of its slow rate of growth and indolent nature, may thin and outwardly displace the cortex but not breach it, and it may provoke either solid, uninterrupted subperiosteal new bone (Fig. 14–2) or none at all.

Correlation of Destructive Pattern with Growth Rate. Bone tumors manifest certain radiographic patterns of destruction that reflect pathologic aggressiveness or quiescence (Table 14–1). These patterns have been analyzed and classified by Lodwick into three basic types (Fig. 14–3).[2] *Geographic destruction* is characterized by a large, well-defined hole with a sharply delineated edge (Fig. 14–3 *A*). The key radiographic feature

Motheaten destruction is characterized by multiple holes that have a tendency to coalesce (Fig. 14–3 *B*). The zone of transition of each hole is not sharp but is instead ill-defined. A motheaten pattern implies severe

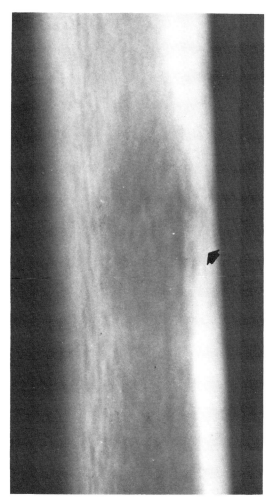

Figure 14–1 Metastasis to the tibia from carcinoma of the uterine cervix in a woman aged 55. Although the destruction occupied almost the entire width of the shaft and extensively involved cancellous bone, it became visible only when destruction extended into the inner cortex (arrow), a late event.

of geographic destruction is a sharp zone of transition between bone that has undergone complete destruction and bone that is completely intact. A geographic pattern implies that the growth rate of the tumor is very slow, resulting in intimate contact between the true edge of the lesion and the visible margin of destroyed bone. A sclerotic rim at the edge of the process signifies quiescence (Fig. 14–4). Slowly growing or quiescent lesions exhibiting a geographic pattern may also manifest coarse trabeculation resulting from irregular ridging of the encompassing host bone. Geographic destruction is characteristic of giant cell tumor (Fig. 14–5).

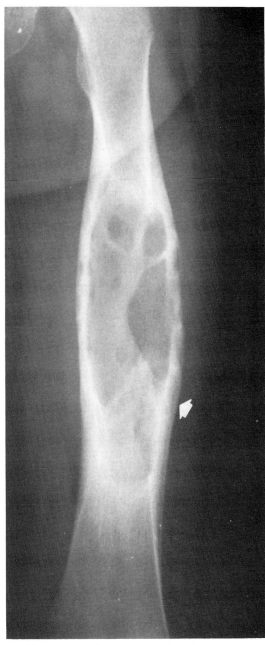

Figure 14–2 Roentgenographic characteristics of a benign tumor: outward displacement of the cortex without breaching it, a sharp interface with the host bone, coarse trabeculation, and solid, uninterrupted subperiosteal new bone (arrow). Eosinophilic granuloma of the femur. [From Vaeth, J. M. (ed.), Frontiers of Radiation Therapy and Oncology. Vol. 10. Basel, S., Karger AG, 1975, pp. 82–107.]

Table 14–1   Primary Malignant Tumors of Bone: Classification According to Patterns of Destruction

Tumor	Peak Age Incidence	Location within Long Bone	Periosteal Reaction	Matrix Mineralization
Geographic Destruction				
Chondrosarcoma	35	Metaphysis or diaphysis, central or periosteal	Expanded shell	Cartilage (flocculent)
Aggressive giant cell tumor (most feature motheaten edge and cortical destruction)	25	Metaphysis and epiphysis	Non-existent or expanded shell	—
Some fibrosarcomas (may also manifest motheaten pattern)	40+	Metaphysis or diaphysis	Scant and amorphous	—
Motheaten Destruction				
Some fibrosarcomas (may also manifest geographic pattern)	40+	Metaphysis or diaphysis	Scant and amorphous	—
Permeated Destruction				
Ewing's sarcoma	15	Diaphysis	Lamellated and/or spiculated	—
Osteosarcoma	15	Metaphysis (occasionally diaphysis)	Lamellated	Osteoid (cumulus cloud, sunburst)
Reticulum cell sarcoma	40+	Diaphysis	Scant and amorphous	—
Sarcoma in Paget's disease	40+	Anywhere	Scant	Not visible in radiograph

cortical destruction and signifies a moderately aggressive lesion. Motheaten destruction is characteristic of most fibrosarcomas.

Permeated destruction is characterized by multiple tiny holes predominating in cortical bone, which gradually diminish in size and number from the center of the lesion to its periphery (Fig. 14–3 *C*). Thus, the zone of transition is broad and ill-defined. Although the cortex is extensively involved, it appears radiographically to be almost intact but with greatly reduced radiodensity. Nevertheless, a permeated pattern implies that the tumor not only has breached the cortex, but probably has extended throughout most or all of the length of the bone. A permeated pattern of destruction implies great aggressiveness and extensive neoplastic infiltration. Permeated destruction is a characteristic feature of primary reticulum cell sarcoma of bone (Fig. 14–6) and of Ewing's sarcoma (Figs. 14–7, 14–10, 14–11, and 14–12). Osteosarcoma also manifests permeated destruction, but the pattern is usually obscured by new tumor bone (Figs. 14–14, 14–16, and 14–21).

Each of the three basic patterns of bone destruction—geographic, motheaten and permeated—may occur alone or in combination with one or both of the other patterns (Fig. 14–8). The motheaten and permeated patterns always signify total penetration of cortex by the tumor, and to distinguish between them is not of critical importance, but to distinguish these two patterns from the geographic pattern is of utmost importance for diagnostic and therapeutic decisions. The importance of making this distinction lies in the fact that the geographic pattern implies a slow rate of growth, the motheaten pattern an intermediate rate, and the permeated pattern the most rapid rate of growth. When the observer recognizes and understands the implications of each pattern, he may then estimate the growth rate of a bone tumor from a single radiographic examination. Unfortunately, estimating the benignancy or malignancy of certain tumors by these criteria is still fraught with risk, especially in the case of giant cell tumors. Another warning is that when one is considering the diagnostic possibilities of primary bone tumors, it is necessary to bear in mind that the lesion may be metastatic (Figs. 14–1 and 14–9). In patients more than 50 years of age, the

Text continued on page 296.

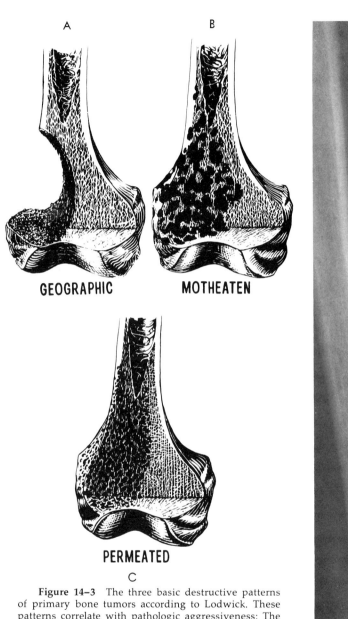

A   B

GEOGRAPHIC   MOTHEATEN

PERMEATED

C

Figure 14-3 The three basic destructive patterns of primary bone tumors according to Lodwick. These patterns correlate with pathologic aggressiveness: The geographic pattern implies a slow rate of growth, the motheaten pattern an intermediate rate, and the permeated pattern a rapid rate. (From Lodwick, G. S., Solitary malignant tumors of bone. The application of predictor variables in diagnosis. Semin. Roentgenol. *1*:293–313, July 1966. By permission of Grune & Stratton, Inc., and the author.)

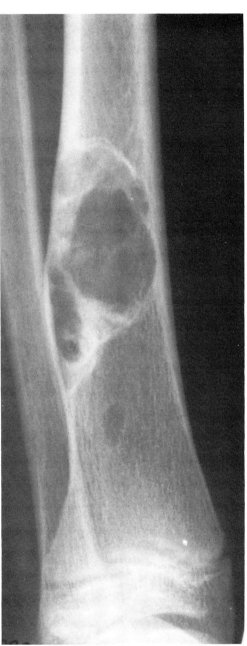

Figure 14-4 Nonossifying fibroma of the tibia. A sclerotic rim at the edge of geographic destruction implies quiescence of the tumor. [From Vaeth, J. M. (ed.), Frontiers of Radiation Therapy and Oncology. Vol. 10. Basel, S. Karger AG, 1975, pp. 82–107.]

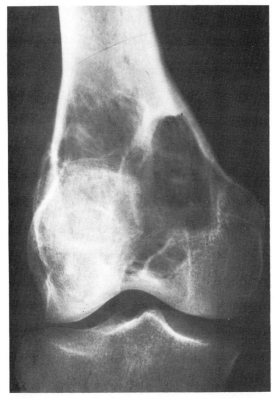

Figure 14–5 Geographic pattern of destruction resulting from a slow-growing giant cell tumor of the distal end of the femur. The sharp zone of transition between bone that has undergone complete destruction and bone that is completely intact implies relative indolence in growth behavior. [From Vaeth, J. M. (ed.), Frontiers of Radiation Therapy and Oncology. Vol. 10. Basel, S. Karger AG, 1975, pp. 82–107.)

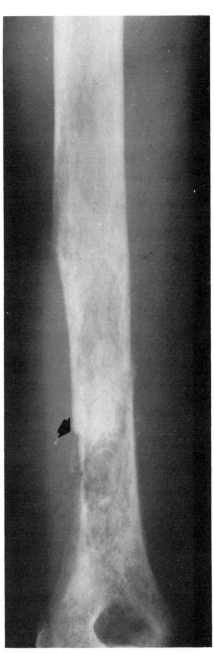

Figure 14–6 Permeated pattern of destruction in the absence of subperiosteal new bone characterizes this primary reticulum cell sarcoma of the humerus. A pathologic fracture has also occurred (arrow). The permeated pattern signifies total penetration of the cortex by the aggressive tumor. [From Vaeth, J. M. (ed.), Frontiers of Radiation Therapy and Oncology. Vol. 10. Basel, S. Karger AG, 1975, pp. 82–107.]

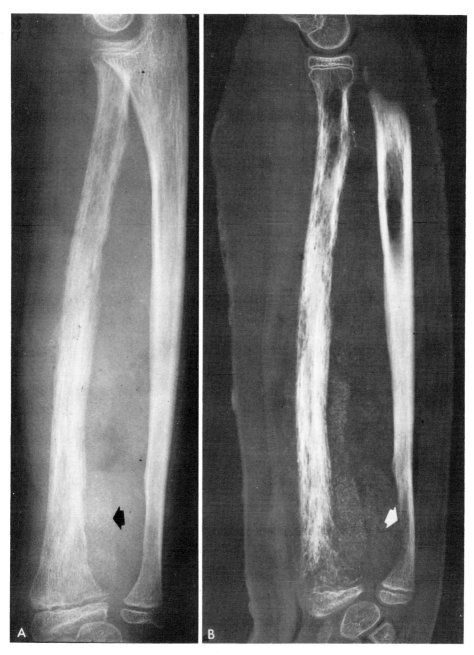

Figure 14–7   *A,* Ewing's sarcoma. Permeated pattern of destruction and multitudinous, delicate, perpendicular spicules of subperiosteal new bone (arrow) characterize this Ewing's sarcoma of the radius. The tumor has infiltrated throughout the length of the bone, a feature typical of aggressive tumors producing permeated destruction. *B,* Radiograph of sagittal section of amputation specimen reveals pressure erosion of the shaft of the ulna by the bulky tumor (arrow). [*A* from Vaeth, J. M. (ed.), Frontiers of Radiation Therapy and Oncology. Vol. 10. Basel, S. Karger AG, 1975, pp. 82–107.]

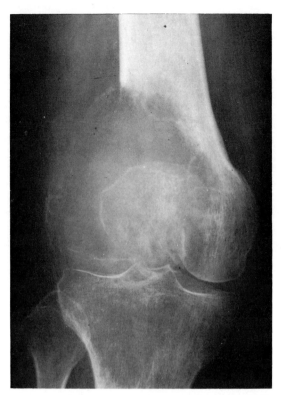

Figure 14–8 Aggressive giant cell tumor. While this tumor has basically a geographic destructive pattern, cortical destruction and an indistinct zone of transition between destroyed and intact bone imply relative aggressiveness. [From Vaeth, J. M. (ed.), Frontiers of Radiation Therapy and Oncology. Vol. 10. Basel, S. Karger AG, 1975, pp. 82–107.]

incidence of metastatic tumor in bone far exceeds that of primary bone tumor.

Age of the Patient as an Aid to Roentgenologic Diagnosis. While clinical history may have limited value in the diagnosis of bone tumors, the age of the patient is an important consideration. As examples, the peak incidence of lytic bone lesions from acute leukemia and neuroblastoma is in the first decade; osteosarcoma and Ewing's sarcoma are most common in the second decade; giant cell tumor is rare before the third decade; metastatic tumor and multiple myeloma are the most frequent malignant tumors of bone in patients more than 50 years of age. Another example of the value of the patient's age in roentgenologic interpretation is in the differentiation between Ewing's sarcoma and reticulum cell sarcoma of a flat bone such as the ilium (Fig. 14–10). Both Ewing's sarcoma and reticulum cell sarcoma cause a perme-

ated pattern of destruction. Despite the similarity of destructive pattern, these two tumors in long bones may be distinguished by the extent of associated periosteal response. Ewing's sarcoma characteristically evokes an extensive, delicately spiculated or lamellated proliferation of subperiosteal new bone (Figs. 14–7, 14–11, and 14–12),

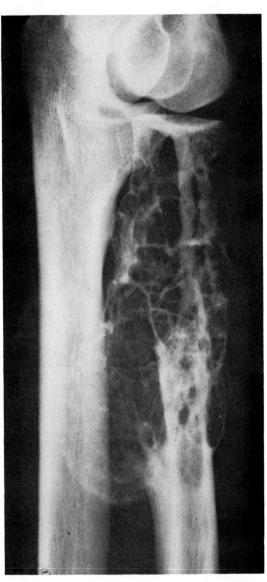

Figure 14–9 Metastatic renal cell carcinoma to the proximal end of the radius, with a bubbly, geographic pattern of destruction simulating benignity. However, it is important to remember that beyond the age of fifty, metastatic tumor in bone occurs far more frequently than primary tumor. [From Vaeth, J. M. (ed.), Frontiers of Radiation Therapy and Oncology. Vol. 10. Basel, S. Karger AG, 1975, pp. 82–107.]

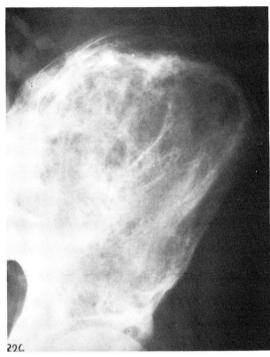

Figure 14–10 Age of the patient can be a diagnostic clue. Permeated destruction is present in the ilium of a 15-year-old boy. Both Ewing's and reticulum cell sarcomas manifest a permeated pattern. In a long bone, Ewing's sarcoma evokes spiculated or lamellated subperiosteal new bone, while reticulum cell sarcoma does not. The periosteum of flat bones, however, does not have a capacity for vigorous production of subperiosteal new bone, resulting in the loss of this important distinguishing feature. Of these two tumors, Ewing's sarcoma seldom occurs beyond the second decade while reticulum cell sarcoma predominates later in life. Thus, the age of this patient is a clue to the diagnosis of Ewing's sarcoma. [From Vaeth, J. M. (ed.), Frontiers of Radiation Therapy and Oncology. Vol. 10. Basel, S. Karger AG, 1975, pp. 82–107.]

while reticulum cell sarcoma does not (Fig. 14–6). However, the periosteum of flat bones, in contrast to that of long bones, does not have a capacity for vigorous new bone production. Thus, in the ilium this paucity of new bone results in the loss of an important distinguishing feature between Ewing's and reticulum cell sarcomas. However, Ewing's sarcoma seldom occurs beyond the second decade of life, while reticulum cell sarcoma predominates in the third through sixth decades. Thus, when two entirely different neoplasms assume identical appearances radiographically, the age of the patient may sometimes permit a logical choice to be made between them (Fig. 14–10).[3]

Mineralization of Tumor Matrix. Recognition of a specific type of tumor matrix by its pattern of mineralization is essential. In general, the greatest degree of mineralization in tumor cartilage or osteoid occurs in the region of its greatest maturity, usually within the center of the tumor. Calcification within tumor cartilage takes the form of rings, flocculant deposits, or sharply defined crystal-like clusters (Figs. 14–13 and 14–20). The *central* predominance of the calcifications aids in distinguishing a cartilage tumor within bone from a medullary bone infarct, in which the calcifications tend to be at the periphery of the lesion. The pattern of mineralization in tumor osteoid is also variable, and depends upon the rate of tumor growth. Rapidly growing

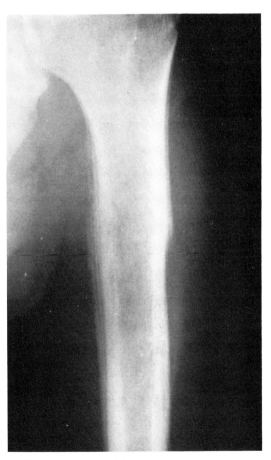

Figure 14–11 Multiple lamellae of subperiosteal new bone occurring in response to a Ewing's sarcoma of the humerus. The lamellae disappear centrally, where the extreme rapidity of tumor growth has destroyed the subperiosteal new bone and hindered its further elaboration.

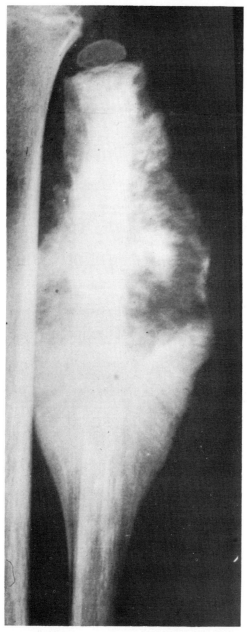

14–15, and 14–21). The resultant poorly-differentiated tumor bone may form a "sunburst" of rays or spicules that may actually be indistinguishable from subperiosteal new bone. Slowly growing tumors such as parosteal osteosarcomas usually produce

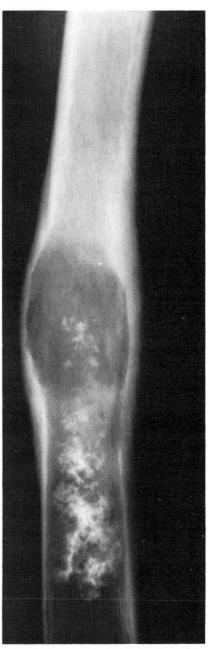

Figure 14–12 Perpendicular spicules of subperiosteal new bone in response to Ewing's sarcoma of the fibula. This type of reaction signifies permeated destruction by a malignant tumor whose growth rate is extremely rapid. A shell of new bone has formed at the periphery of the spicules, implying that the process which was formerly aggressive has at least temporarily become quiescent as the result of recent radiation therapy.

tumors such as osteosarcoma usually produce immature, woven tumor bone in the form of clouds with ill-defined edges and a lack of structured appearance (Figs. 14–14,

Figure 14–13 Characteristic floccules of calcification within tumor cartilage, in a slow-growing chondrosarcoma of the femur. [From Vaeth, J. M. (ed.), Frontiers of Radiation Therapy and Oncology. Vol. 10. Basel, S. Karger AG, 1975, pp. 82–107.]

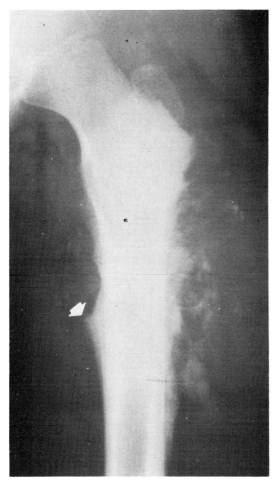

Figure 14–14 Characteristic ill-defined clouds of tumor new bone extending beyond the cortex, in an osteosarcoma of the femur. A Codman triangle is also visible (arrow). [From Vaeth, J. M. (ed.), Frontiers of Radiation Therapy and Oncology. Vol. 10. Basel, S. Karger AG, 1975, pp. 82–107.]

solid, mature tumor bone all the way to their sharply defined periphery.

Heterotopic Bone Simulating Osteosarcoma. Heterotopic bone formation may occur within soft tissues subsequent to trauma, which may have been recognized or unrecognized. Such ossification—called *circumscribed myositis ossificans*—may resemble mineralized tumor osteoid on radiographs. A mistaken roentgenologic diagnosis of osteosarcoma may be made if the heterotopic bone is located near a focus of subperiosteal new bone resulting from a traumatic subperiosteal hemorrhage. However, subperiosteal new bone resulting from hemorrhage is usually solid and uniform,

as befits its benign origin, whereas that secondary to malignancy is characteristically interrupted, spiculated, or lamellated. Initially, heterotopic bone within the soft tissues appears fluffy and is faintly visible in radiographs. As the bone matures over a period of weeks, its density and solidity increase. The bone gradually differentiates into cortical and cancellous elements, and eventually undergoes shrinkage. A clue distinguishing circumscribed myositis ossificans from mineralized tumor osteoid is that the former matures centripetally, and is therefore most dense and solid at its periphery. On the other hand, tumor osteoid matures centrifugally, and thus it tends to be most dense centrally. Microscopically, immature heterotopic new bone may bear a striking similarity to osteosarcoma.

Tumor Size and Potential for Metastasis. In general, the larger a bone tumor, the greater the likelihood of malignancy. However, the assumption of a direct relationship between a tumor's size and its potential for metastasis, while seemingly logical, may at times be erroneous. That tumor size and aggressiveness need not necessarily be interdependent is illustrated by the case of a 13-year-old girl who complained of intermittent sharp pain in the left thigh for three months.[4] Radiographs of the left femur revealed a flocculent, calcific density in the diaphysis of the bone at the junction of the middle and distal thirds (Fig. 14–15). Cortical destruction and subperiosteal new bone proliferation were absent. Tomography confirmed the absence of a fracture line and the lack of cortical destruction. An excision biopsy of the lesion led to a pathologic diagnosis of an osteosarcoma that measured only 2.0 cm in its greatest dimension. Full-chest tomography immediately following the biopsy revealed several small pulmonary metastases that were not visible in the standard preoperative chest radiographs. The metastases enlarged and multiplied rapidly and relentlessly, resulting in death two months after the femoral biopsy. The classic radiographic features of a primary malignant bone tumor may become manifest only when the tumor is far advanced locally. In a child, therefore, osteosarcoma must be considered the prime diagnostic possibility whenever fluffy intramedullary densities merge radiographically

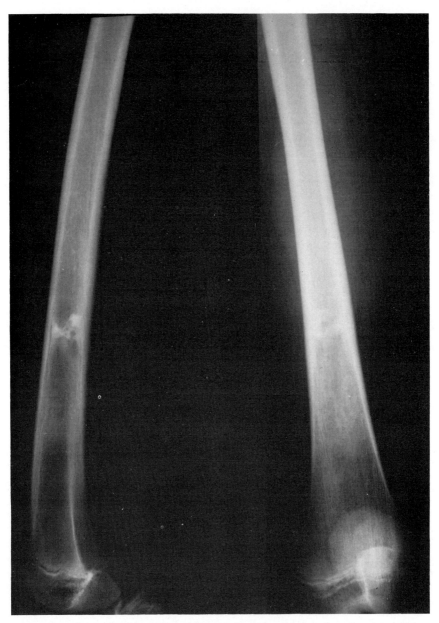

Figure 14–15   Lethal osteosarcoma of the mid-femur. Lateral and anteroposterior views. Pulmonary metastasis had already occurred. The primary tumor measured only 2 cm at pathologic examination and did not result in cortical destruction *or* in subperiosteal new bone proliferation. In a child, osteosarcoma must be considered the prime diagnostic possibility wherever an intramedullary cloudlike shadow, no matter how small, is present radiographically, even in the absence of the classic roentgenologic criteria of malignancy. [From Vaeth, J. M. (ed.), Frontiers of Radiation Therapy and Oncology. Vol. 10. Basel, S. Karger AG, 1975, pp. 82–107. Courtesy of Harvard Ellman, M. D.]

to form a "cumulus cloud" shadow, no matter how small, and even in the absence of other radiographic features of malignancy.

General Considerations in Differential Diagnosis

Significance of Edema in Soft Tissue. The osteosarcoma shown in Figure 14–16 illustrates subtle cortical destruction (open arrow) and another radiographic feature helpful in distinguishing a neoplasm from inflammation: absence of soft-tissue edema.

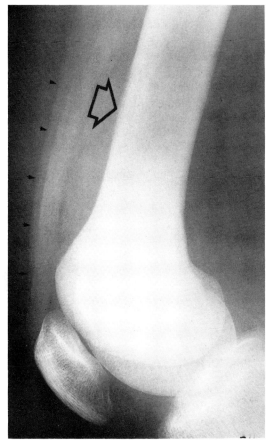

Figure 14–16 A sharp interface between muscle and subcutaneous fat (small arrowheads) signifies an absence of soft-tissue edema, which in turn indicates that the pathologic process involving the bone surface is not inflammatory. This osteosarcoma of the femur manifests subtle cortical destruction (open arrow) and a striking increase in radiographic density, resulting from the intraosseous deposition of tumor bone. [From Vaeth, J. M. (ed.), Frontiers of Radiation Therapy and Oncology. Vol. 10. Basel, S. Karger AG, 1975, pp. 82–107.]

Although the muscle mass is displaced by the tumor, the fatty septa surrounding the muscle bundles remain sharp and the interface between muscle and subcutaneous fat is well defined (arrowheads), indicating a lack of edema and, by inference, *an absence of inflammation.* Situations do arise in which it is difficult to decide roentgenologically and clinically whether a destructive process of bone is inflammatory or neoplastic. In these situations, the absence of soft-tissue edema is a valuable clue that the process is *not* an inflammatory one. It should be remembered, however, that some Ewing's sarcomas do evoke an inflammatory response with associated soft-tissue edema. Moreover, a massive malignant tumor may, by its pressure, obstruct overlying veins, resulting in edema secondary to venous stasis. Thus the *presence* of edema is not as specific as its absence in distinguishing between inflammation and tumor. Hyperemia accompanies both inflammatory *and* malignant neoplastic diseases of bone, with resultant enlargement of overlying superficial veins. Since the veins are outlined by subcutaneous fat, their enlargement may be perceived radiographically.

Significance of Subperiosteal New Bone. Recognition of the benign or malignant origin of subperiosteal new bone is essential in distinguishing a benign lesion from a malignant one. The healthy periosteum, when activated by relatively benign stimuli, produces solid new bone with a smooth outline and, when fully developed, with uniform density. These benign stimuli include hyperemia secondary to overlying soft-tissue inflammation, edema caused by venous stasis, subperiosteal hemorrhage, osteomyelitis, eosinophilic granuloma (Fig. 14–2), benign fracture, hypertrophic pulmonary osteoarthropathy,* osteoid osteoma, and lipid storage disorders such as Gaucher's disease. The resultant newly formed benign subperiosteal bone is separated from the underlying cortex by a thin radiolucent zone. No regular pattern of lamellation or spiculation is observed. The layer of new bone may be thick or thin and of smooth or irregular contour, depending upon the duration of the process and the intensity and uneven-

---

*May be associated with cancer of the lung, however.

ness of the underlying stimulus, but its solid, uniform character remains constant.

By contrast, subperiosteal new bone that is stimulated by an underlying malignant neoplasm is *not* even, uniform, and solid in appearance, but instead appears delicate and interrupted — typically longitudinally lamellated or perpendicularly spiculated. It should be understood, however, that while these are classic periosteal manifestations of malignancy — particularly in osteosarcoma and Ewing's sarcoma — they may occasionally accompany an active, rapidly progressive benign process such as osteomyelitis or repeated subperiosteal hemorrhage. In the benign processes, however, the spicules of new bone are usually more coarse and the lamellations of new bone fewer and thicker than those associated with malignancy.

The characteristic lamellations of subperiosteal new bone in response to Ewing's sarcoma are shown in Figure 14–11. The lamellations disappear centrally, where ultra-rapid tumor growth has actually destroyed the new bone and hindered its further elaboration. The multiplicity of lamellations probably reflects alternating periods of rapid and slow tumor growth. During a period of slow growth, the periosteum is displaced less rapidly, and thus has time to form a layer of new bone, but during rapid growth the periosteum cannot produce an effective encapsulating shell. Instead, the tumor penetrates the thin layers of subperiosteal new bone already formed, displacing the periosteum even further peripherally. Unlike the delicate, thin strips of lamellated new bone laid down in response to Ewing's sarcoma, an aggressive benign process such as osteomyelitis tends to manifest thicker layers that may coalesce at various sites along the shaft.

The perpendicular spicules of new bone that may be elaborated by the periosteum in response to Ewing's sarcoma grow along tiny vascular channels between the periosteum and cortex. This type of reaction signifies extremely rapid growth. A shell of new bone appearing at the periphery of the perpendicular spicules implies that the underlying process was once aggressive and rapidly growing, but has since become quiescent. This type of response may result from radiation therapy (Fig. 14–12).

A *Codman triangle* of new bone is an isolated cuff of subperiosteal new bone at the boundary of a mass that is rapidly elevating the periosteum (Fig. 14–14). The triangle is found most frequently in association with malignant neoplasms of bone, but it sometimes arises in response to rapid displacement of the periosteum by exudate or blood. The triangle may also result from an aggressive aneurysmal bone cyst (Fig. 14–17).

Specific Radiographic Features

Multiple Myeloma (Plasma Cell Myeloma). This tumor of hematopoietic origin is the most common primary malignant tumor involving bone. The *classic* radiographic description of myeloma is one of multitudinous, "punched-out" holes accompanied by cortical destruction and little or no periosteal reaction, predominantly affecting those bones in which the red marrow normally persists throughout adulthood (i.e., vertebrae, ribs, skull vault, and pelvis). An equally frequent but less well-appreciated radiographic presentation of this disease features generalized loss of bone density (simulating osteoporosis), with resultant collapse of multiple vertebrae and pathologic fractures of ribs, in the absence of visible discrete foci of destruction. Occasionally, an expansile focus of myeloma may balloon a segment of affected bone, frequently a rib. Breaching of the cortex with extraosseous extension of tumor is a common occurrence.

Myeloma is usually multicentric but may occasionally begin as a solitary destructive focus — solitary plasmacytoma — only to disseminate eventually throughout the skeleton. Multiple myeloma is rare before the fifth decade of life, and therefore age is a clue to diagnosis. Almost all reported cases of myeloma are entirely osteolytic. Rarely, a sclerotic response occurs that may accompany secondary amyloid deposition within the myeloma lesions. Multiple myeloma, like *diffuse* metastatic disease, may go undetected in radionuclide bone scans because of an absence of visible focal or discrete lesions. The chief problem in roentgenologic differential diagnosis lies in distinguishing multiple myeloma from

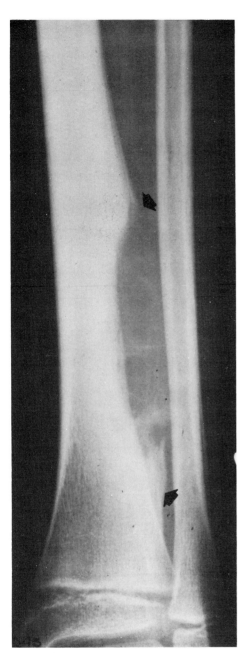

Figure 14–17 Codman triangles (arrows) and multiple lamellae of subperiosteal new bone in response to an aggressive aneurysmal bone cyst of the tibia. Although a Codman triangle is most frequently associated with malignant tumor, it may accompany subperiosteal hemorrhage, infection, or an aggressive aneurysmal bone cyst. The lesion recurred following each incomplete extirpation.

metastatic tumor. Discrete foci of destruction resulting from multiple myeloma are usually very numerous, especially in the skull vault, and being multicentric in origin tend to be of similar size, while metastatic

lesions tend to be fewer in number and of varying size.

Ewing's Sarcoma. This extremely aggressive and infiltrative tumor is aptly reflected radiographically by a permeated pattern of destruction extending throughout much or all of an affected bone (Figs. 14–7, 14–10, 14–11, and 14–12). In long bones, the center of the tumor usually is in the diaphysis. Interrupted, delicately lamellated or spiculated subperiosteal new bone is usually an accompanying feature. The peak age incidence is 15 years. (See also Chapter 17, and Fig. 17–20.)

Osteosarcoma. This tumor manifests the most characteristic roentgenologic feature of all primary bone tumors—a cumulus cloud or sunburst of mineralized tumor osteoid (Figs. 14–14, 14–15, and 14–21). Striking aggressiveness is implied in radiographs by its permeated destructive pattern, but this pattern is frequently masked by mineralized tumor osteoid. In long bones, the center of the lesion is usually in the metaphysis. Osteosarcoma is the second most common primary malignant tumor of bone, being preceded only by multiple myeloma. As with Ewing's sarcoma, the peak age incidence is 15 years. (See also Chapter 17 and Fig. 17–16.) Osteosarcoma may arise occasionally in elderly patients, within a focus of Paget's disease of bone (Fig. 14–18). Furthermore, the increase in bone density and distortion of bone architecture resulting from Paget's disease may lead to difficulty in radiologic recognition of an accompanying osteosarcoma. Radionuclide scans utilizing strontium-85, strontium-87, fluorine-18, or technetium-99m polyphosphate (or diphosphonate) may reveal extraskeletal metastases of osteosarcoma (including the lungs), which themselves may rarely be sufficiently calcified to be visible in radiographs (Fig. 14–19).

Giant Cell Tumor. This tumor arises near the end of a bone, usually at the knee, and predominates in the third decade of life. Histologic grading of giant cell tumor is notoriously unreliable as a guide to its malignant potential. Similarly, unlike most primary bone tumors, it is impossible to predict from the radiographic appearance of a giant cell tumor whether it will pursue a benign or malignant course. The most a radiologist can affirm from the radiograph, when confronted with the possibility of

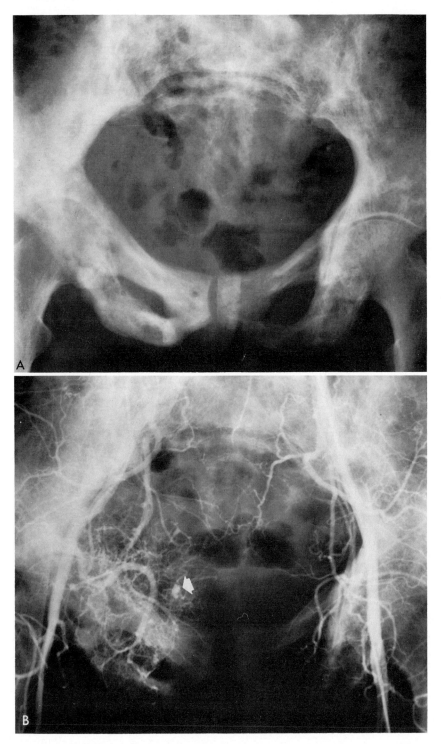

Figure 14–18   Osteosarcoma arising in bone involved by Paget's disease. This 57-year-old woman complained of pain in the region of a clinical right suprapubic mass. *A*, Standard radiograph illustrating proliferative stage of Paget's disease throughout the pelvis, but no evidence of bone destruction by tumor. *B*, Aorto-iliac arteriogram reveals a large, vascular tumor arising from the right pubic bone. Numerous irregularly outlined pelvic vessels on patient's right, which fail to diminish in caliber and which pursue bizarre pathways, signify a malignancy. A "tumor lake" or pool of radiopaque medium is signified by arrow. [From Vaeth, J. M. (ed.), Frontiers of Radiation Therapy and Oncology. Vol. 10. Basel, S. Karger AG, 1975, pp. 82–107.]

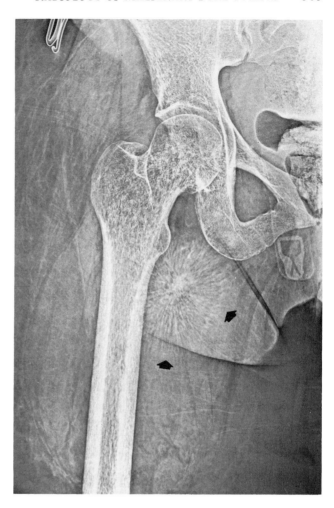

Figure 14-19 Extraosseous metastasis from osteosarcoma. The primary tumor in the distal femur was treated by amputation at the mid-shaft. This *xeroradiograph* discloses a "sunburst" of mineralized tumor osteoid within a lymph node (arrows). [From Wolfe, J.: Xeroradiography: Image content and comparison with film roentgenograms. Am. J. Roentgenol. Radium Ther. Nucl. Med., *117*:690–695, 1973. Courtesy of John Wolfe, M. D., and Charles C Thomas, Publisher.]

giant cell tumor, is its probable aggressiveness or indolence (Figs. 14–5 and 14–8). Nevertheless, it should be understood that a giant cell tumor that appears aggressive may pursue an entirely benign clinical course, while a giant cell tumor that appears benign may quickly undergo metastasis. Thus, the actual clinical course of the patient is the only reliable indicator of a giant cell tumor's malignant potential.

Fibrosarcoma of Bone. This tumor is rare, predominating in patients over the age of 40. It usually arises in the shaft or metaphysis of a long bone and results in a geographic or motheaten pattern of destruction. Fibrosarcoma may provoke a septated or amorphous shell of subperiosteal new bone, but not perpendicularly spiculated new bone.

Chondrosarcoma. This tumor is usually found in patients over the age of 35.

It takes two classic radiographic forms. The first is a slowly growing central tumor, with a geographic destructive pattern expanding a segment of the metaphysis and the adjacent shaft of a long bone (Fig. 14–13); the other is a large, eccentric tumor predominantly occurring at the surface of flat bones such as ribs, pelvis, and scapulae, and only minimally involving the underlying bone (Fig. 14–20). Both forms of chondrosarcoma frequently manifest typical cartilage matrix calcification, but the absence of this calcification does not exclude the diagnosis. These tumors tend to remain relatively circumscribed, unlike Ewing's sarcoma, reticulum cell sarcoma, and osteosarcoma, which usually infiltrate extensively through the length of the affected bone (whether it is evident roentgenologically or not).

Enchondroma, the most common *benign* tumor of bone, occurs predominantly in

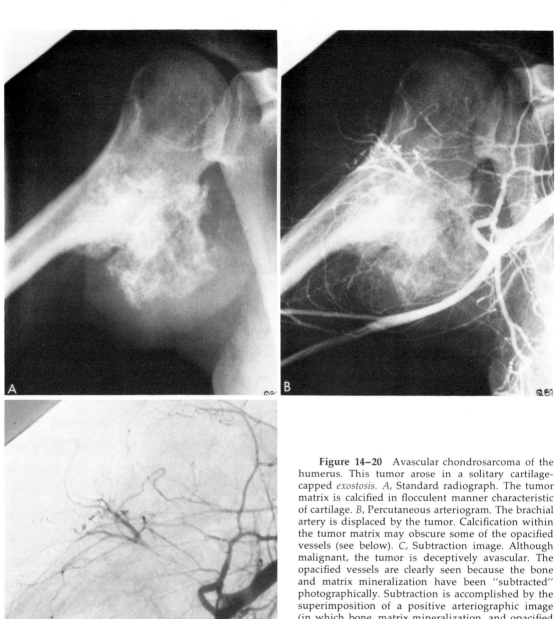

Figure 14–20   Avascular chondrosarcoma of the humerus. This tumor arose in a solitary cartilage-capped *exostosis*. *A*, Standard radiograph. The tumor matrix is calcified in flocculent manner characteristic of cartilage. *B*, Percutaneous arteriogram. The brachial artery is displaced by the tumor. Calcification within the tumor matrix may obscure some of the opacified vessels (see below). *C*, Subtraction image. Although malignant, the tumor is deceptively avascular. The opacified vessels are clearly seen because the bone and matrix mineralization have been "subtracted" photographically. Subtraction is accomplished by the superimposition of a positive arteriographic image (in which bone, matrix mineralization, and opacified vessels appear black) upon a standard negative radiograph exposed immediately prior to the arteriographic injection. [From Vaeth, J. M. (ed.), Frontiers of Radiation Therapy and Oncology. Vol. 10. Basel, S. Karger AG, 1975, pp. 82–107.]

the short tubular bones of the hands and feet. Chondrosarcoma, on the other hand, is rare in the short tubular bones, occurring predominantly in the axial skeleton and proximal ends of the femora and humeri. A benign cartilage tumor within the axial skeleton, especially the ribs, pelvis, and scapulae, or within the proximal ends of the femora and humeri, is far more likely to undergo transformation into chondrosarcoma or fibrosarcoma than is a benign cartilage tumor located within the more peripheral parts of the skeleton. The onset of pain, an enlarging mass, or a change in the radiographic pattern of matrix calcification may signify sarcomatous degeneration within a cartilage tumor that was once benign.

The incidence of chondrosarcoma arising in patients with multiple hereditary cartilage-capped exostoses or multiple enchondromatosis (Ollier's disease) is difficult to ascertain, but is estimated to be less than 10 per cent. However, chondrosarcomatous degeneration in association with multiple enchondromatosis is more frequent in patients with Maffucci's syndrome (multiple enchondromatosis *in combination with* cavernous hemangiomas of soft tissue).

Primary Reticulum Cell Sarcoma of Bone. Primary reticulum cell sarcoma is a rapidly infiltrating tumor occurring predominantly in the long bones of patients 40 years of age and older. As befits its aggressiveness, the pattern of destruction is permeated, and a long segment of bone is usually involved (Fig. 14–6). The periosteal response is typically amorphous, not spiculated or lamellated, and Codman triangles do not usually occur. When a tumor of bone with the pathologic characteristics of reticulum cell sarcoma is discovered concurrently with a known soft-tissue focus of reticulum cell sarcoma (histiocytic lymphoma), it is usually classified as a metastasis from the soft-tissue component. On the other hand, a reticulum cell sarcoma of bone occurring in the absence of a soft-tissue focus of tumor elsewhere has usually been classified as a primary tumor of bone. Lymphography therefore may play a *vital role* in classifying reticulum cell sarcoma that presents in bone. The primary bone tumor is radiosensitive, and long-term survival is not unusual in the localized form of the disease.

Specialized Diagnostic Techniques

Arteriography in the Evaluation of Bone Tumors. While selective arteriography cannot replace biopsy, it is simple to perform, relatively innocuous to the patient, and potentially has much to offer as a guide to the diagnosis and management of bone tumors.[10-16] The merits of arteriography transcend its disadvantages. Since most primary malignant bone tumors manifest arteriographic evidence of malignancy, arteriography may complement pathologic studies in the differentiation of malignant from benign bone tumors. Arteriography may disclose the onset of malignancy within a long-standing benign cartilaginous tumor, or within a focus of Paget's disease (Fig. 14–18) or fibrous dysplasia. Arteriography is sometimes helpful in choosing a biopsy site, since the area of greatest vascularity often represents the most malignant part of the tumor. Lastly, arteriography aids in defining the limits of intraosseous and extraosseous tumor growth. These limits are usually more extensive than may be inferred from the study of standard radiographs. Thus arteriography aids in the planning of surgical or radiotherapeutic treatment, and it may also permit accurate mapping of the arterial blood supply of a tumor prior to perfusion chemotherapy.

Certain disadvantages of arteriography must also be stressed. A normal arteriogram does not exclude malignancy, since some indolent chondrosarcomas, fibrosarcomas, and reticulum cell sarcomas may be deceptively innocent in their arteriographic appearance (Fig. 14–20).[14] Arteriography does not permit differentiation between histologic types of primary malignant tumor, nor between primary and metastatic tumors. Giant cell tumors show great variation in their arteriographic appearance; some aggressive tumors are avascular while others that subsequently pursue a benign course show striking hypervascularity resembling malignancy.[10, 11, 14] Finally, serial arteriographic changes *do not* provide a dependable guide to the response of a tumor to radiotherapy.[14]

Arteriographic Signs of Malignancy. The only pathognomonic arteriographic sign of malignancy is the presence of so-called pathologic vessels or tumor neovascularity. These vessels have been described with precision by Strickland as being "deployed seemingly without purpose, ending their haphazard journey in amorphous spaces in the midst of necrotic tissue."[14] In other words, tumor vessels pursue a bizarre, irregular path and, being in part lined by tumor cells, are ragged in outline and fail to diminish progressively in caliber (in contradistinction to normal or inflammatory vessels). They often terminate as small, scattered "tumor lakes" in which the radiopaque medium pools for a considerable time, because the walls of the lakes have no elasticity with which to expel it. Arteriovenous shunting is another frequently occurring manifestation of malignancy, but one that may sometimes occur also in benign inflammatory processes such as chronic periostitis and chronic synovitis, including pigmented villonodular synovitis.[13, 17] Other arteriographic signs that are characteristic but not diagnostic of malignancy include: abrupt termination of an otherwise normal artery (possibly a result of local thrombosis or infarction within the tumor); straight veins coursing at right angles to the normal flow of venous return; and a myriad of small vessels encircling the periphery of an area of relative avascularity (the avascular area presumably is a mass of necrotic tumor, although an abscess could have a similar appearance). Diffuse staining of tumor by radiopaque medium, while frequently associated with malignancy, is not diagnostic. It occasionally is manifest in benign disease, notably some benign giant cell tumors, some aneurysmal bone cysts, chronic periostitis, and chronic synovitis including pigmented villonodular synovitis.[11, 13, 14, 17]

Xeroradiography and Xeroarteriography in the Evaluation of Bone Tumors. In the early 1940s, a photographic process based upon photoelectric rather than photochemical principles was developed. Because the process was a dry one, it was called xerography. In the radiographic counterpart of the process—xeroradiography—the electrostatic image of an object that is interposed in an x-ray beam is recorded upon a plate coated with a semiconductor, selenium. The electrostatic image is made visible by application to the exposed plate of oppositely charged, blue powder granules. The blue image is then transferred to paper, thereby becoming a finished xeroradiograph.[18, 19]

Although xeroradiography has received wide acclaim as an improved radiographic technique for the earlier detection of breast cancer, it deserves wider acceptance than it has received in the evaluation of skeletal disease. Xeroradiography in many ways excels standard film radiography for evaluating bone tumors. It provides enhanced detail of bone destruction, tumor matrix mineralization, periosteal reaction, and associated soft-tissue changes (Fig. 14–21).[18, 21] Po and Grollman have found in studying bone tumors that xeroradiographic imaging of arteriograms reveals greater vascular detail than has hitherto been recorded, except perhaps through the use of special roentgenographic magnification techniques.[20]

Edge enhancement of small blood vessels filled with radiopaque medium makes xeroradiography a valuable adjunct to arteriography of bone tumors (Fig. 14–22). The small vessels are revealed in exquisite detail, far exceeding that recorded in standard film arteriograms.[23, 24] Two drawbacks of xeroarteriography are: (1) the present inability to perform rapid-sequence serial imaging, thus prohibiting study of hemodynamic factors; and (2) the fact that xeroradiographic study must be confined to a relatively thin anatomic part such as a limb, because the xeroradiographic plate is less sensitive than a film-screen combination. However, when utilized for evaluation of bone tumors in the limbs, xeroarteriography may *complement* the routine rapid-sequence film arteriographic examination.

Lymphography in the Staging of Bone Tumors. Lymphography is rarely performed for staging primary malignant bone neoplasms. Nevertheless, regional lymph node metastases occur in one third of cases of primary malignant bone tumors, and patients harboring lymph node metastases have a significantly shorter period of survival in comparison to patients with tumor-free lymph nodes.[25] In a series of 50 patients with malignant bone tumors, Makai and associates in fact demonstrated lymphographic evidence of node metastases in 19 cases, 14 of which were confirmed by lymph node biopsy. Of 14 patients with osteosarcomas in their series, 7 had lymph node metastases. Similarly, lymph node metastases were complications in 5 of 15

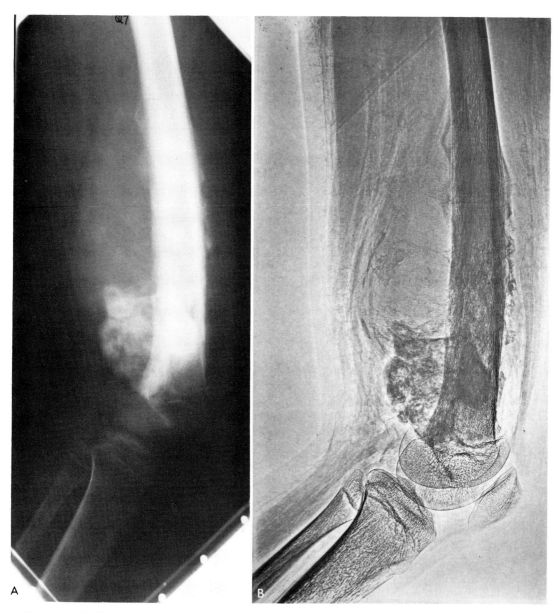

Figure 14–21   Comparison of lateral standard film radiograph (*A*) with corresponding xeroradiograph (*B*). Osteosarcoma of the femur. The xeroradiographs provide enhanced detail of bone destruction, tumor matrix mineralization, periosteal reaction, and overlying soft-tissue changes. [From Vaeth, J. M. (ed.), Frontiers of Radiation Therapy and Oncology. Vol. 10. Basel, S. Karger AG, 1975, pp. 82–107.]

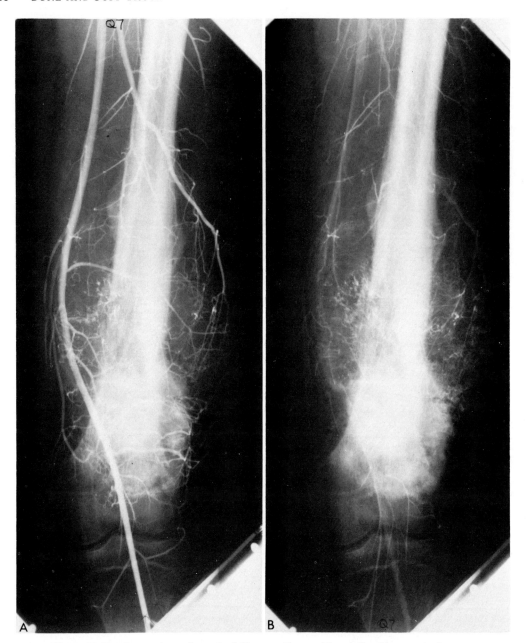

Figure 14–22 Comparison of standard film arteriogram (*A* and *B*) with xeroarteriogram.

patients with fibrosarcomas, 3 of 9 with chondrosarcomas, 3 of 4 with reticulum cell sarcomas, 1 of 5 with Ewing's sarcomas, and none of 3 with giant cell tumors.[25] Thus it would appear that lymphography may be deserving of a more prominent role in staging primary malignant bone tumors than it has occupied heretofore.

RADIOLOGY IN SOFT-TISSUE SARCOMAS OF THE LIMBS

Soft-tissue sarcomas of the limbs—malignant tumors also of mesodermal origin—comprise neoplasms derived from muscle, connective tissue, synovium, and blood

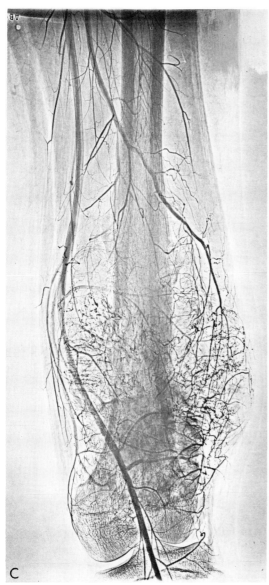

C

Figure 14-22 *Continued (C)* Osteosarcoma of femur (same case as illustrated in Figure 14-21). Edge enhancement of small vessels in the xeroarteriogram results in exquisite detail far exceeding that recorded in the film arteriogram. [From Vaeth, J. M. (ed.), Frontiers of Radiation Therapy and Oncology. Vol. 10. Basel, S. Karger AG, 1975, pp. 82–107. Courtesy of Jonathan Po, M. D., and Julius H. Grollman, Jr., M. D., University of California, Los Angeles.]

vessels. In the limbs, the most common of these relatively uncommon tumors, in descending order of frequency, are: fibrosarcoma, liposarcoma, rhabdomyosarcoma, synovial sarcoma, and neoplasms of blood

vessel supportive tissues including hemangiosarcoma, Kaposi's disease, hemangioendothelioma, and hemangiopericytoma. Lymphomas and tumors of neural supportive tissues have been omitted from this discussion.

Although soft-tissue malignant neoplasms usually appear to be pseudoencapsulated on gross pathologic examination, they frequently infiltrate microscopically into adjacent muscle and subcutaneous fat, resulting in the radiographic findings of loss of the fatty intermuscular septa and blurring of the interfaces between muscle and subcutaneous fat. In contradistinction, malignant neoplasms originating in bone usually are contained by the periosteum, resulting in the *preservation* of overlying soft-tissue structures, even when they are severely displaced outward by a bulky tumor.

Most soft-tissue neoplasms produce few, if any, radiographic clues to their origin. Although well-differentiated *liposarcomas,* like their benign counterpart, may contain enough fat to result in increased radiolucency, undifferentiated liposarcomas may not manifest this radiographic change because of hypercellularity with minimal fat in the tumor. Liposarcoma seldom occurs before age 30 and predominates in the fifth decade. *Synovial sarcoma* predominates in a relatively young age group—between 18 and 35. It usually arises in a lower limb, frequently near a joint capsule insertion but seldom within a joint, and it originates from tendon sheaths or bursae. Amorphous calcification is manifested radiographically in a minority of these tumors. Nearby bone may undergo pressure atrophy with synovial sarcoma, characterized by an extensive, well-marginated ("dished-out") cortical erosion with a sclerotic border; sometimes there is actual tumor invasion, characterized by poorly circumscribed bone destruction. *Pleomorphic rhabdomyosarcoma* seldom occurs before the sixth decade, but *embryonal rhabdomyosarcoma* occurs in infants and children. *Fibrosarcoma* occurs at all ages.

Arteriography. Opinion varies widely as to the usefulness of arteriography in the evaluation of peripheral soft-tissue tumors. Pathologic tumor neovascularity, as described by Strickland and reviewed earlier in this chapter, is frequently absent in malignant soft-tissue neoplasms but is virtually pathognomonic of malignancy *when observed*.[14] The only clinically and histologically benign lesion that manifests classic tumor neovascularity is the glomus tumor.[11] Levin and associates evaluated the arteriograms of 40 patients with peripheral soft tissue masses. Eleven of these 40 manifested coarse tumor neovascularity (as defined by Strickland), and all were histologically and/or clinically malignant. Twenty-three masses manifested only a profusion of fine arterial vessels and, during the capillary phase of the angiogram, a vascular blush. Of these 23 masses, 18 were malignant and 5 inflammatory.[26] Some malignant tumors—notably those of blood vessel supportive tissues—give rise to a characteristic angiographic pattern of strikingly increased vascularity, while others that are even more highly malignant (such as some fibrosarcomas) do not exhibit neovascularity.[27] Hyperemia may also accompany myositis ossificans circumscripta, ischemic necrosis of muscle, and certain soft-tissue inflammatory processes.

Despite the aforementioned diagnostic pitfalls, arteriography may aid in the determination of an appropriate biopsy site in soft-tissue tumors as well as in bone tumors, since the greatest vascular abnormalities tend to reside within the most malignant parts of the tumor. It is also useful in the detection of recurrent tumor after previous excision, and it will disclose the feeding arteries for perfusion or infusion chemotherapy.

References

1. Stewart, J. R., Dahlin, D. C., and Pugh, D. G.: Pathology and radiology of solitary benign bone tumors. Semin. Roentgenol., 1:268–292, 1966.
2. Lodwick, G. S.: Solitary malignant tumors of bone: The application of predictor variables in diagnosis. Semin. Roentgenol., 1:293–313, 1966.
3. Lodwick, G. S.: The Bones and Joints: An Atlas of Tumor Radiology. Chicago, Year Book Medical Publishers, 1971.
4. Ellman, H., Gold, R. H., and Mirra, J. M.: Roentgenologically "benign" but rapidly lethal diaphyseal osteosarcoma: A case report. J. Bone Joint Surg., 56A:1267–1269, 1974.
5. Ackerman, L. V., and Spjut, H. J.: Tumors of bone and cartilage. *In* Atlas of Tumor Pathology. Section II, fasc. 4. Washington, D.C., Armed Forces Institute of Pathology, 1962.
6. Dahlin, D. C.: Bone Tumors: General Aspects and Data on 3,987 Cases. 2nd ed. Springfield, Ill., Charles C Thomas, 1967.
7. Jaffe, H. L.: Tumors and Tumorous Conditions of the Bones and Joints. Philadelphia, Lea & Febiger, 1958.
8. Lichenstein, L.: Bone Tumors. 4th ed. St. Louis, C. V. Mosby, 1972.
9. Netherlands Committee on Bone Tumors. Radiological Atlas of Bone Tumors. Vol. I. Baltimore, Williams & Wilkins, 1967.
10. Herzberg, E. L., and Schreiber, M. H.: Angiography in mass lesions of the extremities. Am. J. Roentgenol. Radium Ther. Nucl. Med., 111:541–546, 1971.
11. Lagergren, C., and Lindbom, A.: Angiography of peripheral tumors. Radiology, 79:371–377, 1962.
12. Ring, S. M., Beranbaum, E. R., Madayag, M. A., et al.: Angiography of aneurysmal bone cyst. Bull. Hosp. Joint Dis., 33:1–7, 1972.
13. Steinbach, H. L.: Angiography of bones and joints. *In* Abrams, H. L. (ed.), Angiography. 2nd ed. Boston, Little, Brown, 1971, pp. 1299–1321.
14. Strickland, B.: Value of arteriography in the diagnosis of bone tumours. Br. J. Radiol., 32:705–713, 1959.
15. Sutton, D.: Percutaneous angiography with special reference to peripheral vessels. Br. J. Radiol., 28:13–25, 1955.
16. Yaghmai, I., Shamsa, A. Z., Shariat, S., et al.: Value of arteriography in the diagnosis of benign and malignant bone lesions. Cancer, 27:1134–1147, 1971.
17. Lagergren, C., Lindbom, A., and Soderberg, G.: Hypervascularization in chronic inflammation demonstrated by angiography: Angiographic, histopathologic, and microangiographic studies. Acta Radiol., 49:441–452, 1958.
18. Wolfe, J. N.: Xeroradiography: Image content and comparison with film roentgenograms. Am. J. Roentgenol. Radium Ther. Nucl. Med., 117:690–695, 1973.
19. Wolfe, J. N.: Xeroradiography of the bones, joints and soft tissues. Radiology, 93:583–587, 1969.
20. Po, J., and Grollman, J. H., Jr.: Personal communication.
21. Campbell, C. J., Roach, J., and Grisolia, A.: Comparative study of xeroroentgenography and routine roentgenography in the recording of roentgen images of bone specimens. J. Bone Joint Surg., 39A:577–582, 1957.
22. Hills, T. H., Stanford, R. W., and Moore, R. D.: Xeroradiography. II. Present medical applications. Br. J. Radiol., 28:545–551, 1955.
23. James, P., Baddeley, H., Boag, J. W., et al.: Xeroradiography–its use in peripheral contrast medium angiography. Clin. Radiol., 24:67–71, 1973.
24. Parsavand, R.: Infusion angiography using xeroradiography. Radiology, 112:739–740, 1974.
25. Makai, F., Belán, A., and Málek, P.: Lymphatic metastases of bone tumors. Lymphology, 3:109–116, 1971.
26. Levin, D. C., Watson, R. C., and Baltaxe, H. A.: Arteriography in diagnosis and management of acquired peripheral soft-tissue masses. Radiology, 103:53–58, 1972.
27. Cockshott, W. P., and Evans, K. T.: The place of soft tissue arteriography. Br. J. Radiol., 37:367–375, 1964.

Chapter Fifteen

INTRACRANIAL NEOPLASMS

Hervey D. Segall, M.D.

CLINICAL CONSIDERATIONS

The first symptom of an intracranial neoplasm is determined more by the site of the lesion than its histology.[1] Overall, headache is the most common single symptom. Complaints referable to disorders of locomotion, speech, sensation, vision, and position sense may be caused by lesions in the posterior half of the cerebral hemispheres. Patients with anterior temporal and frontal lesions often have seizures and an organic brain syndrome as their earliest symptoms. However, increased intracranial pressure from any cause may also lead to impairment of mental function. Deep hemispheric lesions may produce movement disorders. Tumors of the hypothalamic-hypophyseal area cause endocrinopathies and visual loss, while posterior fossa neoplasms are associated with ataxia, dysmetria, clumsiness, or symptoms referable to dysfunction of any of the cranial nerves. Obstruction to the egress of cerebrospinal fluid caused by a neoplasm encroaching on the ventricular system is responsible for accompanying complaints related to a generalized increase in intracranial pressure.[2]

The clinical signs that may be associated with intracranial neoplasms comprise the full spectrum of cerebral hemispheric, cerebellar, and brain stem dysfunctions. Abnormalities may be demonstrable in any part of the neurologic examination including assessment of mental status, tests of the motor, sensory, reflex, and speech patterns, and evaluation of the cranial nerves and cerebellar and parietal lobes, as well as the neuro-endocrine evaluation.[3]

The following conditions most commonly simulate tumors and are the most frequent differential considerations: (1) developmental anomalies, including cysts, Arnold-Chiari malformations, and aqueductal stenosis; (2) vascular disorders, including thromboembolic disease, aneurysm, arteriovenous malformation, and hematoma (acute intracerebral hematomas can also be a manifestation of an intracerebral neoplasm); (3) post-traumatic sequelae, particularly an extracerebral hematoma of the chronic subdural type; (4) infectious and granulomatous disorders, including intracerebral and subdural abscess, encephalitis, lues, tuberculosis, parasitic and sarcoid lesions; (5) toxic and metabolic disorders, particularly those related to renal, hepatic, or endocrine dysfunctions, and (6) degenerative and demyelinating disorders, particularly Alzheimer's disease, Pick's disease, and multiple sclerosis. In addition, the syndromes of "normal"-pressure hydrocephalus and pseudotumor cerebri often merit consideration.[4]

Since it would require several volumes to describe in detail the clinical and radiologic features of intracranial tumors and the differential possibilities that must be considered, the emphasis of this chapter will be placed on the *types of radiologic examinations* now available, from the simple skull series to some of the most complex diagnostic modalities now employed in medicine. Examples will be cited of their respective contributions (and limitations) in practical decision making and clinical care.

313

SKULL ROENTGENOGRAPHY

A plain skull series, which should comprise multiple projections (including postero-anterior and Towne views, both lateral projections, and a standard base projection), is an innocuous study that should be obtained routinely for patients suspected of having an intracranial neoplasm. More information will be derived from the plain skull series, if the examination is monitored by a radiologist who is aware that additional special projections beyond the more conventional views may prove useful in a given patient. Tomography (body-section radiography) may also be indicated in special situations, particularly in the examination of anatomically intricate areas such as the petrous bone, where overlapping structures may impede plain film interpretation.

A negative plain skull examination by no means *excludes* an intracranial neoplasm. In one series, for example, almost one half of children with brain tumors also had normal skull roentgenograms.[5] However, as a result of an intracranial tumor, any of the following radiographic findings may become evident: skull manifestations of intracranial hypertension (see below), displacement of the pineal body and other normally calcified structures, enlargement of the sella turcica, enlargement or destruction of certain cranial foramina and canals, bone thinning or destruction, hyperostosis, enlargement of cranial vascular channels, a soft-tissue "mass" bulging into an air-containing paranasal sinus, focal swelling of the soft tissues, and pathologic calcifications. However, there are also benign, non-neoplastic causes of *any* of the above findings on plain skull films. Thus, in addition to being relatively insensitive for detecting tumors, the plain skull roentgenogram findings are often quite *nonspecific.*

Increased intracranial pressure may result from the mass effect of a neoplasm (including the associated edema), its obstruction of the ventricular and subarachnoid pathways, or a combination of both. In children in the first decade of life who have intracranial hypertension, plain skull roentgenograms may demonstrate widening of the cranial sutures. However, one must also be alert to the fact that abnormally wide sutures may occasionally occur in the absence of intracranial hypertension (for

example, with delayed ossification because of cretinism, or during rapid brain growth following recovery from malnutrition).

With increasing age, other skull film manifestations of elevated pressure are more likely to be observed, including erosion of the floor and dorsum of the sella (these changes occur only after *at least six weeks* of elevated intracranial pressure). The "beaten-silver" appearance of the inner table of the skull is rarely seen today, since it is a manifestation of very long-standing intracranial hypertension. Digital markings on the inner table of the skull, which simulate the "beaten-silver" appearance of long-standing cranial hypertension, may be rather pronounced in normal children, adolescents, and young adults, and they may be interpreted erroneously as a manifestation of increased pressure by the inexperienced observer.[12]

Plain skull film tumor *calcifications* are rarely seen with gliomas, but are more frequent with oligodendrogliomas and ependymomas. A focus of intracerebral calcium in a suspected tumor, however, may be impossible to differentiate from calcium within a granuloma, hematoma, vascular malformation, or other *non*-neoplastic condition. Occasionally, various types of calcifications are also demonstrated roentgenologically in meningiomas. The pattern of calcifications is usually not diagnostic, but deposits found in areas where meningiomas are common (e.g., the parasaggital area, sphenoid ridge and suprasellar region, or posterior fossa) are very suggestive. When bone changes typical of a meningioma are also found adjacent to a focus of calcium within one of these areas, a correct diagnosis of meningioma is virtually assured. Enlarged meningeal vascular channels in the skull leading toward such abnormal foci provide additional confirmatory information.

Abnormal roentgenographic calcification is common within intrasellar and suprasellar craniopharyngiomas and is almost invariably found in these lesions when the patient is a child. In fact, in a child, nodular or curvilinear calcification within or above an enlarged sella (the sella having an intact bony cortex, which itself may be increased in density) is unlikely to be caused by anything but a craniopharyngioma (Fig. 15–1).[17,18]

Plain film calcification is observed not

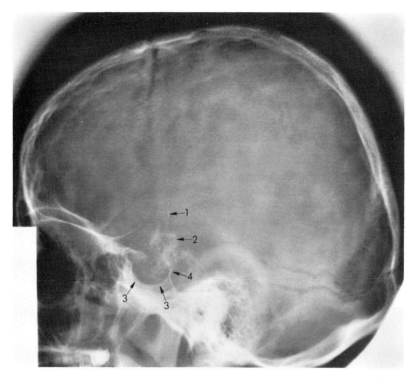

Figure 15–1   Lateral skull radiograph. Craniopharyngioma, with calcifications and sellar enlargement. 1, faint curvilinear calcification (vertical) that delimits the margin of a cystic portion of the tumor. 2, amorphous calcification within a solid portion of the tumor. 3, the intact sellar floor. 4, the thinned dorsum sellae.

infrequently within pinealomas and chordomas.[19] Intracranial chondromas of the inner table or skull base are rare, but are likely to calcify. Rare lipomas of the corpus callosum are readily diagnosed by the combination of curvilinear calcium and a localized fatty lucency on skull films, as well as by their typical location. Infrequently, calcifications are seen in slowly growing intracranial metastases and in pituitary adenomas and dermoids. It may be most helpful to review carefully with the neuroradiologist all films suspected of showing abnormal intracranial calcifications, because *artifacts* produced by hair braids, electroencephalogram paste, and other foreign materials will sometimes be found to be responsible for these densities.

Bone destruction may be seen on plain skull films in the presence of meningioma, neurinoma, chordoma, and other intracranial tumors as well as with metastases, solitary myeloma, and multiple myeloma involving the calvarium.[7,20–23] Necrosis of calvarial bone following intensive radiation therapy for a brain tumor may give a roentgeno-graphic appearance similar to some of these lesions, but it is usually characterized by its restriction to the area of the radiotherapy portal. Bone destruction may also be produced by benign lesions such as eosinophilic granuloma, osteomyelitis, or leptomeningeal cyst. On the other hand, some meningiomas incite the formation of *new* bone (sclerosis) within the adjacent skull table, or in the sphenoid or petrous ridges.

Enlargement or destruction of the various neurovascular skull foramina and canals may be produced by lesions such as optic glioma, glomus jugulare tumor, and neurinomas of the fifth, seventh, eighth, ninth, and eleventh nerves.[6–8,11]

Pituitary adenomas and the less common pituitary carcinoma may enlarge the sella turcica. Eosinophilic pituitary adenomas may be associated with other skull findings that indicate acromegaly, such as thickening of the skull tables, enlargement of the paranasal sinuses, and prognathism. Enlargement of the sella can be caused by non-neoplastic conditions (see also the earlier discussion of intracranial hypertension), such as a carotid aneurysm or an "empty" sella (herniation of the subarachnoid space into the sella). This emphasizes the potential importance of angiography and pneumoencephalography in the examination of the patient with sellar enlargement (see below).[18,24]

Findings on the plain skull roentgenograms may occasionally contribute to a decision regarding subsequent steps in the diagnostic examination. A calcified pineal body that has shifted away from an expanded cerebral hemisphere may indicate the side that will be shown at arteriography to harbor an intracranial lesion. (However, it should be remembered that unilateral cerebral atrophy can also cause a pineal shift toward the *atrophic* side.) Recognition of pressure changes on skull films may cause lumbar puncture and pneumoencephalography to be deferred or avoided, because of the increased danger associated with these procedures in patients who have intracranial hypertension.

Plain skull roentgenograms obtained *after* surgery may indicate how much of a calcified tumor has been removed. A bulging bone flap on skull films made after a craniotomy may give evidence that a hematoma is present or that hydrocephalus or tumor recurrence has developed. Displacement of metallic surgical clips may also indicate new growth of a neoplasm or development of a complicating lesion. In patients treated with ventricular shunts for hydrocephalus secondary to an obstructing tumor, plain skull films may indicate whether or not placement of the shunt tubing is satisfactory and may also reveal the appearance of pressure changes when shunt dysfunction occurs.

It may be appreciated from the above illustrations that the skull series may demonstrate a variety of useful findings in the presence of intracranial tumors and following their treatment. Frequently, the observed changes are not specific enough to permit a diagnosis, but the findings on skull roentgenography may indicate useful directions for further clinical and radiologic study.[25,26]

RADIONUCLIDE BRAIN SCANNING

Increased radionuclide uptake within an intracranial neoplasm is explained by breakdown of the normal "blood-brain barrier," by increased vascularity of the tumor, or by active accumulation of radionuclide within the tumor. A tumor thereby may be detectable as a "hot spot" on the brain scan (Figs. 15–2 and 15–7B). The scanning technique requires prior intravenous injection of a radiopharmaceutical, but this examination is safe and may be requested with less trepidation than angiography or other invasive neuroradiologic procedures. Technetium-99m pertechnetate and its chelates are now the standard preparations, with other radionuclides being useful in certain circumstances. Scanning for tumors is best delayed at least several hours following intravenous injection of radionuclide.[29–32]

Another noninvasive examination, computerized axial tomography (see the next section), only recently developed, generally offers more information than the radionuclide scan. As a result, it now appears that the radionuclide brain scan will have a diminished role in the future.

Intracranial neoplasms are frequently picked up by the brain scan (in 80 to 85 per cent of cases); however, the brain scan lacks the ability of angiography to provide specific anatomic information or vascular detail suggesting the pathologic nature of the lesion. Abscesses, encephalitis, hematomas, infarcts, cerebral contusions, vascular malformations, multiple sclerosis, and lesions of the cranium can all produce "hot spots" identical to those of neoplasms on the brain scan.[33–38]

The configuration and location of a "hot spot" or the available clinical information may nevertheless suggest that one is dealing with cerebral infarction or hematoma rather than neoplasm. In such cases, *serial* brain scans showing resolution over a period of weeks may confirm the probability of a non-neoplastic process, thus averting craniotomy.

Serial scintiangiography (dynamic vascular flow studies, requiring serial images of the brain during and immediately following radionuclide injection) has been useful in suggesting that a specific lesion found on a standard brain scan might be an arteriovenous malformation.[7,30,35,39,40] Early vascular accumulation of the radionuclide within the malformation, with subsequent rapid "washout," is characteristic. It should be pointed out, however, that a similar appear-

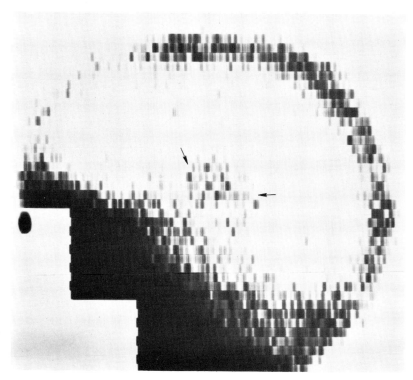

Figure 15–2 Radionuclide brain scan using technetium-99m pertechnetate; left lateral scan. The arrows indicate an abnormal area of radionuclide uptake. This scan result was an indication for performing further neuroradiologic procedures. Craniotomy finally revealed an ependymoma. (Courtesy of Shelby Miller, M. D.)

ance may also occur with certain vascular tumors, although the vascular washout is usually not as fast. The rapid appearance of an abnormality on the dynamic study, combined with the subsequent persistence of this abnormality on the delayed standard scan, will point toward a diagnosis of a meningioma or a vascular glioma.[41] Most other intracranial tumors are not shown during the dynamic vascular flow phase of the study.

Correlation of the plain skull films with the brain scan may help to identify those few "positive" scans that result from cranial osseous lesions.[42] Technetium-99m polyphosphate (a bone scanning agent) will delineate early neoplasms involving the calvarium, even when the plain skull films still appear normal. Technetium-99m polyphosphate may also demonstrate sphenoid wing meningiomas undetected by the technetium-99m pertechnetate brain scan.

Because the radionuclide brain scan is simple and noninvasive, it has traditionally been an important *screening test* for patients with a suspected intracranial neoplasm. A negative brain scan might terminate, for the time being, the diagnostic tumor ex-

amination of a patient for whom the index of clinical suspicion already is low. However, because of the relatively high false-negative rate of scans for intracranial tumors, the examination should certainly proceed even if the brain scan is "normal" when the clinical findings and other diagnostic information warrant it.

A "positive" brain scan may help to direct further examination. It may assist in determining which vascular system should be injected at angiography, and it may also indicate for the neuroradiologist those areas of the brain that merit the most careful scrutiny when angiographic or other special study abnormalities are not readily apparent. The scan may assist the neurosurgeon to decide which section of a cerebral neoplasm would be best for a biopsy by indicating areas of highest tumor "activity." The presence of multiple "hot" areas on the brain scan suggest that one may be dealing with metastatic intracranial disease. Although the radionuclide brain scan is considered a screening test for angiography, it may be diagnostically superior in an occasional case, depicting a lesion that is not demonstrable angiographically.

Certain neoplasms are depicted with greater accuracy on scans than others: glioblastomas and meningiomas are detected by brain scanning in 90 to 95 per cent of cases, perhaps because of extensive alteration of the blood-brain barrier (in glioblastomas) or profuse tumor vascularity with retention of radionuclide within the tumor. Metastatic deposits are detected with less accuracy (about 75 to 80 per cent), while only two thirds of low-grade astrocytomas are visualized. The location of the tumor is another factor affecting diagnostic accuracy. A lesion is more difficult to diagnose when it cannot be separated easily from large vascular structures normally seen on the brain scan, such as the dural sinuses. Lesions close to the skull base, such as intrasellar tumors and brain stem tumors, can be very difficult to detect on scans. Tumor size is another variable; for example, acoustic tumors over 2 cm in size often can be detected despite their proximity to the petrous bone, whereas smaller neuromas of the eighth nerve escape detection on the technetium brain scan.

In patients who have undergone craniotomy, a combination of the radionuclide gallium-67 citrate (which tends to localize within residual or recurring cerebral neoplasms, but not in bone) and bone-seeking technetium-99m polyphosphate (which often outlines the periphery of the craniotomy) may prove useful. Because uptake of radionuclide does occur postoperatively around the margins of the craniotomy defect, it may be useful to obtain a brain scan within two or three months after resection of the brain tumor as a *baseline* for later scans. An increase in nuclide uptake on later scans, particularly at some distance from the margins of the craniotomy, may indicate recurrent tumor.[43]

COMPUTERIZED AXIAL TOMOGRAPHY*

A completely new technique for examining the brain and related structures has recently become available. By giving considerably more information than radionu-

clide brain scanning and permitting diagnoses that sometimes elude even cerebral angiography and pneumography, computerized axial tomography (CT) is making a remarkable impact on the field of neuroradiology. These examinations may be performed with or without intravenous contrast materials and with little hazard or discomfort to the patient. A complete CT examination gives an x-ray dose to the patient roughly equivalent to a conventional skull series.

This new imaging technique is based on the fact that various tissues within the body, including those which differ only slightly in physical density and atomic number, absorb different quantities of incident x-ray photons. The cerebral tissues and cerebrospinal fluid also differ slightly in their x-ray absorption coefficients; while these small differences in x-ray absorption are not appreciated with conventional radiographic techniques, they can be exploited with computerized axial tomography.[44-46]

With this new technique, a narrow beam of x-rays is rotated slowly about the patient's head, which is inserted into a latex cap within a plastic water-containing box. Thousands of x-ray readings are recorded by extremely sensitive detectors moving in parallel and rotating with the x-ray tube, over a period of several minutes.

After a mini-computer within the machine processes the recorded information, a picture is constructed on a cathode ray tube that represents a "mosaic" of relative absorption values within tiny individual zones of tissue in the patient's head. A Polaroid picture is then made from the cathode ray tube that illustrates a single transaxial "slice" or cross-section through the skull and brain (Figs. 15–3 and 15–4). Usually, eight or more different "slices" (8 or 13 mm thick) are obtained during the course of a complete CT examination. Locations of the cross-sections range from the skull base and posterior fossa, upward to the skull vertex.

Using a standard gray-scale display for depicting intracranial anatomy, the cerebral ventricles and subarachnoid cisterns appear black (Fig. 15–4*A*) or dark gray. In fact, air or fatty tissue produces the blackest of tones; cerebral soft tissues appear as light gray, while tissues with a higher coefficient of

---

*Sometimes referred to as "EMI" or "ACTA" scanning, by association with some of the prototype units used for CT scanning.

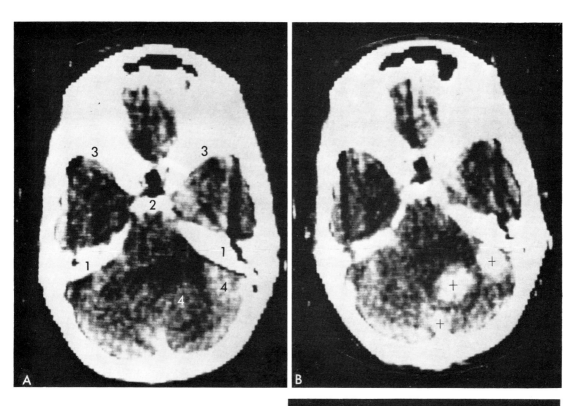

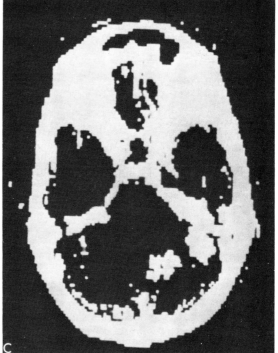

Figure 15–3 Computerized tomographic (CT) scan. Cerebellar metastases. *A,* Without intravenous contrast. This "slice" shows the normal bony anatomy of the petrous ridges (1), the dorsum sellae (2), and sphenoid ridges (3). In addition, two areas of slightly increased tissue absorption are seen involving the right part of the cerebellum (4); however, it might be difficult to be certain that these are true abnormalities without the subsequent injection of intravenous contrast material (as demonstrated in *B*). *B,* following the injection of iodinated contrast material intravenously, three metastases within the cerebellum are clearly demonstrated. These are indicated by +. *C,* By changing the machine "window level" and "window width," the three metastases shown in *A* and *B* are demonstrated even more dramatically in the posterior fossa. (All scans courtesy of Robert Levis, M. D.)

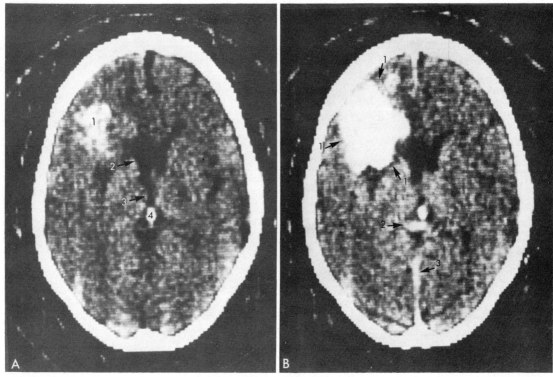

Figure 15–4 *A,* CT scan prior to injection of intravenous contrast material. Calcified meningioma. 1, a high-density area is due to calcification *within* the tumor, but the actual margins of the tumor are not demonstrated. 2, there is some displacement of the fluid-filled frontal horns (shown in black) from left to right. 3, the third ventricle is also slightly displaced from left to right. 4, the slightly displaced, calcified (shown in white) pineal gland. *B,* CT scan following the intravenous injection of iodinated contrast material; the true dimensions of this vascularized meningioma are indicated by arrows (1). Furthermore, as a result of intravenous injection of contrast material, vasculature in the region of the pineal (2, showing large veins in the pineal region) and in the region of the straight sinus (3) has now become apparent. (Both scans courtesy of Phillip Shiu, M. D.)

absorption, such as bone or the calcified pineal body (Fig. 15–4*A*) or choroid plexus glomera, appear white on the scan. Calcium-containing brain lesions, as well as clotted blood, also appear in white on the Polaroid print. Extremely white densities are produced by residual Pantopaque and metallic surgical clips. At present, these expensive computized tomographic units are generally being installed only in larger hospitals. A prototype, the EMI Scanner, has been marketed for close to $500,000.

While the CT examination falls in the category of noninvasive tests without risk to the patient, an intravenous injection of iodine-containing contrast material may also be performed in conjunction with this examination to demonstrate the vascularity of lesions and to enhance the contrast between a lesion and normal tissue. With intravenous contrast infusion, it is also sometimes possible to demonstrate or to confirm certain lesions not readily appreciated on the standard CT scan (Fig. 15–3*B*).[46]

Not only has the new CT scan been useful in the demonstration of neoplastic lesions (Figs. 15–3*B* and 15–4*B*), but it also gives additional information about a tumor and its effects on the brain and the ventricular system. Cystic areas within a neoplasm and edema of the brain surrounding it may be visualized, and hydrocephalus resulting from a tumor is also readily apparent. When more than one tumor nodule is present, CT scanning will readily denote multiplicity, a finding again strongly suggesting metastatic disease.

Even without intravenous contrast material, it is possible to diagnose (or at least to suggest) other *non*-tumorous conditions such as hematoma, cerebral infarct, pseudotumor cerebri, and cerebral atrophy.

The CT scan method can identify hemorrhagic areas associated with aneurysms and arteriovenous malformations, but angiography will still remain paramount in the investigation of these conditions.[44]

Gliomas

Results with CT scans have been impressive, and it appears that very few (about 3 per cent) symptomatic gliomas are being missed. Intravenous contrast enhancement may be useful in separating some tumors from infarcts or non-neoplastic cysts, and it may also be helpful in identifying small neoplasms earlier. CT scans appear to be superior to radionuclide scans in detecting intracerebral lesions, and they are often superior to angiography in suggesting the actual type and extent of a lesion.

Low-or intermediate-grade astrocytomas appear on the CT scan (without intravenous contrast) as irregularly marginated, gray-black lesions that are more lucent (having lesser x-ray absorption) than normal brain. Glioblastomas may have a similar appearance, but they commonly also have poorly defined patches of increased density (white areas) caused by intra-tumoral hemorrhage or by the aggregates of densely packed tumor cells themselves. Calcific foci within these tumors may also be readily observed on the CT scan. Cystic changes within cerebral tumors may sometimes be recognized on the scan but are not always apparent (inasmuch as the highly proteinaceous neoplastic cyst fluid may be similar in density to brain). In the brain stem, the demonstration of a cystic component within a tumor may encourage palliative surgery that might otherwise not be attempted. Although it may be difficult in this location to differentiate inflammatory lesions, encephalomalacia, and infarcts from gliomas, the *exclusion* of a cyst, abscess, or blood clot may permit nonsurgical treatment. Small hypothalamic and optic chiasm gliomas may be missed by the CT scan, but they can be demonstrated subsequently by air-contrast examinations (see below).

As indicated previously, brain infarcts may also have reduced x-ray absorption, appearing darker than normal brain tissue on the CT scan, but often differentiation from a tumor can be made on the basis of the smoother contours and lesser mass effect of an infarct. Intra-lesional areas of greater density mimicking a glioblastoma may be seen with a hemorrhagic brain infarction. When there is a problem in the differential diagnosis, re-examination in ten to fourteen days often helps: the neoplasm is usually static or larger, while edema accompanying an infarction may have subsided to some degree.

Metastases

Metastases as small as 6 to 9 mm can be visualized on CT scans.[46] Intravenous contrast enhancement has made it easier to identify these smaller nodules when they are vascular. Experience thus far indicates that the CT scan is more effective than the radionuclide brain scan in demonstrating metastatic lesions. This new method is also superior to angiography in diagnosing the presence, size, and distribution of intra-cerebral metastases. In general, the CT scan appears always to be superior to other neuroradiologic modalities and to radio-nuclide brain scanning, in particular, in demonstrating multiple lesions. Patients shown to have multiple intracranial metastases on CT scans may be referred for radiotherapy, thus circumventing difficult angiographic and pneumographic studies, if it is felt that other lesions which may be multiple (such as abscesses) can be ruled out.[47,48]

Meningiomas

Although some meningiomas reportedly have not been shown on CT scans, New and associates believe that the accuracy rate of CT scan diagnosis of meningioma is close to 100 per cent when the technique is utilized with skill and care.[46] Meningiomas frequently appear on the CT scan as homogeneous whitish (high-absorption) lesions near the inner skull table or skull base, having a density similar to hematomas. Although the history and clinical findings with these two types of lesions differ, distinction on the CT scans may also be made utilizing an injection of intravenous contrast material that will increase the density of meningiomas

(Fig. 15–4*B*) (the scan density of hematomas remains unchanged). Calcification within meningiomas (Fig. 15–4*A*) can also be recognized (in these cases, the lesional density or whiteness is extremely high), but the calcified regions of course show little or no increase in density following the injection of contrast material. Some meningiomas have a CT scan density only slightly higher than that of normal brain. In these patients, contrast infusion is most useful, effecting an increase in density associated with the vascularity of the tumor.

In meningiomas, plain skull films and tomograms may yield additional correlative information. The peculiar *texture* of meningioma calcification is better appreciated on standard skull films than on CT scans, and areas of cranial hyperostosis and bone lysis are also better demonstrated. Enlarged vascular grooves and pressure changes may also be shown with the standard roentgenograms. It appears, however, that radionuclide brain scanning will assume a less important role in the diagnosis of suspected meningiomas and may be deleted from the examination of most of these patients in the future. However, angiography will still be useful in some cases and occasionally will give additional diagnostic information, particularly in the region of the sella.

Tumors Close to the Skull Base

For a number of technical reasons, lesions close to the skull base are situated less favorably for CT scan demonstration and analysis. In the diagnosis of acoustic neuromas and other *cerebellopontine angle tumors,* high-quality plain skull films and tomography are essential. CT scans in these cases (including intravenous contrast enhancement) will be an important supplemental technique. However, tiny acoustic neuromas will be missed by CT scanning and will still require Pantopaque cisternography for diagnosis. Even with larger tumors, some neurosurgeons will undoubtedly also desire preoperative angiographic evaluation to demonstrate the vascular anatomy; in addition, pneumography and brain scanning will probably still play a role, particularly when CT scans are equivocal or negative.

Pituitary adenomas and *craniopharyngio-*

mas are less advantageously situated for CT scan evaluation because of their proximity to the skull base. However, cystic collections within these lesions can often be shown on a CT scan, particularly when the absorption coefficient of the cyst fluid is sufficiently low (high-lipid fluid contents have low x-ray absorptions and are especially suitable for CT scan demonstration). In this regard, CT scanning has a considerable advantage over other neuroradiologic techniques and may be of fundamental importance in determining the appropriate surgical approach and treatment (cyst drainage, attempted removal, or other).

From the above, it is apparent that computerized axial tomography is having, and will continue to have, an enormous impact in the diagnosis of intracranial neoplasms. However, as with all diagnostic modalities, this new method has limitations. CT scanning does not obviate the need for a complete skull series, which should be interpreted along with the CT scan. Details of changes in the bone (erosions, hyperostotic areas, pressure changes) are appreciated on the skull series but not on the CT scan. Likewise, the image resolution of a CT scan is not yet sufficiently detailed to ascertain the texture and pattern of intracranial calcifications, even while the CT scan is more sensitive to the *presence* of intracerebral calcium than the plain skull radiograph. As with any other radiographic technique, movement of the patient may prevent a satisfactory examination. This problem is even more germane to CT scanning, however, since each scan requires several minutes to perform.* As indicated above, only angiography can demonstrate precisely the vascular anatomy that will be encountered at surgery, as well as the vessels actually feeding a tumor and the morphology of vessels within a tumor or malformation.

It should be apparent that the CT scan, by virtue of its great safety and high information yield, will be invaluable as a follow-up diagnostic method after therapy. It will be useful in ascertaining tumor regression or recurrence, and it may also be used to follow ventricular size in postoperative patients. It

---

*Newer equipment, currently becoming available, promises to decrease individual CT scan times considerably, to 20 seconds or even less. Improved spatial resolution is also being offered now.

will also be helpful in the diagnosis of post-operative complications, including hematomas and fluid collections.

In summary, CT scanning carries no risk except when intravenous contrast enhancement is used (in which case the risk can be regarded as minimal, about the same as for an intravenous pyelogram). This remarkable new technique permits clear visualization of the ventricles, subarachnoid spaces, and other intracranial structures. Because of differences in density from the normal brain, tumors of various kinds can be demonstrated with a high degree of accuracy. Cystic as well as hemorrhagic or calcific foci within tumors may also be appreciated because of density differences in the lesions. Multiple intracranial lesions that are characteristic of metastatic disease are depicted with greater accuracy by CT scanning than by any other technique.

ULTRASOUND

In general, cerebral ultrasound examination[49, 50] does not add much to the information that can be derived from other modalities discussed in this chapter. However, there are important individual exceptions, as in the case of the patient who lacks a calcified pineal body and whose clinical status alone may not warrant or permit more difficult studies; in this case, A-mode ultrasound measurement for determining midline displacement can occasionally be helpful (provided the examination is performed and interpreted by an expert).[50] Ultrasound is apparently without risk (unlike the examinations employing contrast materials), and the equipment is relatively inexpensive, particularly when compared to that needed for computerized tomography. Ultrasound may also be used for measurement of third and lateral ventricle size, for the characterization of space-occupying lesions as cystic or solid, and the anatomic localization of the brain stem. For a fuller discussion of these applications, the reader is referred to the article by Tenner and associates.[50]

CEREBRAL ANGIOGRAPHY

Following the injection of iodinated contrast materials into the carotid or vertebral arteries, the immediate serial demonstration of intracranial arteries and veins in various projections may be accomplished. The details of various angiographic techniques are important to the neuroradiologist but will not be considered here.

Although serious complications resulting from cerebral angiography are not common, they unfortunately do occur; therefore, one does not subject the patient to cerebral angiography without good reason.[51, 52] Because of their specialized knowledge and experience, the neurologist or neurosurgeon should first be consulted; it is their prerogative to initiate arrangements for angiographic examinations, which are best performed under the direction of a trained neuroradiologist.

In some cases, the diagnosis of an intracranial neoplasm can be made with certainty on the basis of a cerebral angiogram (Figs. 15–5 and 15–6). The angiographic demonstration of characteristic tumor vessels within the brain substance may permit the diagnosis of a malignant intra-axial neoplasm with virtual certainty. Irregular, dilated, and tortuous tumor vessels occurring in wild tangles and irregular meshworks usually indicate a grade III or IV glioblastoma, although hypervascular metastases, angioblastic meningiomas, meningeal sarcomas, and choroid plexus neoplasms occasionally may present similar angiographic appearances.[53–59] There is a rough correlation between the degree of vascularity on the angiogram and the malignant grade of a tumor.[58]

Meningiomas, the majority of which are benign, nevertheless demand surgical intervention if lasting control is to be expected. A confident angiographic diagnosis can often be made preoperatively in these cases. A characteristic, well-defined and homogenous juxtameningeal tumor blush, lasting into the venous phase of the angiogram, may be demonstrated. Radially arranged vessels supplying the meningioma are also characteristic. *External* carotid vessels feeding the tumor have diagnostic significance and favor a meningioma; they also need to be reckoned with at surgery. The extra-axial location (growing outside of the brain substance) of this particular lesion may be evident angiographically.[60–66]

It is evident, therefore, that very specific diagnostic information may sometimes be

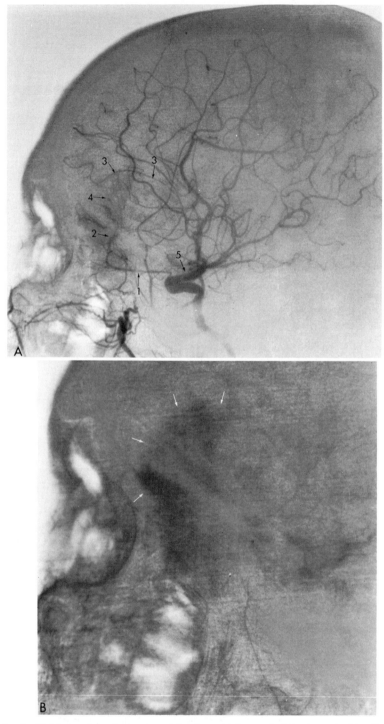

Figure 15–5   *A,* Right carotid arteriogram, lateral projection arterial phase (subtraction film). Subfrontal meningioma. The ophthalmic artery (1) gives rise to abnormally large posterior ethmoidal branches (2) that supply the tumor. This subfrontal tumor elevates and stretches the frontopolar artery (3). 4, a very early *arterial* tumor "stain." 5, depression and posterior displacement of the supraclinoid portion of the internal carotid artery, with resultant closing of the carotid siphon. *B,* Several seconds later, during the *capillary phase,* a somewhat homogeneous "stain" (arrows) is visible within this subfrontal meningioma.

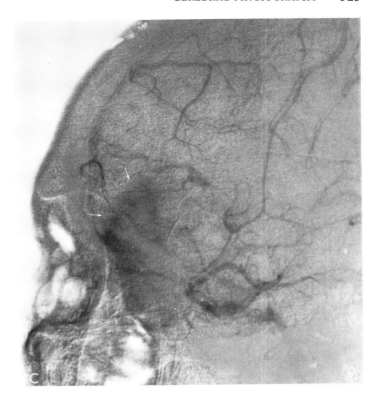

Figure 15–5 *Continued C,* the meningioma "stain" (arrows) persists also into the *venous phase* of the carotid arteriogram (several seconds after *B*).

obtainable only with angiography. On the other hand, it should be pointed out that the astrocytoma and the meningioma by no means always show characteristic angiographic findings. In fact, they occasionally may share certain angiographic features, so that one may be confused with the other.[67] The experienced neuroradiologist seldom has difficulty differentiating a neoplasm from an arteriovenous malformation. As an example of differential diagnostic difficulties that can arise, however, it may be hard to be certain angiographically that a cerebellar arteriovenous malformation with a "mass" caused by an associated hematoma is not in fact a hemangioblastoma.

With new improvements in angiographic techniques it has become apparent that pituitary adenomas can also "stain" on angiograms; this may mean that an air-contrast study will not be needed in some patients. Craniopharyngiomas may also exhibit tumor vascularity, on occasion, as may some teratomatous tumors. Neurinomas (arising most commonly from the eighth and fifth cranial nerves) are also occasionally vascular, and vascular glomus tumors may be situated intracranially. With some tumors, even some highly malignant glioblastomas,

only a mass will be demonstrated, without evident tumor vessels (Fig. 15–7 *A*): these lesions cannot be differentiated angiographically from a number of other lesions producing a mass effect, such as abscess, hematoma, benign cyst, and even encephalitis. Early filling of cerebral veins draining a lesion or a nonspecific angiographic stain may suggest a neoplasm, but these findings are also less diagnostic than the presence of tumor vessels; these findings can be seen, for example, in cerebral contusions, infarcts, and cerebritis.[68–70] Tumor vessels demonstrated in two or more separate locations of the brain suggest metastatic disease, although multifocal gliomas can occur rarely. Multiple cerebral lesions without the characteristic angiographic signature of a neoplasm may well be metastases, but it is important to keep in mind that other nonneoplastic lesions, such as abscesses, may also be multifocal.

In addition to providing a diagnosis of neoplasm, the angiogram may permit precise tumor localization and therefore assist in determining operability. It depicts the vascularity of a tumor and delineates the supplying vessels, with implications for developing the appropriate surgical strategy. The

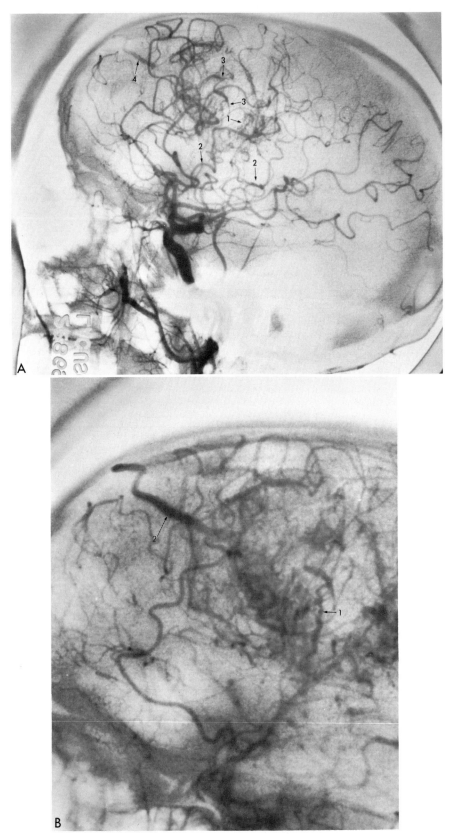

Figure 15–6 *See legend on the opposite page.*

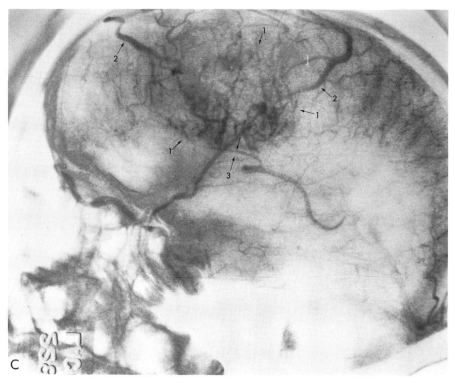

Figure 15–6 *A,* Lateral view left carotid arteriogram, *arterial phase* (subtraction technique). Glioblastoma multiforme. 1, irregular vessels within the tumor. 2, depression of the "sylvian triangle" of middle cerebral vessels. 3, the abrupt narrowing of some vessels in the region of the tumor due to tumor encasement. 4, premature filling of a vein due to abnormal arterial-venous shunting within the tumor. *B,* Several seconds later in arterial phase (same patient as in *A*). 1, an irregular and abnormal vessel within this frontal lobe glioblastoma. 2, further early filling of the draining vein (compare with 4 in *A*). *C,* Lateral projection, *venous phase* (several seconds after *B*). 1, the margins of abnormal vascularity outlining the tumor. 2, large veins draining the tumor. 3, depression of a vein (the anterior caudate vein) within the right frontal horn, caused by this large frontal lobe tumor.

preoperative angiogram also shows valuable vascular landmarks for the neurosurgeon; it may be useful in this regard even when it is "normal" and when the diagnosis of tumor has been established by other studies.[71]

Superior sagittal sinus invasion or occlusion by a meningioma can be recognized angiographically. This also is important in planning surgical treatment. On the other hand, an arteriogram may disclose that the patient's symptoms are *not* due to a neoplasm, but rather are caused by an aneurysm, an arteriovenous malformation, or a subdural blood or fluid collection.

Angiography may also be informative as a follow-up examination after operation or radiotherapy for a tumor.[72] An angiogram of a patient who is doing poorly after surgery may, for example, disclose the development of a subdural hematoma, hydrocephalus, or

a vascular occlusion (occasionally caused by a misplaced surgical clip). The likelihood that tumor recurrence accounts for deterioration in a patient's clinical status may also be evaluated angiographically. Severe cerebral arteritis with occlusive vascular disease after intensive radiotherapy has also been observed.[73] Residual or recurrent tumor, subdural blood or fluid collections, and ventricular dilatation also can be diagnosed with computerized tomography, but post-treatment vascular complications will still be depicted best with arteriography.

In summary, cerebral angiography carries some risk but may offer unique information that is unobtainable by other means. Lesions can be accurately localized, meningiomas or malignant intracerebral neoplasms can be confidently diagnosed, the vascular anatomy in the area of a lesion can be well outlined, and other information, such

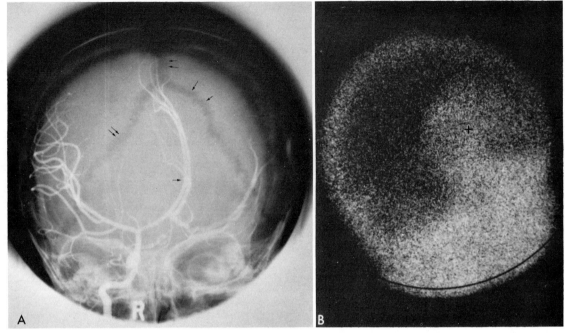

Figure 15–7 *A,* Right carotid arteriogram, anteroposterior projection, arterial phase. Right frontal mixed glioma. As a result of the large frontal lobe tumor, there is a right to left displacement of the more anterior part of the anterior cerebral artery from its usual midline location (the "round" shift is indicated by the single arrow). The paired arrows indicate the abnormal widening of the sagittal and lambdoidal sutures resulting from increased intracranial pressure caused by the tumor. *B,* Technetium-99m pertechnetate brain scan, right lateral projection. The "+" indicates an area of increased radionuclide uptake associated with this right frontal mixed glioma. (Courtesy of Shelby Miller, M. D.)

as the size of the cerebral ventricles or the presence of sagittal sinus invasion by tumor, can be ascertained. Vascular non-tumorous conditions that sometimes simulate a tumor clinically can also be diagnosed. Angiography may be useful in the follow-up of selected patients who have already been treated for tumor.

PNEUMOENCEPHALOGRAPHY AND VENTRICULOGRAPHY

Careful radiologic evaluation with specialized studies of the ventricular system and the subarachnoid cerebrospinal fluid pathways provides morphologic data concerning the adjacent brain tissue, as well as an anatomic delineation of the channels themselves. Computerized tomography may provide much of the same information without risk or discomfort to the patient, which accounts in part for its current meteoric impact on neuroradiology and its related clinical specialties (see earlier section). In

fact, in institutions where experience with CT scanning is now substantial, there has been a significant decrease in the number of pneumoencephalograms and ventriculograms performed, while arteriography has been less affected.

The images presently produced by computerized tomography, however, are less detailed and lack the fine definition that is possible with x-ray film studies utilizing air as the contrast material to outline the ventricles and subarachnoid spaces. Therefore, CT scanning in its present form is not likely to replace air studies entirely for smaller tumors, particularly when they are near the skull base (for example, optic and hypothalamic gliomas). *Positive* contrast ventriculography (using Conray or Pantopaque) is not used routinely by most neuroradiologists, but is still employed with generally good results by some neurosurgeons working with limited time and equipment. Occasionally, lesions have been demonstrated with the use of positive contrast media that could not be seen on air-contrast examinations (see below).[74, 75]

Lumbar puncture may be dangerous, leading to brain herniations in patients with greatly increased intracranial pressures; hence, a decision to perform pneumoencephalography by means of lumbar puncture, rather than by direct injection of air into the lateral ventricles, should be based upon detailed information about the patient derived from clinical as well as radiologic studies. The consulting neurologist, neurosurgeon, and neuroradiologist must individualize their approach in each case when choosing between pneumoencephalography and ventriculography. Space does not permit a discussion sufficient to encompass all possibilities, but it may be stated that lumbar puncture for pneumoencephalography is less likely to be performed (1) when there is papilledema or other clinical findings indicative of intracranial hypertension, (2) when there is radiologic evidence of intracranial hypertension, or (3) when there is CT scan or arteriographic evidence of hydrocephalus. Initial brain scan evidence of an intracranial neoplasm may in itself be a relative deterrent to lumbar puncture and pneumoencephalography until more diagnostic information is assembled. When there is angiographic evidence for a large supra-

tentorial mass with hippocampal herniation, or a clear-cut cerebellar mass with tonsillar hernation, lumbar puncture is definitely contraindicated. In patients who have severe hydrocephalus and an intracranial mass that could well cause a cerebral herniation, angiography may be employed initially with much less trepidation than pneumoencephalography. When there is no hydrocephalus, valuable information may be obtained by pneumography, particularly with tumors in difficult areas such as the cerebellopontine angle, brain stem, and immediate suprasellar region.[76-78] The ability of the pneumoencephalogram to distinguish between a mass within the brain stem (Fig. 15–8), as opposed to one within the subarachnoid cisterns and outside of the brain stem, is also of fundamental importance.[77] Surgery may be indicated in the latter situation, whereas radiotherapy alone may be advisable with the intrinsic brain stem tumor. In the evaluation of a child with a probable brain stem tumor, computerized tomography again is expected to alter the approach in many cases.

Air study has proved essential in demonstrating the site of a ventricular or subarachnoid block, as well as in suggesting the

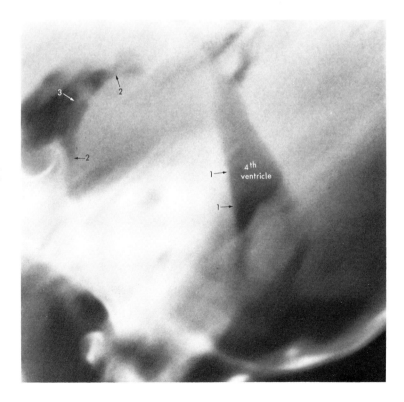

Figure 15–8 Pneumoencephalogram, lateral projection. Brain stem glioma. Note air within the fourth ventricle. Its floor (1) is displaced posteriorly by pontine mass. 2, the anterior and superior margins of the pons, which is enlarged by the tumor (sella is to left of lower arrow). The basilar artery (3) is outlined by air in the pontine and interpeduncular cisterns.

nature of the obstructing lesion in many individuals in whom arteriography and CT scanning have revealed dilated ventricles but have not convincingly demonstrated a mass.[79] When hydrocephalus has been demonstrated by angiography or CT scanning, it is important to establish that all the dilated chambers are in communication if a single shunt is to suffice as treatment; this can be done with ventriculography. We have shown that it is possible for the midline structures to remain undisplaced, even in certain cases where only *one* foramen of Monro is obstructed by tumor.[79] Primary intraventricular tumors, as well as tumor implants that have seeded there from a primary tumor situated elsewhere in the central nervous system, will be depicted graphically with an air study.

When there has been pneumographic or ventriculographic delineation of a "mass" and its vascularity is not known, one should remember at least to consider an aneurysm, a vascular malformation, or another highly vascular lesion before embarking on a course of treatment. Arteriographic delineation of the lesion may therefore be important prior to surgical intervention. Known instances of radiation therapy having been delivered to unoperated vein of Galen malformations that were thought to be pinealomas, or to vertebrobasilar aneurysms thought to be brain stem tumors, underline the importance of considering the possibility of a vascular lesion in the differential diagnosis. On the other hand, avascular masses demonstrated by arteriography, particularly in children, could still represent fluid-filled diverticula or cysts (which *may* fill with air at pneumography), rather than tumors.[80, 81] The fluid content of these lesions should usually be recognizable with CT scanning. However, when dealing with a space-occupying lesion in the pineal region, it is still important to differentiate an acquired diverticulum (arising from a dilated lateral ventricle) from a non-communicating cyst, inasmuch as surgical exploration of the pineal region would not be appropriate for "Dyke's diverticulum."[81] The diagnosis of a ventricular diverticulum is based on demonstration of its filling with air at pneumography, whereas ordinary CT scanning cannot make this distinction.

For the delineation of lesions within and immediately adjacent to the cerebral ventricles, air examinations are unrivaled.

The precise anatomic information derived from these studies may be of considerable value to the neurosurgeon and radiotherapist. *After* surgery or radiotherapy, air studies may also prove valuable in follow-up evaluations.[82, 83] The response of a hypothalamic tumor to radiotherapy, for example, can be shown by diminution in size of the mass. Cerebral atrophy following radiotherapy has also been documented by pneumography.[83]

In summary, it will be apparent from these examples that air-contrast studies (ventriculograms and pneumoencephalograms) have considerable information to offer in the evaluation of patients with tumors in certain locations, and in evaluating those with hydrocephalus in whom the exact site and nature of a suspected obstructing lesion (possibly a tumor) must be demonstrated. Nevertheless, the risks of lumbar puncture (and, therefore, of pneumoencephalography) in a patient with intracranial hypertension associated with severe hydrocephalus or with large tumors that threaten to cause brain herniation, should be appreciated.[84, 85] As a result, pneumoencephalography is being performed less now and, when performed, it is generally the last examination done. Ventriculography is also performed less, because other procedures frequently are as useful—or more useful—and are safer, avoiding the necessity to cannulate or needle the ventricle through the brain. Air examinations, however, will continue to be performed for the demonstration of lesions not well shown by angiography, computerized tomography, or brain scans, and to complement these examinations in selected cases.

POSTERIOR FOSSA POSITIVE CONTRAST CISTERNOGRAPHY

Positive contrast medium (Pantopaque) can be instilled into the lumbar subarachnoid space by a lumbar puncture and maneuvered into the posterior cranial fossa (Fig. 15–9), utilizing a tilt table with fluoroscopic control.

The single most important indication for Pantopaque cisternography is the need to demonstrate or exclude a small mass (usually a neurinoma) within the internal auditory canal or meatus.[86–88] This may be the only satisfactory radiologic technique

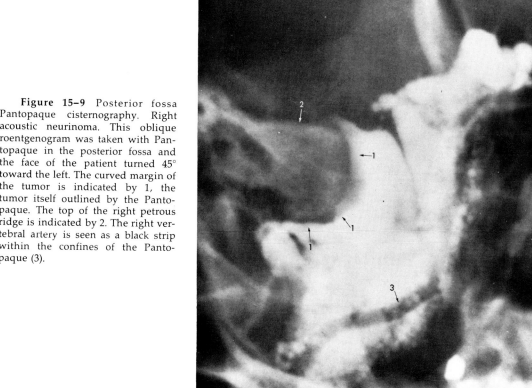

Figure 15–9 Posterior fossa Pantopaque cisternography. Right acoustic neurinoma. This oblique roentgenogram was taken with Pantopaque in the posterior fossa and the face of the patient turned 45° toward the left. The curved margin of the tumor is indicated by 1, the tumor itself outlined by the Pantopaque. The top of the right petrous ridge is indicated by 2. The right vertebral artery is seen as a black strip within the confines of the Pantopaque (3).

for evaluating such a very early lesion. Occasionally, slightly larger lesions protruding outside the canal and into the cerebellopontine angle cistern might also be demonstrated only by positive contrast; however, more sizable cerebellopontine angle masses, especially those over 2 cm, can frequently be demonstrated by radionuclide brain scanning, CT scanning, arteriography, or pneumography, and the use of these techniques may be preferred.

Acknowledgments: The author wishes to thank Michael L. J. Apuzzo, M.D. (Department of Neurosurgery, University of Southern California School of Medicine) for his revision of the clinical comments, Michael S. Tenner, M.D., and Jan K. Siemsen, M.D., for reviewing the chapter and for their helpful comments, and Marilyn Odor for her secretarial assistance.

References

1. Matson, D. D.: Neurosurgery of Infancy and Childhood. 2nd Ed. Springfield, Ill., Charles C Thomas, 1969.
2. Zimmerman, H. M.: The ten most common types of brain tumor. Semin. Roentgenol., *6*:48–58, 1971.
3. Gilroy, J., and Meyer, J. S.: Medical Neurology. London, Macmillan, 1969.
4. Taveras, J. M., and Wood, E. H.: Diagnostic Neuroradiology. Baltimore, Williams & Wilkins, 1964.
5. Grossman, H., Winchester, P. H., Deck, M., et al.: Brain tumors in children with normal skull roentgenograms. Am. J. Roentgenol. Radium Ther. Nucl. Med., *112*:329–331, 1971.
6. Azar-Kia, B., Schechter, M. M., Liebeskind, A., et al.: The enlarged foramen ovale. Am. J. Roentgenol. Radium Ther. Nucl. Med., *118*: 420–425, 1973.
7. Bartal, A. D., Djaldetti, M. M., Mandel, E. M., et al.: Dumb-bell neurinoma of the hypoglossal nerve. J. Neurol. Neurosurg. Psychiatry, *36*:592–595, 1973.
8. Britton, B. H.: Glomus tympanicum and glomus jugulare tumors. Radiol. Clin. North Am., *12*: 543–551, 1974.
9. El Gammal, T., and Allen, M. B.: Further consideration of sellar changes associated with increased intracranial pressure. Br. J. Radiol., *45*:561–569, 1972.
10. Kahn, E. A., Gosch, H. H., Seeger, J. F., et al.: Forty-five years experience with the craniopharyngiomas. Surg. Neurol., *1*:5–12, 1973.
11. Mountjoy, J. R., Dolan, K. D., and McCabe, B. F.: Neurilemmoma of the ninth cranial nerve

masquerading as an acoustic neuroma. Arch. Otolaryngol., *100*:65–67, 1974.

12. Newton, T. H., and Potts, D. G.: Radiology of the Skull and Brain. Vol. 1. St. Louis, C. V. Mosby, 1971.

13. Segall, H. D., Segal, H. L., Teal, J. S., et al.: Calcifying cerebral cavernous hemangioma with brain scan and angiographic findings. Neuroradiology, *7*:133–138, 1974.

14. Yuhl, E. T., and Schmitz, A. L.: Occipital emissary channel and increased intracranial pressure. Acta Radiol. (Diagn.), *9*:124–127, 1969.

15. Segall, H. D., Mikity, V. G., Rumbaugh, C. L., et al.: Cranial sutures in the first two years of life: Normal measurements and the "spring suture." Neuroradiology, *4*:124, 1972.

16. Tabaddor, K., Shulman, K., and Dal Canto, M. D.: Neonatal craniopharyngioma. Am. J. Dis. Child., *128*:381–383, 1974.

17. Chynn, K.: Neuroradiologic exploration in intra- and parasellar conditions. Radiol. Clin. North Am., *4*:93–115, 1966.

18. Hilal, S. K.: Angiography of juxtasellar masses. Semin. Roentgenol., *6*:75–88, 1971.

19. Schechter, M. M., Liebeskind, A. L., and Azar-Kia, B.: Intracranial chordomas. Neuroradiology, *8*:67–82, 1974.

20. Meszaros, W. T.: The many facets of multiple myeloma. Semin. Roentgenol., *9*:219–228, 1974.

21. Kutcher, R., Ghatak, N. R., and Leeds, N. E.: Plasmacytoma of the calvaria. Radiology, *113*:111–115, 1974.

22. Renner, R. R., and Smith, J. R.: Plasma cell dyscrasias (except myeloma). Semin. Roentgenol., *9*:209–218, 1974.

23. Gifford, R. D., Goree, J. A., and Jimenez, J. P.: Tumor bulge into the sphenoid sinus. A roentgen sign of parasellar meningioma. Am. J. Roentgenol. Radium Ther. Nucl. Med., *112*: 324–328, 1971.

24. Kaufman, B., and Chamberlin, W. B.: The ubiquitous "empty" sella turcica. Acta Radiol., *13*:413–425, 1972.

25. Kirkwood, J. R., Margolis, M. T., and Newton, T. H.: Prostatic metastasis to the base of the skull simulating meningioma en plaque. Am. J. Roentgenol. Radium Ther. Nucl. Med., *112*: 774–778, 1971.

26. Minagi, H., and Newton, T. H.: Cartilaginous tumors of the base of skull. Am. J. Roentgenol. Radium Ther. Nucl. Med., *105*:308–313, 1969.

27. Holman, B. L.: The brain scan. Postgrad. Med., *54*:143–149, 1973.

28. Jones, A. E., Frankel, R. S., Di Chiro, G., et al.: Brain scintigraphy with 99m Tc pertechnetate, 99mTc polyphosphate, and 67Ga citrate. Radiology, *112*:123–129, 1974.

29. Kinser, J. A., Rosler, H., and Stalder, A.: Type-specific tumor patterns in the combined early and late cerebral scintigrams. Neuroradiology, *6*:27–31, 1973.

30. Penning, L., Front, D., Bechar, M., et al.: Factors governing the uptake of pertechnetate by human brain tumours: A scintigraphic study. Brain, *96*:225–234, 1973.

31. Ramsey, R. G., and Quinn, J. L.: Comparison of accuracy between initial and delayed 99mTc-

pertechnetate brain scans. J. Nucl. Med., *13*: 131–134, 1972.

32. Webber, M. M.: Technetium 99m normal brain scans and their anatomic features. Am. J. Roentgenol. Radium Ther. Nucl. Med., *94*: 815–818, 1965.

33. Gize, R. W., and Mishkin, F. S.: Brain scans in multiple sclerosis. Radiology, *97*:297–299, 1970.

34. Maynard, C. D., Hanner, T. G., and Witcofski, R. L.: Positive brain scans due to lesions of the skull. Arch. Neurol., *18*:93–97, 1968.

35. Landman, S., and Ross, P.: Radionuclides in the diagnosis of arteriovenous malformations of the brain. Radiology, *108*:635–639, 1973.

36. Segall, H. D., Rumbaugh, C. L., Bergeron, R. T., et al.: Neuroradiology in infections of the brain and meninges. Surg. Neurol., *1*:178–186, 1973.

37. Brooks, W. H., Mortara, R. H., and Preston, D.: The clinical limitations of brain scanning in metastatic disease. J. Nucl. Med., *15*:620–621, 1974.

38. Binet, E. F., and Loken, M. K.: Scintiangiography of cerebral arteriovenous malformations and aneurysms. Am. J. Roentgenol. Radium Ther. Nucl. Med., *109*:707–713, 1970.

39. Cowan, R. J., Maynard, C. D., Meschan, I., et al.: Value of the routine use of the cerebral dynamic radioisotope study. Radiology, *107*:111–116, 1973.

40. Sheldon, J. J., Smoak, W. M., Gargano, F. P., et al.: Dynamic scintigraphy in intracranial meningiomas. Radiology, *109*:109–115, 1973.

41. McQuade, S., and Higgins, H. P.: 99mTc-polyphosphate in diagnosing meningiomas of the sphenoid wing. J. Nucl. Med., *15*:1205–1206, 1974.

42. Bernstein, J., and Hoffer, P. B.: Use of the delayed brain scan in differentiating calvarial from cerebral lesions. J. Nucl. Med., *15*:681–684, 1974.

43. Wilkins, R. H., Pircher, F. J., and Odom, G. L.: The value of postoperative brain scan in patients with supratentorial intracranial tumors. J. Neurosurg., 111–118, 1966.

44. Baker, H. L., Campbell, J. K., Houser, D. W., et al.: Computer assisted tomography of the head: An early evaluation. Mayo Clin. Proc., *49*:17–28, 1974.

45. Davis, D. O., and Pressman, B. D.: Computerized tomography of the brain. Radiol. Clin. North Am., *12*:297–313, 1974.

46. New, P. F. J., Scott, W. R., Schnur, J. A., et al.: Computed tomography with the EMI scanner in the diagnosis of primary and metastatic intracranial neoplasms. Radiology, *114*:75–87, 1975.

47. Deutsch, M., Parsons, J. A., and Mercado, R.: Radiotherapy for intracranial metastases. Cancer, *34*:1607–1611, 1974.

48. Posner, J. B.: Diagnosis and treatment of metastases to the brain. Clin. Bull., *4*:47–57, 1974.

49. Pendl, G., and Kratochwil, A.: Two-dimensional echoencephalography in the young child. Neuroradiology, *4*:36–40, 1972.

50. Tenner, M. S., Wodraska, G., and Adapon, B. D.: Newer ultrasound techniques in the evaluation of neurologic disorders. Radiol. Clin. North Am., *12*:283–295, 1974.

51. Wishart, D. L.:Complications in vertebral angiography as compared to non-vertebral cerebral angiography in 447 studies. Am. J. Roentgenol. Radium Ther. Nucl. Med., 113:527–537, 1971.

52. Field, J. R., Lee, L., and McBurney, R. F.: Complications of 1000 brachial arteriograms. J. Neurosurg., 36:324–332, 1972.

53. Cassady, J. R., and Wilner, H.: The angiographic appearance of intracranial sarcomas. Radiol., 88:258–263, 1967.

54. Cronqvist, S.: Angiography and cerebral blood flow in malignant glioma. Acta Radiol. (Ther.), 8:78–85, 1969.

55. Goree, J. A., and Dukes, H. T.: The angiographic differential diagnosis between the vascularized malignant glioma and the intracranial arteriovenous malformation. Am. J. Roentgenol. Radium Ther. Nucl. Med., 90:512–521, 1963.

56. Leeds, N. E., and Goldberg, H. I.: Abnormal vascular patterns in benign intracranial lesions: Pseudotumors of the brain. Am. J. Roentgenol. Radium Ther. Nucl. Med., 118:576–585, 1973.

57. Leeds, N. E., and Rosenblatt, R.: Arterial wall irregularities in intracranial neoplasms. Radiology, 103:121–124, 1972.

58. Scatliff, J. H., Guinto, F. C., and Radcliffe, W. B.: Vascular patterns in cerebral neoplasms and their differential diagnosis. Semin. Roentgenol., 6:59–69, 1971.

59. Scatliff, J. H., Radcliffe, W. B., Pittman, H. H., et al.: Vascular structure of glioblastomas. Am. J. Roentgenol. Radium Ther. Nucl. Med., 105: 795–805, 1969.

60. Finn, J. E., and Mount, L. A.: Meningiomas of the tuberculum sellae and planum sphenoidale: A review of 83 cases. Arch. Ophthalmol., 92:23–27, 1974.

61. Kieffer, S. A., Larson, D. A., Gold, L. H. A., et al.: Rapid circulation in intracranial meningiomas. Radiology, 106:575–580, 1973.

62. Marc, J. A., and Schechter, M. M.: Cortical venous rerouting in parasagittal meningiomas. Radiology, 112:85–92, 1974.

63. Merten, D. F., Gooding, C. A., and Newton, T. H.: The radiographic features of meningiomas in childhood and adolescence. Pediatr. Radiol., 2:89–96, 1974.

64. Salamon, G. M., Combalbert, A., Raybaud, C., et al.: An angiographic study of meningiomas of the posterior fossa. J. Neurosurg., 35:731–741, 1971.

65. Sansregret, A., and Ledoux, R.: Lesser wing meningiomas: A few unfamiliar differential diagnoses. Neuroradiology, 2:9–14, 1971.

66. Schechter, M. M., Zingesser, L. H., and Rosenbaum, A.: Tentorial meningiomas. Am. J. Roentgenol. Radium Ther. Nucl. Med., 104 123–131, 1968.

67. Henry, J. M., Schwartz, F. T., Sartawi, M. A., et al.: Cystic meningiomas simulating astrocytomas. J. Neurosurg., 40:647–650, 1974.

68. Hooshmand, I., Rosenbaum, A. E., and Stein, R. L.: Radiographic anatomy of normal cerebral deep medullary veins: Criteria for distinguishing them from their abnormal counterparts. Neuroradiology, 7:75–84, 1974.

69. Zulch, K. J., Behrend, R. C., and Finkemeyer, H.: The "early filling vein:" Is "early venous filling" in an angiogram really a reliable sign of malignancy? Neuroradiology, 5:111–113, 1973.

70. Segall, H. D., Rumbaugh, C. L., Bergeron, R. T., et al.: Brain and meningeal infections in children: Radiological considerations. Neuroradiology, 6:8–16, 1973.

71. Segall, H. D., Kurze, T., Rumbaugh, C. L., et al.: Selected experiences with strategic neuroradiology. Bull. Los Angeles Neurol. Soc., 38: 1–12, 1973.

72. Kramer, S., and Lee, K. F.: Complications of radiation therapy: The central nervous system. Semin. Roentgenol., 9:75–83, 1974.

73. Kagan, A. R., Bruce, D. W., and Di Chiro, G.: Fatal foam cell arteritis of the brain after irradiation for Hodgkin's disease: Angiography and pathology. Stroke, 2:232–238, 1971.

74. Andreussi, L., Clarisse, J., Jomin, M., et al.: Ventriculography with watersoluble contrast in the diagnosis of posterior fossa tumors (107 Cases). Neuroradiology, 8:25–38, 1974.

75. Steiner, G. M.: Positive contrast ventriculography with dimer X in hydrocephalus. Clin. Radiol., 25:517–523, 1974.

76. Schain, R. J., and Wilson, G.: Brainstem encephalitis with radiographic evidence of medullary enlargement. Neurology, 21:537–539, 1971.

77. Pribram, H. F. W.: The differentiation of extrinsic from intrinsic intracranial tumors with particular reference to posterior fossa tumors. Am. J. Roentgenol. Radium Ther. Nucl. Med., 98: 542–549, 1966.

78. Liliequist, B.: Pontine angle tumor: Encephalographic appearances. Acta Radiol. (Suppl.), 186:1–96, 1959.

79. Segall, H. D., Pitts, F. W., Rumbaugh, C. L., et al.: Foramen of Monro obstruction in children: Intra-axial lesions. Radiology, 110:125–134, 1974.

80. Segall, H. D., Hassan, G., Ling, S. M., et al.: Suprasellar cysts associated with isosexual precocious puberty. Radiology, 3:607–616, 1974.

81. Dyke, C. S.: Acquired subtentorial pressure diverticulum of a cerebral lateral ventricle. Radiology, 39:167, 1942.

82. Stein, B. M., Tenner, M. S., and Fraser, R. A. R.: Hydrocephalus following removal of cerebellar astrocytomas in children. J. Neurosurg., 36: 763–768, 1972.

83. Wilson, G. H., Byfield, J., and Hanafee, W. N.: Atrophy following radiation therapy for central nervous system neoplasms. Acta Radiol. (Ther.), 11:361–368, 1972.

84. Weisberg, L. A.: The syndrome of increased intracranial pressure without localizing signs: A reappraisal. Neurology, 25:85–88, 1975.

85. Bergeron, R. T., and Rumbaugh, C. L.: Problems incident to pneumographic and other non-angiographic radiologic contrast studies of the brain. Bull. Los Angeles Neurol. Soc., 36:1–10, 1971.

86. Kurze, T., Keim, R. J., and Segall, H. D.: Surgical Removal of an Acoustic Neuroma. New York, Avens, 1974.

87. Scanlan, R. L.: Positive contrast medium (iophendylate) in diagnosis of acoustic neuroma. Arch. Otolaryngol., 80:698–706, 1974.

88. Long, J. M., Kier, E. L., and Hilding, D. A.: Pitfalls of posterior fossa cisternography using 2 ml of iophendylate (Pantopaque). Radiology, 102: 71–75, 1972.

Chapter Sixteen

SPINAL CORD

Hervey D. Segall, M.D.

CLINICAL CONSIDERATIONS

The symptoms and signs of neoplastic lesions of the spinal canal or spinal cord are usually relentlessly progressive, with no evidence of the remission or exacerbation that may be evident in multiple sclerosis or degenerative disc disease.[1] Symptoms of pain, paresthesia, and dysesthesia are often more severe during the nocturnal hours. It is not unusual for a spinal tumor to cause pain simulating an abnormality of a viscus in the abdomen or thorax. In other patients, insidious progression of weakness or clumsiness of one or more limbs may occur. Unless the conus medullaris is involved, complaints referable to bowel and bladder dysfunction are not conspicuous features of the early symptomatology of spinal cord neoplasms.

Localized tenderness over the involved vertebral segment may be evident. Peripheral motor manifestations may include atrophy, fasciculations, and weakness, and may indicate the anatomic level of the spinal lesion. Spastic paresis or paralysis is a manifestation of corticospinal motor tract dysfunction. Diffuse, patchy, or segmental hypalgesia or anesthesia is a common sensory finding; the distribution of the sensory deficit may also suggest the level of the involved cord segment. Hyperreflexia and pathologic alterations of plantar and abdominal reflexes are indicative of corticospinal tract dysfunction, while hyporeflexia or loss of deep tendon reflexes may be evident with nerve root or segmental motor neuron involvement. Anhidrosis often has great localizing value in establishing the level of cord involvement. The neurologic findings often indicate correctly the level of a tumor when it is intramedullary; however, the actual location of a spinal canal block on myelography and the level of neurologic findings in *extradural* (often metastatic) tumors may differ. Signs related to the lower cranial nerves may result from cervical or cervicomedullary junction lesions; these include Horner's syndrome, nystagmus (especially of the "down-beat" type), and facial sensory loss.[2] Papilledema has also been described with spinal cord neoplasms.[3]

Finally, gross skeletal or cutaneous anomalies may be apparent in association with spinal cord tumors; these include scoliosis, foot deformities, cutaneous dimples, dermal sinuses, hair tufts, hemangiomas,[5] lipomas[6] and other dysmorphic manifestations of various neurocutaneous syndromes, most notably von Recklinghausen's disease (neurofibromatosis).

Many neurologic disorders may mimic spinal neoplasms, and the neuroradiologist plays a cardinal role in the evaluation of the patient to establish the presence of benign tumors and other potentially correctable lesions. The most commonly encountered structural or developmental alterations that should be considered in the differential diagnosis are basilar invagination of the skull, platybasia, and other skeletal abnormalities at the atlanto-occipital junction. Also to be considered is the Arnold-Chiari malformation or a cervicomedullary syrinx, which itself may be associated with an intramedullary tumor. In children, diastematomyelia and congenital tethering of the distal spinal cord should be considered; degenerative spinal disease, with or without midline disc protrusion, may also be an occasional source of diagnostic difficulty. Demyelinating diseases including primary degenerative diseases of the central nervous system, particularly amyotrophic lateral sclerosis, are frequent considerations.[7] Systemic disease accompanying pernicious anemia, lues, radiation myelopathy, spinal arteriovenous malformation, and parasaggital cerebral neoplasms, as well as neoplastic, infectious, or metabolic osseous lesions of the spine, are other differential possibilities.

COMMON RADIOLOGIC TECHNIQUES

Plain Films and Tomograms

Plain films and tomograms of the spine are often valuable in patients suspected of having intraspinal pathology,[8] although many tumors involving the spinal cord or its investments may be unassociated with changes on the plain spine film. Destruction and compression of a vertebra is commonly seen with metastatic tumor (Fig. 16–1), including myeloma, but isolated lytic changes can also occur with histiocytosis-X and with Paget's disease. Spinal infections usually cause destructive changes in the vertebral end-plate and narrowing of the intervertebral disc space. Consequently, spinal inflammatory lesions can generally be differentiated

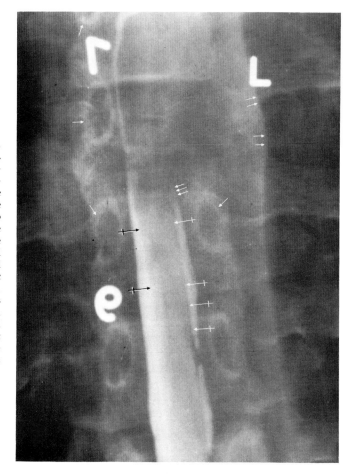

Figure 16–1 Pantopaque myelogram. Vertebral body and pedicular destruction, with partial spinal "block" due to metastatic neoplasm. There is a paraspinal soft tissue mass on the left side at the level of the eighth thoracic vertebra, as indicated by the double arrows (top right). There is also malignant destruction of a portion of the eighth thoracic vertebral body and of the left pedicle of the same vertebra. A normal right pedicle of the eighth, and normal pedicles of the seventh and ninth thoracic vertebrae are indicated by single arrows. The tumor is extradural and therefore is shown displacing the Pantopaque column away from the margins of the spinal canal (three adjacent arrows). Note left to right displacement of the spinal cord lower in the thoracic spinal canal (spinal cord margins are indicated by the cross-hatched arrows).

from vertebral (osseous) neoplasms roentgenographically. Osteoblastic forms of metastic disease (especially from breast and prostatic carcinomas) must also be differentiated from benign conditions affecting the vertebra (i.e., Paget's disease).[9, 10] Primary bone tumors of the vertebral column may also be detectable on plain spine radiographs.[11, 12]

Intraspinal neurofibromas can cause flattening and erosion of the adjacent pedicles (Fig. 16–2), as well as enlargement of the spinal neuroforamina; however, similar changes can be caused (infrequently) by meningiomas and other lesions, including meningoceles and vertebral artery aneurysms.[13–15] Tumors that may enlarge the bony spinal canal include ependymomas and astrocytomas, but syringomyelia, hydromyelia, or dural ectasia can also do this. Roentgenographically observable changes in vertebral alignment, including scoliosis or kyphosis, may also be associated with an intraspinal neoplasm. A visible paraspinal soft tissue mass may be seen on plain films in the presence of a tumor (Fig. 16–1), but a similar finding may also be associated with an intraspinal hematoma or infection. Although plain spine films are frequently unrevealing in patients with spinal meningiomas, roentgenologically visible calcification can sometimes occur within these lesions. From time to time, calcifications may also be identified on plain films within neuroblastomas, ganglioneuromas, neurolemmomas, chordomas, and other neoplasms.[8, 9]

Finally, *non*-neoplastic conditions, such as anomalies at the atlanto-occipital junction (which, as mentioned above, may produce clinical findings simulating tumor), should be searched for carefully on plain spine films of the patient suspected of having a tumor.

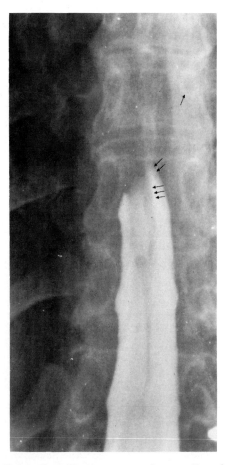

Figure 16–2 Pantopaque myelogram. Extradural thoracic neurofibroma. A neurofibroma has partly eroded one pedicle inferiorly on the left side, as indicated by single arrow. This tumor has also displaced the Pantopaque column (two arrows) away from the margins of the spinal canal and has pushed the spinal cord itself (triple arrows) to the right.

Contrast Myelography

Because plain films and tomograms alone seldom give enough information about suspected pathology within the spinal canal on which to base treatment, special radiologic methods for demonstrating the intraspinal contents with injected contrast media have been devised. Myelography entails the injection of positive (Pantopaque) or negative (gas) contrast materials into the subarachnoid space, following a needle puncture (usually lumbar) under local anesthesia.[16–54] Iophendylate (Pantopaque) myelography is performed by manipulating this hyperbaric, iodine-containing oily material under fluoroscopic control to all portions of the spinal canal with the patient on a tilt table.

Utilizing myelography, it is possible to determine whether or not a neoplasm is present within the spinal canal. Generally, one can also tell if a neoplasm originates within the spinal cord substance or outside the cord, and whether an extramedullary lesion is intradural or extradural. The size, level, and exact location (anterior, posterior, right, left) of an intraspinal mass can also be determined, and this information is essential to the neurosurgeon who will attempt to perform a biopsy of or to excise the lesion. For example, knowing that an intraspinal meningioma is *ventrally* situated may lead him to modify his surgical approach accordingly. The dural incision itself should be made directly over the site of the intradural lesion.

Pantopaque myelography involves some discomfort (mostly local, at the injection site) to the patient; serious reactions are rare. Pantopaque is removed through the same spinal needle at the completion of the examination, except in a patient with a high-grade block of the spinal canal caused by a neoplasm or other lesion. In these patients, any reduction of the intraspinal pressure caudal to a block by removal of fluid may aggravate cord compression, with resultant further neurologic deterioration. For the same reason, cerebrospinal fluid is not removed at the start of the myelographic examination of a patient in whom a block is suspected. At the completion of the examination, the site of a demonstrated spinal block should be marked utilizing fluoroscopy, so that subsequent laminectomy can be performed at the correct level. When a complete block is present, it might be desirable also to demonstrate for the neurosurgeon the *upper* margin of an intraspinal lesion and whether or not higher lesions exist. To this end, Pantopaque may also be injected from above the lesion, by means of a lateral cervical puncture. When radiation therapy is to be delivered to radiosensitive lymphomas or metastatic oat cell carcinomas in the spinal canal without surgical exploration, the lesions need to be outlined radiographically for precise treatment planning. The myelographic method obviously is not limited to the diagnosis or exclusion of neoplasms, and other differential considerations such as arteriovenous malformation, herniated intervertebral disc, epidural abscess, arachnoiditis, meningocele, diastematomyelia, tethering of the lower spinal cord, and the Arnold-Chiari malformation may also be diagnosed or inferred by this means.

The late development of myelopathy in a patient who has received intensive radiation therapy to an area of tissue including the spinal cord could be explained by the presence of either metastatic disease or radiation myelitis. A normal myelogram, or one that shows segmental atrophy of the spinal cord in such a patient, might imply a radiation lesion. Metastatic disease within the spinal canal will usually become manifest as a visible epidural mass; the occasional *intra*dural but extramedullary metastatic deposit(s) may also be demonstrable by myelography. Rarely metastases involve the spinal cord itself, resulting in cord widening on the myelogram (radiation myelopathy, it should be noted, can also result very rarely in widening of the cord during its acute, edematous phase[16]). Although not routinely used in post-treatment cases, selective spinal arteriography has been reported to assist in the differential diagnosis of postirradiation myelomalacia, demonstrating arterial occlusive changes.[17]

In depicting the exact relationship of an intraspinal tumor to the cord and meninges, two (or more) different roentgenographic projections are required. *Intramedullary tumors* will expand the cord from side to side as well as from front to back, correspondingly narrowing the Pantopaque stream on all sides of the cord (Fig. 16–3). Most intramedullary neoplasms are gliomas (many are ependymomas), but carcinomatous metastases, lipomas, leukemia, hemangioblastomas, and rarely epidermoids can also widen the cord. Hematomyelia or inflammatory lesions can occasionally widen the cord and may simulate a cord tumor; syringomyelia and hydromyelia can also simulate or coexist with one of the larger spinal cord neoplasms. In a patient with a uniformly enlarged spinal cord (involving a long segment), direct puncture is recommended by some clinicians for chemical and cytologic analysis of cyst fluid as well as for decompression. When a cyst accompanies a suspected cord tumor, subsequent endomyelography (direct injection of contrast material into the cord cavity) may localize a tumor nodule for surgical exploration.[18]

Neoplasms *outside the cord but within the dural membranes* (intradural but extramedullary) almost always are either neurofibromas or meningiomas (Fig. 16–4). Patients with intracranial tumors (especially medulloblastomas, pinealomas, and ependymomas) may develop distal metastases borne by cerebrospinal fluid (seeding) that involve the spinal cord and the roots of the cauda equina.[19] These deposits may also

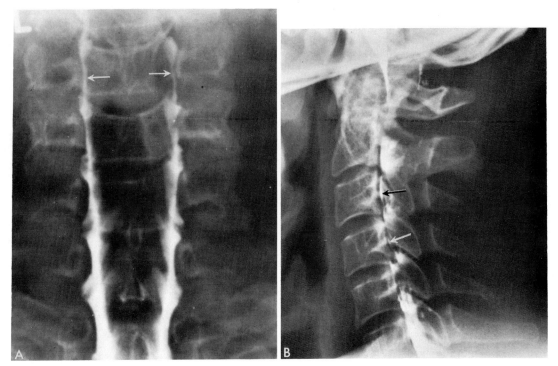

Figure 16–3 *A,* Pantopaque myelogram. Cervical ependymoma of spinal cord. An anteroposterior film taken during Pantopaque myelography shows the enlargement of the cervical portion of the spinal cord (central cylindrical defect in the contrast column). Cord is enlarged from side to side, so that the Pantopaque-filled gutters appear narrowed on either side (single arrows). *B,* Lateral view enlargement of the cervical spinal cord by the ependymoma has also produced narrowing of the ventral gutter, so that only a thin layer of Pantopaque is evident anteriorly. The arrows point to the ventral edge of the enlarged spinal cord, as outlined by a thin layer of Pantopaque in the ventral gutter.

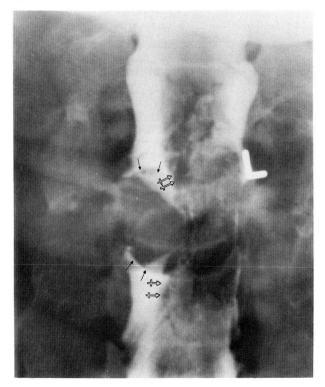

Figure 16–4 Pantopaque myelogram. Anteroposterior projection in cervical region, showing an intradural extramedullary tumor (a meningioma). The oval tumor (single arrows) is seen as a filling defect within the Pantopaque column on the right side, displacing the spinal cord from right to left. The white arrows indicate points of maximum displacement of the right margin of the cord.

be demonstrated intradurally at myelography. Primary epidermoidomas and lipomas in the spinal canal may be demonstrated outside the cord but within the dural membranes, and vertebral artery aneurysms rarely may be encountered myelographically in the cervical region. Intradural cholesteatomas are discovered rarely in the lumbar region, as a late complication of a spinal puncture performed months or years earlier.

Extradural tumors demonstrated myelographically within the spinal canal are usually metastatic, although the benign tumors that are usually situated intradurally (see above) can also appear extradurally. Extradural lesions displace the myelographic contrast column away from the bony margins of the spinal canal (Figs. 16–1 and 16–2). Accompanying changes in the adjacent bony structures, alluded to earlier, may be of considerable diagnostic value in localizing and confirming extradural lesions. Epidural abscess can simulate a tumor, but may be diagnosed roentgenographically because of simultaneous inflammatory narrowing of the disc interspace(s) or vertebral end-plate destruction (see above). Herniated discs are almost always localized myelographically to a specific intervertebral disc level, and are seldom difficult to differentiate from neoplasms. On occasion, hematomas and cysts can also be situated extradurally.

Gas myelography (using air) is a useful alternative method for demonstrating neoplasms and other masses within the spinal canal. Hydromyelia may be differentiated readily from solid intramedullary lesions using gas myelography. On Pantopaque examination, both types of lesions will appear simply as an enlarged cord, but in a patient with hydromyelia the cord may be observed to "collapse" readily during gas myelography. On the other hand, the gas myelogram will show *persistent* cord enlargement with a solid intramedullary lesion. Occasionally in hydromyelia, however, Pantopaque can be maneuvered directly into the dilated central canal of the cord by way of the foramen cecum, establishing the diagnosis.[20] There are some disadvantages to gas myelography: it requires the use of sophisticated laminographic equipment, and spinal arteriovenous malformations and certain other non-neoplastic conditions may not be demonstrable by this technique.

SPECIALIZED RADIOLOGIC TECHNIQUES

Compared to plain spine roentgenography and to contrast myelography, the following techniques are infrequently performed for patients with known or suspected neoplasms in the spinal canal. The first two categories (intravenously injected radionuclide and computerized tomographic studies) are relatively innocuous. Spinal arteriography, a much more precise anatomic procedure, carries some risk.

Radionuclide Studies

Although they have not achieved universal popularity, rapid blood flow studies, using an external radiation detector over the spine after the intravenous injection of a radionuclide, have been successful in demonstrating some hemangioblastomas of the spinal cord. Radionuclide angiography, obviously, is not as definitive as selective catheter angiography (see the section on arteriography), but it merits consideration as a screening test for vascular spinal cord lesions. In some cases, it has led directly to a decision to perform catheter angiography, obviating the need for prior myelography. Radionuclide angiography has also been recommended as a simple follow-up modality to demonstrate successful extirpation of a cord hemangioblastoma.[55] Other reports concerning the utilization of radionuclides to demonstrate spinal tumors have appeared in the literature.[56,57]

Radionuclide bone scans may also be utilized to reveal metastatic lesions within the spine.[58] Occasionally, lesions may be delineated by bone scanning that cannot be seen radiographically. It should be remembered, however, that non-neoplastic disorders (such as Paget's disease or osteoarthritis) can also be associated with focal increases in radionuclide uptake on bone scans.

Computerized Axial Tomography

Computerized axial tomographic devices are now becoming available that permit cross-sectional radiographic studies of the entire body, including the spine, and this may facilitate noninvasive screening of patients with spinal cord disease. At least one case is now on record in which demonstration of the cystic portion of a cord ependymoma was possible with this new modality.[59] (See also Chapter 15.)

Arteriography

Selective spinal arteriography has been employed in patients with intraspinal mass lesions, and it is primarily useful in delineating spinal cord arteriovenous malformations.[60-71] Pathognomonic angiographic features may also be present with hemangioblastomas, but angiography may not succeed in reliably differentiating some of these from arteriovenous malformations. Diffuse, nodular "staining" of the cord without rapid arteriovenous shunting is characteristic of hemangioblastomas at arteriography.[60] Reported findings have been relatively meager in the glioma group, although arteriographic abnormalities with possible surgical significance have been reported with a number of cord ependymomas.[61]

Selective angiography to delineate a tumor that involves the osseous portion of the spinal column (for example, an aneurysmal bone cyst) may prove rewarding, whether or not the spinal canal is compromised by the tumor.[62] At the same examination, especially with tumors involving certain critical levels of the spine, it may be of great importance to establish whether any of the nearby normal segmental vessels also provide direct vascular supply to the spinal cord. Obviously, interruption of this segmental vascular supply during a surgical procedure to the spine *could* result in a significant neurologic deficit.

The great majority of reported spinal cord complications following angiography, including paraplegias, have occurred following *unintentional* and uncontrolled introduction of contrast material into the spinal cord branch vessels (as during aortography, etc.);[63] instances of permanent cord complications related to an intentional selective spinal arteriogram are quite rare. Other complications of spinal angiography have also occurred.[64, 65]

Acknowledgments: The author wishes to express thanks to Michael L. J. Apuzzo, M.D. (Department of Neurosurgery, University of Southern California School of Medicine), who reviewed this chapter and revised the clinical comments.

References

1. Gilroy, J., and Meyer, J. S.: Medical Neurology. London, Macmillan, 1969.
2. Aring, C. D.: Lesions about the junction of medulla and spinal cord. J.A.M.A., *229*:1879, 1974.
3. Ammerman, B. J., and Smith, D. R.: Papilledema and spinal cord tumors. Surg. Neurol., *3*:55–57, 1975.
4. Raynor, R. B.: Papilledema associated with tumors of spinal cord. Neurology, *19*:700–704, 1969.
5. Nassar, S. I., and Correll, J. W.: Subarachnoid hemorrhage due to spinal cord tumors. Neurology, *18*:87–94, 1968.
6. Matson, D. D.: Neurosurgery of Infancy and Childhood. 2nd ed. Springfield, Ill., Charles C Thomas, 1969.
7. Taveras, J. M., and Wood, E. H.: Diagnostic Neuroradiology. Baltimore, Williams and Wilkins, 1964.
8. Paul, L. W., and Juhl, J. H.: Essentials of Roentgen Interpretation. 2nd ed. New York, Harper and Row, 1965.
9. Feldman, F., and Seaman, W. B.: The neurologic complications of Paget's disease in the cervical spine. Am. J. Roentgenol. Radium Ther. Nucl. Med., *105*:375–382, 1969.
10. Siegelman, S. S., Levine, S. A., and Walpin, L.: Paget's disease with spinal cord compression. Clin. Radiol., *19*:421–425, 1968. Am. J. Roentgenol. Radium. Ther. Nucl. Med., *105*:375, 1969.
11. Ramani, P. S.: Chondromyxoid fibroma: A rare cause of spinal cord compression. J. Neurosurg., *40*:107–109, 1974.
12. Vinstein, A. L., and Franken, E. A.: Hereditary multiple exostoses. Am. J. Roentgenol. Radium Ther. Nucl. Med., *112*:405–407, 1971.
13. Anderson, R. E., Shealy, C. N.: Cervical pedicle erosion and rootlet compression caused by a tortuous vertebral artery. Radiology, *96*:537–538, 1970.
14. Zimmerman, H. B., and Farrell, W. J.: Cervical vertebral erosion caused by vertebral artery tortuosity. Am. J. Roentgenol. Radium Ther. Nucl. Med., *108*:767–770, 1970.
15. Fagan, C. J., and Swischuk, L. E.: Dumbbell neuroblastoma or ganglioneuroma of the spinal canal. Am. J. Roentgenol. Radium Ther. Nucl. Med., *120*:453–460, 1974.
16. Marty, R., and Minckler, D. S.: Radiation myelitis simulating tumor. Arch. Neurol., *29*:352–354, 1973.
17. DiChiro, G., and Herdt, J. R.: Angiographic demonstration of spinal cord arterial occlusion in postradiation myelomalacia. Radiology, *106*:317–319, 1973.
18. Kendall, B., and Simon, L.: Cyst puncture and endomyelography in cystic tumours of the spinal cord. Br. J. Radiol., *46*:198–204, 1973.

19. Pecker, J., Simon, J., Guy, G., et al.: Radiological features of the meningoradicular metastases of tumors of the central nervous system: Report of two cases. J. Neurosurg., 38:627–630, 1973.

20. Heinz, E. R., and Goldman, R. L.: The role of gas myelography in neuroradiologic diagnosis. Radiology, 102:629–634, 1972.

21. Autio, E., Suolanen, J., Norrback, S., et al.: Adhesive arachnoiditis after lumbar myelography with meglumine iothalamate (Conray). Acta Radiol. (Diag.), 12:17–24, 1972.

22. Bender, J. L., Van Landingham, J. H., and Manno, N. J.: Epidural lipoma producing spinal cord compression: Report of two cases. J. Neurosurg., 41:100–103, 1974.

23. Bergeron, R. T., and Rumbaugh, C. L.: Problems incident to pneumographic and other non-angiographic radiologic contrast studies of the brain. Bull. Los Angeles Neurol. Soc., 36:1–10, 1971.

24. Bergeron, R. T., Rumbaugh, C. L., Fang, H., et al.: Experimental pantopaque arachnoiditis in the monkey. Radiology, 99:95–101, 1971.

25. Bobroff, L. M., and Leeds, N. E.: Minimal terminal irregularities of the distal subarachnoid space as a sign of epidural seeding. Am. J. Roentgenol. Radium Ther. Nucl. Med., 118:601–604, 1973.

26. Brinker, R. A.: Lumbar spinal puncture for neuroradiology procedures. Am. J. Roentgenol. Radium Ther. Nucl. Med., 118:674–676, 1973.

27. Bryan, P.: CSF seeding of intra-cranial tumours: A study of 96 cases. Clin. Radiol., 25:355–360, 1974.

28. Calogero, J. A., and Moossy, J.: Extradural spinal meningiomas: Report of four cases. J. Neurosurg., 37:442–447, 1972.

29. Chait, A., and Gannon, W. E.: Schistosomiasis of the spinal cord. Am. J. Roentgenol. Radium Ther. Nucl. Med., 105:400–403, 1969.

30. Chynn, K. Y.: Painless myelography: Introduction of a new aspiration cannula and review of 541 consecutive studies. Radiology, 109:361–367, 1973.

31. Davis, D. O., and Rumbaugh, C. L.: Pantopaque myelography. Semin. Roentgenol., 7:197–215, 1972.

32. Edelson, R. N., Deck, M. D. F., and Posner, J. B.: Intramedullary spinal cord metastases. Neurology, 22:1222–1231, 1972.

33. Epstein, B. S.: Spinal canal mass lesions. Radiol. Clin. North Am., 4:185–202, 1966.

34. Fox, J. L.: Redundant nerve roots in the cauda equina. J. Neurosurg., 30:74–75, 1969.

35. Freidberg, S. R.: Removal of an ossified ventral thoracic meningioma. J. Neurosurg., 37:728–730, 1971.

36. Gardner, R. C.: Intradural cholesteatoma (pearly tumor): A rare complication of myelography or spinal puncture. South. Med. J., 66:1070–1071, 1973.

37. Heinz, E. R., Schlesinger, E. B., and Potts, D. G.: Radiologic signs of hydromyelia. Radiology, 86:311–318, 1966.

38. Hinck, V. C., and Sachdev, N. S.: Myelographic findings in hypertrophic interstitial neuritis. Am. J. Roentgenol. Radium Ther. Nucl. Med., 95:947–948, 1965.

39. Howe, J. R., and Taren, J. A.: Foramen magnum tumors: Pitfalls in diagnosis. J.A.M.A., 225:1061–1066, 1973.

40. Hughes, J. T.: Pathology of the Spinal Cord. Philadelphia, J. B. Lippincott, 1966.

41. Jefferson, A.: Localized enlargement of the spinal canal in the absence of tumour: A congenital abnormality. J. Neurol. Neurosurg. Psychiatry, 18:305–309, 1955.

42. Johnson, R. E., and Roberson, G. H.: Subpial lipoma of the spinal cord. Radiology, 3:121–125, 1974.

43. Kelly, D. L., and Alexander, E.: Lateral cervical puncture for myelography. Technical note. J. Neurosurg., 29:106–110, 1968.

44. Kirks, D. R., and Newton, T. H.: Sarcoidosis: A rare cause of spinal cord widening. Radiology, 102:643, 1972.

45. Mayher, W. E., Daniel, E. F., and Allen, M. B.: Acute meningeal reaction following Pantopaque myelography. J. Neurosurg., 34:396–404, 1971.

46. McRae, D. L., and Standen, J.: Roentgenologic findings in syringomyelia and hydromyelia. Am. J. Roentgenol. Radium Ther. Nucl. Med., 98:695–703, 1966.

47. Parker, J. J., and Anderson, W. B.: Myelitis simulating spinal cord tumor. Am. J. Roentgenol. Radium Ther. Nucl. Med., 95:942–946, 1965.

48. Prentice, W. B., Kieffer, S. A., Gold, L. H. A., et al.: Myelographic characteristics of metastasis to the spinal cord and cauda equina. Am. J. Roentgenol. Radium Ther. Nucl. Med., 118:682–689, 1973.

49. Salcman, M., Quest, D. O., and Mount, L. A.: Histiocytosis-X of the spinal cord: Case report. J. Neurosurg., 41:383–386, 1974.

50. Shapiro, R.: Myelography. 2nd ed. Chicago, Year Book Medical Publishers, 1968.

51. Southworth, L. E., Jimeniz, J. P., and Goree, J. A.: A practical approach to cervical air myelography. Am. J. Roentgenol. Radium Ther. Nucl. Med., 107:486–490, 1969.

52. Tenner, M. S.: Myelography of nonmass lesions in the spinal canal. Semin. Roentgenol., 7:277–296, 1972.

53. Traub, S. P.: Mass lesions in the spinal canal. Semin. Roentgenol., 7:240–259, 1972.

54. Young, D. A., and Burney, R. E.: Complication of myelography—Transection and withdrawal of a nerve filament by the needle. N. Engl. J. Med., 285:156–157, 1971.

55. DiChiro, G., Jones, A. E., Johnston, G. S., et al.: Value and limits of radionuclide angiography of the spinal cord. Radiology, 109:125–130, 1973.

56. Fazio, C., Agnoli, A., Bava, G. L., et al.: Demonstration of spinal tumors with intravenously injected 99m Tc-Pertechnetate. J. Nucl. Med., 10:508–510, 1969.

57. Ljass, F. M.: Radioisotope myelography with ^{133}Xe. Neuroradiology, 7:29–35, 1974.

58. Legge, D. A., Tauxe, W. N., Pugh, D. G., et al.: Radioisotope scanning of metastatic lesions of bone. Mayo Clin. Proc., 45:755–761, Dec., 1970.

59. DiChiro, G., Axelbaum, S. P., Schellinger, D., et al.: Computerized axial tomography in syringomyelia. N. Engl. J. Med., 292:13–16, 1975.

60. DiChiro, G., and Doppman, J. L.: Differential angiographic features of hemangioblastomas

and arteriovenous malformations of the spinal cord. Radiology, 93:25–30, 1969.

61. DiChiro, G., and Wener, L.: Angiography of ependymomas of the spinal cord and filum terminale. Am. J. Roentgenol. Radium Ther. Nucl. Med., 122:628–633, 1974.

62. Billings, K. J., and Werner, L. G.: Aneurysmal bone cyst of the first lumbar vertebra. Radiology, 104:19–20, 1972.

63. DiChiro, G.: Unintentional spinal cord arteriography: A warning. Radiology, 112:231–233, 1974.

64. DiChiro, G., and Wener, L.: Angiography of the spinal cord: A review of contemporary techniques and applications. J. Neurosurg., 39:1–29, 1973.

65. Teal, J. S., Rumbaugh, C. L., Segall, H. D., et al.: Acute renal failure following spinal angiography with methylglucamine iothalamate: Case report. Radiology, 104:561–562, 1972.

66. Albertson, K. W., Doppman, J. L., and Ramsey, R.: Spinal seizures induced by contrast media: A new method of comparing neurotoxicity of radiopaque agents. Radiology, 107:349–351, 1973.

67. DiChiro, G.: Recent successes and failures in radiographic and radioisotopic angiography of the spinal cord. Br. J. Radiol., 45:553–560, 1972.

68. Djindjian, R.: Arteriography of the spinal cord. Am. J. Roentgenol. Radium Ther. Nucl. Med., 107:461–478, 1969.

69. Doppman, J. L.: Arteriography of the spinal cord. Semin. Roentgenol., 7:231–239, 1972.

70. Herdt, J. R., DiChiro, G., and Doppman, J. L.: Combined arterial and arteriovenous aneurysms of the spinal cord. Radiology, 99:589–593, 1971.

71. Herdt, J. R., Shimkin, P. M., Ommaya, A. K., et al.: Angiography of vascular intraspinal tumors. Am. J. Roentgenol. Radium Ther. Nucl. Med., 115:165–170, 1972.

Chapter Seventeen

PEDIATRIC NEOPLASMS

Michael T. Gyepes, M.D., and Lorraine E. Smith, M.D.

CLINICAL CONSIDERATIONS

Presenting Signs and Symptoms

Leukemia, brain tumors, and lymphomas (including Hodgkin's disease) cause the major proportion of cancer fatalities in children under the age of 14 years. Over 50 per cent of children with non-leukemic cancer present initially with disseminated disease.[1] Most diagnoses of cancer are made within three to five months of the initial symptoms, with the result that the delay is no greater, and is often less, than it is with cancer in adults.[2]

In children, lumps of unknown cause that are rapidly growing or painful, cause neurologic deficit, or are persistent for two to three months should be suspected of possible malignancy. Examples are growths in the parotid (mucoepidermoid cancer), cervical lymph nodes (lymphomas, including Hodgkin's disease), and thyroid (which sometimes occurs in a patient with a history of previous irradiation of benign disease, in the thymus or adenoids); growing tumors of the chest wall ("always" malignant); and localized swelling in the soft tissues of the head, trunk, and extremities. All soft-tissue sarcomas may be more extensive locally than the clinical examination suggests.[3-9]

Retinoblastoma is a congenital tumor, but it is rare for it to be diagnosed within the first three months of life. Over three fourths of retinoblastomas are diagnosed before the patient is 3 years old. An ab-normal light reflex in the pupil means that more than one-half the retina is involved and that there may already be accompanying retinal detachment. Regional lymph node metastasis occurs when the periorbital tissues have become involved. Bilateral retinoblastomas must be regarded and treated as two distinct tumors.[10] In addition to this tumor, it should be remembered that the pupillary "white reflex" can also be caused by retrolental fibroplasia, or by vitreous or organized retinal hemorrhages.

Gliomas of the optic nerve occur in older children (around 10 years of age), and the main symptom is a progressive deficit in vision that leads to blindness.

Within the chest, benign cysts, thymomas, benign or malignant teratomas, and lymphosarcomas can cause pain, pressure, dyspnea, or superior caval compression by virtue of their position in the anterior or middle mediastinum.[11] A posterior mediastinal mass in a child is assumed to be a neuroblastoma or ganglioneuroma until proven otherwise; these tumors are often found incidentally on a chest radiograph taken for another condition, unless they are associated directly with spinal cord compression.[12]

In the abdomen, an enlarging mass in the right upper quadrant may be a liver tumor rather than a Wilms' tumor. Liver tumors are usually painless, jaundice is rare, and liver function can often be normal. Liver tumors often occur before a child is 1 year of age and sometimes occur neonatally. Hemangiomas of the liver may be large enough to obstruct bowel. Alternative-

343

ly, arteriovenous shunting may lead to neonatal congestive heart failure. Malignant liver tumors (angiosarcoma, hepatoblastoma, hepatocarcinoma) are associated with pallor, *weight loss,* and sometimes hemihypertrophy. Abdominal pain and an age at onset of over 2 years are poor prognostic signs.[13] (See Chapter 9.)

Massive and rapidly enlarging neonatal hepatomegaly from metastatic neuroblastoma can present as a clinical emergency. Treatment on the basis of elevated catecholamine levels only, with appropriate clinical findings, is justified. Both neuroblastoma and Wilms' tumor have a better prognosis if diagnosed in a child under 1 year of age, and both usually present clinically as a firm non-tender palpable abdominal mass.[14] Over 80 per cent of patients over the age of 2 with neuroblastoma have radiographic bone metastases. Fever, anemia, malaise, or gastrointestinal symptoms can be of such magnitude that the clinician is distracted initially from making the correct diagnosis. Skin, liver, and microscopic bone-marrow invasion are still compatible with an excellent survival rate (similar to that expected in stage I and II; see section on staging), as long as the primary tumor is not large and *the patient is under 1 year of age.*[15-19]

Wilms' tumor may be associated with aniridia, cryptorchidism, or hemihypertrophy. Unlike infant "visceral" neuroblastoma, visceral metastases in a patient with Wilms' tumor are always associated with a poorer survival rate when compared to that of stage I and II (regionally localized) disease. Most metastases occur in the first year following treatment, and the overwhelming majority are manifest within two years.[20, 21]

Vaginal and prostaticovesical myosarcomas usually present with orificial bleeding, infection, pain, or urinary retention. Retroperitoneal and sacrococcygeal teratomas can present with genitourinary symptoms or constipation associated with a palpable abdominopelvic mass. Metastases to lymph nodes, bones, or lungs usually occur within one year of diagnosis in these childhood tumors, but they may occur later.[22]

Brain tumors occur most commonly in children between 5 and 8 years of age.[23] Tumors occurring at an age when the cranial sutures are still open behave more treacher-

ously. Headache and vomiting are the only "early" symptoms. Focal neurologic signs and symptoms occur later. The brain stem (which occupies less than 10 per cent of the brain's area) is the location for over 80 per cent of these malignant tumors. Irritability, malaise, or awkwardness, which may result from so many other childhood diseases, can also be the first sign of a brain tumor. These tumors may be congenital, and it may be to the discredit of the physician that he sometimes fails to heed parental concerns concerning minor degrees of behavioral change or a failure to achieve developmental milestones, which could facilitate an earlier diagnosis.[24, 25]

Differential Diagnosis

On occasion, massive tumors presumed to be hepatomas have been resected, only to find they are hamartomas or hemangiomas. Almost all benign abdominal cysts and tumors eventually cause pressure on contiguous structures, or cause symptoms by rupturing or becoming infected. Retroperitoneal teratomas can be cystic and are sometimes malignant (the latter in less than 10 per cent of cases, however).[26] Although Wilms' tumors are usually painless, they can become traumatized during a fall, and some may subsequently cause symptoms that simulate those of appendicitis. In an infant, a mass in the right upper abdomen that is associated with jaundice is usually a choledochal cyst. The extremely rare childhood cystoadenocarcinoma of the pancreas, Meckel's diverticulum or other duplication involving the gastrointestinal tract, large cyst of the spleen, or mesenteric or omental cyst can all cause obstruction with increasing abdominal girth and nausea and vomiting.[27-29]

Solitary cysts or multiple cysts may occur in the liver in association with renal polycystic disease. Hemangioma is the most common *primary* hepatic tumor in childhood, but metastatic tumors (leukemia, lymphoma, neuroblastoma, and Wilms' and gonadal tumors) are more common than primary tumors. Over 50 per cent of all perinatal abdominal masses are caused by hydronephrosis or multicystic kidney.[28]

Enlarged lymph nodes in the neck may

be metastatic from lymphoma, leukemia, thyroid carcinoma, or neuroblastoma; occasionally they may be confused with primary soft-tissue sarcomas.

Malignant lesions occurring in the lungs of children are practically all metastases from Wilms' tumors, bone or thyroid malignancies, or soft-tissue tumors. Primary bronchial carcinoid tumor and anaplastic carcinoma of the lung have been reported in children, but are extremely uncommon. The superior-anterior mediastinum contains the normal thymus, which can simulate a malignant tumor, and may harbor teratomas (including dermoid cysts) and substernal extensions of cervical lymphangiomas and goiters. The middle mediastinum may become enlarged with lymphomas, vascular anomalies, and foregut cysts, but infectious lymphadenopathy is much more common. The posterior mediastinum can contain meningeal and neurenteric cysts as well as neurogenic tumors. All benign or neoplastic cysts in the chest can cause pressure symptoms or become infected.

Malignant tumors of the paranasal sinuses can cause swelling of the face, nose, and eye with visual disturbances, proptosis, and extraocular muscle paralysis. If these symptoms are caused by a myosarcoma of the orbit the prognosis is excellent, and this tumor must therefore be differentiated from other extensive intraocular tumors.[30]

Filling defects in the bladder can be caused by ectopic ureteroceles and inflammatory polyps as well as by myosarcomas. Myosarcomas of the bladder may extend submucosally to involve the ureters and urethra, simulating primary disease at these sites.

Primary sarcomas of the soft tissues of the extremities infiltrate widely and are always much more extensive than they seem clinically. Myosarcomas and synovial sarcomas of the soft tissues metastasize to regional lymph nodes and the lungs, and they also recur locally after simple surgical excision. Soft-tissue fibrosarcomas (often well differentiated) rarely metastasize and can be cured by surgery alone if care is taken to excise them widely in three dimensions. Angiomas and lipomas can be locally invasive like fibrosarcomas, but metastasis is rare.[8, 9, 30-32] Any "benign" soft-tissue tumor that rapidly recurs after excision must be regarded as a sarcoma, although so-called

benign fibroblastic and lipoblastic proliferations may demonstrate this facility. The differential diagnosis of soft-tissue masses includes neurofibromas, lipomas, hemangiomas, and myositis ossificans.

In bone lesions, differential considerations including a benign healing fracture, a fracture through a benign lytic lesion, osteomyelitis, a bone infarct, a benign cartilaginous lesion, or fibrous dysplasia can all complicate or delay the diagnosis of a malignant tumor of bone. It is critical to remember that, on occasion, a short-term follow-up roentgenogram can be indispensable in demonstrating tell-tale growth of a subtle malignant childhood tumor involving bone.

Therapeutic Decisions and Staging

The staging systems for adrenal neuroblastomas and Wilms' tumors are similar (see Table 17–1). If the radiologist can establish preoperatively that the regional lymph nodes are involved (or there is further intra-abdominal or extra-abdominal spread), that there is infiltration of major vessels (aorta, vena cava, superior mesenteric, renal, adrenal), or that the tumor is multiple (neuroblastoma or bilateral Wilms' tumor), he can be of considerable help in treatment planning. One per cent of neuroblastomas are multiple, and 10 per cent of Wilms' tumors are bilateral.

Chest radiographs and skeletal survey are important for all childhood malignancies, with the exception of retinoblastoma. A patient with a retinoblastoma that is 4 to 10 disc diameters in size and is behind the

Table 17–1 Staging System

Stage I	Confined to the organ of origin (completely resectable)
Stage II	Local extension of the tumor (most are resectable)
Stage III	Distant spread confined to the abdomino-pelvic cavity (or mediastinum, for neuroblastoma)
Stage IV	"Deep" parenchymal involvement and/or extra-abdominal spread (lung, liver, bone, etc.)

equator has a very favorable prognosis.[33] Microscopic extension along the optic nerve to the brain can only be appreciated by careful pathologic examination of serial sections. Bilaterality is common if there is a family history of retinoblastoma.[34]

Often, patients with malignant hepatomas have dissemination (mostly to the lung) at the time of diagnosis. Bone and soft-tissue tumors rarely metastasize to the liver; they spread much more often to the lungs (and occasionally to other bones). Regional nodes are involved in 10 per cent of patients with a sarcoma in an extremity, and some centers include the regional nodes routinely in the treatment regimen. Myosarcomas as well as Ewing's tumors may present with minimal bone involvement and a very large soft-tissue component. Wide resection followed by irradiation is usually recommended for myosarcoma, and irradiation only is used for Ewing's sarcoma and reticulum cell sarcoma of the bone. Amputation is the treatment of choice for osteosarcoma in the periphery.

Noninvasive radiographic techniques are especially important in staging Hodgkin's disease, since splenectomy is not universally recommended in patients less than 10 years old, and intestinal obstruction may be caused by adhesions that occur following exploratory laparotomy.

Clinical Follow-up

When one is dealing with children one looks forward to a prolonged survival. Finding a solitary metastasis (usually in the lung) in a patient with Wilms' tumor, myosarcoma, and osteosarcoma is important because it may not preclude a cure.[35, 36] Cure of tumor recurrence at the primary site has also been reported in myosarcomas and medulloblastomas. Unfortunately, cure of a local recurrence in retinoblastoma after surgery is rare enough to be anecdotal, but the contralateral eye should be followed for the development of a second tumor up to five years after diagnosis.

Another general aspect of post-treatment follow-up of patients with tumors is the recognition of treatment-induced injury, such as a radiation stricture or a postoperative fistula. Approximately 2 per cent of children who survive a first malignancy will develop a second malignancy, and the second tumor is not always in the irradiated field (i.e., not "radiation induced").[37] Structural alterations of the spine, ilium, ribs, and face within the portal of irradiation will occur in children.[38, 39] Spinal curvature may be detected as early as six months after irradiation for Wilms' tumor or neuroblastoma. The length of the long bones can be severely affected if the metaphysis and epiphysis must be included within a radiation portal. Occasionally osteochondrosarcomas and exostoses also occur 1 to 20 years following intensive irradiation of another tumor.[40, 41]

Intestinal obstruction can be caused by vincristine therapy, by postoperative adhesions, or by recurrent tumor. Intensive total abdominal irradiation has been employed with combined therapy (radiation therapy and actinomycin D) and severe enteritis has resulted. Abdominal irradiation above 3500 rads to portals including the liver, chemotherapy alone (methotrexate, BCNU), and "immunotherapy" (BCG) can cause hepatitis. It must not be forgotten that metastases and hepatitis can both occur in the liver at the same time.[42]

Delayed cancer of the thyroid, hypoplasia of the aorta, alteration in the progress of dentition, and breast hypoplasia have all been implicated as sequelae to curative radiation treatment in children.

RADIOLOGIC CONSIDERATIONS

Retinoblastoma

Retinoblastomas constitute a small percentage of childhood tumors, but because of their location and their great tendency for bilaterality, they are of special importance. They represent the most common orbital tumor in children, and the therapeutic approaches are complex and require careful diagnostic assistance.[43-46]

PRESENTING RADIOGRAPHIC SIGNS

A child with a retinoblastoma usually has visual difficulties (often a "squint" noted by the parent), proptosis, or abnormal

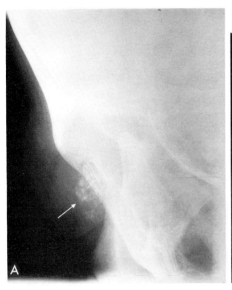 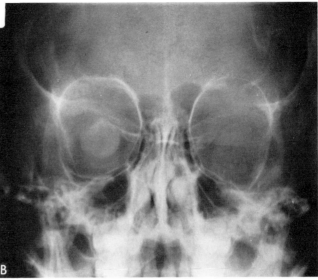

Figure 17–1   Large, rapidly growing retinoblastoma in a 5-year-old male. *A,* Oblique view of the right orbit demonstrates a small area of speckled calcification (arrow) within the tumor that is projected over the zygoma. *B,* This anteroposterior film, taken three and one-half weeks after the one in *A,* shows marked increase in the amount of calcification.

eye appearance or movement. Anteroposterior, oblique, and lateral views of the orbits should be the first radiographs to be taken. Many retinoblastomas show some calcification. Additional oblique views, exposed with soft-tissue technique, demonstrate the anterior portion of the eyeball, particularly in patients with proptosis (Fig. 17–1*A*). Erosion of the bony walls of the orbit (Fig. 17–2*A*) and involvement of the optic foramina are relatively uncommon early radiologic signs.

DIFFERENTIAL DIAGNOSIS

The diagnosis of retinoblastoma is rarely in doubt. Few other orbital lesions that calcify occur in children. Retinal hemorrhage and retinal angiomatosis may have calcifications, but their appearance on ophthalmologic examination is quite different. Further studies including brain scans, skull and sinus radiographs, or special neuroradiologic procedures may be necessary to ascertain the local extent of the tumor as well as to establish or rule out the presence of bilateral tumors. An important diagnostic consideration is that adrenal neuroblastomas are notorious for metastasizing to the orbital region, and an intravenous pyelogram should be part of the initial workup for an orbital neoplasm in a child. In patients who

present with proptosis, the differential diagnosis must include other orbital tumors (primarily the various sarcomas, including rhabdomyosarcomas), mucoceles, histiocytosis, angiomatous malformations, and leukemic infiltrates.

LOCALIZATION AND STAGING

In addition to the anteroposterior and oblique orbital views, special views of the optic foramina must also be obtained.[47] Since extension along the optic nerves is always a possibility, if there is any doubt about the size, shape, or margins of the optic foramina, tomograms of the optic canals in the basal projection should also be obtained.

If there is any question about bony erosion of the walls of the orbits, tomographic studies should be performed without hesitation or delay (Fig. 17–3). In addition to tomograms in the anteroposterior projection, basal tomograms might be of considerable assistance in fully delineating the bony confines of the orbits, particularly the posterior portions. Tomograms may also be of help in detecting small soft-tissue (tumoral) calcifications.

When the patient presents with proptosis and an orbital mass, the advisability of an orbital venogram should also be consid-

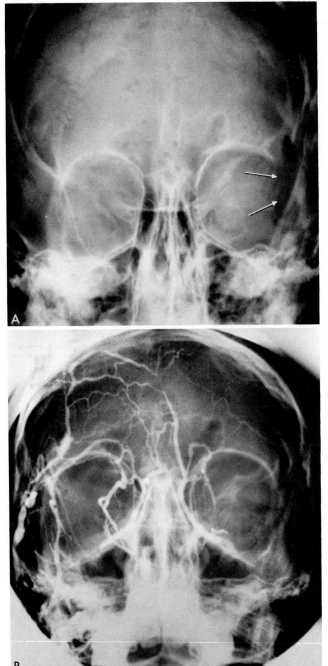

Figure 17–2   *A,* Retinoblastoma with orbital erosion in a 12-year-old female with a large and expansile tumor in the left orbit. The calcification is faint. Destruction of the lateral wall of the left orbit is apparent (arrows). *B,* Orbital venogram of the same patient. The patient's right side is normal, but on the left the venous plexus in the medial portion of the orbit is effaced and distorted by tumor.

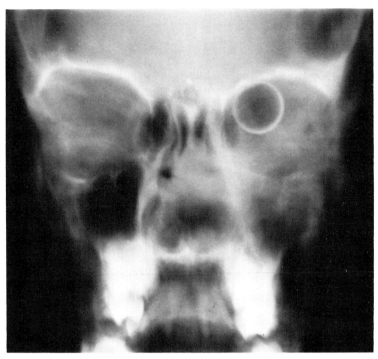

Figure 17-3 Retinoblastoma with local extension, which recurred after enucleation in a 12-year-old female. The prosthetic device is clearly seen in the left orbit. It is displaced by the recurrent tumor which has pushed it medially and upwards. The tomogram also shows tumor extension into the left maxillary antrum and into the left nasal passage. The inferior orbital wall is irregular and mottled, secondary to tumor invasion.

ered (Fig. 17-2 *B*) Orbital venography is an excellent tool in visualizing medial and superomedial extension of soft-tissue tumors, including vascular malformations, in and around the orbit.[48-50] There appears to be little indication for retrobulbar air or radiologic positive-contrast studies in retinoblastomas, particularly since orbital venography is simpler and safer.[51] Special ultrasound studies, when available, may be of further value for delineating extrabulbar tumor extension.*

Skull roentgenograms, including the basal projection, should be part of the initial examination. Intracranial extension of a retinoblastoma is one avenue of regional spread (Fig. 17-4). If there is a serious possibility of intracranial spread, then of course appropriate pneumoencephalographic or neuroarteriographic studies should be performed.

---

*At the time of this writing, computerized tomographic (CT) scanning is assuming increased importance and may prove to be *the* best technique for delineating intra-orbital masses. ED.

Although retinoblastomas usually spread by local and regional extension, distant metastases do occur.[52] For this reason, chest radiographs and a skeletal survey should also be included in the staging of retinoblastomas.

RADIOLOGIC FOLLOW-UP

The primary concern in the follow-up of the successfully treated patient is the early detection of local recurrence and regional spread. Views of the orbit and optic foramina should be part of the routine follow-up. The additional studies mentioned above need only be used if there is a serious clinical suspicion of local extension (Fig. 17-3). Chest roentgenograms should be part of the follow-up, but the need for skeletal surveys is somewhat controversial; certainly, routine skeletal surveys, as with neuroblastomas, seem to be unnecessary unless clinical and laboratory findings suggest the presence of systemic metastases.

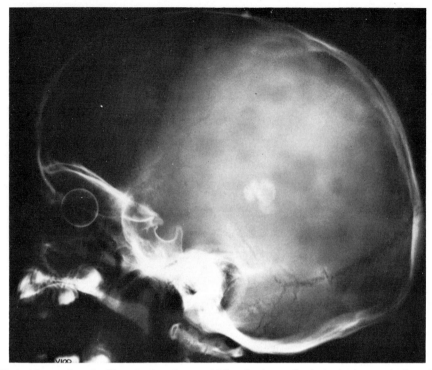

Figure 17–4 Metastatic retinoblastoma in a 3-year-old female. A prosthetic device is seen in the orbit, and there is a large, discrete calcification in the middle fossa. The diagnosis of intracranial metastasis, in the area of the calcification, was proved by cerebral angiography. The patient also had extension of tumor into the spinal subarachnoid space. Final confirmation of extensive distant metastases was made at autopsy.

Retroperitoneal Malignant Tumors

PRESENTING RADIOGRAPHIC SIGNS

Wilms' tumors and neuroblastomas are the most common malignant abdominal tumors in young children, and the survival rate has steadily improved in the past two decades.[53, 54] New diagnostic imaging tools and the better use of older techniques have played an important part in achieving these results.[55]

Palpable abdominal tumors in infants and small children are usually detected either during a routine physical examination or during handling by the mother. The subsequent plain film examination of the abdomen often confirms the presence of a soft-tissue mass. Calcification in the mass is characteristic of (although not exclusive to) neuroblastomas (Fig. 17–5), while Wilms' tumors rarely calcify. Since neuroblastomas tend to metastasize to the regional lymph nodes more readily than Wilms' tumors, widening of the para-aortic stripe on the plain abdominal film suggests the presence of neuroblastoma rather than Wilms' tumor.

The first examination, after the chest roentgenograms and abdominal film, should be an abdominal ultrasound B-scan.[56, 57] There is increasing evidence that this method will permit differentiation between solid (malignant) and cystic (usually benign) masses. Extensive experience is not yet available. Every effort should be made to explore fully the possibilities of this non-invasive technique, which does not require the catheterization of vessels or the potentially hazardous introduction of contrast materials. The next radiologic examination should be an intravenous pyelogram (Fig. 17–6). In an infant with an abdominal mass, this should be a modified version of the intravenous pyelogram involving so-called total body opacification (TBO) (Fig. 17–7).[58] By injecting approximately 4 cc of contrast material per kg of body weight into an infant or small child and by obtaining films immediately after the injection of the contrast material, one can usually "catch" the con-

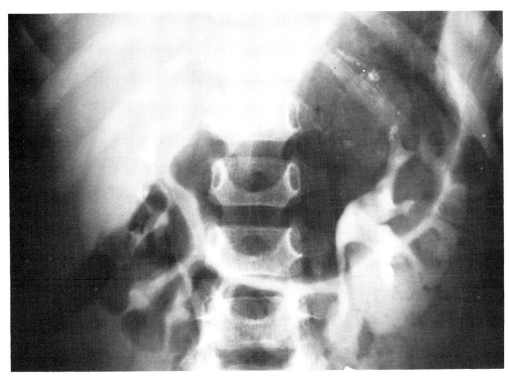

Figure 17–5 Left adrenal neuroblastoma. The intravenous pyelogram shows a roughly triangular area containing numerous calcifications in the region of the left adrenal. The pelvocalyceal system on the left is only minimally distorted and is not displaced. The right pelvocalyceal system, although faintly seen, is normal. At surgery, the patient had a large intra-adrenal neuroblastoma.

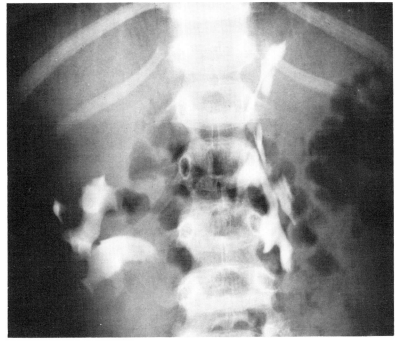

Figure 17–6 Bilateral Wilms' tumor in a 4½-year-old male with a hard abdominal mass. The intravenous pyelogram shows marked distortion of both kidneys. On the left, the pelvocalyceal system is displaced towards the midline. The calyces are compressed and splayed apart, while on the right the infiltrating tumor appears to have rotated the pelvocalyceal system around its vertical axis. (Approximately 10 per cent of Wilms' tumors are bilateral.)

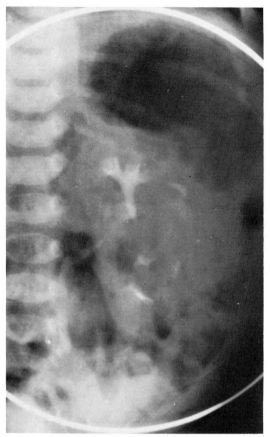

Figure 17–7 Fetal renal hamartoma in a 1-month-old female. The total body opacification (TBO) modification of the intravenous pyelogram (see text) shows enlargement of the left kidney with spreading and distortion of the calyces. The metal ring is part of a compression device which was used to displace the bowel loops from in front of the kidney. (Fetal renal hamartoma is a benign tumor which simulates Wilms' tumor in infancy radiographically, and to a lesser extent, histologically as well.)

trast material in the capillaries of the various parenchymal organs. Thus one can visualize not only the nephrogram phase of the intravenous pyelogram, but also a comparable hepatogram,'' a splenogram,'' and capillary visualization of the tumor in question.[59] Those masses that do not take up contrast material appear to be radiolucent (i.e., cystic) and therefore almost surely benign in this age group. Masses that do take up the contrast material, however, are often malignant. This simple but excellent technique has withstood the test of time and has been used to good advantage in a large number of patients in many centers.

A further simple modification of the intravenous pyelogram is derived by in-

jecting the contrast material into one of the *foot* veins, in preference to one in the arm, and attempting thereby to obtain visualization of the inferior vena cava. Blockage of the inferior vena cava or its displacement may assist in determining the regional extent of retroperitoneal tumor.[60]

DIFFERENTIAL DIAGNOSIS

The most important considerations in differential diagnosis are benign masses. Hydronephrosis, with or without duplication of the collecting systems, benign cystic renal teratomas (the so-called multicystic kidney), various abdominal cysts (mesenteric or omental), duplications, and actual benign tumors, such as "fetal renal hamartoma"[61, 62] in infancy, are the important differential diagnostic considerations (Fig. 17–7). Total body opacification will assist in differentiating solid tumors from cystic lesions (see previous section).[63] Intrinsic distortion of the pelvocalyceal systems on the later films of the total body opacification examination or the intravenous pyelogram usually indicates the presence of an intrarenal tumor (often Wilms'), while displacement of the pelvocalyceal systems without gross distortion of their normal architecture indicates either a tumor or displacement by an unopacified duplication of the renal pelvis or an extrarenal mass (para-aortic nodes or an adrenal tumor). In special problem situations angiograms, including selective renal or adrenal arteriograms, may be performed,[64, 65] but these procedures are not routine in children.[66]

LOCALIZATION AND STAGING

The basic radiologic studies utilized in the localization of these abdominal tumors have been discussed already in the previous section. Since both Wilms' tumors and neuroblastomas have high metastatic potentials (Fig. 17–8), it is important to obtain chest roentgenograms and full skeletal surveys at the time of initial diagnosis (Fig. 17–9). Liver involvement is a potential problem in both of these tumors but particularly in neuroblastoma. Usually liver and spleen scans are the methods of choice for investigating this problem initially by imaging techniques. Bone scans might have

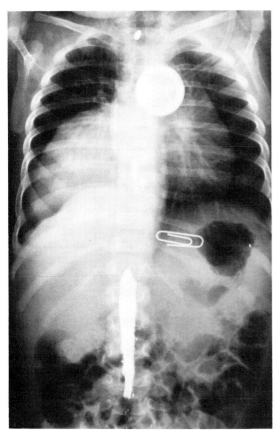

Figure 17–8 Intrathoracic neuroblastoma with extension into the spinal canal in a 6-month-old male. The presenting symptom was increasing paresis of the lower extremities. The radiograph shows a large intrathoracic neuroblastoma in the right hemithorax; radiologic contrast material also outlines the lower margin of a block in the spinal subarachnoid space at the level of the twelfth thoracic vertebra.

potential usefulness for detecting early bone metastases in neuroblastomas,[67] although the rapidly growing metaphyses of normal children might be misinterpreted

as "hot spots" and falsely suggest the presence of metastases. Involvement of the lymphatic system has already been discussed, and indeed lymphograms have been performed and reported both in Wilms' tumors and neuroblastomas. Undoubtedly, metastatic involvement of the lymphatic system can be demonstrated by this technique. However, since we found it of relatively limited practical assistance in treatment planning, we have not used lymphograms routinely for patients with these tumors.

RADIOLOGIC FOLLOW-UP

Chest roentgenograms, skeletal surveys, and abdominal films are the basic tools in the radiologic follow-up of Wilms' tumors and neuroblastomas. Chest roentgenograms and skeletal surveys are, of course, done for the purpose of detecting occult metastases. We have found chest tomograms of somewhat limited use in young uncooperative children, although in special situations they may be of help. Follow-up abdominal films may be of considerable assistance if metal surgical clips have been placed into the tumor or tumor bed at the time of surgery. Displacement of the clips can easily be detected radiographically and can serve as an early warning sign of recurrence. Clearly, the intravenous pyelogram is the ideal method for following the status of the kidney and other retroperitoneal organs. However, the number of "routine" follow-up intravenous pyelograms in children must be limited, and in certain situations we have performed so-

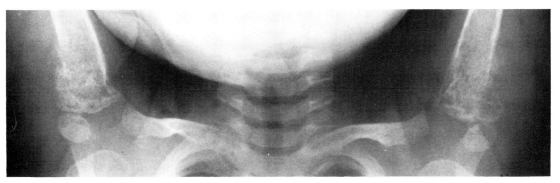

Figure 17–9 Metastatic neuroblastoma in a 1½ year-old female. Symmetrical, infiltrative destruction is present in the metaphyseal ends of both humeri, and there were many other bony metastases. The primary tumor was an adrenal neuroblastoma. (Metaphyseal metastases, frequently symmetrical in character, are common in disseminated neuroblastomas.)

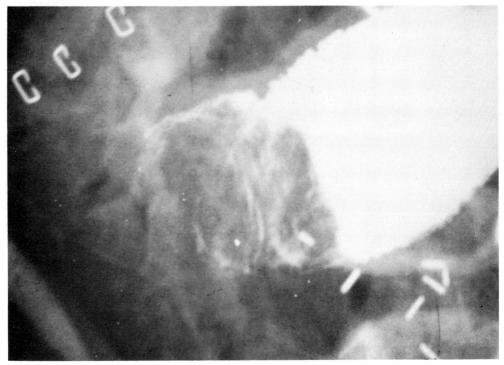

Figure 17-10 Postoperative intussusception. This 2-year-old male had surgery for a left-sided Wilms' tumor several days before this barium enema film was made. The study was undertaken because of cramping abdominal pain. Spot films show the intussusception in the transverse portion of the colon.

called "limited" intravenous pyelograms in which only one or two films are taken, usually at about 15 minutes after injection.

Treatment of Wilms' tumors and neuroblastomas may require extensive intervention. Complications are therefore not uncommon. Postoperative intussusception following extensive abdominal and retroperitoneal surgery is a known complication. Awareness of the potential complication should be helpful in facilitating early and definitive diagnosis by barium enema examination (Fig. 17–10).

Other acute complications involve the kidneys and adrenals, and the possibility of postoperative infections in this region (either in acute or subacute form) will on occasion create differential diagnostic difficulties because of the ever-present possibility of tumor recurrence. Actinomycin and vincristine may cause a nonobstructive ileus that is corroborated on plain abdominal films. Other types of acute complications caused by chemotherapy, such as hemorrhagic cystitis and enteritis, rarely require radiologic studies for diagnosis.

Delayed complications, or more correctly late sequelae of therapy, may relate to radiation therapy (Fig. 17–11) and, to some extent, to chemotherapy. Pulmonary fibrosis in the irradiated field is a late complication that one can expect when the radiation dose is above certain levels, although its presence is not always diagnosable on the follow-up chest roentgenograms. Certainly, radiation of the developing axial skeleton may be unavoidable, and late changes in the vertebral column (scoliosis) and ileum (hypoplasia) are well known following radiation therapy. Less well known is the potential for late damage to the *un*involved kidney and other parenchymal organs, primarily the liver, inasmuch as these organs tend to respond to radiation less acutely than the bowel. Chronic radiation damage in the form of malabsorption, segmental stenoses, or fistulae unfortunately still occurs. Finally, one must remember that the spinal cord is also sensitive to radiation, although gross changes in the thoracolumbar cord or the subarachnoid space have been reported relatively rarely.

Lymphomas

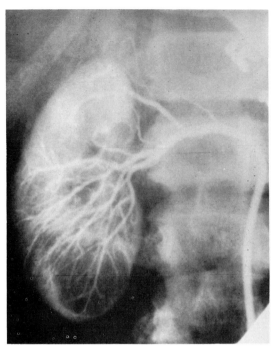

Figure 17–11 Seventeen years following postoperative abdominal radiation for a *left*-sided Wilms' tumor. The right kidney, which was included in the radiation field, is seen to be small on the arteriogram with loss of cortex throughout and a cyst in the lower pole. The vertebral changes were also secondary to radiation therapy.

PRESENTING RADIOGRAPHIC SIGNS

The lymphomas represent the most frequent cause of death from malignant disease in children, and the presence of the Burkitt's type of lymphoma is increasingly being recognized in North America as well as in Africa where it was first described. The lymphomas (including Hodgkin's) are protean in their radiologic and clinical manifestations, and therefore we will necessarily restrict our comments now to general observations. (See also Chapters 1 and 2.)

The non-Hodgkin's lymphomas in children originate in many sites, and thus it is difficult to offer any specific comments on the presenting radiologic signs. The Burkitt's type of lymphoma, for example, frequently originates within bony sites such as the mandible (Fig. 17–12), or viscera such as the kidney, the ovary, the gastrointestinal tract, and the retroperitoneal and intraperitoneal lymph nodes.

Most children with Hodgkin's disease present with an abnormal chest roentgenogram. Mediastinal widening caused by

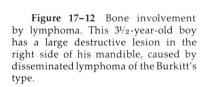
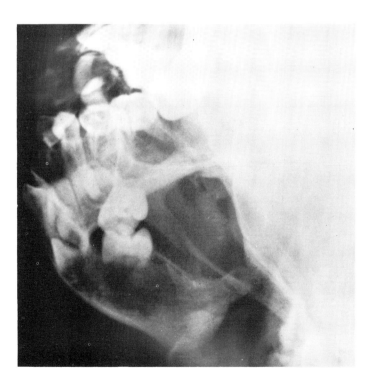

Figure 17–12 Bone involvement by lymphoma. This 3½-year-old boy has a large destructive lesion in the right side of his mandible, caused by disseminated lymphoma of the Burkitt's type.

lymphadenopathy is the most common presentation for Hodgkin's disease in this age group, just as it is in young adults. Hilar lymphadenopathy may or may not be present, but it is far less frequent than strictly mediastinal involvement.

DIFFERENTIAL DIAGNOSIS

In Hodgkin's disease in adolescents the differential diagnosis is usually that of a mediastinal mass. Of teratoma, substernal thyroid, and thymoma, the first two are less common in children, but usually occur at an earlier age than thymoma. Thymic hyperplasia, as it occurs in association with hyperthyroidism or myasthenia gravis, may on occasion create difficulties with the differential diagnosis. Although thymomas usually have sharp and rather clearly defined margins in all three dimensions (i.e., in the lateral plane as well), the differential diagnosis may be difficult. On rare occasions, a mediastinal abscess or congenital vascular abnormality might be mistaken for mediastinal lymphadenopathy. Mediastinal widening from hyperplasia of the adipose tissues, in association with long-term steroid administration in various chronic diseases, is a more recently recognized entity. The *normal* thymus has often been mistaken radiographically for a "mediastinal mass" in infants.

LOCALIZATION AND STAGING

Once the diagnosis of a lymphoproliferative disorder is established, a mediastinal mass virtually always requires further delineation.[68] As implied earlier, in an infant or small child the normal thymus might be difficult to differentiate from a mediastinal tumor. In these cases, chest fluoroscopy is usually sufficient to establish the true nature of the mediastinal mass (i.e., the normal thymus is pliable and will change markedly in size and configuration with the changing intrathoracic pressure induced by inspiration and expiration).

Older children with a true mediastinal mass need chest tomograms in the anteroposterior and lateral projections. Angiography is rarely necessary except in patients who are suspected of having superior vena

cava obstruction. In these children, visualization of the superior vena cava by injecting contrast in both antecubital veins will establish the diagnosis readily.

The skeletal survey is an integral part of staging. In patients with Hodgkin's disease or regional non-Hodgkin's lymphoma, the lymphogram is important in establishing or ruling out the presence of retroperitoneal disease (Fig. 17–13).[69] It is important to recognize that lymphograms are not substantially more difficult to perform in children than they are in adults. In younger children, we perform them under heavy sedation or light general anesthesia, but in children over 12 years of age they can usually be done with local anesthesia. Although all patients with Hodgkin's disease not known to be stage IV should be staged surgically,[70-72] the staging operation will usually not extend down to the lower para-aortic and iliac nodes; thus, the lymphogram is of considerable help in visualizing this region.

We rarely perform inferior vena cavograms routinely, but when they are part of

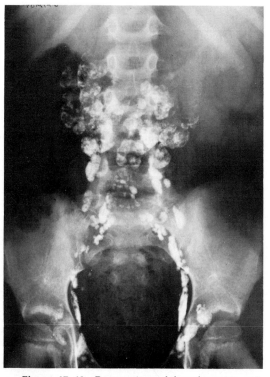

Figure 17–13 Retroperitoneal lymphoma in a 7-year-old boy. The lymphangiogram shows massive involvement of the para-aortic nodes on both sides. They are large and foamy in appearance and extend far lateral to their normal paravertebral location.

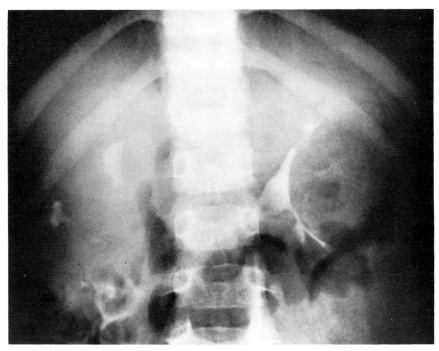

Figure 17–14   Bilateral renal involvement by an undifferentiated lymphoma in a 4-year-old boy. Distortion of the pelvocalyceal systems is apparent on both sides. (Lymphomatous involvement of the kidneys might simulate Wilms' tumor; the similarity between this case and the one shown in Figure 17–6 is a good example.)

the staging procedure they are best done after the lymphangiogram so that the relationships of the opacified lymph nodes, cava and ureters can easily be assessed. The intravenous pyelogram, of course, will also be helpful to confirm or rule out the presence of a lymphomatous infiltration of the kidneys (Fig. 17–17). Arteriography is rarely necessary, although in special situations, such as in suspected but unconfirmed liver involvement, it can occasionally be of some assistance.[73] In most cases, the noninvasive liver and spleen scan will be sufficient.

RADIOLOGIC FOLLOW-UP

Chest roentgenograms and abdominal films are most important as follow-up tools in patients treated for Hodgkin's disease or lymphoma. The mediastinal changes must be followed carefully. Also, the presence or absence of lung involvement or a potential pulmonary sensitivity reaction to chemotherapy (bleomycin or methotrexate, for example) can be assessed on the follow-up chest roentgenograms. The abdominal film is of considerable help because of the rela-

tively slow elution of contrast material from the lymph nodes.[74] Even though the rate of disappearance of nodal contrast is faster in children than in adults, the opacified nodes and the position of surgical clips placed at the time of staging laparotomy are of great assistance in detecting extension or recurrence of disease. Skeletal surveys are not part of the routine follow-up procedure in lymphomas, although with proper indication bone films are frequently obtained because bone (particularly periosteal) involvement is not uncommon in the more undifferentiated tumors (Fig. 17–15).

Malignant Tumors of the Extremities and Limb Girdles

PRESENTING RADIOGRAPHIC SIGNS

These tumors arise from almost any mesodermal tissue element (Fig. 17–16). Osteogenic sarcomas and, to a lesser extent, chondrosarcomas, myosarcomas, liposarcomas, fibrosarcomas, and the small "round-cell" tumors such as Ewing's sarcoma are the

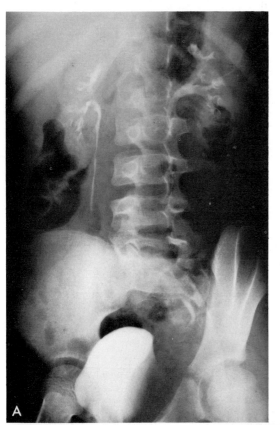

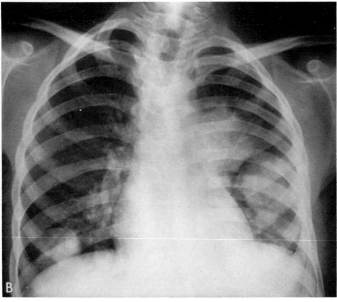

Figure 17–15 *A,* Undifferentiated sarcoma of the pelvis. Oblique film from the intravenous pyelogram shows a large soft tissue mass indenting the left inferolateral aspect of the bladder. (On coned-down films, periosteal new bone formation was also evident on the superior margin of the left pubis). *B,* Chest roentgenogram of the same patient, showing multiple metastases in both lungs. (This patient had an undifferentiated sarcoma. Neither rhabdomyosarcoma nor Ewing's tumor originating in the pubic bone could be proven conclusively, although the radiographic appearance and behavior of the tumor would be compatible with either diagnosis.)

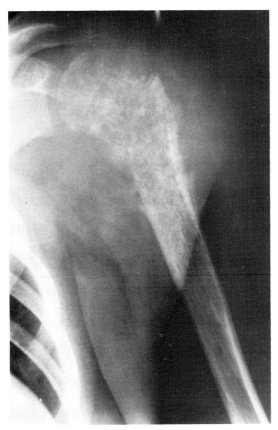

Figure 17–16 Osteogenic sarcoma in a 9-year-old female. Irregular lytic destruction of the humeral head and upper shaft predominates in this case, with irregular, spiculated subperiosteal new bone formation. An associated soft tissue mass in the axilla is not clearly defined on the film but was evident clinically. (This figure illustrates an osteosarcoma that does *not* have the "typical" appearance. See text and Fig. 14–14).

lesions most commonly encountered in this age group. (See also Chapter 14.) Children with malignant limb lesions usually present because of pain or nonspecific swelling in the involved extremity. Occasionally, a palpable mass or limping (in the case of a lower extremity lesion) is the presenting sign. The radiologic presentation varies with the site and tissue of origin of the tumor. Osteosarcomas have a characteristic appearance if they produce "tumor bone." Similarly, the so-called laminated type of periosteal new bone formation is frequently found in (although it is not diagnostic of) Ewing's tumors.

While most osteogenic sarcomas produce new "tumor bone" and therefore have a characteristic appearance, a minority do not—as illustrated in Figure 17–16. In the latter variety, differentiation from other tumors, such as Ewing's sarcoma, rests primarily on tumor localization. Osteogenic sarcomas tend to be metaphyseal, whereas Ewing's sarcomas often occur in the tubular portions of the bones (i.e., the diaphyses).

The associated soft-tissue changes will also depend on the type and aggressiveness of the tumor. Sharply defined soft tissue masses on radiographs of an extremity, as may be seen in some rhabdomyosarcomas, can be associated with malignancy just as frequently as irregular or ill-defined soft-tissue infiltrates. The latter may be encountered with or without dystrophic calcifications, in the more infiltrative types of tumors (Fig. 17–17 and 17–18).

Clearly, good quality radiographs of the bone and soft tissue of the involved extremity are a basic requirement for arriving at an accurate radiologic diagnosis. At times radiographic magnification films or special xeroradiograms may be of assistance in defining details of bone destruction or the outlines of a soft-tissue mass.

There is every reason to attempt to make

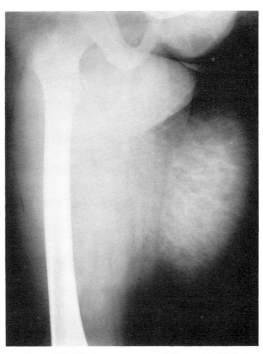

Figure 17–17 Liposarcoma of the right thigh in a 9-year-old boy. A large soft tissue tumor originates from the medial portion of the right thigh. Denser connective tissue strands are clearly seen within the large and relatively lucent (i.e., *fat*-containing) tumor mass. Biopsy confirmed the suspected presence of a liposarcoma.

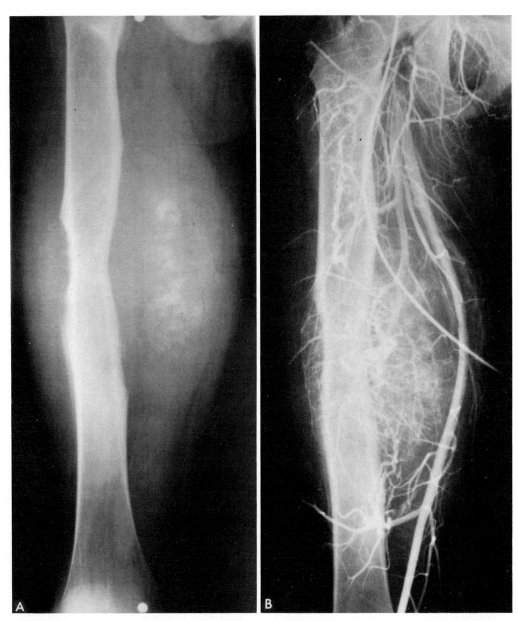

Figure 17–18 *A,* Ewing's tumor in a 10-year-old girl. A destructive lesion is located in the diaphysis of the right femur. Linear subperiosteal new bone formation is particularly well seen on the distal lateral aspect of the femur. Speckled, dystrophic calcification is also evident in the deep thigh muscles, quite separate from the periosteal new bone formation. *B,* Femoral arteriogram on the same patient. The arteriogram for catheter placement was undertaken prior to a planned selective arterial infusion of adriamycin. The large tumor mass is highly vascular, and the primary source of vascular supply appears to be the deep femoral artery. The superficial femoral artery is displaced medially but is not directly invaded; however, it supplies a few of the inferior branches feeding the tumor.

the radiologic diagnosis as definitively as possible. The differential diagnosis of extremity lesions is frequently difficult for the pathologist as well as for the radiologist. Percutaneous bone biopsy utilizing a Craig-type needle (under fluoroscopic control and guidance) is an excellent diagnostic tool, particularly for establishing a suspected metastasis prior to palliative radiotherapy. Diagnostic studies with bone or tumor seeking radionuclides have been utilized extensively as screening procedures for metastatic lesions.[75, 76]

DIFFERENTIAL DIAGNOSIS

Almost all the component radiologic abnormalities found in malignant tumors of the extremities can be mimicked by inflammatory and other benign lesions. Some of the benign (or at least "more benign") bone lesions, such as giant cell tumors in late adolescence or eosinophilic granulomas may imitate the widely destructive radiologic bone changes that are associated with malignancies. It is also of the greatest importance to search for a primary tumor elsewhere if there is the slightest possibility that the presenting bone lesion might be associated with a neuroblastoma, thyroid carcinoma, or leukemia, or is a metastasis from another osseous tumor (Ewing's, reticulum cell, or osteogenic sarcoma).

Periosteal new bone formation and adjacent soft-tissue calcifications, often of the non-proliferative or "inert" type, can appear ominous but may be caused solely by trauma, and in those suspect situations one is obliged to search carefully for a possible occult (and benign) fracture underlying the obvious periosteal new bone. Tomograms may be of great value in this situation, and if necessary the studies can be repeated in several weeks. Swelling caused by hematomas, and soft-tissue calcifications associated with dermatomyositis or other collagen diseases are not infrequently observed, and the final diagnosis is often impossible to make by radiologic means alone.

The classic differential diagnostic problem between a bone malignancy and osteomyelitis is somewhat less difficult today than in the days prior to antibiotics. Because of the widespread (and early) use of antibiotics, the progressive or advanced radiologic changes of osteomyelitis rarely develop. Nevertheless, perhaps it is necessary to

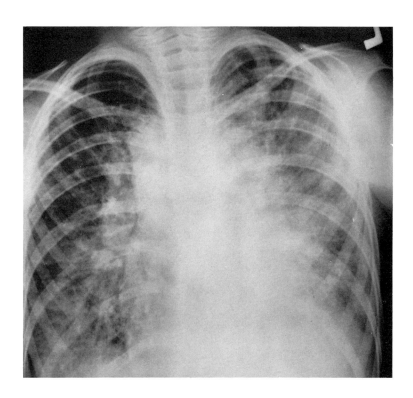

Figure 17–19 Metastatic osteogenic sarcoma in a 7-year-old male. The chest roentgenogram shows lymphangitic (or interstitial) pulmonary spread, as well as massive nodal metastases. The primary tumor was in the forearm. (Most osteogenic sarcomas give rise to round, blood-borne metastases in the lungs, but lymphangitic spread, as in this case, is also seen occasionally).

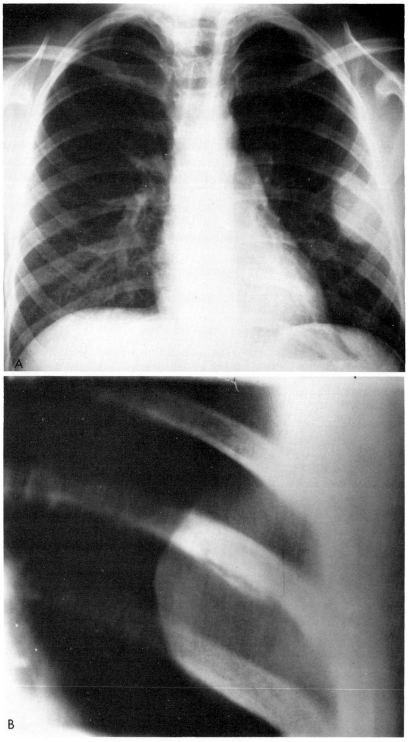

Figure 17–20 *A*, Ewing's tumor originating from the left sixth rib in a 10-year-old girl. The chest roentgenogram shows a soft tissue mass beneath the rib. *B*, Tomograms of the same patient clearly show the osseous involvement, with periosteal new bone formation and the associated soft tissue mass.

re-emphasize that a virulent or incompletely treated osteomyelitis may imitate malignant bone tumors in the extremities to a frightening degree. Except for occasional tomograms, further studies of the lesions themselves are rarely necessary. On occasion, angiograms or lymphograms must be done in order to evaluate the vascularity of a lesion (prior to biopsy) or the involvement of regional nodes, or as a prelude to local infusion therapy (Fig. 17–18). Careful examination of the soft tissue density on plain films may also be helpful (Figs. 17–17 and 17–18 *A*).

LOCALIZATION AND STAGING

Chest roentgenograms, whole-lung tomograms, skeletal survey examinations, and intravenous pyelograms are the most important radiologic examinations in the staging of extremity lesions. Bone scans are highly recommended if these techniques are available in a particular institution, but direct bone-marrow examination must not be neglected before treatment in those lesions that have a tendency to infiltrate the marrow (i.e., rhabdomyosarcoma).

RADIOLOGIC FOLLOW-UP

The radiologic methods of follow-up are much the same as described in the section on localization and staging. Chest roentgenograms (Figs. 17–19), skeletal surveys, and various scanning procedures are our most important tools. In the evaluation of suspected metastases, as in the liver, more complex angiographic studies are occasionally needed.

Acknowledgment: We are most grateful to Robert Neerhout, M.D. (Department of Pediatrics, University of California, Los Angeles) for reviewing this chapter and for his excellent suggestions.

References

1. Miller, R. W.: Fifty-two forms of childhood cancer: United States mortality experience, 1960–1966. J. Pediatr., 75:685–689, 1969.
2. Wells, H. G.: Congenital tumors. Arch. Pathol., 30:535–601, 1940.
3. Balsaver, A. M., Butler, J. J., and Martin, R. G.: Congenital fibrosarcoma. Cancer, 20:1607–1616, 1967.
4. Ehrlich, F. E., Haas, J. E., and Kiesewetter, W. B.: Rhabdomyosarcoma in infants and children: Factors affecting long-term survival. J. Pediatr. Surg., 6:571–577, 1971.
5. Hays, D. M., Mirabal, V. Q., Karlan, M. S., et al.: Fibrosarcomas in infants and children. J. Pediatr. Surg., 5:176–183, 1970.
6. Kauffman, S. L., and Stout, A. P.: Congenital mesenchymal tumors. Cancer, 18:460–476, 1965.
7. Levkoff, A. H., Gonzalez, C. G., and Neher, J. L.: Congenital diffuse fibromatosis—A case report. Pediatrics, 35:331–333, 1965.
8. Nixon, H. H., and Scobie, W. G.: Congenital lipomatosis: A report of four cases. J. Pediatr. Surg., 6:742–745, 1971.
9. Stout, A. P.: Fibrosarcoma in infants and children. Cancer, 15:1028–1040, 1962.
10. Ellsworth, R. M.: The practical management of retinoblastoma. Trans. Am. Ophthalmol. Soc., 67:462–534, 1969.
11. Haller, J. A., Mazur, D. O., and Morgan, W. W., Jr.: Diagnosis and management of mediastinal masses in children. J. Thorac. Cardiovasc. Surg., 58:385–392, 1969.
12. Filler, R. M., Traggis, D. G., Jaffe, N., et al.: Favorable outlook for children with mediastinal neuroblastoma. J. Pediatr. Surg., 7:136–143, 1972.
13. Ishak, K. G., and Glunz, P. R.: Hepatoblastoma and hepatocarcinoma in infancy and childhood. Cancer, 20:396–422, 1967.
14. Bolande, R. P.: Benignity of neonatal tumors and concept of cancer repression in early life. Am. J. Dis. Child., 122:11–14, 1971.
15. Becker, J. M., Schneider, K. M., and Krasna, I. H.: Neonatal neuroblastoma. Pediatrics, 36:359–366, 1965.
16. Ehrensperger, J., and Genton, N.: Cancer in the newborn. *In* Saegesser, F., and Pettavel, J. (eds.), Surgical Oncology. Baltimore, Williams & Wilkins, 1971.
17. Shown, T. E., and Durfee, M. F.: Blueberry muffin baby: Neonatal neuroblastoma with subcutaneous metastases. J. Urol., 104:193–195, 1970.
18. Breslow, N., and McCann, B.: Statistical estimation of prognosis for children with neuroblastoma. Cancer Res., 31:2098–2103, 1971.
19. Leiken, S., Evans, A. E., Heyn, R., et al.: The impact of chemotherapy on the survival of children with advanced neuroblastoma—An analysis of patients diagnosed in 1956, 1962 and 1966–1968. J. Pediatr., 84:131–134, 1974.
20. Wolff, J. A., D'Angio, G. J., Hartmann, J., et al: Long-term evaluation of single versus multiple dose actinomycin therapy of Wilms' tumor. N. Engl. J. Med., 290:84–86, 1974.
21. Vietti, T. J., Sullivan, M. P., Haggard, M. E., et al.: Vincristine sulfate and radiation therapy in metastatic Wilms' tumor. Cancer, 25:12–30, 1970.
22. Chretien, P. B., Milam, J. D., Foote, F. W., et al.: Embryonal adenocarcinomas (a type of malignant teratoma) of the sacrococcygeal region. Cancer, 26:522–535, 1970.
23. Bloom, H. J. G.: Combined modality therapy for intracranial tumors. Cancer, 35:111–120, 1975.
24. Lin, S., Lee, K. F., and O'Hara, A. E.: Congenital astrocytomas: The roentgenographic manifesta-

tions. Am. J. Roentgenol. Radium Ther. Nucl. Med., *115*:78–85, 1972.

25. Fessard, C.: Cerebral tumors in infancy. Am. J. Dis. Child, *115*:302–308, 1968.

26. Engel, R. M., Elkins, R. C., and Fletcher, B. D.: Retroperitoneal teratoma. Cancer, *22*:1068–1073, 1968.

27. Greene, R. E.: Abdominal mass in infancy. J.A.M.A., *202*:121–123, 1967.

28. Raffensperger, J., and Abousleiman, A.: Abdominal masses in children under one year of age. Surgery, *63*:514–521, 1968.

29. Shafie, M. E., Spitz, L., and Ikeda, S.: Malignant tumors of the small bowel in neonates presenting with perforation. J. Pediatr. Surg., *6*:61–64, 1971.

30. Sagerman, R. H., Tretter, P., and Ellsworth, R. M.: The treatment of orbital rhabdomyosarcoma of children with primary radiation therapy. Am. J. Roentgenol. Radium Ther. Nucl. Med., *114*: 31–34, 1972.

31. Horne, C. H. W., Slavin, G., and McDonald, A. M.: Late recurrence of juvenile fibrosarcoma. Br. J. Surg., *55*:102–103, 1968.

32. Jensen, A. R., Martin, L. W., and Longino, L. A.: Digital neurofibrosarcoma in infancy. J. Pediatr., *51*:566–670, 1967.

33. Reese, A. B., and Ellsworth, R. M.: Management of retinoblastoma. Ann. N.Y. Acad. Sci., *114*:958, 1964.

34. Jensen, R. D., and Miller, R. W.: Retinoblastoma: Epidemiologic characteristics. N. Engl. J. Med., *285*:307–711, 1971.

35. Martini, N., Huvos, A. G., Mike, V., et al.: Multiple pulmonary resection in treatment of osteogenic sarcoma. Ann. Thorac. Surg., *12*:271–280, 1971.

36. Heyn, R. M., Holland, R., Newton, W. A., Jr., et al.: The role of combined chemotherapy in the treatment of rhabdomyosarcoma in children. Cancer, *34*:2128–2142, 1974.

37. Tefft, M., Vawter, G. F., and Mitus, A.: Second primary neoplasms in children. Am. J. Roentgenol. Radium Ther. Nucl. Med., *103*:800–821, 1968.

38. Rutherford, H., and Dodd, G. D.: Complications of radiation therapy: Growing bone. Semin. Roentgenol., *9*:15–27, 1974.

39. Forrest, A. W.: Tumors following radiation about the eye. Trans. Am. Acad. Ophthalmol. Otolaryngol., *65*:694–717, 1961.

40. Altman, D. H., and Piccinini, M. T.: The radiodiagnostic follow-up of patients with Wilms' tumor. *In* Kaufmann, H. J. (ed.), Progress in Pediatric Radiology. Vol. 3. Chicago, Year Book Medical Publishers, 1970.

41. Veraguth, P.: Les séquelles de la radiothérapie chez l'enfant. Radiol. Clin. Biol., *41*:285–297, 1972.

42. Fellows, K. E. Jr., Vawter, G. F., and Tefft, M.: Hepatic effects following abdominal irradiation in children: Detection by Au¹⁹⁸ scan and confirmation by histologic examination. Am. J. Roentgenol., Radium Ther. Nucl. Med., *103*: 422–431, 1968.

43. Arger, P. H., Mishkin, M. M., and Nenninger, R. H.: An approach to orbital lesions. Am. J. Roentgenol. Radium Ther. Nucl. Med., *115*: 595–606, 1972.

44. Evans, R. A., Schwartz, J. F., and Chutorian, A. M.:

Radiologic diagnosis in pediatric ophthalmology. Radiol. Clin. North Am., *1*:459–495, 1963.

45. Hepler, R. S.: Clinical diagnosis of orbital tumors. Radiol. Clin. North Am., *10*:3–10, 1972.

46. Kirkpatrick, J. A., and Capitanio, M. A.: Radiology of the orbit in infancy and childhood. Radiol. Clin. North Am., *10*:143–166, 1972.

47. Potter, G. M.: Tomography of the orbit. Radiol. Clin. North Am., *10*:21–38, 1972.

48. Hanafee, W. N.: Orbital venography. Radiol. Clin. North Am., *10*:63–81, 1972.

49. Russell, D. B., and Miller, J. D.: Orbital venography. Radiology, *103*:267–273, 1972.

50. Vignaud, J., Clay, C., and Aubin, M. L.: Orbital arteriography. Radiol. Clin. North Am., *10*:39–61, 1972.

51. Lombardi, G.: Orbital pathology and contrast media. Radiol. Clin. North Am., *10*:115–128, 1972.

52. Carbajal, U. M.: Metastases in retinoblastoma. Am. J. Ophthalmol., *48*:47–69, 1959.

53. Aaron, B. S.: Wilms' tumor—A clinical study of eighty-one patients. Cancer, *33*:637–646, 1974.

54. Koop, C. E.: The neuroblastoma. Progr. Pediatr. Surg., *4*:1–28, 1972.

55. Tank, E. S., Poznanski, A. K., and Holt, J. F.: The radiologic discrimination of abdominal masses in infants. J. Urol., *109*:128–132, 1973.

56. Bearman, S., Sanders, R. C., and Oh, K. S.: B-scan ultrasound in the evaluation of pediatric abdominal masses. Radiology, *108*:111–117, 1973.

57. King, D. L.: Renal ultrasonography: An aid in the clinical evaluation of renal masses. Radiology, *105*:633–640, 1972.

58. O'Connor, J. F., and Neuhauser, E. B. D.: Total body opacification in conventional and high dose intravenous urography in infancy. Am. J. Roentgenol. Radium Ther. Nucl. Med., *90*: 63–71, 1963.

59. Griscom, N. T.: The roentgenology of neonatal abdominal masses. Am. J. Roentgenol. Radium Ther. Nucl. Med., *93*:447–463, 1965.

60. Gammill, S., Puyau, F., and Neitzschman, H.: Phlebo-arterio-urography in the assessment of abdominal masses in children. Am. J. Roentgenol. Radium Ther. Nucl. Med., *120*:389–397, 1974.

61. Berdon, W. E., Baker, D. H., and Wigger, J. H.: Benign fetal hamartoma: The renal tumor of the newborn. Paper presented at the meeting of the American Roentgen Ray Society, Washington, D. C., 1972.

62. Berdon, W. E., Wigger, H. J., and Baker, D. H.: Fetal renal hamartoma—A benign tumor to be distinguished from Wilms' tumor. Am. J. Roentgenol. Radium Ther. Nucl. Med., *118*: 18–27, 1973.

63. Rose, J., Berdon, W. E., Sullivan, R. J., et al.: Prolonged jaundice as presenting sign of massive adrenal hemorrhage in newborn. Radiographic diagnosis by IVP with total body opacification. Radiology, *98*:263–272, 1971.

64. Clark, R. E., Moss, A. A., deLormier, A. A., et al.: Arteriography of Wilms' tumor. Am. J. Roentgenol. Radium Ther. Nucl. Med., *113*:476–490, 1971.

65. McDonald, P., and Hiller, H. G.: Angiography in abdominal tumor in childhood with particular

reference to neuroblastoma and Wilms' tumor. Clin. Radiol., *19*:1–18, 1968.

66. Bron, K. M., Riley, R. R., and Girdany, B. R.: Pediatric arteriography in abdominal and extremity lesions. Radiology, *92*:1241–1255, 1969.

67. Helson, L., Watson, R. C., Benua, R. S., et al.: F-18 radioisotope scanning of metastatic bone lesions in children with neuroblastoma. Am. J. Roentgenol. Radium Ther. Nucl. Med., *115*: 191–199, 1972.

68. Brower, A. C., and Seale, D. L.: A critical appraisal of radiographic studies employed in the staging of patients with Hodgkin's disease. Radiology, *110*:97–101, 1974.

69. Lee, K. F.: Lymphography in malignant lymphomas —An analysis of 400 cases. CRC Crit. Rev. Radiol. Sci., *3*:45–79, 1972.

70. Elias, E. G., Park, J. S., and Mittelman, A.: Exploratory laparotomy for staging of lymphomas. Surgery, *72*:590–595, 1972.

71. Kaplan, H. S., Dorfman, R. F., Nelson, T. S., et al.: Staging laparotomy and splenectomy in Hodgkin's disease. Analysis of indications and patterns of involvement in 285 consecutive, unselected patients. Natl. Cancer Inst. Monogr., *36*:291–301, 1973.

72. Mitchell, R. I., and Peters, M. V.: Lymph node biopsy during laparotomy for the staging of Hodgkin's disease. Ann. Surg., *178*:698–702, 1973.

73. Jonsson, K., and Lunderquist, A.: Angiography of the liver and spleen in Hodgkin's disease. Am. J. Roentgenol. Radium Ther. Nucl. Med., *121*: 789–792, 1974.

74. Castellino, R. A., Fuks, Z., Blank, N., et al.: Roentgenologic aspects of Hodgkin's disease: Repeat lymphangiography. Radiology, *109*:53–58, 1973.

75. Kolarz, G., Salzer, M., Salzer-Kuntschik, M., et al.: Die bedeutung der knochenszintigraphie fur diagnose und therapie des osteosarkoms der langen rohrenknochen. Arch. Orthop. Unfallchir., *76*:333–344, 1973.

76. McNeil, B. J., Cassady, J. R., Geiser, C. F., et al.: Fluorine-18 bone scintigraphy in children with osteosarcoma or Ewing's sarcoma. Radiology, *109*:627–631, 1973.

Index

Page numbers in *italics* indicate illustrations. Page numbers followed by (t) indicate tables.